Practical Anatomic Pathology

Series Editors

Fan Lin, Geisinger Health System
Danville, PA, USA

Ximing J. Yang, Feinberg School of Medicine
Northwestern University
Chicago, IL, USA

This Book Series is designed to provide a comprehensive, practical and state-of-the-art review and update of the major issues and challenges specific to each subspecialty field of surgical pathology in a question and answer (Q&A) format. Making an accurate diagnosis especially from a limited sample can be quite challenging, yet crucial to patient care. This Book Series, using the most current and evidence-based resources 1) focuses on frequently asked questions in surgical pathology in day-to-day practice; 2) provides quick, accurate, terse, and useful answers to many practical questions encountered in daily practice; 3) emphasizes the importance of a triple test (clinical, radiologic, and histologic correlation); 4) delineates how to appropriately utilize immunohistochemistry, in situ hybridization and molecular tests; and 5) minimizes any potential diagnostic pitfalls in surgical pathology. These books also include highly practical presentations of typical case scenarios seen in an anatomic pathology laboratory. These are in the form of case presentations with step-by-step expert analysis. Sample cases include common but challenging situations, such as evaluation of well-differentiated malignant tumors vs. benign/reactive lesions; distinction of two benign entities; sub-classification of a malignant tumor; identification of newly described tumor and non-tumor entities; workup of a tumor of unknown origin; and implementation of best practice in immunohistochemistry and molecular testing in a difficult case. The Q&A format is well accepted, especially by junior pathologists, for several reasons: 1) this is the most practical and effective way to deliver information to a new generation of pathologists accustomed to using the Internet as a resource and, therefore, comfortable and familiar with a Q&A learning environment; 2) it's impossible to memorialize and digest massive amounts of new information about new entities, new and revised classifications, molecular pathology, diagnostic IHC, and the therapeutic implications of each entity by reading large textbooks; 3) sub-specialization is a very popular practice model highly demanded by many clinicians; and 4) time is very precious for a practicing pathologist because of increasing workloads in recent years following U.S. health care reforms. This Book Series meets all of the above expectations. These books are written by established and recognized experts in their specialty fields and provide a unique and valuable resource in the field of surgical pathology, both for those currently in training and for those already in clinical practice at various skill levels. It does not seek to duplicate or completely replace other large standard textbooks; rather, it is a new, comprehensive yet concise and practical resource on these timely and critical topics.

Haodong Xu • Robert W. Ricciotti
Jose G. Mantilla
Editors

Practical Lung Pathology

Frequently Asked Questions

Springer

Editors
Haodong Xu
Department of Laboratory Medicine and Pathology
University of Washington Medical Center
Seattle, WA, USA

Robert W. Ricciotti
Department of Laboratory Medicine and Pathology
University of Washington Medical Center
Seattle, WA, USA

Jose G. Mantilla
Department of Laboratory Medicine and Pathology
University of Washington Medical Center
Seattle, WA, USA

ISSN 2629-3692 ISSN 2629-3706 (electronic)
Practical Anatomic Pathology
ISBN 978-3-031-14401-1 ISBN 978-3-031-14402-8 (eBook)
https://doi.org/10.1007/978-3-031-14402-8

This Springer imprint is published by the registered company Springer Nature Switzerland AG
The registered company address is: Gewerbestrasse 11, 6330 Cham, Switzerland

Aim and Scope

This text consists of neoplastic and nonneoplastic lung pathology. The aim is to discuss frequently encountered issues and diagnostic problems using a Q&A format and case presentations. Emphasis is placed on differentiating one from another based on histopathological features, ancillary tests including immunohistochemical and molecular analyses, and clinical and radiologic correlation. In particular, clinical-radiologic-pathologic correlation is emphasized in the diagnosis of interstitial lung disease (ILD).

This text addresses the issues and diagnostic criteria in segregating a reactive process from adenocarcinoma, poorly differentiated adenocarcinoma from poorly differentiated squamous cell carcinoma, small cell carcinoma from other types of neuroendocrine tumors, large cell carcinoma from large cell neuroendocrine carcinoma, spindle cell/sarcomatoid carcinoma from sarcomatoid mesothelioma, and carcinoma from epithelioid mesothelioma in small biopsy specimens. It also discusses key features useful for differentiating usual interstitial pneumonia (UIP) pattern from non-UIP patterns of ILD such as hypersensitivity pneumonitis, nonspecific interstitial pneumonia, and organizing pneumonia patterns in wedge biopsy specimens as well as highlights the differential diagnosis in granulomatous inflammation.

As a whole, this text answers many of the difficult questions relevant to daily practice of lung pathology. Each chapter is well written and addresses a specific diagnostic question significantly related to patients' treatment options.

Audience: Practicing pathologists and pathology trainees including residents, fellows, and medical students, as well as trainees in other medical specialties.

Preface

The practice of pulmonary pathology usually encompasses a wide variety of findings beyond the histologic features. Behind every case there is a milieu of clinical signs and symptoms, radiographic characteristics, and measurable functional alterations, which lend accuracy to our diagnostic interpretation. In addition, the continuous expansion of our understanding of human genetics has offered us a variety of novel tools to aid in the diagnosis and treatment of both neoplastic and nonneoplastic diseases.

In this textbook we discuss common and rare diagnostic dilemmas that we experience in the practice of neoplastic and nonneoplastic lung pathology. We use a Q&A format with a comprehensive focus that includes clinical, radiologic, and histopathologic findings, as well as ancillary studies such as immunohistochemistry and molecular analysis, aiming to bring answers relevant to each patient's treatment. The topics we cover are varied and include neoplasms, interstitial lung disease, infection and vascular processes, among others.

As a whole, the objective of this text is to answer many of the difficult questions relevant to the daily practice of lung pathology. We hope that it will be useful for practicing pathologists and trainees, as well as physicians practicing in other specialties that diagnose and treat pulmonary diseases.

Seattle, WA Haodong Xu
Seattle, WA Robert W. Ricciotti
Seattle, WA Jose G. Mantilla

Contents

Part I

Neoplastic Lung Pathology

Bronchial Squamous Cell Papilloma Versus Squamous Cell Carcinoma

1

Ari Kassardjian and Gregory A. Fishbein

Case Presentation

A 61-year-old man was referred to our institution for investigation of recent cough and hemoptysis. The patient was previously healthy, with a history of smoking (15 pack-years) and no significant occupational exposures. A computed tomography (CT) scan revealed a single lobulated and exophytic endobronchial nodule with no definitive infiltrative features. Bronchoscopy performed on admission revealed a single nodule, partially obstructing the left main stem bronchus, located at 2.5 cm from the carina (Fig. 1.1). An excisional endobronchial biopsy was submitted for pathologic evaluation.

Grossly, the nodule was tan-white, friable, and polypoid. Histologic sections revealed a lesion composed of papillae containing fibrovascular cores lined by stratified squamous epithelium with orderly maturation and focal viral cytopathic changes (Fig. 1.2a). No features of invasive squamous cell carcinoma were seen. RNA in situ hybridization for both low-risk and high-risk human papilloma virus (HPV) was positive for low-risk HPV (Fig. 1.2b).

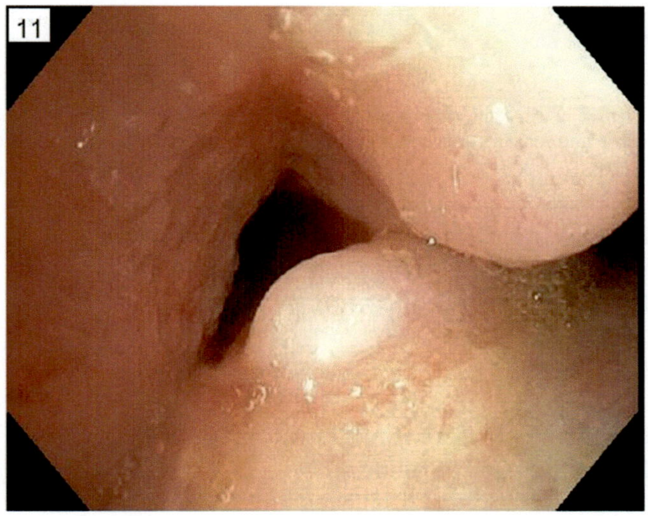

Fig. 1.1 Bronchoscopy showing a single, white-tan, glistening, polypoid nodule within the left main stem bronchus

A. Kassardjian · G. A. Fishbein (✉)
Department of Pathology and Laboratory Medicine, David Geffen School of Medicine at UCLA, Los Angeles, CA, USA
e-mail: gfishbein@mednet.ucla.edu

H. Xu et al. (eds.), *Practical Lung Pathology*, Practical Anatomic Pathology, https://doi.org/10.1007/978-3-031-14402-8_1

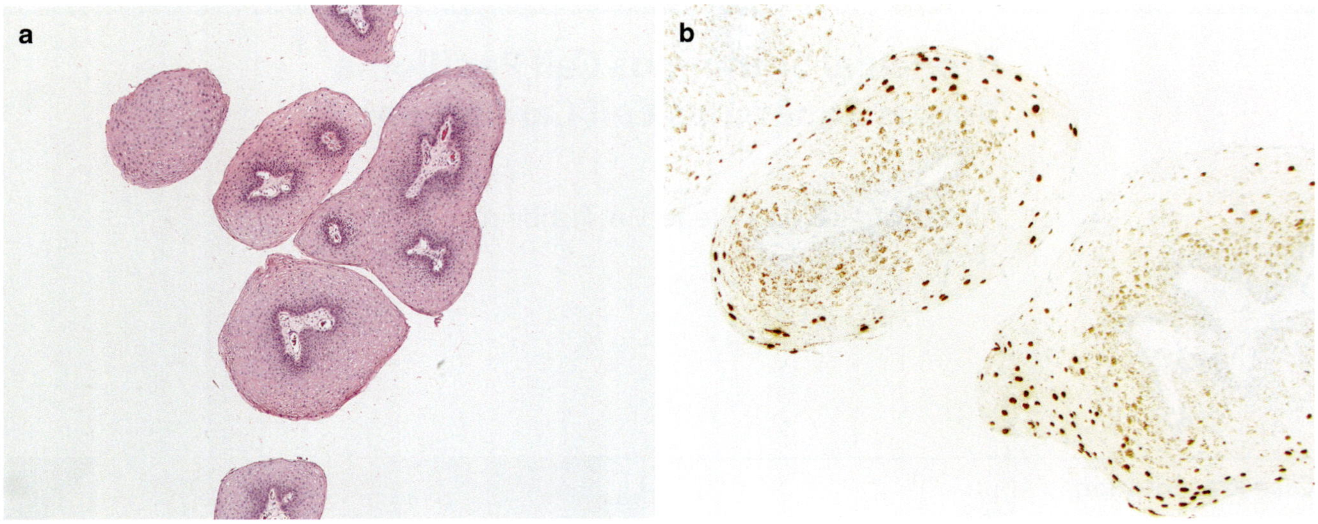

Fig. 1.2 Histologic examination shows a lesion composed of papillae having fibrovascular cores lined by squamous epithelium with orderly maturation and focal viral cytopathic effect (**a**). The tumor cells were found to harbor low-risk HPV RNA by in situ hybridization (**b**)

Pathologic Diagnosis: Bronchial Squamous Cell Papilloma—Negative for Severe Dysplasia and Malignancy

Key Points

What Is the Differential Diagnosis for Bronchial Squamous Cell Papilloma?

In general, bronchial papillomas are classified according to the number of lesions, location, and histologic type. Solitary papillomas of the bronchus are divided into three types: squamous cell papilloma (the most common), glandular papilloma, and mixed squamous cell and glandular papillomas. Squamous cell papilloma may be further subclassified as exophytic or inverted. The main differential diagnosis of bronchial squamous papilloma includes papillary squamous cell carcinoma and endobronchial inflammatory polyps. Multiple papillomas within the trachea or bronchus may represent either recurrent respiratory papillomatosis or endobronchial inflammatory polyps. It is important to note that endobronchial inflammatory polyps, despite having focal squamous metaplasia, lack true papillary architecture and fibrovascular cores.

How Do I Differentiate Bronchial Squamous Cell Papilloma from Papillary Squamous Cell Carcinoma?

In the setting of endobronchial papillary lesions with squamous differentiation in patients with clinical symptoms (hemoptysis, dyspnea, and fever), important diagnostic considerations include bronchial squamous papilloma or papillary squamous cell carcinoma.

Bronchial squamous papillomas feature arborizing fibrovascular cores with stratified squamous epithelium. The squamous epithelium typically has orderly maturation with surface keratinization. Parakeratosis, acanthosis, and intraepithelial neutrophils can be commonly seen (Fig. 1.3). HPV viral cytopathic effects including large, hyperchromatic, wrinkled nuclei and perinuclear halos are seen in a majority of cases which correlate with the presence of HPV RNA that can be detected by in situ hybridization. Squamous papillomas can show epithelial dysplasia. The dysplasia is graded according to the current World Health Organization (WHO) guidelines as mild, moderate, and severe (Fig. 1.4) [1].

As opposed to benign bronchial squamous cell papilloma, papillary squamous cell carcinoma of the lung shows malignant cytologic features, even when stromal invasion and desmoplastic reaction are not evident. Recognizing even focal invasion within a papillary squamous lesion warrants a diagnosis of squamous cell carcinoma; however, it may be difficult to determine invasion in small biopsy specimens. A diagnosis of squamous cell carcinoma should be made in the setting of a clinically appreciable exophytic mass with lack of squamous maturation, marked atypia, pleomorphism, and increased mitotic figures, even without definitive stromal invasion. Immunohistochemistry does not play a role in differentiating bronchial squamous papilloma versus papillary squamous cell carcinoma.

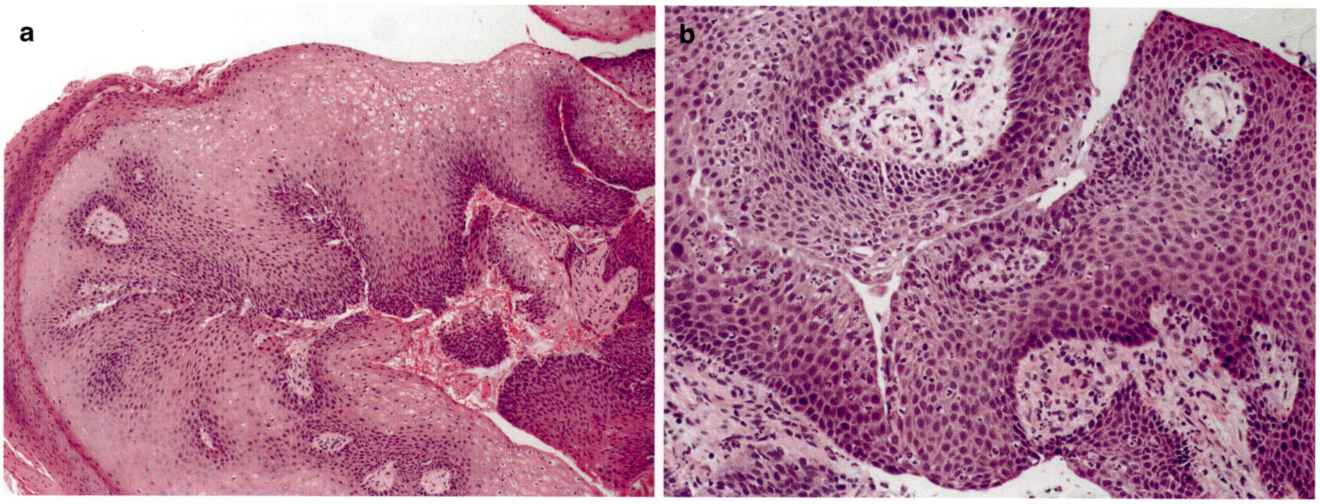

Fig. 1.3 Squamous papilloma with parakeratosis, acanthosis, and viral cytopathic effect (**a**) and intraepithelial neutrophils (**b**)

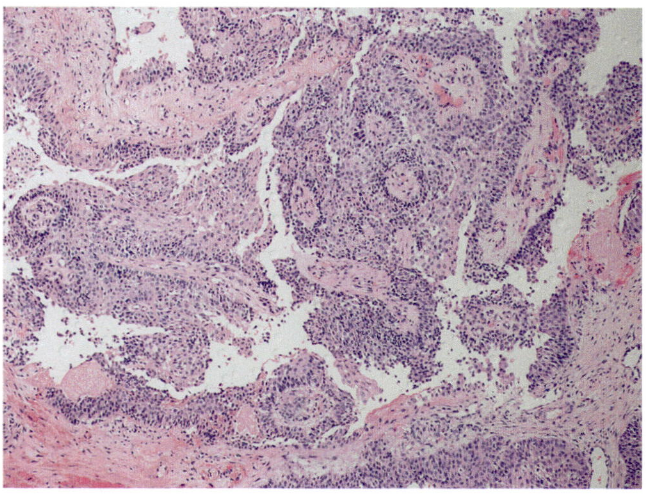

Fig. 1.4 Squamous papilloma with arborizing fibrovascular cores, loss of maturation, cellular crowding, and increased nuclear-to-cytoplasmic ratio consistent with severe dysplasia

Are Bronchial Squamous Papilloma and Squamous Cell Carcinoma Associated with Viral Infection?

There is a strong association between HPV and bronchial squamous papilloma [2–4]. HPV appears to play a pathogenic role in both solitary papillomas and respiratory papillomatosis. The possibilities for acquiring the virus are as a latent birth infection with delayed presentation or as an acquired infection from infected secretions. Both high-risk (e.g., types 16, 18, 31, 33, and 35) and low-risk HPV (e.g., types 6 and 11) have been associated with malignant transformation [4, 5]. In situ hybridization can be used to confirm the presence of HPV RNA in bronchial squamous papillomas. HPV does not appear to play a significant role in the development of primary lung squamous cell carcinomas [6].

Are There Radiographic Differences Between Bronchial Squamous Cell Papilloma and Papillary Squamous Cell Carcinoma?

A solitary squamous papilloma can be an incidental finding on imaging. These lesions usually present as an endobronchial mass in the segmental bronchi with a lobulated appearance on CT scan. The presence of a lobulated contour on imaging aids in distinguishing benign papillomas from infiltrating carcinomas [7]. These features correlate well with the gross findings of solitary bronchial papillomas, which have an exophytic and papillary/lobulated surface with no ulceration or bleeding.

Bronchial papillomas show a significantly lower fluorodeoxyglucose (FDG) uptake compared to squamous cell carcinomas. Careful study of FDG uptake by positron emission tomography (PET)/CT at the site of bronchial obstruction can be helpful in distinguishing benign from malignant endobronchial lesions. PET scan is also helpful in evaluating for lymph node metastasis, the presence of which would support malignancy [8].

Chest X-rays often show no significant findings in patients with solitary bronchial papillomas; however, if the lesion is large and expansile, they can form a hilar mass which causes airway obstruction, consolidation, and lobar collapse and can mimic squamous cell carcinoma [9].

What Are the Clinical and Epidemiologic Differences Between Bronchial Squamous Papillomas and Primary Lung Squamous Cell Carcinomas?

Similar to squamous cell carcinoma, bronchial squamous papillomas are much more common in males than in females. Patients usually present in their fifth to sixth decade of life. Although the majority of patients with squamous papillomas are tobacco smokers, a direct etiological role of smoking has not been firmly established. Unlike conventional primary squamous cell carcinomas of the lung, solitary bronchial squamous papillomas and recurrent respiratory papillomatosis are caused by HPV infection. Most patients present with nonspecific, obstructive, symptoms that include coughing, wheezing, and dyspnea. Hemoptysis and fever are also often symptoms which bring the patient to medical attention [2].

References

1. Travis WD, Brambilla E, Nicholson AG, Yatabe Y, Austin JHM, Beasley MB, et al. WHO classification of tumours of the lung, pleura, thymus and heart. J Thorac Oncol. 2015;10(9):1243–60. https://doi.org/10.1097/JTO.0000000000000630.
2. Tryfon S, Dramba V, Zoglopitis F, Iakovidis D, Sakkas L, Kontakiotis T, et al. Solitary papillomas of the lower airways: epidemiological, clinical, and therapeutic data during a 22-year period and review of the literature. J Thorac Oncol. 2012 Apr;7(4):643–8. https://doi.org/10.1097/JTO.0b013e3182468d06.
3. Syrjänen K, Syrjañen S. Solitary bronchial squamous cell papilloma - another human papillomavirus (HPV)-associated benign tumor: systematic review and meta-analysis. Contemp Oncol (Pozn). 2013;17(5):427–34. https://doi.org/10.5114/wo.2013.38565.
4. Popper HH, Wirnsberger G, Jüttner-Smolle FM, Pongratz MG, Sommersgutter M. The predictive value of human papilloma virus (HPV) typing in the prognosis of bronchial squamous cell papillomas. Histopathology. 1992;21(4):323–30. https://doi.org/10.1111/j.1365-2559.1992.tb00402.x.
5. Popper HH, El-Shabrawi Y, Wöckel W, Höfler G, Kenner L, Jüttner-Smolle FM, et al. Prognostic importance of human papilloma virus typing in squamous cell papilloma of the bronchus: comparison of in situ hybridization and the polymerase chain reaction. Hum Pathol. 1994;25(11):1191–7. https://doi.org/10.1016/0046-8177(94)90036-1.
6. Bishop JA, Ogawa T, Chang X, Illei PB, Gabrielson E, Pai SI, et al. HPV analysis in distinguishing second primary tumors from lung metastases in patients with head and neck squamous cell carcinoma. Am J Surg Pathol. 2012;36(1):142–8. https://doi.org/10.1097/PAS.0b013e3182395c7b.
7. Kang H, Kim TS, Han J, Kim H. Fibroepithelial polyp of the bronchus: CT and histopathologic findings. Korean J Radiol. 2012;13(3):355–7. https://doi.org/10.3348/kjr.2012.13.3.355.
8. Cho A, Hur J, Kang WJ, Cho HJ, Lee JH, Yun M, et al. Usefulness of FDG PET/CT in determining benign from malignant endobronchial obstruction. Eur Radiol. 2011;21(5):1077–87. https://doi.org/10.1007/s00330-010-2006-1.
9. Inoue Y, Oka M, Ishii H, Kimino K, Kishikawa M, Ito M, et al. A solitary bronchial papilloma with malignant changes. Intern Med. 2001;40(1):56–60. https://doi.org/10.2169/internalmedicine.40.56.

Pulmonary Hamartoma Versus Chondroid Neoplasms

2

Sofia Liou and Gregory A. Fishbein

Case Presentation

A 67-year-old man with a 54 pack-year smoking history presents for evaluation of a 1 cm lung nodule found on routine lung cancer screening. He has no respiratory symptoms aside from an intermittent cough that is sometimes productive. Chest computed tomography (CT) also shows emphysema. The lesion resides in the parenchyma of the right middle lobe and is a smoothly marginated solid nodule.

A CT-guided biopsy of the nodule shows predominantly cartilage and myxoid connective tissue with benign-appearing epithelial elements. No overt features of malignancy are identified. Conservative management is favored, and the patient is scheduled for repeat CT in 1 year.

Pathologic Diagnosis: Pulmonary Hamartoma

What Is the Definition of a Pulmonary Hamartoma? What Are Its Clinical and Prognostic Features?

Pulmonary hamartomas, which represent the majority of benign pulmonary neoplasms, are composed of a disorganized mixture of benign mesenchymal and epithelial components that arise from embryological rests [1]. Formally, they consist of at least two mesenchymal elements—cartilage, fat, smooth muscle, or connective tissue—with entrapped clefts of respiratory epithelium. These lesions are most often found in adults between 40 and 60 years of age, affecting men more commonly than women with a 3:1 ratio [2, 3]. The geographic distribution is such that peripheral lesions are much more common than central endobronchial lesions (less than 10%) [3].

The prognosis of pulmonary hamartomas is excellent. Most lesions are clinically observed and do not need to be excised given their benign and slow-growing nature. However, they can enlarge over time, and those in an endobronchial location (Fig. 2.1) can cause obstructive symptoms such as cough, dyspnea, and hemoptysis as well as result in pneumonia [4]. Complete surgical excision via enucleation or segmental resection is curative; the lesions tend to "shell out" easily upon surgical manipulation. Recurrence and malignant transformation are rare [5].

What Are the Radiographic Features of Pulmonary Hamartomas?

Pulmonary hamartomas are usually discovered incidentally on imaging as "coin" lesions and can be often diagnosed radiographically. They comprise 6% of all solitary pulmonary nodules [6, 7]. In cases where radiographic evaluation is

S. Liou · G. A. Fishbein (✉)
Department of Pathology and Laboratory Medicine, David Geffen School of Medicine at UCLA, Los Angeles, CA, USA
e-mail: gfishbein@mednet.ucla.edu

H. Xu et al. (eds.), *Practical Lung Pathology*, Practical Anatomic Pathology, https://doi.org/10.1007/978-3-031-14402-8_2

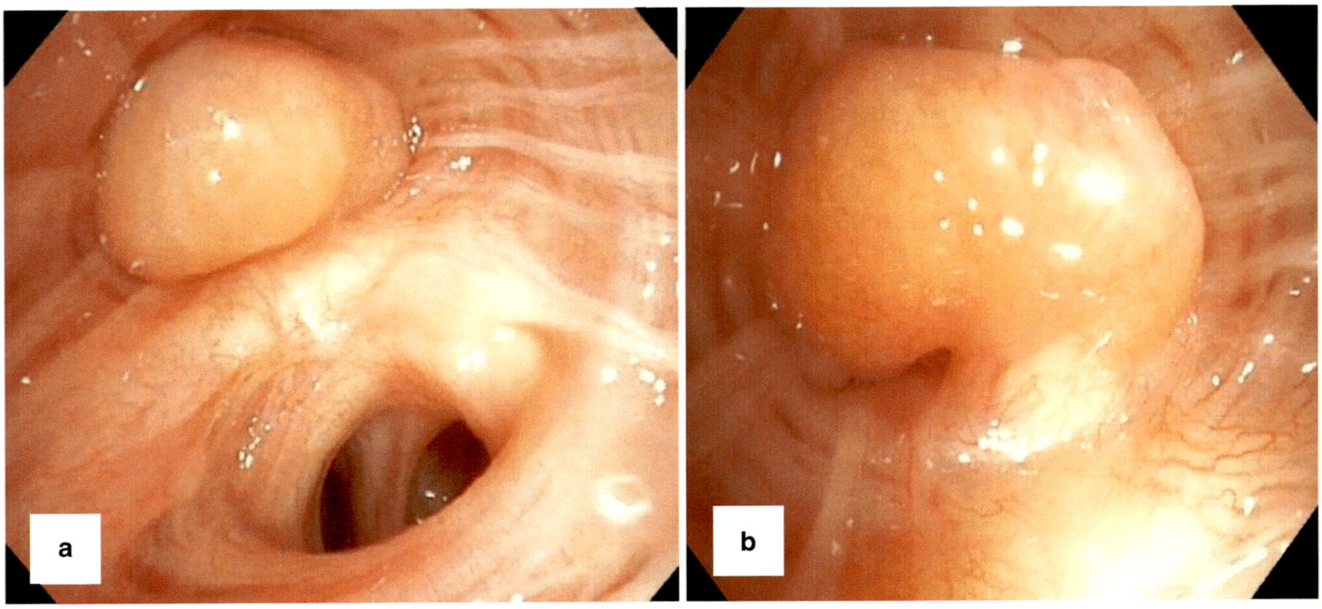

Fig. 2.1 Bronchoscopic visualization of an obstructing left upper lobe endobronchial hamartoma. Biopsy of the lesion revealed benign hyaline cartilage and mature adipose tissue

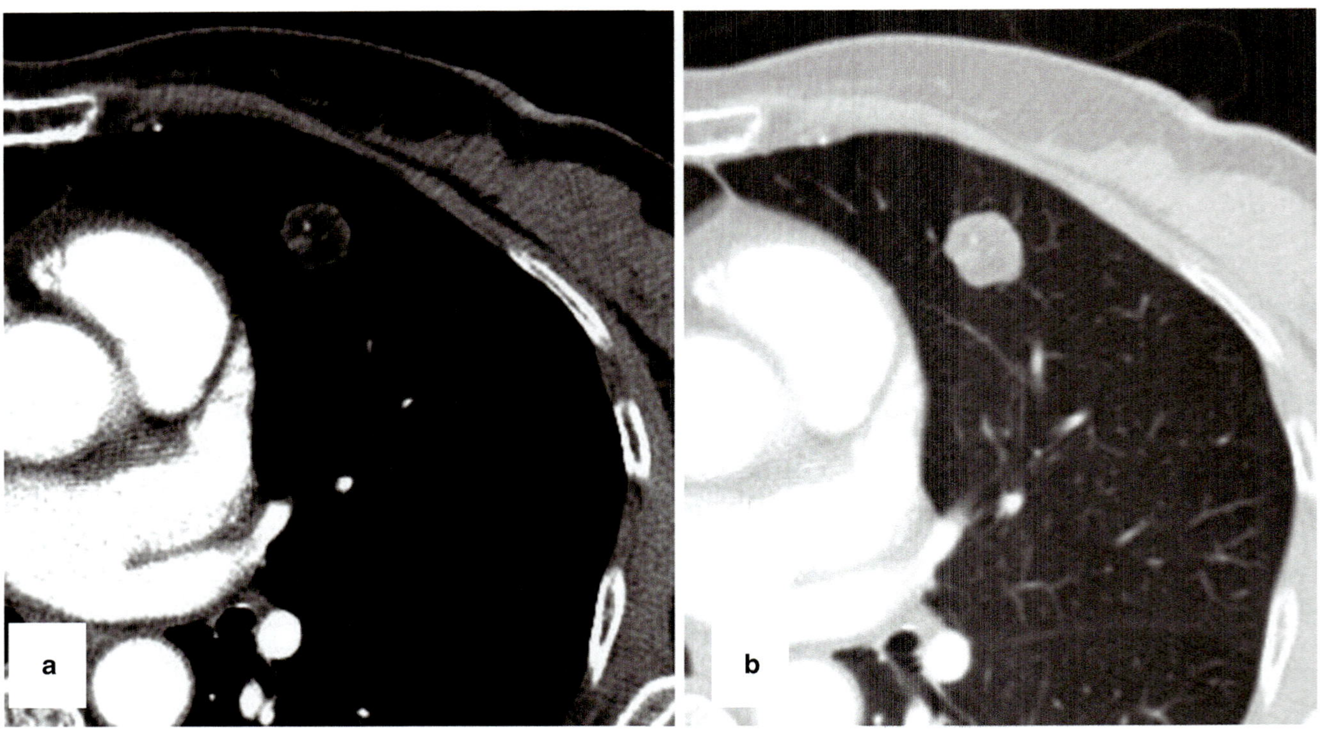

Fig. 2.2 Computed tomography (CT) image showing a 1.7 cm lobulated, smoothly marginated fatty nodule with punctate calcification in the anterior left upper lung lobe, consistent with a pulmonary hamartoma

indeterminate, fine-needle aspiration or core biopsy can assist and obviate the need for surgical intervention. Consistent with their benign nature, pulmonary hamartomas are slow-growing, well-circumscribed, and solitary on radiologic imaging. The lesions appear as heterogeneous nodules with smooth-to-lobulated borders and a signature composition of nodular "popcorn" calcifications and adipose tissue [8] (Fig. 2.2). While the presence of calcifications is helpful for radiologic diagnosis, in practice they are present in only 10–30% of cases [3, 9].

What Are the Pathologic Features of Pulmonary Hamartomas?

Macroscopically, pulmonary hamartomas are firm, solitary, round-to-lobulated lesions that usually measure less than 4 cm in diameter (Fig. 2.3). Cut surfaces are tan-white to gray with glistening chondroid and mucoid areas. Cartilaginous areas of the tumor may be difficult to cut and require decalcification.

Histologically, lung hamartomas are composed of varying proportions of mature hyaline cartilage, adipose tissue, and smooth muscle, as well as entrapped clefts of respiratory epithelium which may be ciliated or non-ciliated (Fig. 2.4). Descriptors such as lipomatous, fibroleiomyomatous, or chondromatous are used to further characterize the lesion. Of note, most pulmonary hamartomas have a predominantly chondroid or chondromyxoid component, which can make the differentiation between hamartomas and pure chondromas challenging (Table 2.1). Rarely, the bone as well as bone marrow may be present in pulmonary hamartoma.

Immunohistochemistry is not necessary for diagnosis, as morphologic diagnoses can be made on routine staining alone. However, mesenchymal markers and immunohistochemical stains for sex steroid hormone receptors have shown positive reactivity in pulmonary hamartomas [10].

Molecular and cytogenetic studies on pulmonary hamartomas suggest a neoplastic origin. Translocation t(3;12)(q27–28;q14–15) is present at high frequencies in pulmonary hamartomas, which results in fusion of the *HMGA2* and *LPP* genes. The *HMGA2–LPP* fusion gene usually consists of exons 1–3 of *HMGA2* and exons 9–11 of *LPP* and is expressed in all tumors with this translocation [11–14].

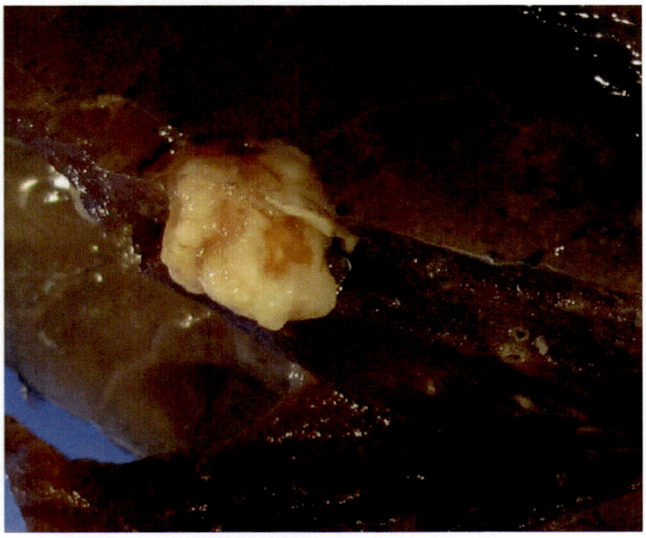

Fig. 2.3 Gross image of an incidentally found pulmonary hamartoma (1.0 cm) from a pneumonectomy specimen. The lesion has lobulated borders and a firm cartilaginous component which required decalcification prior to histologic sectioning. Image contributed by Fereidoun Abtin, MD from UCLA Department of Radiology

What Is the Differential Diagnosis for Pulmonary Hamartomas?

The differential includes granulation tissue, intrapulmonary metastases, synchronous primary carcinomas, leiomyosarcoma, benign metastasizing leiomyoma, lymphangioleiomyomatosis, mesenchymal cystic hamartoma, and chondroid neoplasms.

How Does One Differentiate a Predominately Chondroid Pulmonary Hamartoma from a Chondroid Neoplasm?

Chondroid neoplasms contain only one type of tissue and lack epithelial inclusions, whereas pulmonary hamartomas consist of multiple types of connective tissue and invaginations of respiratory epithelium [3]. If core-needle biopsy consists of only cartilaginous material, limitations in sampling are possible, and both entities remain in the differential. Of note, chondroid neoplasms contain areas of endochondral ossification more frequently than hamartomas. If mature adipose tissue is seen interspersed in a predominantly cartilaginous lesion, the findings favor a pulmonary hamartoma over a purely chondroid entity.

Are Either Chondromas or Pulmonary Hamartomas Associated with Other Conditions?

Pulmonary chondromas may be part of the Carney triad, a rare nonfamilial syndrome that is characterized by the coexistence of three types of neoplasms: pulmonary cartilaginous tumors, gastric stromal tumors, and extra-adrenal paragangliomas. 75% of patients with Carney triad have one or more pulmonary chondroma. Morphologically, pulmonary hamartomas have some overlapping features with pulmonary chondromas of the Carney triad; both are circumscribed, lobulated, and have cartilaginous components. However, chondromas in the Carney triad tend to be multiple and have a fibrous pseudocapsule, unlike hamartomas which are typically solitary and unencapsulated [15, 16]. In addition, syndromic chondromas lack entrapped respiratory epithelium and more often have areas of osseous metaplasia.

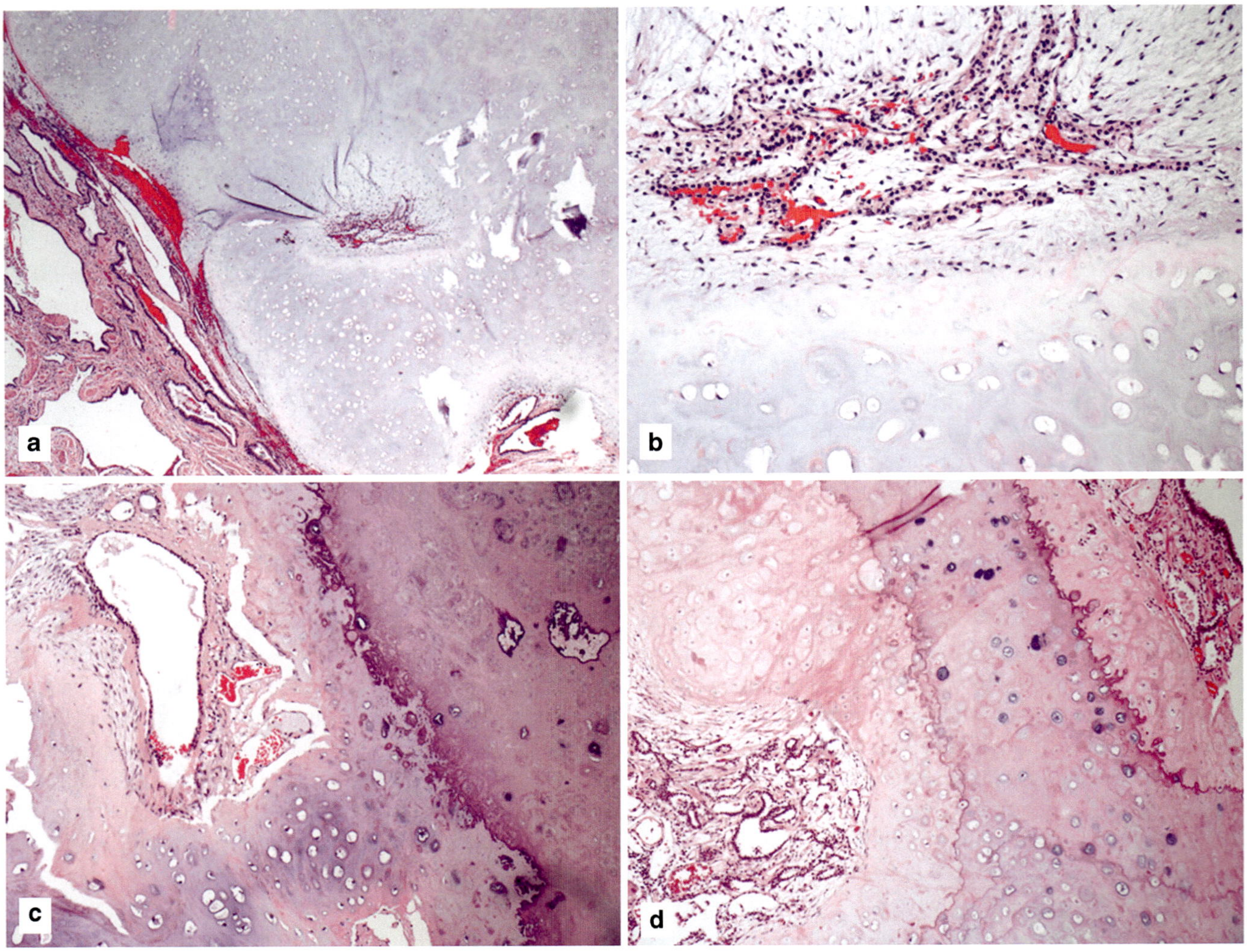

Fig. 2.4 (**a**) Pulmonary hamartoma with a predominantly chondroid appearance. (**b**) Clefts of entrapped respiratory epithelium are seen adjacent to mature hyaline cartilage. (**c**) and (**d**) are two foci of an incidentally found hamartoma showing mature hyaline cartilage with entrapped respiratory epithelium

Table 2.1 Predominant tissue type in a Dutch series of 154 pulmonary hamartomas [3]

Predominant tissue type	Parenchymal hamartomas (n = 142) (%)	Endobronchial hamartomas (n = 12) (%)
Chondroid	80	50
Fibroblastic	12	8
Fatty	5	34
Osseous	3	8

Are There Demographic Differences Between Patients with Pulmonary Chondroma and Patients with Hamartoma?

The vast majority (80%) of patients affected by the Carney triad are young women with a mean age of 20 years [15, 16]. Thus, most chondromas are found in young females. Chondromas may occur sporadically as well, though rare, and these occur mostly in men with a mean age of 53 years [15]. Pulmonary hamartomas afflict older adults with incidence peaking in the sixth decade.

How Does One Differentiate Pulmonary Hamartoma from Chondrosarcoma?

Primary pulmonary chondrosarcoma is exceedingly rare [17–19]; however, the lungs are a common site for metastatic skeletal chondrosarcoma. Knowledge of a prior history of skeletal chondrosarcoma is key. If no such established history exists for a patient with chondrosarcoma affecting the lung(s), then clinical and radiologic investigation is warranted to search for another primary site.

The distinction between low-grade chondrosarcoma (grade 1 of 3) and hamartoma may be difficult in limited biopsy samples given the deceptively bland cytologic features of the former. Identification of an invasive pattern of growth is necessary to make this diagnosis, and extensive sampling may therefore be needed [20, 21]. Intermediate- and high-grade (grades 2 and 3) chondrosarcomas typically demonstrate increased cellularity and cytologic atypia and, in the case of the latter, overt nuclear pleomorphism and conspicuous mitotic activity [20].

References

1. Umashankar T, Devadas AK, Ravichandra G, Yaranal PJ. Pulmonary hamartoma: cytological study of a case and literature review. J Cytol. 2012;29(4):261–3.
2. Ge F, Tong F, Li Z. Diagnosis and treatment of pulmonary hamartomas. Chin Med J. 1998;13:61–2.
3. Van den Bosch JM, Wagenaar SS, Corrin B, et al. Mesenchymoma of the lung (so called hamartoma): a review of 154 parenchymal and endobronchial cases. Thorax. 1987;42:790–3.
4. Cosio BG, Villena V, Echave-Sustaeta J, et al. Endobronchial hamartoma. Chest. 2002;122:202–5.
5. Basile A, Gregoris A, Antoci B, et al. Malignant change in a benign pulmonary hamartoma. Thorax. 1989;44:232–3.
6. Siegelman SS, Zerhouni EA, Leo FP, et al. CT of the solitary pulmonary nodule. Am J Roentgenol. 1980;135:1–13.
7. Madewell JE, Feigin DS. Benign tumours of the lung. Semin Roentgenol. 1977;12:175–86.
8. Gleeson T, Thiessen R, Hannigan A, et al. Pulmonary hamartomas: CT pixel analysis for fat attenuation using radiologic-pathologic correlation. J Med Imaging Radiat Oncol. 2013;57:534–43.
9. Whyte RI, Donington JS. Hamartomas of the lung. Semin Thorac Cardiovasc Surg. 2003;15:301–4.
10. Pelosi G, Rosai J, Viale G. Immunoreactivity for sex steroid hormone receptors in pulmonary hamartomas. Am J Surg Pathol. 2006;30:819–27.
11. Dal Cin P, Kools P, De Jonge I, et al. Rearrangement of 12q14-15 in pulmonary chondroid hamartoma. Genes Chromosomes Cancer. 1993;8:131–3.
12. Fletcher JA, Longtine J, Wallace K, et al. Cytogenetic and histologic findings in 17 pulmonary chondroid hamartomas: evidence for a pathogenetic relationship with lipomas and leiomyomas. Genes Chromosomes Cancer. 1995;12:220–3.
13. Kazmierczak B, Wanschura S, Rosigkeit J, et al. Molecular characterization of 12q14-15 rearrangements in three pulmonary chondroid hamartomas. Cancer Res. 1995;55:2497–9.
14. von Ahsen I, Rogalla P, Bullerdiek J. Expression patterns of the LPP-HMGA2 fusion transcript in pulmonary chondroid hamartomas with t(3;12)(q27 approximately 28;q14 approximately 15). Cancer Genet Cytogenet. 2005;163:68–70.
15. Carney JA. Carney triad: a syndrome featuring paraganglionic, adrenocortical, and possibly other endocrine tumors. J Clin Endocrinol Metab. 2009;94:3656–62.
16. Rodriguez FJ, Aubrey MC, Tazelaar HD, et al. Pulmonary chondroma: a tumor associated with Carney triad and different from pulmonary hamartoma. Am J Surg Pathol. 2007;31:1844–53.
17. Travis WD, et al. WHO classification of tumours of the lung, pleura, thymus and heart. 4th ed. Lyon: IARC; 2015.
18. Shah ND, Diwanji SR. Primary chondrosarcoma of the lung with cutaneous and skeletal metastases. Singap Med J. 2007;48(7):e196–9.
19. Rees GM. Primary chondrosarcoma of lung. Thorax. 1970;25(3):366–71.
20. Kim MJ, Cho KJ, Ayala AG, Ro JY. Chondrosarcoma: with updates on molecular genetics. Sarcoma. 2011;2011:405437.
21. Eefting D, Schrage YM, Geirnaerdt MJ, Le Cessie S, Taminiau AH, Bovee JV, et al. Assessment of interobserver variability and histologic parameters to improve reliability in classification and grading of central cartilaginous tumors. Am J Surg Pathol. 2009;33(1):50–7.

3 Reactive Type II Pneumocyte Hyperplasia Versus Adenocarcinoma

Jiqing Ye

Case Presentation

A 41-year-old man with history of heavy smoking presented at the emergency department with chest pain and hemoptysis. A computed tomography (CT) scan demonstrated a 5.3 × 4.8 × 4.0 cm left hilar mass and possible left adrenal metastasis. Also identified was an associated opacity in the left upper lobe and lingula which could represent post-obstructive atelectasis, pneumonia, hemorrhage, or tumor. The CT scan also demonstrated narrowing of the left pulmonary artery. Clinically, the tumor was unresectable. A transbronchial biopsy was attempted and yielded only benign bronchial mucosa. A decision was made to obtain a diagnostic specimen by wedge biopsy. By gross examination, the wedge biopsy specimen contained an ill-defined gray and firm, 3.2 × 1.2 × 0.9 cm mass. A touch preparation at the time of frozen section showed predominantly pigmented macrophages and scattered clusters of epithelial cells with mild atypia (Fig. 3.1a, b). At low-power magnification, the frozen sections showed foci of necrosis and atypical epithelial cells (Fig. 3.2a, b). The atypical cells were more striking in the areas adjacent to necrosis. The cells are relatively uniform in size and the N/C ratio. No desmoplasia was identified. Adenocarcinoma was favored at the time of frozen section. The surgery was stopped assuming that diagnostic material was obtained. Permanent sections of the mass showed extensive geographic necrosis with reactive fibrosis (Fig. 3.3a). There were multiple foci of small arteries with almost completely obliterated lumen and organizing thrombus (Fig. 3.3b). In the areas away from necrosis, atypical reactive type II pneumocyte hyperplasia was noted (Fig. 3.4a, b). The alveolar lining cells have a hobnail appearance without nuclear overlapping or any secondary structures such as multilayers, papillae, micropapillae, or solid/large nest formation. The nuclei were enlarged with some showing vesicular chromatin and prominent nucleoli, and a rim of cytoplasm could be appreciated. No atypical mitotic figures were noted. In the areas of necrosis, the nuclear atypia is more pronounced (Fig. 3.4c, d), and the squamous metaplasia was present and exhibited striking reactive atypia (Fig. 3.4d, upper right corner). Yet, the nuclear size is relatively uniform. The septa are mildly thickened with reactive stromal cells (Fig. 3.4e); however, the overall alveolar architectures were maintained, and they were better appreciated on a TTF-1 immunostain (Fig. 3.4f). Small foci of organizing pneumonia pattern of injury were also noted. The differential diagnosis included reactive type II pneumocyte hyperplasia and adenocarcinoma in situ (AIS). The clinical setting and the exuberant epithelial proliferation with cytological atypia made the interpretation difficult. Additional expert consultation was obtained. Ultimately, a diagnosis of atypical type II pneumocyte proliferation was rendered, and a reactive process rather than a neoplastic process is favored. Shortly after, the patient underwent MRI studies, which demonstrated multiple ring-enhancing lesions in the brain. A core biopsy of a lesion showed poorly differentiated adenocarcinoma (Fig. 3.5). In addition, the tumor cells from the brain biopsy were CK7 positive, CK20 negative, TTF-1 negative, and CDX-2 weakly positive. The proliferating cells in the wedge biopsy of the lung were positive for TTF-1. Taken together, the most likely scenario was that the primary tumor in the left hilum was a TTF-1-negative poorly differentiated adenocarcinoma, which was not sampled by the wedge biopsy. Unfortunately, the patient died shortly after the diagnosis of metastatic lung adenocarcinoma to the brain was made.

J. Ye (✉)
Department of Pathology and Laboratory Medicine, Rochester Regional Health System, Rochester, NY, USA
e-mail: jiqing.ye@rochesterregional.org

H. Xu et al. (eds.), *Practical Lung Pathology*, Practical Anatomic Pathology, https://doi.org/10.1007/978-3-031-14402-8_3

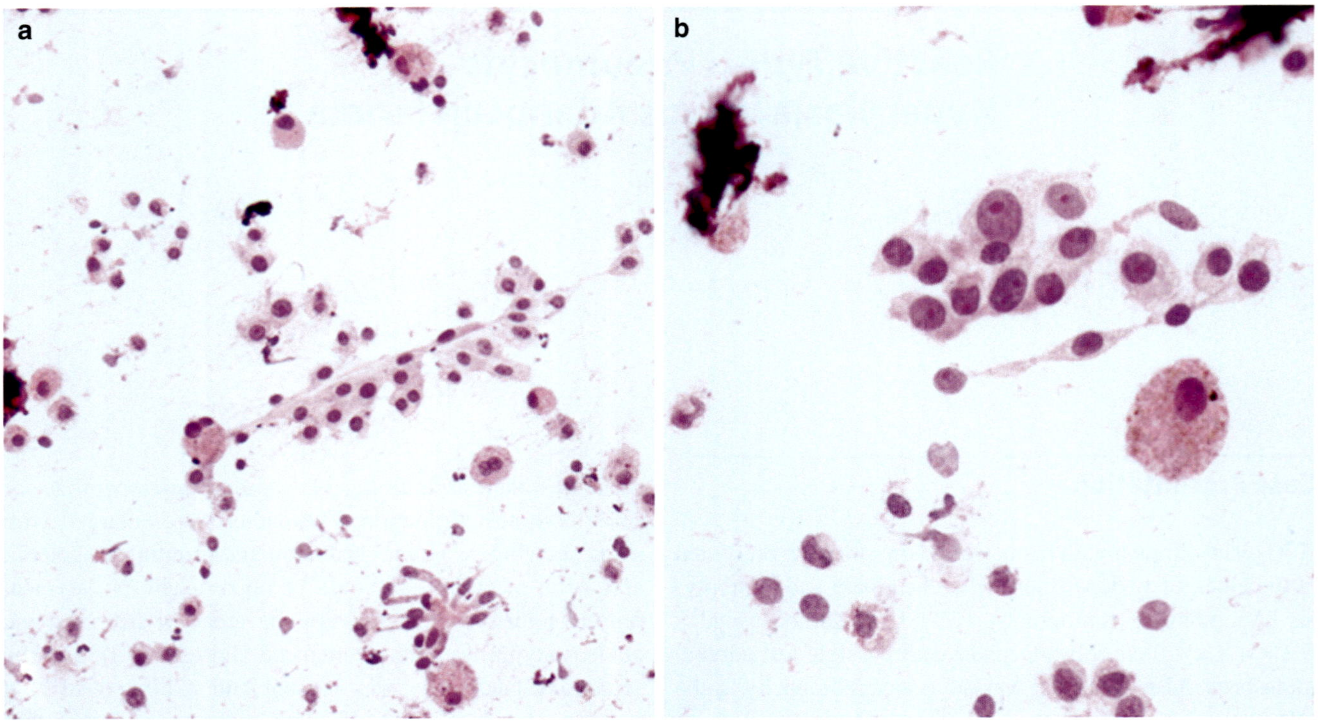

Fig. 3.1 Scrape preparation during frozen section showed pigmented macrophages and scattered clustered of epithelial cells with mild atypia and low N/C ratio. (**a**) 200×; (**b**) 400×

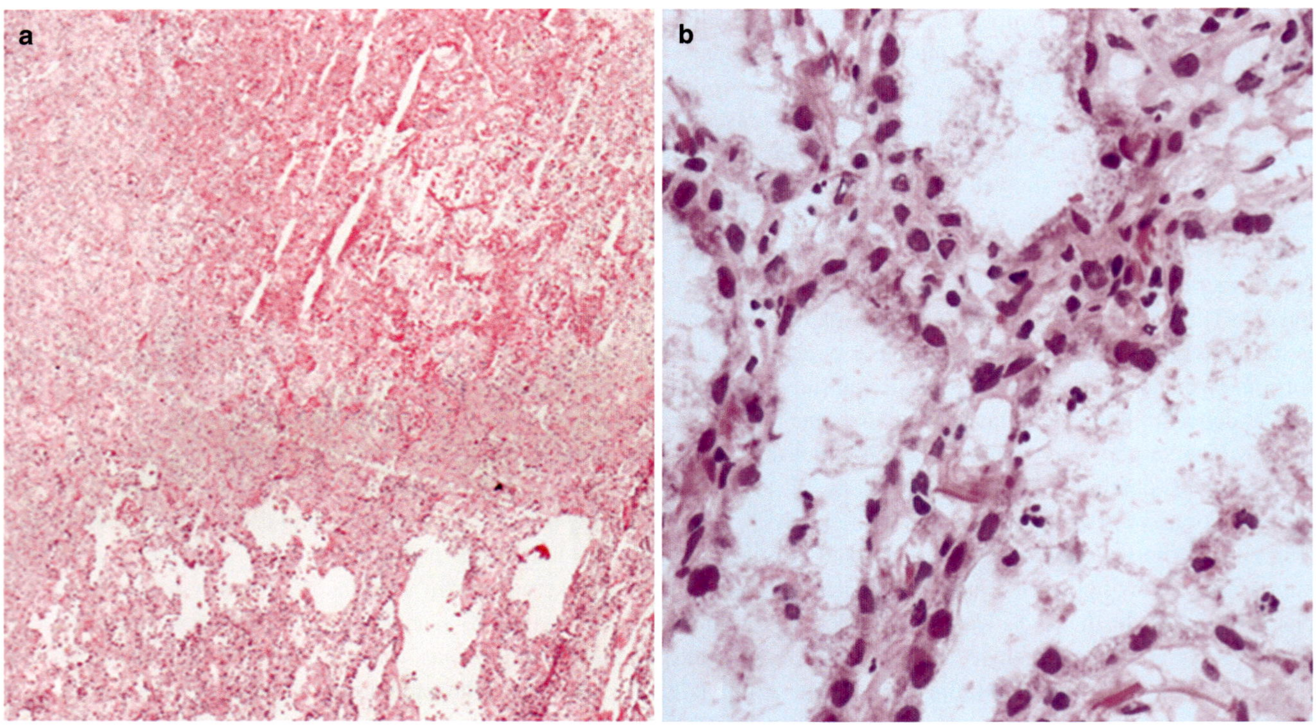

Fig. 3.2 Frozen sections. (**a**) Fibrinoid necrosis and eosinophilic appearance at 40× magnification. (**b**) Type II pneumocyte proliferation with atypia at 400×

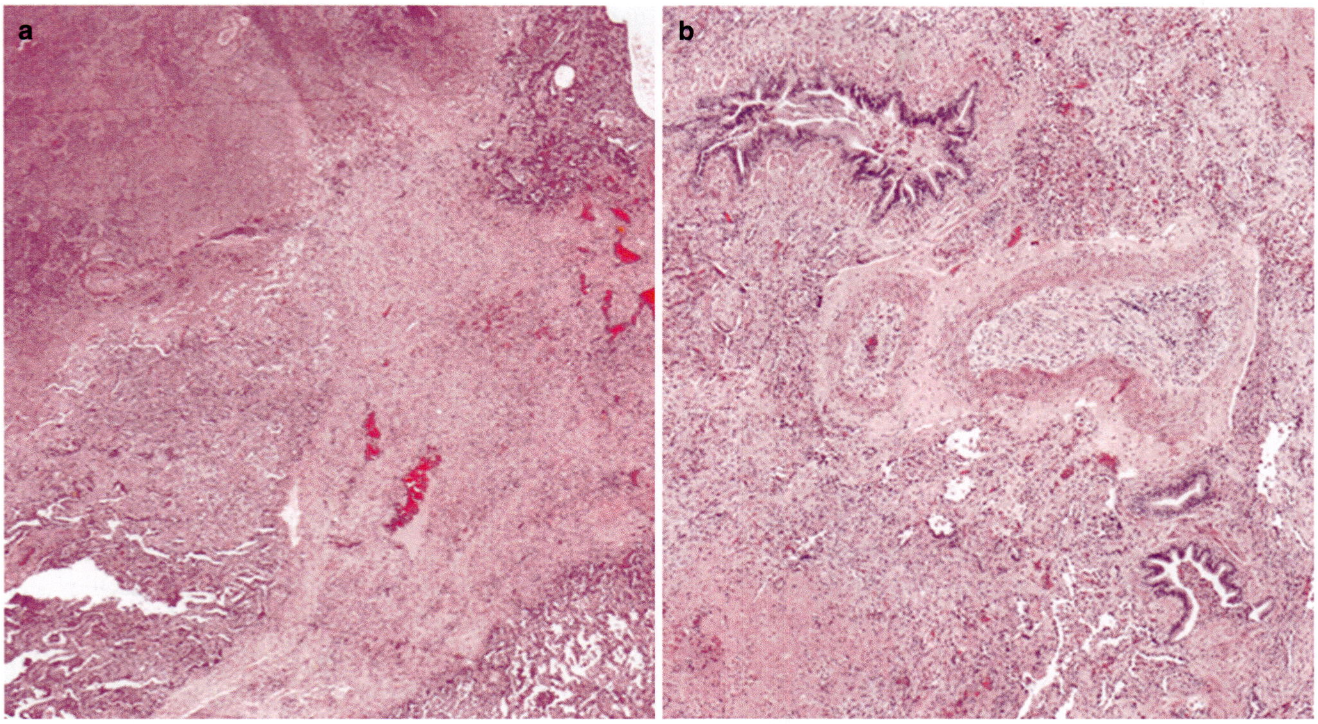

Fig. 3.3 Permanent H&E sections. (**a**) Geographic necrosis at 200×. (**b**) Small arteries with marked intimal hyperplasia and organizing thrombus at 400×

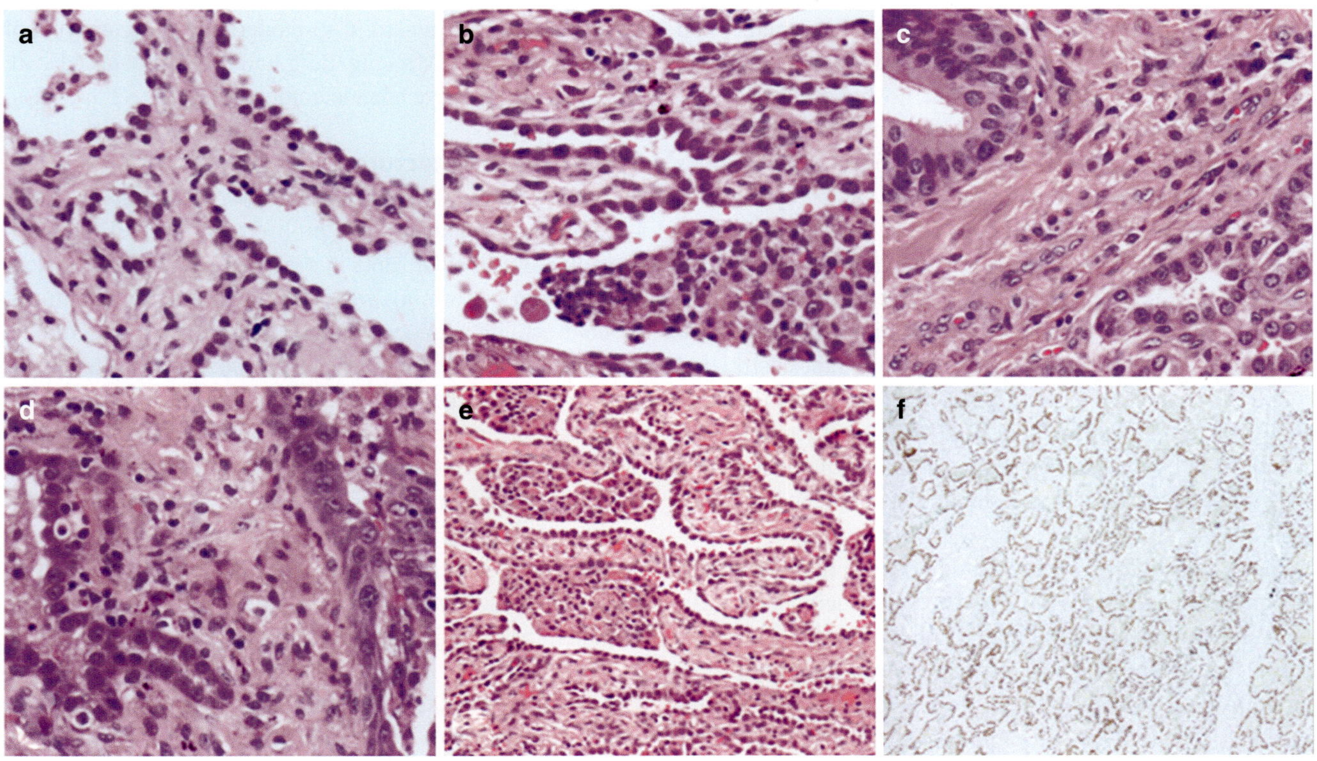

Fig. 3.4 (**a**) and (**b**) Reactive type II pneumocyte hyperplasia away from the necrotic area. (**c**) and (**d**) Proliferating type II pneumocytes with cytological atypia adjacent to the necrotic areas. Reactive ciliated bronchiolar epithelium (**c**) and squamous metaplasia (**d**). (**e**) Alveolar architecture was maintained with thickened septa, reactive fibroblasts, reactive endothelial cells, and inflammatory infiltrate. (**f**) TTF-1 immunostain showed type II pneumocyte positivity highlighting maintained alveolar architecture. Original magnification, H&E (**a**–**d**) 400×; (**e**) 200×; IHC (**f**) 200×

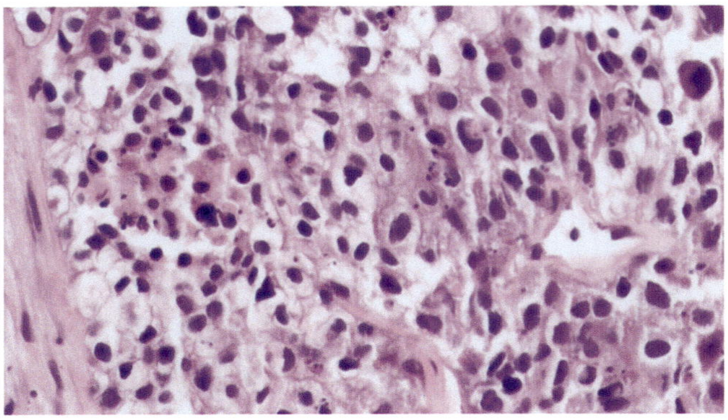

Fig. 3.5 Metastatic carcinoma in the brain at original magnification, 400×

Final Pathologic Diagnosis: Reactive Type II Pneumocyte Hyperplasia in the Wedge Biopsy

Differentiation Features of Reactive Type II Pneumocyte Hyperplasia and Adenocarcinoma

Reactive Type II Pneumocyte Hyperplasia

Alveoli of the lung are lined with type I and II pneumocytes. Type I pneumocyte is very large, thin, and flat stretched over a very large area, while type II pneumocyte is a smaller cell (Fig. 3.6a) [1]. In the setting of acute and chronic lung injuries, type II pneumocytes can undergo hyperplastic/metaplastic changes including type II pneumocyte hyperplasia, bronchiolar metaplasia, intestinal/Goblet cell/mucinous metaplasia, squamous metaplasia, and basal cell hyperplasia (Fig. 3.6b–d) [2–6]. Reactive type II pneumocyte hyperplasia is a nonspecific reactive process that has been observed in many types of lung injuries including pneumothorax, diffuse alveolar damage, organizing pneumonia, lipogranuloma/aspiration pneumonia, necrotizing or non-necrotizing granulomas, and benign lung parenchyma adjacent to a neoplastic process, among others [2, 7]. When reactive type II pneumocyte hyperplasia exhibits marked cytological atypia, one might be misled to the diagnosis of adenocarcinoma [6–9].

In most cases, the differentiation between reactive type II pneumocyte hyperplasia and non-mucinous well-differentiated adenocarcinoma is straightforward. However, in some situations exemplified by the above case, the differentiation between the two can be challenging. The distinguishing features between reactive type II pneumocyte hyperplasia and adenocarcinoma are summarized in Table 3.1 [7–9]. The evaluation process can be artificially broken down into three aspects: cytomorphology of the proliferation cells, secondary architecture, and identification of underlying lung injury and the background stroma and inflammatory infiltrates. A correct diagnosis can usually be reached based on the integrated evaluation of all aspects.

Cytomorphology

In reactive type II pneumocyte hyperplasia, similar to a reactive process seen in any other organ system, the nuclei are usually not hyperchromatic. The N/C ratio is usually relatively low. The presence of cytoplasm prevents the nuclei from overlapping with each other. The nuclei are usually vesicular, each with a single prominent nucleolus. They are usually relatively uniform in size, lack of nuclear pleomorphism, and have regular and smooth nuclear contour. The pneumocytes typically maintain their attachment to the alveolar base membrane and may have tombstone-like configuration. In a sense, the apical-basal orientation is maintained (Fig. 3.7a–d) [8, 9]. In contrast, in adenocarcinoma, the neoplastic cells have abnormal nuclear features such as size variation, nuclear pleomorphism, high N/C ratio, nuclear overlapping, irregular contours, hyperchromasia, abnormally prominent nucleoli, and unevenly stained chromatin pattern. Atypical mitotic figures can also be seen (Fig. 3.7g, h). When a lesion is small, ≤0.5 cm with lepidic architecture, and mild-to-moderate cytologic atypia of pneumocytes, it is designated as atypical adenomatous hyperplasia (AAH) (Fig. 3.7e, f). When a lesion is >0.5 cm but ≤3.0 cm with lepidic architecture and mild-to-moderate cytologic atypia of pneumocytes, it is AIS (Fig. 3.7g and h). AAH and AIS are precursors of invasive adenocarcinoma.

Secondary Architectures

In reactive type II pneumocyte hyperplasia, the alveolar structure is maintained. The proliferating type II pneumocytes line the alveolar septa in a single layer without nuclear stratification or forming any complex secondary structures. In contrast, in adenocarcinoma, the alveolar structure is maintained only in lepidic growth pattern. In the acinar growth pattern, the acini usually vary in size and shape exhibiting an infiltrating pattern (Fig. 3.8c) [7–9]. In more obviously malignant cases, there may be other secondary structures such as papillae and micropapillary formation or solid/large, nested growth patterns. Of note, epithelioid histiocytes or detached pneumocytes in a desquamated fashion in alveolar spaces in a reactive process should not be mistaken for solid growth pattern.

The Underlying Lung Injury, Background Stroma, and Inflammatory Cell Infiltrates

The background stroma and pattern of injury usually offer clues whether it is a reactive process or neoplastic process. In reactive type II hyperplasia, the underlying etiology should be present. The underlying patterns of lung injury

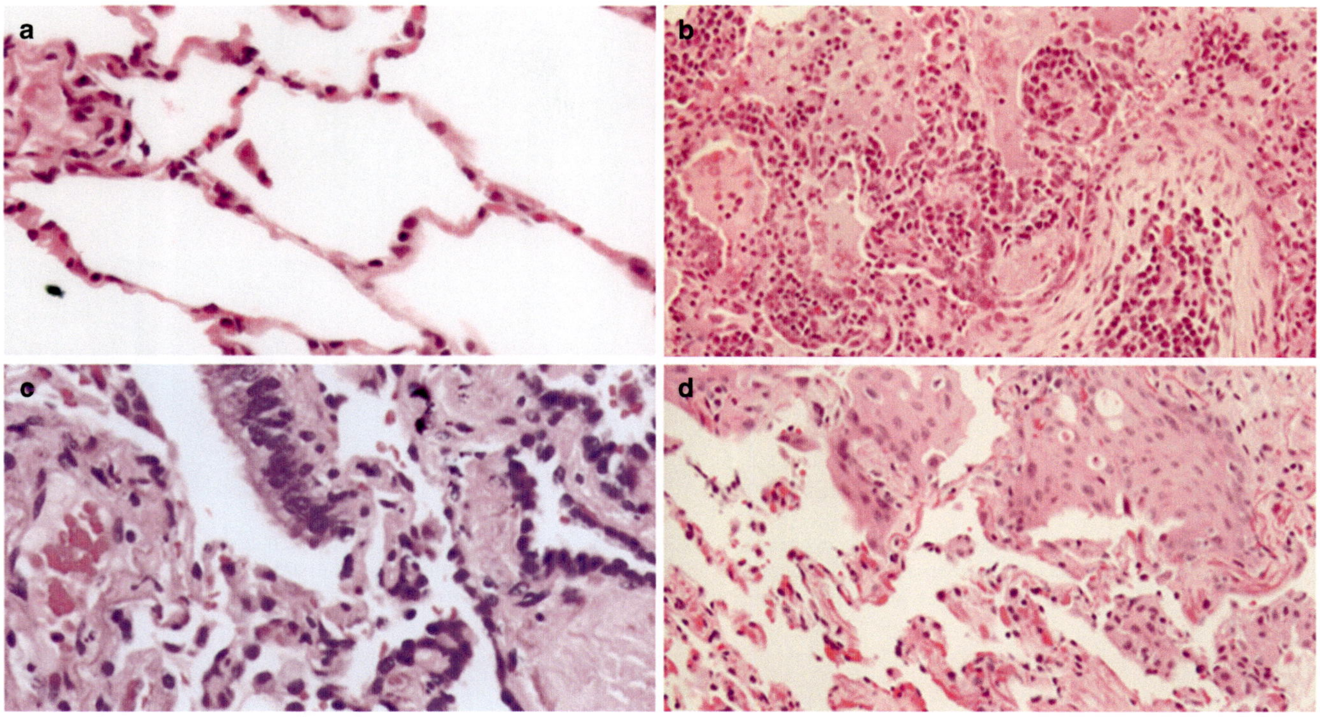

Fig. 3.6 (**a**) Normal lung alveoli are lined by flat type I pneumocytes and cuboidal type II pneumocytes. (**b**) Reactive type II pneumocyte hyperplasia associated with organizing pneumonia. (**c**) Bronchiolar metaplasia. (**d**) Squamous metaplasia. Original magnification 400×

Table 3.1 Diagnostic features used to separate reactive type II pneumocyte hyperplasia from others

	Reactive type II pneumocyte hyperplasia	Invasive adenocarcinoma	Atypical adenomatous hyperplasia	Adenocarcinoma in situ
Size	Any size	Any size	≤ 0.5 cm	> 0.5 cm but ≤3.0 cm
CT	Mass lesion	Mass lesion	Undetectable/ ground glass	Ground-glass mass lesion
Cytomorphology	Uniformly enlarged nuclei; non-hyperchromatic, single prominent nucleoli; regular nuclear membrane; nonoverlapping nuclei; low N/C ratio; and maintained apical-basal polarity	Variably enlarged nuclei, hyperchromasia, overlapping nuclei, irregular nuclear membrane, and loss of apical-basal polarity	Nuclear enlargement; features in between reactive and neoplastic	Similar to invasive adenocarcinoma
Architecture	Lepidic pattern; no nuclear stratification, no papillary, micropapillary, or solid pattern	Nuclear stratification; lepidic pattern; acinar pattern with variable sized, angulated, infiltrating acini; additional papillary, micropapillary, and solid patterns	Lepidic pattern	Lepidic pattern
Underlying acute injury and background stroma	Bluish cellular septa stroma; additional findings of underlying acute lung injuries such as organizing pneumonia, necrotizing granulomas, infarction, acute inflammatory exudate, and macrophages in alveoli	Fibroelastotic stroma or desmoplastic stroma; may have superimposed acute lung injuries such as necrosis, granulomas, organizing pneumonia, or acute inflammatory infiltrate	May have mildly thickened fibrotic septa	May have mildly thickened fibrotic septa
Axillary studies p53 EGFR mutations	Usually negative Negative	May be positive May be positive	May be positive May be positive	May be positive May be positive

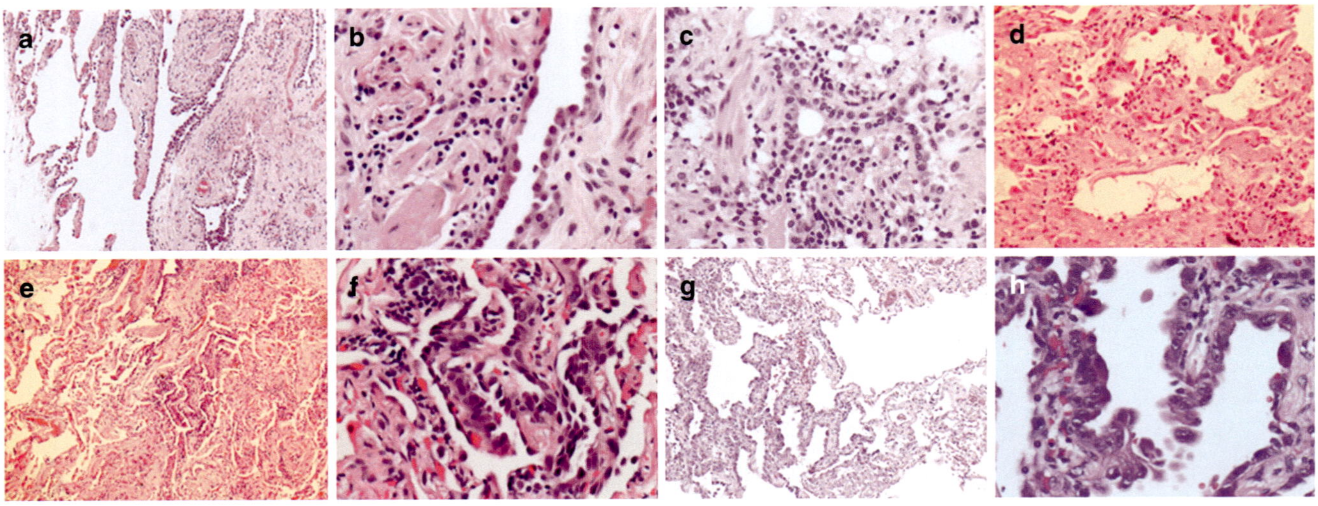

Fig. 3.7 (**a**) and (**b**) Type II pneumocyte hyperplasia in pneumothorax, respectively. Type II pneumocyte hyperplasia in lipogranuloma (**c**) and in diffuse alveolar damage (**d**). (**e**) and (**f**) atypical adenomatous hyperplasia, respectively. (**g**) and (**h**) Adenocarcinoma with lepidic growth pattern. Original magnification, (**a**, **e**, and **g**) 100×; (**b**, **c**, **d**, and **h**) 400×

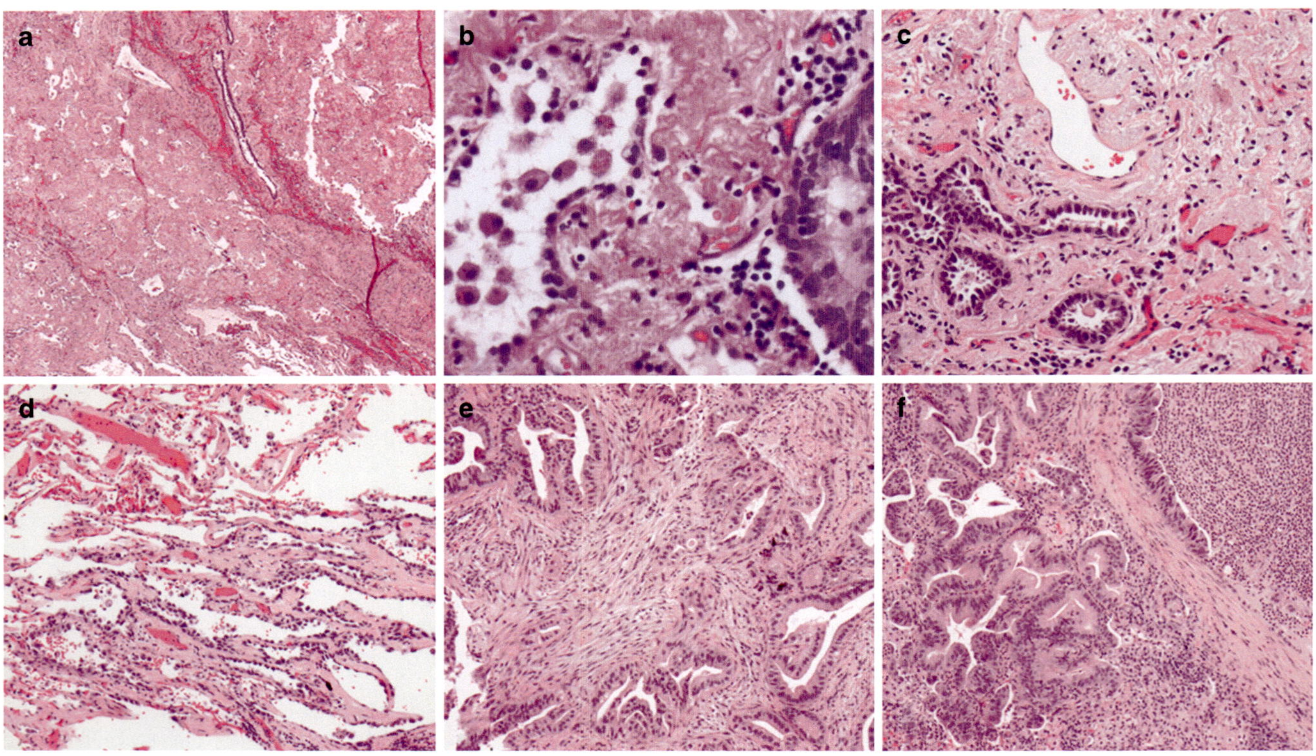

Fig. 3.8 (**a**) Fibroelastotic stroma seen in a benign scar with (**b**) entrapped acini lined by reactive type II pneumocytes and bronchiolar epithelium. (**c**) Fibroelastotic scar in the center of an acinar adenocarcinoma. Tumor acini/glands are seen. (**d**) Lepidic growth pattern is seen at the periphery. (**e**) Acinar adenocarcinoma with desmoplastic stroma. (**f**) Acute inflammatory infiltrate and other types can be seen in adenocarcinoma. (**a** and **f**) 100×; (**b**, **c**, **d**, **e**, and **h**) 400×

include, but are not limited to, pneumothorax, necrotizing granulomas, lipogranuloma, organizing pneumonia, infarction, diffuse alveolar damage, and acute bronchiolitis/pneumonia [2, 6, 7].

In adenocarcinoma without superimposed necrosis or infection, two variations of the stroma may be seen: fibroelastotic scar-like stroma and desmoplastic stroma. The fibroelastotic scar-like stroma can be seen in a benign scar

(Fig. 3.8a, b) or the center of an adenocarcinoma (Fig. 3.8c). Usually, adenocarcinoma with lepidic growth pattern can be appreciated at the periphery of the fibroelastotic scar (Fig. 3.8d). The identification of an invasive component within the fibroelastotic stroma is diagnostic of invasive adenocarcinoma. In adenocarcinomas with acinar pattern, the tumor acini usually exhibit variation of size and shape. They appear to be infiltrative. Entrapped benign bronchioles should not be mistaken for invasive component. The second variety of stroma is desmoplastic type stroma (Fig. 3.8e). It consists of dense myofibroblastic proliferation with a myxoedematous appearance. Usually, there are infiltrative angulated malignant acini of varying sizes haphazardly arranged in the stroma.

It is also worthy of pointing out that acute lung injury can be seen in the setting of adenocarcinoma as a result of obstruction, vascular occlusion, or superimposed infection. In this setting, acute lung injury is not usually the dominant finding (Fig. 3.8f). It should be kept in mind that in some situations as exemplified by our case, diagnostic material may not be present in a core biopsy or even a wedge biopsy.

Ancillary Studies

In most cases, a final diagnosis is still based on histopathologic findings. P53 immunostain has been proposed to differentiate reactive atypia from adenocarcinoma. In one study, using 10% positive cells as a cutoff value, 94% reactive atypia are negative for p53, whereas 86% of adenocarcinomas are positive for p53 [10]. In some difficult cases, p53 may lend some support towards the favored diagnosis based on histopathologic evaluation. Immunostain using EGFR mutation-specific antibody has also been proposed to aid the differential diagnosis [11] (Table 3.1).

References

1. Leslie KO, Yousem SA, Colby TV. Lung. In: Mills SE, editor. Histology for pathologists. Philadelphia: Lippincott Williams & Wilkins; 2012. p. 505–39.
2. Travis WD, Colby TV, Koss MN, et al. Non-neoplastic disorders of the lower respiratory tract. In: King DW, editor. Atlas of nontumor pathology. Washington, DC: American Registry of Pathology and Armed Forces Institute of Pathology; 2002.
3. Dacic S. Pulmonary preneoplasia. Arch Pathol Lab Med. 2008;132(7):1083–8.
4. Ogino S, Franks TJ, Yong M, Koss MN. Extensive squamous metaplasia with cytologic atypia in diffuse alveolar damage mimicking squamous cell carcinoma: a report of 2 cases. Hum Pathol. 2002;33(10):1052–4. https://doi.org/10.1053/hupa.2002.128246.
5. Hayashi T, Kumasaka T, Mitani K, Yao T, Suda K, Seyama K. Loss of heterozygosity on tuberous sclerosis complex genes in multifocal micronodular pneumocyte hyperplasia. Mod Pathol. 2010;23(9):1251–60. https://doi.org/10.1038/modpathol.2010.114.
6. Butnor KJ. Avoiding underdiagnosis, overdiagnosis, and misdiagnosis lung carcinoma. Arch Pathol Lab Med. 2008;132(7):1118–32.
7. Shilo K, Colby TV, Travis WD, Franks TJ. Exuberant type 2 pneumocyte hyperplasia associated with spontaneous pneumothorax: secondary reactive change mimicking adenocarcinoma. Mod Pathol. 2007;20(3):352–6. https://doi.org/10.1038/modpathol.3800744.
8. Grotte D, Stanley MW, Swanson PE, Henry-Stanley MJ, Davies S. Reactive type II pneumocytes in bronchoalveolar lavage fluid from adult respiratory distress syndrome can be mistaken for cells of adenocarcinoma. Diagn Cytopathol. 1990;6(5):317–22. https://doi.org/10.1002/dc.2840060506.
9. Idowu MO, Powers CN. Lung cancer cytology: potential pitfalls and mimics - a review. Int J Clin Exp Pathol. 2010;3(4):367–85.
10. Cagle PT, Fraire AE, Greenberg SD, Cox A, Brown RW. Potential utility of p53 immunopositivity in differentiation of adenocarcinomas from reactive epithelial atypias of the lung. Hum Pathol. 1996;27(11):1198–203. https://doi.org/10.1016/s0046-8177(96)90315-9.
11. Mimori T, Kobayashi S, Tanaka A, Sasada S, Yoshida A, Izumo T, et al. Novel use for an EGFR mutation-specific antibody in discriminating lung adenocarcinoma from reactive pneumocyte hyperplasia. Histopathology. 2015;66(6):816–23. https://doi.org/10.1111/his.12516.

Atypical Adenomatous Hyperplasia Versus Peribronchiolar Metaplasia

4

Christopher M. Chandler and Haodong Xu

Case Presentation

A 71-year-old woman with a 27 pack-year smoking history, history of COPD, and chronic productive cough was found to have a slowly enlarging, spiculated 22 × 19 mm right middle lobe opacity on screening CT scan. She had additional subtle ground-glass opacity (GGO) nodules in her right lower lobe and right upper lobe (Fig. 4.1). A PET-CT scan was negative for any evidence of metastatic disease. She underwent right thoracotomy with right middle lobectomy and wedge resections of the right lower lobe.

Gross pathologic evaluation of the middle lobectomy specimen revealed a tan-white, well-circumscribed mass measuring 2.0 × 1.8 × 0.7 cm abutting the pleura. No gross lesions were identified in the lower lobe specimens. Microscopic examination of the mass revealed a proliferation of highly atypical, cuboidal cells forming well-defined glands (<5 mm) within a fibrous stroma and background of similar cells lining the existing alveolar spaces (lepidic growth) consistent with a minimally invasive adenocarcinoma. Additionally, the right lower lobe harbored multifocal proliferations of large, atypical cells lining the thickened alveolar septa (10 mm and 7 mm) with associated multifocal proliferations of less atypical cuboidal cells with hobnail-like growth along thin alveolar septa (less than 5 mm).

After diagnosis, the patient's course was uncomplicated, and she is scheduled for continued surveillance via imaging.

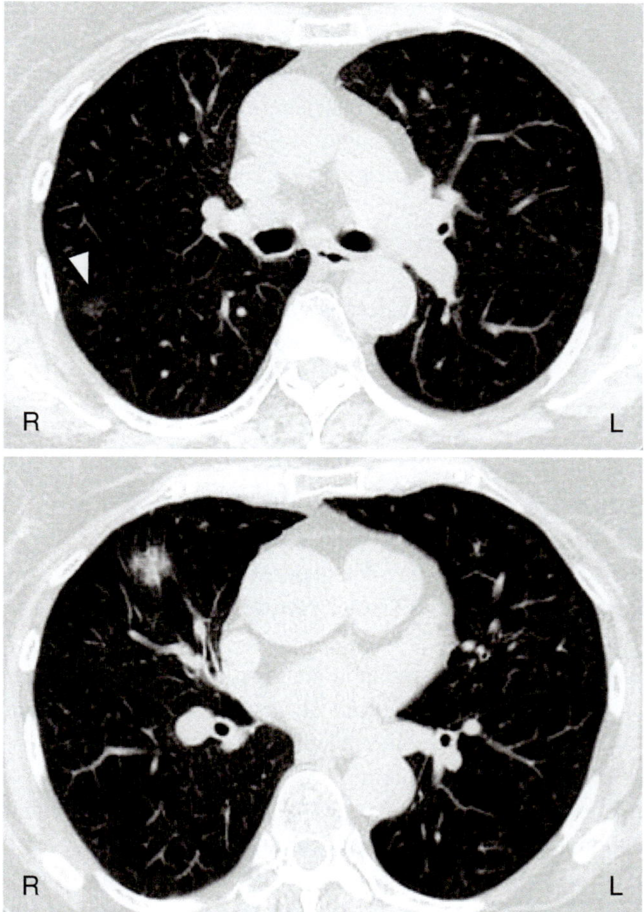

Fig. 4.1 Axial cuts from high-resolution CT scan showing a subtle ground-glass opacity nodule (GGO) in the right lower lobe (arrowhead, top panel) and spiculated 22 x 19 mm right middle lobe opacity (bottom panel)

C. M. Chandler (✉) · H. Xu
Department of Laboratory Medicine and Pathology, University of Washington Medical Center, Seattle, WA, USA
e-mail: cchandl@uw.edu

H. Xu et al. (eds.), *Practical Lung Pathology*, Practical Anatomic Pathology, https://doi.org/10.1007/978-3-031-14402-8_4

Pathologic Diagnosis: Minimally Invasive Adenocarcinoma, Acinar Pattern with Associated Lepidic Component in the Right Middle Lobe, Multifocal Adenocarcinoma In Situ, and Atypical Adenomatous Hyperplasia (AAH) in the Right Lower Lobe

What Are the Radiographic Features of Atypical Adenomatous Hyperplasia, and How Do They Differ from Peribronchiolar Metaplasia?

As illustrated in the above case, AAH is often undetectable by imaging and incidentally discovered in microscopic sections associated with surgical resection of a larger tumor. However, the lepidic growth pattern of AAH can create a hazy GGO nodule lacking a solid component on high-resolution helical CT imaging [1]. The imaging appearance is similar to adenocarcinoma in situ (AIS) consistent with the proposed stepwise progression of AAH to AIS and then invasive adenocarcinoma (the Noguchi Classification) [2]. PBM does not have a distinct appearance on imaging but often occurs within the context of fibrotic or inflammatory lung diseases, the imaging characteristics of which are heterogeneous.

What Are the Gross Pathologic Features of Atypical Adenomatous Hyperplasia and Peribronchiolar Metaplasia, and in What Gross Context Are They Found?

AAH is often not appreciable on gross exam but can appear as a small, less than 5 mm lacy, white to yellow nodular lesion with ill-defined borders often located in the periphery of the lung near the pleura [3–5]. The gross context of AAH is important. The incidence of AAH in the lungs that harbor carcinoma (particularly adenocarcinoma) has been reported to be 5–20% [5, 6], a finding often cited as evidence of possible "field cancerization," the theory that accrued somatic mutations create a cancer-primed cell population that can progress to a malignant lesion upon further insult [7]. PBM does not typically present as a grossly identifiable lesion, and the gross context is distinct from that of AAH. As a reactive lesion, PBM is often associated with fibrotic lung parenchyma and is often seen when examining histologic sections of the lung from patients with a history of smoking or other fibrosing chronic lung diseases including bronchiectasis, chronic hypersensitivity pneumonitis, and constrictive bronchiolitis [8].

What Are the Microscopic Features of Atypical Adenomatous Hyperplasia and Peribronchiolar Metaplasia? Is Immunohistochemistry or Molecular Testing Useful to Distinguish these Entities from One Another?

Microscopically, AAH presents a proliferation of atypical alveolar type II pneumocytes lining the existing alveolar spaces (lepidic growth pattern). The atypical cells often have a hobnail appearance with gaps between adjacent cells along the basement membrane (Fig. 4.2, **panels A–C**). These gaps are a useful histologic feature in distinguishing AAH from AIS, since the latter tends to be more cellular with a continuous proliferation of cells along the existing alveolar structures and thickened alveolar septa (Fig. 4.2, **panel D**). The atypia seen in AAH represents an early phase of neoplasia that may progress along a continuum to invasive adenocarcinoma. The cells have increased nuclear-to-cytoplasmic ratios, hyperchromatic nuclei, and variably prominent nucleoli [3]. The degree of atypia tends to increase with lesion size. These lesions notably lack significant tufting, papillary structures, or high cellularity [4]. Grading of atypia is not recommended in AAH [9]. In keeping with a neoplastic process, there is an abrupt transition from normal pneumocytes to atypical cells which are often at least double the size of neighboring normal cells [10]. The underlying alveolar septa may be slightly thickened but lack significant fibrosis.

PBM may resemble AAH from low-power magnification—a proliferation of columnar to cuboidal cells along existing alveolar spaces. At higher magnification, however, the cells lining the alveolar walls lack significant atypia and show features of normal respiratory epithelium (Fig. 4.3). Indeed, the process was previously termed "Lambertosis" after the canals of Lambert which connect bronchioles to neighboring alveoli (Fig. 4.3). Helpfully, the cells are often ciliated with terminal bars, which is not a typical feature of AAH (Fig. 4.4, **inset**). In contrast to AAH, the surrounding alveolar support network associated with PBM is often fibrotic, distorted, and thickened with focal smooth muscle hyperplasia and chronic inflammatory infiltrates [11]. As it is a result of prior small airway injury/scarring, PBM is usually bronchiolocentric.

PBM itself may have a morphology indistinct from that of bronchiolar adenoma (BA), distal-type, which was recently suggested as a benign lung neoplasm arising from the respiratory epithelium of bronchioles [12]. However, PBM is often seen in a background of interstitial lung disease or inflammatory processes. If presented with a small, solitary, well-circumscribed, bland-appearing ciliated lesion in a background of relatively unremarkable lung, BA, distal-type

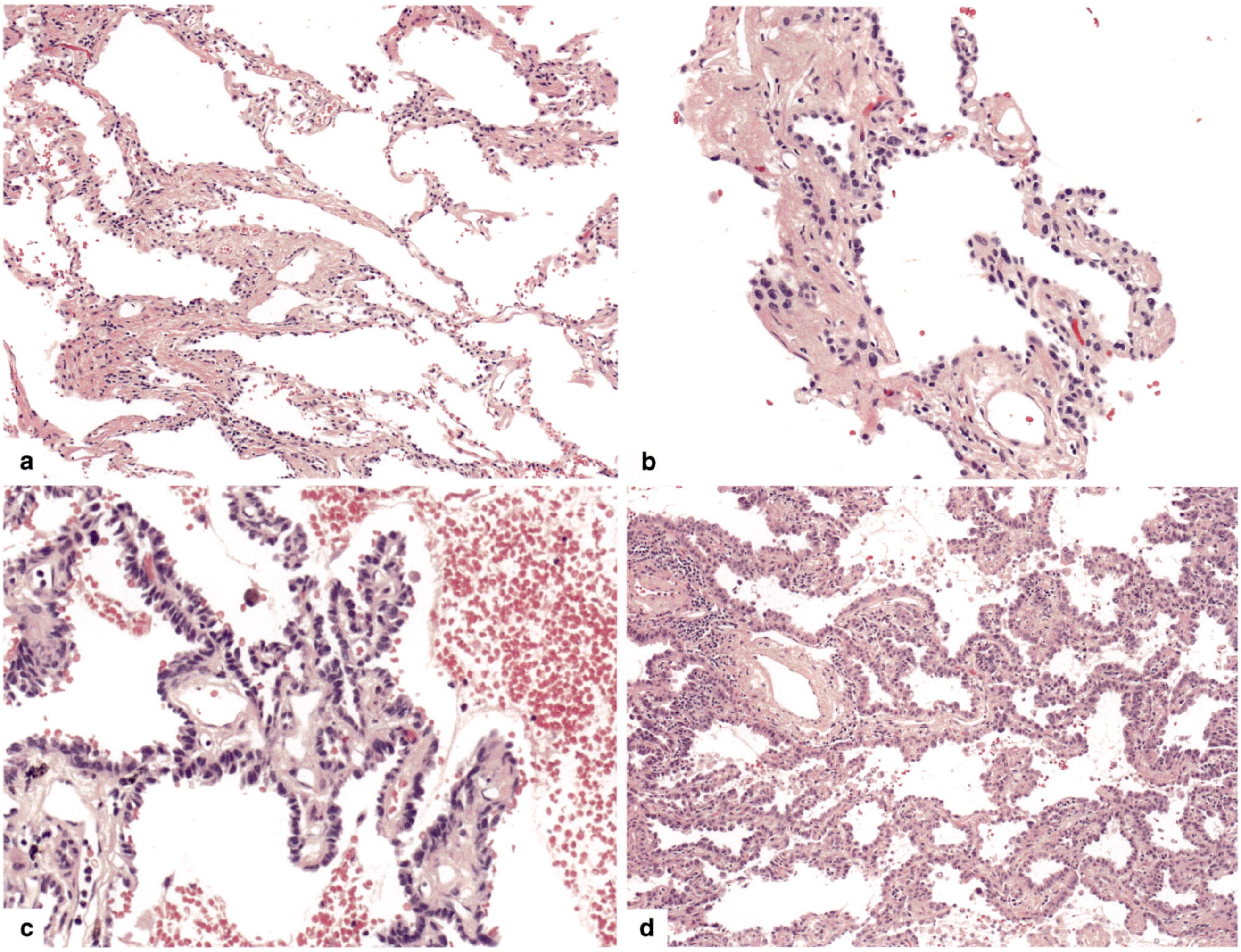

Fig. 4.2 (**a–d**) Atypical adenomatous hyperplasia (AAH). Focal proliferation of atypical type II pneumocytes along the existing alveolar structures. Note that the alveolar septa are not thickened and there are gaps between cells along the basement membrane. (**a**, **b**) mild atypia (100× and 200×, respectively, hematoxylin and eosin), (**c**) severe atypia (200×, hematoxylin and eosin). (**d**) Adenocarcinoma in situ (AIS). The atypical cells are larger, crowded, and focally overlapping and form a continuous proliferation along slightly thickened alveolar septa

and, if a prominent papillary component is present with abundant intra-alveolar mucin, BA, proximal-type, previously named as ciliated muconodular papillary tumor (CMPT), should be considered.

Immunohistochemistry is not typically used to distinguish between AAH and PBM. However, research into the progression of lung adenocarcinoma has established that AAH is immunoreactive for TTF-1, cytokeratins (including CAM5.2 and AE1/AE3), and CEA as well as other markers of Clara cell and/or type II pneumocyte differentiation such as surfactant apoprotein [2, 10, 13, 14]. PBM has been reported to maintain the staining pattern of normal airways by p63 immunohistochemistry, principally cells with nuclear reactivity along the basal layers of the epithelium. AAH and adenocarcinoma can also be positive for p63 but at a much lower frequency (three of five cases of AAH and 12% of adenocarcinoma in one study) [15]. Supportive of its premalignant status, AAH has been found to often harbor mutations in *K-ras*, *EGFR*, and *p53*, the most frequently mutated genes in lung cancer [16–20].

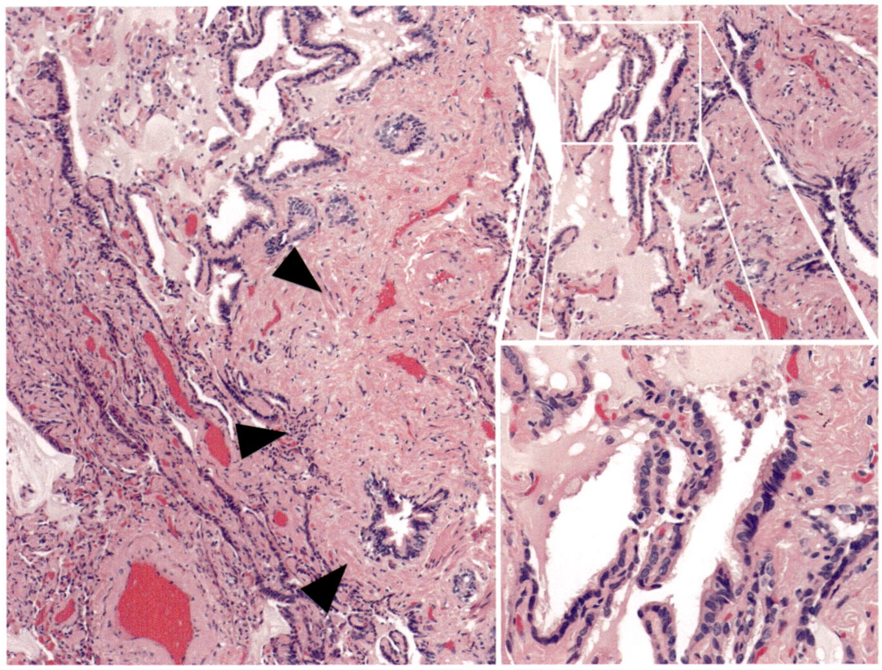

Fig. 4.3 Peribronchiolar metaplasia (PBM). The epithelial lining of alveoli surrounding a terminal bronchiole (arrowheads) is replaced with ciliated, respiratory-type epithelium (inset) as a reactive response to airway inflammation. Note the background bronchiolocentric fibrosis and chronic inflammatory cell infiltrates (100× and 400×, inset, hematoxylin and eosin)

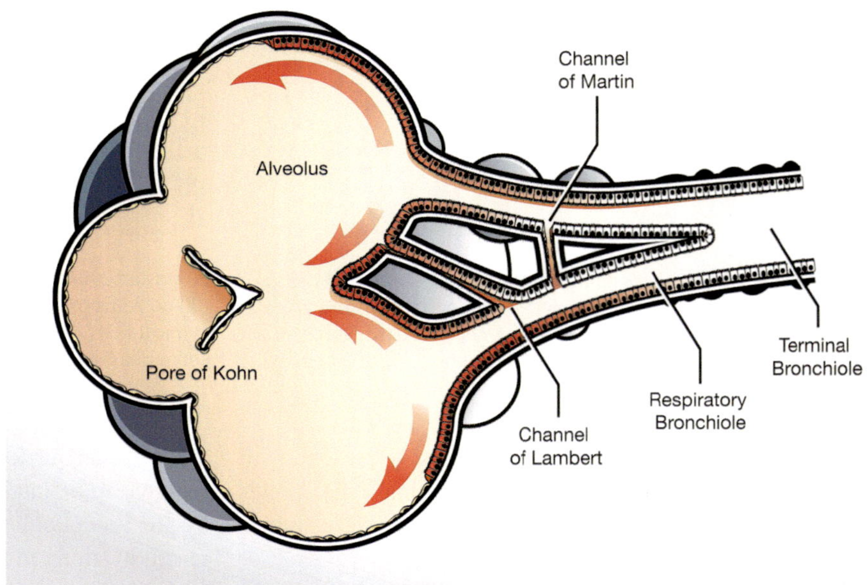

Fig. 4.4 Peribronchiolar metaplasia (PBM) was previously referred to as "Lambertosis" after the canals of Lambert (also called the channels of Lambert) which connect terminal bronchioles to adjacent alveoli. The usual, thin squamous and cuboidal epithelium of the alveolar wall is replaced by metaplastic columnar to cuboidal, ciliated respiratory-type epithelium (pink)

References

1. Lee HY, Lee KS. Ground-glass opacity nodules: histopathology, imaging evaluation, and clinical implications. J Thorac Imaging. 2011;26(2):106–18.
2. Noguchi M. Stepwise progression of pulmonary adenocarcinoma--clinical and molecular implications. Cancer Metastasis Rev. 2010;29(1):15–21.
3. Mori M, Rao SK, Popper HH, Cagle PT, Fraire AE. Atypical adenomatous hyperplasia of the lung: a probable forerunner in the development of adenocarcinoma of the lung. Mod Pathol. 2001;14(2):72–84.
4. Miller RR. Bronchioloalveolar cell adenomas. Am J Surg Pathol. 1990;14(10):904–12.
5. Chapman AD, Kerr KM. The association between atypical adenomatous hyperplasia and primary lung cancer. Br J Cancer. 2000;83(5):632–6.
6. Nakanishi K. Alveolar epithelial hyperplasia and adenocarcinoma of the lung. Arch Pathol Lab Med. 1990;114(4):363–8.
7. Curtius K, Wright NA, Graham TA. An evolutionary perspective on field cancerization. Nat Rev Cancer. 2018;18(1):19–32.
8. Allen TC. Pathology of small airways disease. Arch Pathol Lab Med. 2010;134(5):702–18.

9. Travis WD, Brambilla E, Noguchi M, Nicholson AG, Geisinger KR, Yatabe Y, et al. International association for the study of lung cancer/american thoracic society/european respiratory society international multidisciplinary classification of lung adenocarcinoma. J Thorac Oncol. 2011;6(2):244–85.
10. Rao SK, Fraire AE. Alveolar cell hyperplasia in association with adenocarcinoma of lung. Mod Pathol. 1995;8(2):165–9.
11. Couture C, Colby TV. Histopathology of bronchiolar disorders. Semin Respir Crit Care Med. 2003;24(5):489–98.
12. Chang JC, Montecalvo J, Borsu L, Lu S, Larsen BT, Wallace WD, et al. Bronchiolar adenoma: expansion of the concept of ciliated muconodular papillary tumors with proposal for revised terminology based on morphologic, immunophenotypic, and genomic analysis of 25 cases. Am J Surg Pathol. 2018;42(8):1010–26.
13. Klebe S, Henderson DW. Facts and fiction: premalignant lesions of lung tissues. Pathology. 2013;45(3):305–15.
14. Mori M, Tezuka F, Chiba R, Funae Y, Watanabe M, Nukiwa T, et al. Atypical adenomatous hyperplasia and adenocarcinoma of the human lung: their heterology in form and analogy in immunohistochemical characteristics. Cancer. 1996;77(4):665–74.
15. Sheikh HA, Fuhrer K, Cieply K, Yousem S. p63 expression in assessment of bronchioloalveolar proliferations of the lung. Mod Pathol. 2004;17(9):1134–40.
16. Westra WH, Baas IO, Hruban RH, Askin FB, Wilson K, Offerhaus GJ, et al. K-ras oncogene activation in atypical alveolar hyperplasias of the human lung. Cancer Res. 1996;56(9):2224–8.
17. Kerr KM, Carey FA, King G, Lamb D. Atypical alveolar hyperplasia: relationship with pulmonary adenocarcinoma, p53, and c-erbB-2 expression. J Pathol. 1994;174(4):249–56.
18. Kitamura H, Kameda Y, Nakamura N, Inayama Y, Nakatani Y, Shibagaki T, et al. Atypical adenomatous hyperplasia and bronchoalveolar lung carcinoma. Analysis by morphometry and the expressions of p53 and carcinoembryonic antigen. Am J Surg Pathol. 1996;20(5):553–62.
19. Sartori G, Cavazza A, Bertolini F, Longo L, Marchioni A, Costantini M, et al. A subset of lung adenocarcinomas and atypical adenomatous hyperplasia-associated foci are genotypically related: an EGFR, HER2, and K-ras mutational analysis. Am J Clin Pathol. 2008;129(2):202–10.
20. Sakamoto H, Shimizu J, Horio Y, Ueda R, Takahashi T, Mitsudomi T, et al. Disproportionate representation of KRAS gene mutation in atypical adenomatous hyperplasia, but even distribution of EGFR gene mutation from preinvasive to invasive adenocarcinomas. J Pathol. 2007;212(3):287–94.

Adenocarcinoma In Situ Versus Atypical Adenomatous Hyperplasia

5

Marie Perrone and Robert W. Ricciotti

Case 1

Clinical Presentation

The patient is a 56-year-old female who presented with a persistent cough for approximately 3 weeks. She was initially treated with a course of antibiotics without improvement. In addition, she noted a 4–5 lb. weight loss over the past 1–2 months. She denies shortness of breath, hemoptysis, fever, chills, or night sweats.

Imaging Studies

A chest X-ray demonstrated a subtle reticular airspace opacity, concerning for possible infiltrate or scarring. A follow-up computed tomography (CT) scan showed a spiculated mass within the upper lobe of the right lung composed of a ground-glass opacity measuring approximately 2.9 × 2.5 × 1.6 cm. A positron emission tomography (PET)-CT scan demonstrated mild metabolic activity in the right upper lobe mass (standardized uptake value, SUV 1.9) with no evidence of intrathoracic or extrathoracic metastasis. The patient underwent biopsy and subsequent wedge resection of the lesion.

Pathologic Findings

Gross Examination

Gross examination revealed a lobectomy specimen with a solitary 2.8 × 2.5 × 1.8 cm well-circumscribed, firm, pink-tan parenchymal mass. The mass partially surrounded a bronchus, but no extension into the bronchus was grossly identified. There was no gross evidence of pleural invasion. The remaining lung parenchyma showed mild patchy anthracotic pigment deposition but was otherwise unremarkable.

Histologic Examination

Histologic examination of the lesion revealed a neoplasm showing a purely lepidic/in situ growth pattern (see Fig. 5.1) in which architecturally normal, but slightly thickened, alveolar septa were lined by atypical neoplastic pneumocytic cells. There was no parenchymal, pleural, or lymphovascular invasion and no STAS (spread through air spaces). There was no papillary or micropapillary growth pattern. Lymph nodes collected at the time of the lobectomy contained no metastatic disease.

Final Diagnosis: Adenocarcinoma in Situ (AIS)

Adenocarcinoma in situ (AIS) of the lung is a neoplasm of the glandular cells of the lung without evidence of invasive disease. AIS was a diagnostic term introduced to the World Health Organization's classification of lung tumors in 2015 (Austin JHM, et al.) [1], replacing bronchoalveolar carcinoma (BAC). To diagnose AIS, the neoplasm must be no greater than 3.0 cm, and it must have a purely lepidic growth pattern (no papillary or micropapillary architecture) in which the neoplastic cells grow along alveolar structures which have retained their architecture. STAS should be absent. Additionally, there must be no evidence of invasive disease, including stromal invasion, lymphovascular invasion, or pleural invasion, and there must be no necrosis. Lesions greater than 3.0 cm in size, even in the absence of definite histologic evidence of invasion, or with non-lepidic growth patterns are considered adenocarcinoma and should have the predominant growth pattern(s) specified. For example, a tumor with purely in situ (lepidic) growth that exceeds 3.0 cm should be classified as lepidic-predominant adenocarcinoma.

AIS is most often non-mucinous, but may rarely be mucinous [1]. The non-mucinous type shows Clara cell or type II pneumocyte differentiation, whereas the mucinous type typically shows differentiation toward distal bronchiolar glandu-

M. Perrone · R. W. Ricciotti (✉)
Department of Laboratory Medicine and Pathology, University of Washington Medical Center, Seattle, WA, USA
e-mail: ricciott@uw.edu

H. Xu et al. (eds.), *Practical Lung Pathology*, Practical Anatomic Pathology, https://doi.org/10.1007/978-3-031-14402-8_5

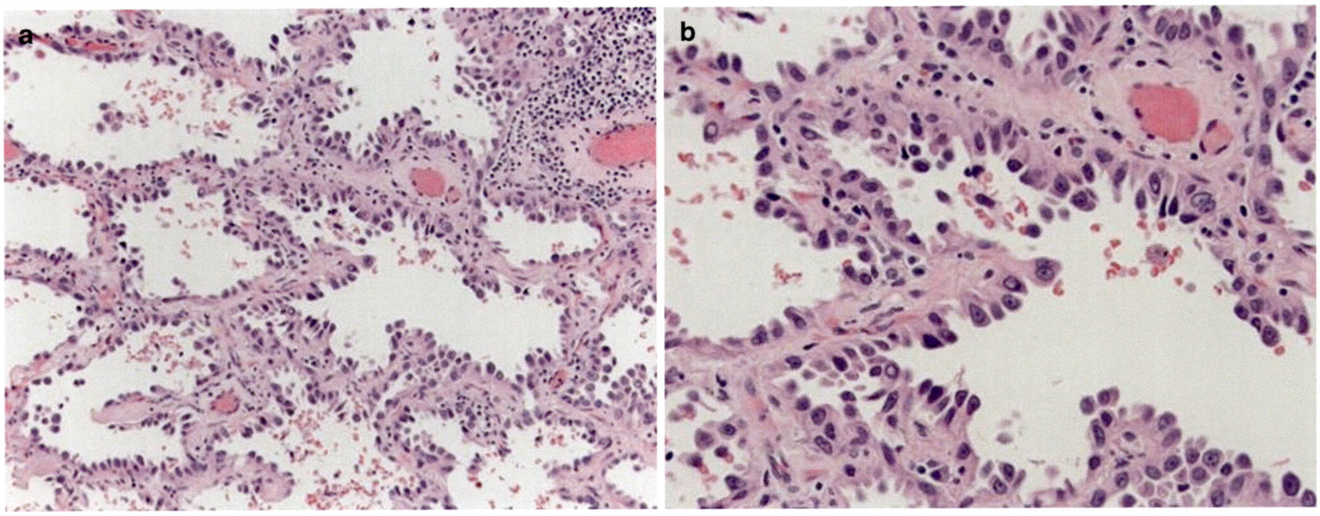

Fig. 5.1 (**a**) Alveolar septa are slightly thickened with maintained architecture and are lined by plump, atypical, neoplastic pneumocytic cells (lepidic pattern). No invasion or papillary/micropapillary architecture is seen. (**b**) Higher-power (400×) magnification demonstrating striking cytologic atypia of the neoplastic cells

lar cells. Non-mucinous AIS will usually express TTF-1, whereas mucinous AIS often will not [2]. There are no known immunohistochemical stains or molecular markers that will distinguish AIS from invasive disease.

These lesions have genetics similar to that of adenocarcinoma of the lung [2], lending support to the neoplastic continuum hypothesis. In smokers, adenocarcinoma in situ has complex genetics. In nonsmokers, these lesions are more likely to have alterations in one of a small subset of genetic drivers, including EGFR, KRAS, ALK, ROS1, and Her2.

The prognosis for patients that undergo resection for AIS is excellent with studies showing a 100% disease-free 5-year survival [3–5].

Case 2

Clinical Presentation

The patient is a 66-year-old female who initially presented with symptoms of an upper respiratory tract infection, including shortness of breath and an intermittent cough. She denied hemoptysis, changes in appetite, unintentional weight loss, fever, chills, and night sweats. As part of her evaluation, she underwent a CT of the chest.

Imaging

A CT of the chest revealed a 1.1 × 0.9 cm solid spiculated mass in the left upper lobe with numerous additional subsolid ground-glass nodules throughout both lungs (<0.5 cm each). A follow-up PET-CT revealed an FDG-avid spiculated nodule with surrounding ground-glass opacity in the left upper lobe with max SUV of 3.7 measuring 1.1 × 1.1 cm. Similar scattered subsolid/ground-glass nodules that are too small to characterize by PET. These findings were concerning for malignancy. The patient underwent left upper lobectomy.

Pathology

Gross Examination

Upon gross examination of the lobectomy specimen, the pleural surface was focally puckered and sectioning revealed an underlying well-defined, tan-white, 1.5 × 1.1 × 0.8 cm mass. The remainder of the lung parenchyma was unremarkable with no other discrete masses or lesions.

Histology

Histologic examination of the 1.5 cm spiculated mass showed destruction of normal alveolar architecture with replacement by fibrous/desmoplastic stroma containing highly atypical neoplastic epithelial cells forming irregular and poorly formed glandular structures (Fig. 5.2a). Examination of the remaining lung parenchyma revealed multiple foci of alveolar structures lined by plump cuboidal to columnar cells with hyperchromatic, mildly atypical nuclei with small nucleoli. These foci ranged in size from 0.2 to 0.4 cm and were distinct and sharply demarcated from the surrounding normal lung parenchyma with no evidence of an invasive component (see Fig. 5.2b–d).

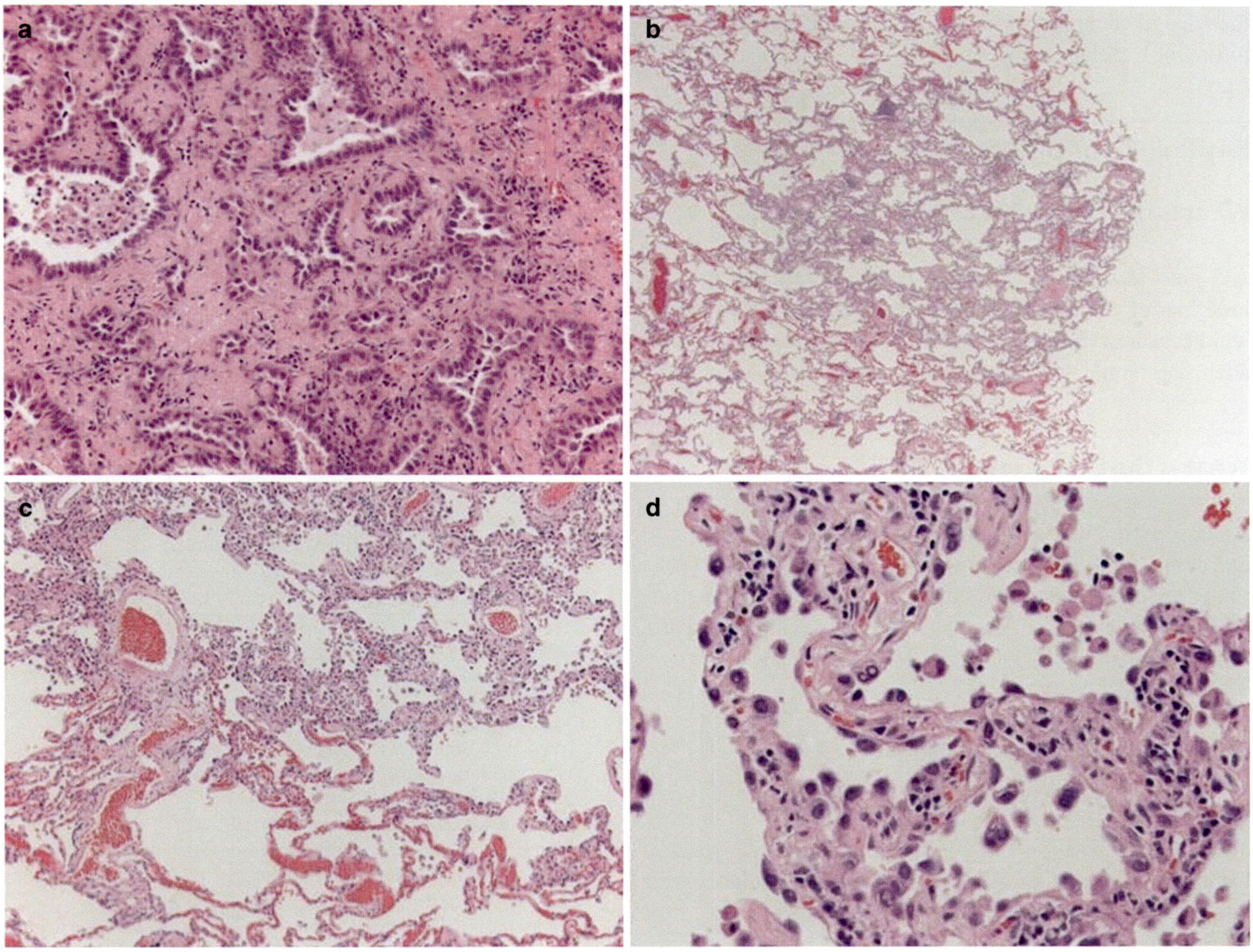

Fig. 5.2 (**a**) Representative area from the 1.5 cm lung mass showing fibrous stroma containing irregular glandular structures comprised of neoplastic epithelial cells. (**b–d**) Separate parenchymal lesions ranging in size from 0.2 to 0.4 cm. (**b**) Low-magnification (20×) view showing a well-circumscribed, roughly circular area that appears more basophilic than the background alveolar parenchyma. (**c**) Medium-power (100×) magnification reveals alveolar structures lined by atypical cells and slightly thickened septa (upper half of image) in comparison with the normal parenchyma (lower half of image). (**d**) High-magnification (400×) view shows plump, atypical cells lining slightly thickened alveolar septa with lymphocytic infiltrate. In comparison with case #1 above, the cytologic atypia is less severe

Final Diagnosis: Invasive Adenocarcinoma, Acinar Pattern Predominant, with Synchronous Foci of Atypical Adenomatous Hyperplasia (AAH)

Atypical adenomatous hyperplasia (AAH) is considered a preinvasive neoplastic lesion by the World Health Organization classification of lung tumors [1, 6]. AAH is frequently diagnosed concurrently with a synchronous malignancy [7–10] and, in that context, given its lepidic growth pattern, should NOT be considered intra-lobar metastasis for pathologic tumor staging purposes. AAH is often asymptomatic and diagnosed incidentally in specimens resected for lung cancer [8, 11]. The genetics of AAH are similar to that of adenocarcinoma [12], and thus, it is thought to be a precursor lesion to adenocarcinoma [2, 9].

On imaging, AAH can appear as a round ground-glass opacity with smooth, distinct borders [11, 13]. However, this appearance is not unique to AAH, and imaging cannot distinguish between AAH and carcinoma [11, 13]. Chest X-rays usually cannot detect AAH [11]. Additionally, AAH can be difficult to identify macroscopically in lung resection specimens.

By histology, AAH is a distinct population of atypical cells growing along the existing alveolar walls in an often discontinuous monolayer, frequently with a "hobnail" appearance. The cells are cuboidal to columnar, with enlarged nuclei relative to the surrounding normal cells, nuclear hyperchromasia, and may have prominent nucleoli. The transition between the atypical cells and the surrounding normal pneumocytes should be abrupt. The alveolar walls upon which these cells are growing may be somewhat thickened and fibrotic. The cytologic atypia is generally less striking than that of adenocarcinoma or AIS. There should not be any tufting or papillary architecture [9, 11].

Key Points for Differentiating AIS from AAH

What Is the Definition of AIS?

AIS must show a purely lepidic growth pattern and must be less than or equal to 3.0 cm in size. Tumors with a purely lepidic pattern that are larger than 3.0 cm are classified as adenocarcinoma, lepidic pattern.

What Is the Definition of AAH?

AAH is a preinvasive lesion that is small in size (≤0.5 cm) and composed of atypical type II pneumocytes or Clara cells lining the alveolar septa. It is well demarcated from the surrounding lung parenchyma, and the cells typically have a mild degree of atypia.

What Is the Relationship Between AAH and AIS?

AIS and AAH have similar genetic profiles. The genetics have given support to a possible multistep carcinogenesis hypothesis (AAH ➔ AIS ➔ carcinoma).

How Can Radiologic Features Help Distinguish AAH and AIS?

AAH is often multifocal. It usually cannot be seen on chest X-ray, but can be seen on a CT as persistent, well-defined, oval or round, nodular GGOs without solid components. AAH is often diagnosed incidentally on a resection specimen for a concurrent malignancy. AIS is usually seen as a pure ground-glass nodule >0.5 cm and <3 cm. However, partly solid nodules require pathologic examination to be categorized as AIS. In those cases, the solid areas seen on CT have been correlated with alveolar collapse, fibrosis, or mucinous components.

What Is the Difference in Prognosis Between AAH and AIS?

The prognosis for AAH and AIS is the same with complete surgical resection. Both lesions in and of themselves have a 100% progression-free 5-year survival; however, any separate concurrent malignancy, as is often seen with AAH, will follow it's own characteristic clinical course.

References

1. Travis WD, Brambilla E, Nicholson AG, Yatabe Y, Austin JHM, Beasley MB, et al. WHO Panel. The 2015 World Health Organization classification of lung tumors: impact of genetic, clinical and radiologic advances since the 2004 classification. J Thorac Oncol. 2015;10(9):1243–60.
2. Inamura K. Clinicopathological characteristics and mutations driving development of early lung adenocarcinoma: tumor initiation and progression. Int J Mol Sci. 2018;19(4):1259. https://doi.org/10.3390/ijms19041259.
3. Russell PA, Wainer Z, Wright GM, Daniels M, Conron M, Williams RA. Does lung adenocarcinoma subtype predict patient survival? A clinicopathologic study based on the new International Association for the Study of Lung Cancer/American Thoracic Society/European Respiratory Society international multidisciplinary lung adenocarcinoma classification. J Thorac Oncol. 2011;6(9):1496–504.
4. Gu J, Lu C, Guo J, Chen L, Chu Y, Ji Y, Ge D. Prognostic significance of the IASLC/ATS/ERS classification in Chinese patients-a single institution retrospective study of 292 lung adenocarcinoma. J Surg Oncol. 2013;107(5):474–80. https://doi.org/10.1002/jso.23259; Epub 2012 Sep 5.
5. Travis WD, Brambilla E, Riely GJ. New pathologic classification of lung cancer: relevance for clinical practice and clinical trials. J Clin Oncol. 2013;31(8):992–1001.
6. WHO classification of tumours editorial board. Thoracic tumours. Lyon (France): international agency for research on cancer, 5th ed., vol. 5. WHO classification of Tumours Series; 2021. https://publications.iarc.fr/595.
7. Butnor KJ. Avoiding underdiagnosis, overdiagnosis, and misdiagnosis of lung carcinoma. Arch Pathol Lab Med. 2008;132(7):1118–32.
8. Park CM, Goo JM, Lee HJ, Lee CH, Kim H, Chung DH, Im J. CT findings of atypical adenomatous hyperplasia in the lung. Korean J Radiol. 2006;7(2):80–6.
9. Mori M, Rao SK, Popper HH, Cagle PT, Fraire AE. Atypical adenomatous hyperplasia of the lung: a probable forerunner in the development of adenocarcinoma of the lung. Mod Pathol. 2001;14(2):72–84.
10. Nakahara R, Yokose T, Nagai K, et al. Atypical adenomatous hyperplasia of the lung: a clinicopathological study of 118 cases including cases with multiple atypical adenomatous hyperplasia. Thorax. 2001;56:302–5.
11. Kawakami S, Sone S, Takashima S, Li F, Yang ZG, Maruyama Y, et al. Atypical adenomatous hyperplasia of the lung: correlation between high-resolution CT findings and histopathologic features. Eur Radiol. 2001;11(5):811–4.
12. Sartori G, Cavazza A, Bertolini F, Longo L, Marchioni A, Costantini M, et al. A subset of lung adenocarcinomas and atypical adenomatous hyperplasia-associated foci are genotypically related: an EGFR, HER2, and K-ras mutational analysis. Am J Clin Pathol. 2008;129(2):202–10.
13. Kim HY, Shim YM, Lee KS, Han J, Yi CA, Kim YK. Persistent pulmonary nodular ground-glass opacity at thin-section CT: histopathologic comparisons. Radiology. 2007;245(1):267–75.

Invasive Adenocarcinoma Versus Adenocarcinoma In Situ

6

Sofia Liou and Gregory A. Fishbein

Case Presentation

A 75-year-old male with no history of smoking presents for evaluation of a left upper lobe pulmonary nodule that was identified on screening. The patient recalls one episode of chest tightness on exertion 1 month ago; he denies any other respiratory symptoms. Chest computed tomography (CT) shows a 2.7 cm subpleural nodule with mixed solid and ground-glass components. The patient undergoes left upper lobe segmentectomy and lymph node dissection, which reveals a 2.3 cm adenocarcinoma with primarily acinar growth pattern and a small component of lepidic growth (Fig. 6.1). The bronchovascular and parenchymal margins are negative, and the tumor is seen invading up to but not through the visceral pleura. All lymph nodes are negative for malignancy.

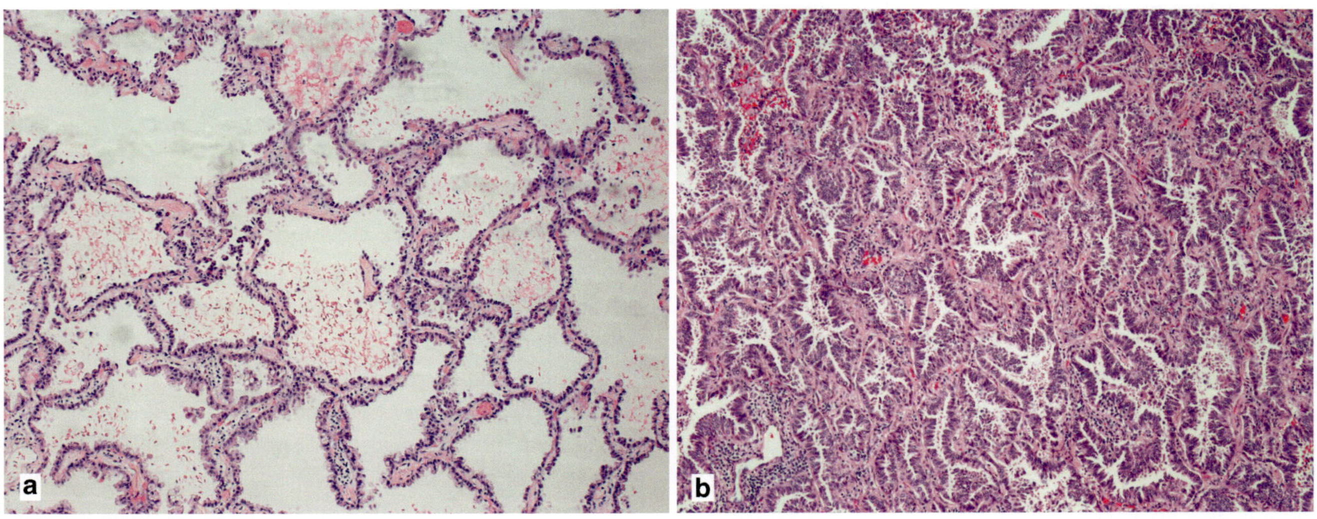

Fig. 6.1 Histologic sections of tumor showing (**a**) lepidic growth pattern and (**b**) acinar growth pattern

S. Liou · G. A. Fishbein (✉)
Department of Pathology and Laboratory Medicine, David Geffen School of Medicine at UCLA, Los Angeles, CA, USA
e-mail: gfishbein@mednet.ucla.edu

H. Xu et al. (eds.), *Practical Lung Pathology*, Practical Anatomic Pathology, https://doi.org/10.1007/978-3-031-14402-8_6

Pathologic Diagnosis: Invasive Lung Adenocarcinoma, Acinar Predominant

What Are the Clinical and Prognostic features of Lung Adenocarcinoma?

Lung cancer is the most common cause of cancer death worldwide, of which lung adenocarcinomas are the predominant histologic subtype [1]. Of all non-small-cell lung carcinomas, which make up 85% of lung cancers, lung adenocarcinomas comprise at least half [2]. The World Health Organization defines lung adenocarcinoma as a malignant epithelial neoplasm with glandular differentiation, mucin production, or expression of pneumocyte markers [3]. Although lung adenocarcinomas are the most prevalent subtype of lung cancer seen in never-smokers, tobacco use is associated with a twofold risk. Demographically, this tumor is most frequently found in adults in their sixth to seventh decade.

Clinically, patients can present with a wide variety of pulmonary symptoms (i.e., cough, hemoptysis, chest pain, shortness of breath) or no symptoms at all, depending on the extent of disease. Obstructive symptoms, secondary to mass effect or local invasion, may occur.

Surgical excision can be curative and may be followed by adjuvant therapy, which includes radiation, chemotherapy, and/or targeted therapy based on immunohistochemical or molecular findings. For example, a high tumor expression of PD-L1 can qualify patients for pembrolizumab, while ALK-driven tumors can be targeted with tyrosine kinase inhibitors. The prognosis depends on the stage at time of diagnosis, histologic pattern, presence of targetable mutations, and underlying comorbidities.

What Are the Radiologic Features of Lung Adenocarcinoma?

Imaging studies are paramount in the detection and diagnosis of lung cancer. Chest radiography and computed tomography studies are most frequently used. Lung adenocarcinomas initially manifest as small, solitary, spherical nodules with borders that range from smooth and lobulated to irregular and spiculated (Fig. 6.2). Tumors may have both solid and nonsolid (so called "ground-glass") components, with the solid component corresponding to invasive adenocarcinoma and the nonsolid component corresponding to lepidic growth (Fig. 6.3) [4–6]. The size of the solid—usually invasive—component generally correlates with the prognosis [7]. Tumors have a geographical predilection for peripheral over hilar regions [8, 9].

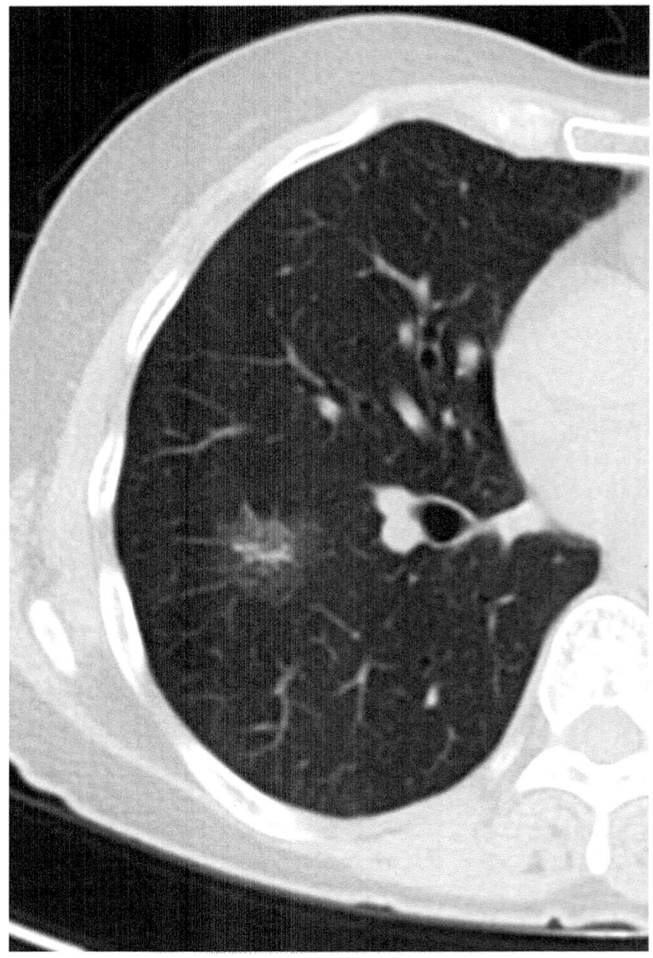

Fig. 6.2 CT imaging shows a 24 × 22 mm mostly ground-glass nodule with spiculated margin in the superior segment of the right lower lobe extending to and tethering the major fissure

What Are the Pathologic Features of Lung Adenocarcinoma?

Macroscopically, lung adenocarcinomas are relatively demarcated, nonencapsulated lesions with yellow-tan cut surfaces that may show central scarring, necrosis, and/or hemorrhage. Visceral pleural involvement is crucial for staging, so care must be taken during gross examination to identify areas of pleural invasion, which often show overlying pleural fibrosis or puckering. As mentioned earlier, the macroscopic heterogeneity of these tumors is significant, as solid areas correspond to invasive adenocarcinoma, while the less opaque and poorly defined areas, often at the periphery of the tumor, correspond to lepidic growth (Fig. 6.4). Areas with lepidic growth may have grossly preserved alveolar spaces. Tumors vary widely in size, ranging from subcentimeter nodules to greater than 10 cm.

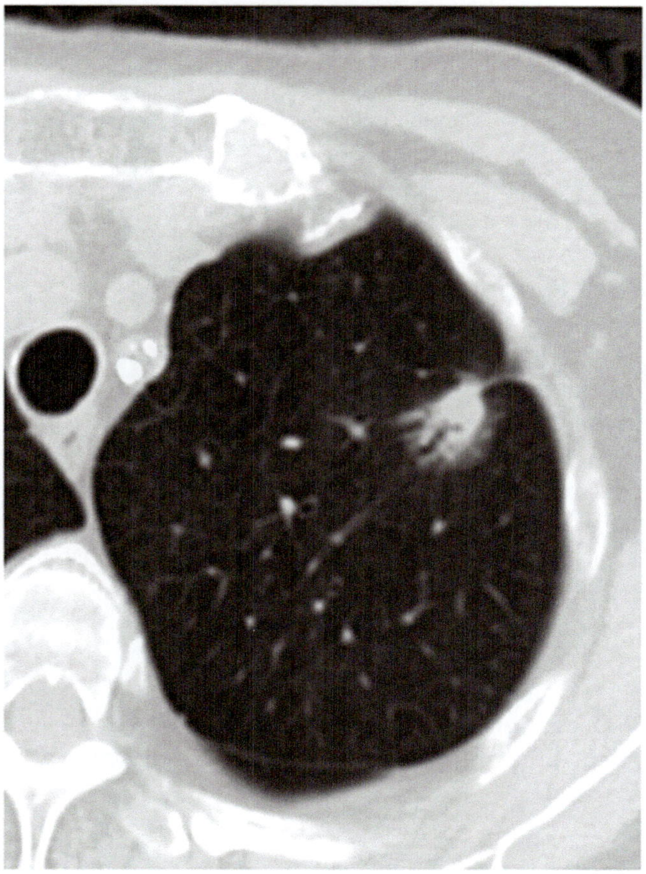

Fig. 6.3 CT imaging shows a mixed solid and ground-glass nodule in the left upper lobe measuring 27 × 12 × 31 mm

Microscopically, lung adenocarcinomas often have a dominant histologic subtype but can show a mixture of different growth patterns, which should be reported and quantified in 5% increments. The most common histologic patterns are lepidic, acinar, papillary, micropapillary, and solid. Additionally, adenocarcinoma cells may show non-mucinous (most common) or mucinous differentiation. Cribriform pattern was recently recognized, which corresponds to more aggressive and poorer prognosis than tumors with acinar growth pattern [10]. The histologic subtype carries prognostic value, as lepidic-predominant adenocarcinoma has a 5-year survival upwards of 90%, whereas micropapillary- and solid-predominant adenocarcinomas have a 5-year survival of 67–70% [9, 11, 12].

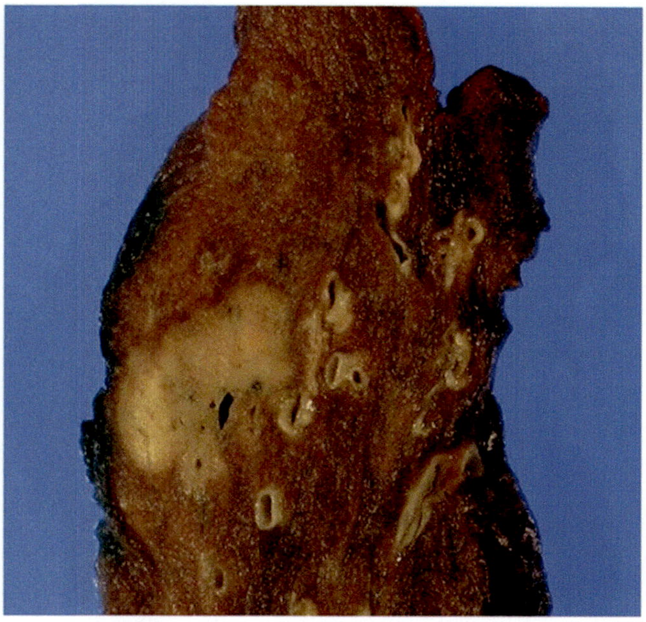

Fig. 6.4 Pulmonary lesion consisting of mixed solid and ground-glass areas, the former corresponding to invasive adenocarcinoma and the latter corresponding to lepidic growth

How Are Special Stains and Immunohistochemistry Used in the Diagnosis of Lung Adenocarcinoma? How About Genetic/Molecular Findings?

Pneumocyte markers that are widely used include TTF-1 (nuclear staining) and napsin A (cytoplasmic staining). 75% of invasive adenocarcinomas are positive for TTF-1 [13]. Lung adenocarcinomas also typically express cytokeratin 7 and lack cytokeratin 20 expression. Special stains that can be used to assess for pleural invasion include Masson's trichrome and Verhoeff's elastic stain. In addition, mucicarmine, Kreyburg, or periodic acid-Schiff with diastase stain can confirm that the entity in question is mucin-producing.

Ancillary studies, such as molecular and fluorescence in situ hybridization (FISH) testing, are a crucial component of tumor assessment. Gene alterations in *EGFR*, *ALK*, and *ROS1* are particularly significant as there is targeted molecular therapy available [14]. Additional oncogenic driver mutations associated with lung adenocarcinoma include *KRAS*, *BRAF*, *ERBB2* (*HER2*), *RET*, *MET*, and *NTRK1*. In general, *EGFR* mutations, which are present in 10–15% of lung adenocarcinomas, are more common in never-smokers, females, and non-mucinous tumors [15, 16]. *KRAS* mutations, which are present in 20–25% of lung adenocarcinomas, are more common in smokers and invasive mucinous adenocarcinomas [6].

What Are the Diagnostic Criteria for Adenocarcinoma In Situ (AIS), Minimally Invasive Adenocarcinoma (MIA), and Invasive Adenocarcinoma?

See Table 6.1.

How Is "Invasion" Defined in Invasive Lung Adenocarcinoma?

First and foremost, any histologic pattern other than lepidic—for example, acinar, papillary, micropapillary, and/or solid—is classified as invasive adenocarcinoma. In addition, extension into the lymphatics, blood vessels, visceral pleura, or alveoli is confirmation of an invasive tumor. Last but not least, the presence of tumor cells infiltrating myofibroblastic stroma counts as invasion. However, the interpretation of stromal reaction can be subjective, such as distinguishing desmoplastic stroma from benign scarring or fibroelastosis [17]. Indeed, there is significant interobserver variability in identifying the presence of invasion.

What Is the Prognosis for Adenocarcinoma In Situ (AIS) and Minimally Invasive Adenocarcinoma (MIA) Versus Invasive Adenocarcinoma?

AIS and MIA have a 5-year disease-free survival of 100%, according to a study that looked at 514 cases of pathologic stage I adenocarcinoma [12]. Invasive adenocarcinoma can be broken down into an intermediate prognosis category (including lepidic, acinar, and papillary predominant patterns) and a poor prognosis category (including solid and micropapillary predominant patterns); the former has a 5-year disease-free survival between 83 and 90% and the latter between 67% and 76% [12].

What Percentage of Resected Lung Adenocarcinomas Are Classified as Adenocarcinoma In Situ (AIS) and Minimally Invasive Adenocarcinoma (MIA) Versus Invasive Adenocarcinoma?

In a study that looked at 514 cases of stage I adenocarcinoma, greater than 90% of cases were classified as invasive adenocarcinoma. Only a small fraction (2%) was classified as AIS and MIA [12].

How Does Tumor Size Play a Role in the Staging of Lung Adenocarcinoma According to the Eighth Edition AJCC Staging Manual?

The tumor size that is reported depends on the histologic subtype. For non-mucinous adenocarcinomas with a lepidic component, the size of the invasive component is paramount to staging, as opposed to the entire tumor size (inclusive of both invasive and lepidic components). This is because the invasive size has been shown to be a greater prognostic indicator of high-stage malignancy than whole tumor size [18, 19]. In tumors where the invasive component cannot be measured in a single focus, an estimation of invasive tumor size can be calculated by multiplying the estimated percentage of tumor that is invasive by the total tumor size. For all other histologic subtypes, including invasive mucinous lung adenocarcinomas, the size of the entire tumor is used to assign a T stage [20].

Table 6.1 Diagnostic criteria for lung adenocarcinoma

	Adenocarcinoma in situ (AIS)	Minimally invasive adenocarcinoma (MIA)	Invasive adenocarcinoma
Tumor size (in greatest dimension)	≤3 cm	≤3 cm	>3 cm
Tumor pattern	Purely lepidic	Predominantly lepidic	Any pattern other than lepidic
Invasion	None	≤5 mm invasion in any dimension in any one focus	>5 mm invasion
Pleural, lymphatic, or vascular invasion	Never	Never	Possible
Spread through air spaces	Never	Never	Possible
Mucinous or non-mucinous	Usually non-mucinous	Usually non-mucinous	Either

What Does Lepidic Pattern Look like? Where Does the Word "Lepidic" Come from?

The term *lepidic* is defined as noninvasive surface alveolar growth of tumor cells, wherein the normal architecture of lung parenchyma is undisturbed, and tumor cells proliferate along the walls of intact alveolar spaces without infiltrating the stroma. First proposed by Canadian pathologist John George Adami in 1902, *lepidic* described tumors derived from surface-lining cells, with origins of the word meaning "a rind, skin, or membrane" [21].

Adenocarcinomas showing lepidic growth have a characteristic look: macroscopically, these areas are ill-defined and less solid and may show preserved alveolar spaces that permit aeration; microscopically, the alveolar walls are expanded by tumor cells, but the parenchymal architecture is entirely preserved (Fig. 6.5). Importantly, there is no lymphovascular or pleural invasion. Lung adenocarcinomas with a lepidic pattern have the most favorable prognosis.

How Are Acinar, Solid, Papillary, and Micropapillary Patterns of Lung Adenocarcinoma Defined?

Acinar growth pattern is characterized by round-to-oval or angulated glands with central lumina typically within desmoplastic stroma (Fig. 6.6). Solid growth pattern consists of sheets or nests of back-to-back tumor cells with little to no recognizable gland formation (Fig. 6.7). Papillary growth is characterized by tumor with at least 75% true papillae with fibrovascular cores, whereas micropapillary pattern is composed of small projections or cellular tufting without fibrovascular cores (Figs. 6.8 and 6.9). In the micropapillary pattern, cells may appear to "float" in the alveolar spaces either singly or in rings. Because papillary and micropapillary patterns have some overlap and it is difficult to fully represent a three-dimensional structure on two-dimensional imaging, there is room for interpretation which makes objective classification challenging.

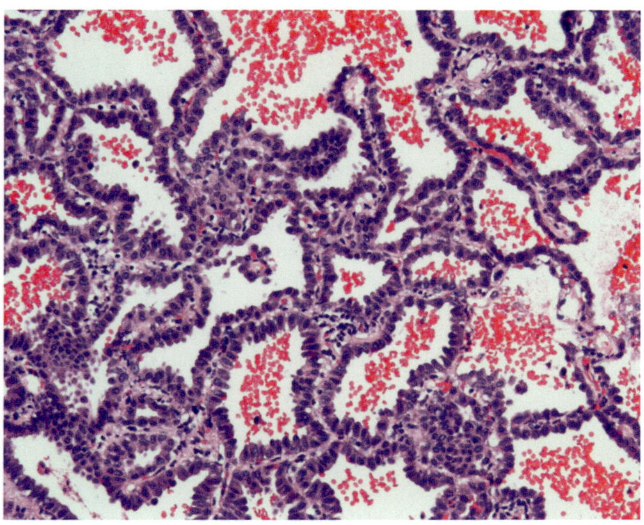

Fig. 6.5 Lepidic growth pattern, characterized by the growth of tumor cells along the surface of alveolar septa with overall preservation of lung architecture

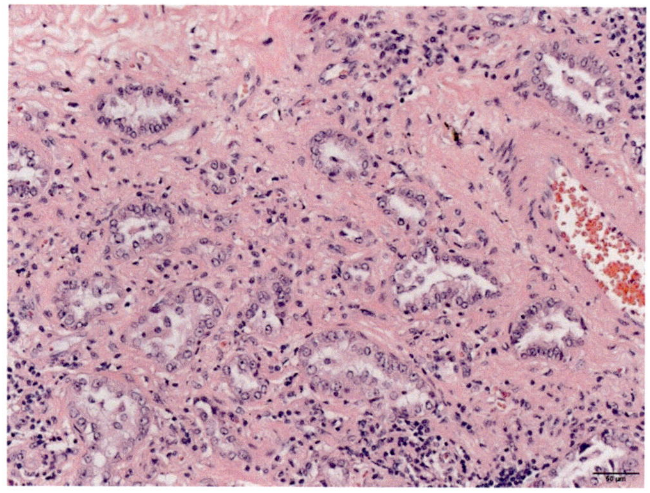

Fig. 6.6 Acinar growth pattern is characterized by a proliferation of round-to-oval or angulated glands with central lumina

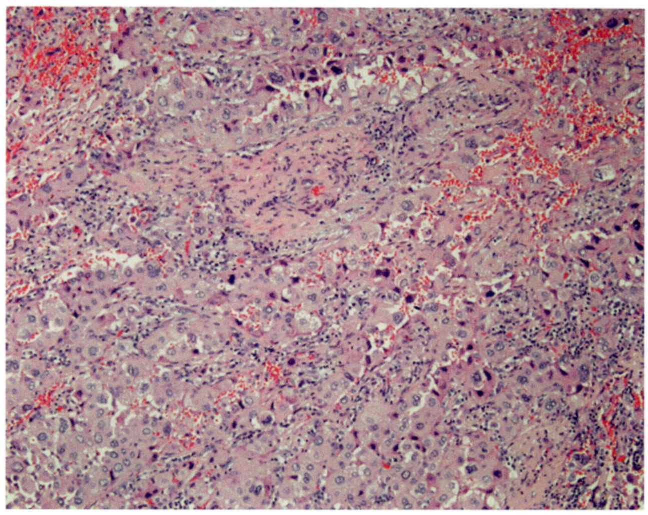

Fig. 6.7 Solid growth pattern, characterized by cords and sheets of back-to-back tumor cells

How Does One Approach a Small Biopsy Specimen that Shows Only Non-mucinous adenocarcinoma with Lepidic Growth Pattern?

Because the biopsy may not be representative of the entire lesion, the tumor should be characterized as "adenocarci-

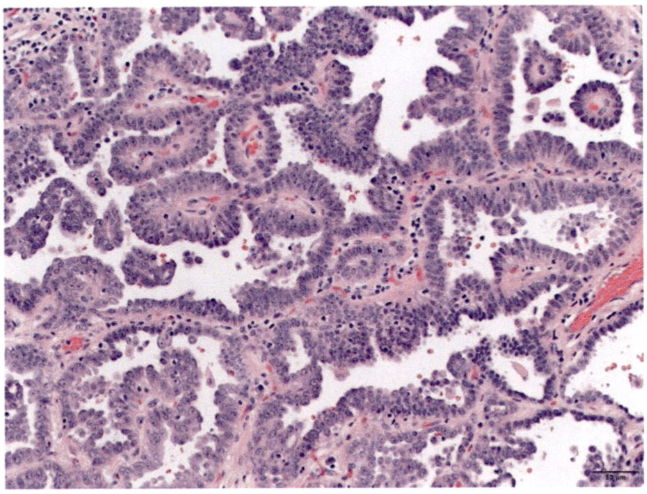

Fig. 6.8 Papillary growth pattern, showing true papillae containing fibrovascular cores

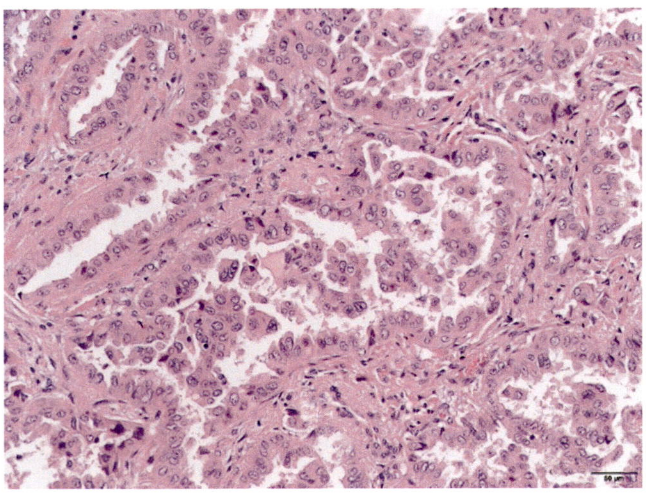

Fig. 6.9 Micropapillary growth pattern, characterized by papillary tufting without fibrovascular cores, as well as nests of cells that appear to "float" in the alveolar spaces

noma with lepidic pattern" without committing the lesion to adenocarcinoma in situ [4]. A definitive diagnosis can only be made on resection specimens, as the entire tumor needs to be evaluated for an invasive component. Should further sampling reveal any of the following, a diagnosis of lepidic-predominant lung adenocarcinoma can be made: (a) tumor invading pleura or lymphovasculature, (b) tumor necrosis, or (c) spread through air spaces.

How Does One Approach a Case with Multiple Lepidic-Predominant Lesions, for Example, a Lobectomy Specimen with Multiple Discrete Foci of Lepidic-Prominent Adenocarcinoma, Minimally Invasive Adenocarcinoma, and Adenocarcinoma In Situ?

The designation applied to such cases is *multifocal lung adenocarcinoma with lepidic features*. The T assignment corresponds to the highest T lesion and is followed by the suffix "m" (for multiple) or the number of discrete tumors in parentheses (i.e., T1b(m) or T1b(3)). A single N and M category is used for the lesions collectively. The prognosis is favorable as this pattern of disease demonstrates a low frequency of nodal or extra-thoracic metastases. Retrospective studies suggest that these represent synchronous primary tumors rather than intrapulmonary metastases [22–24].

What Is the Differential Diagnosis for Lung Adenocarcinoma?

The differential is broad and includes atypical adenomatous hyperplasia, large cell neuroendocrine carcinoma, poorly differentiated squamous cell carcinoma, adenoid cystic carcinoma, papillary thyroid carcinoma, mesothelioma, and adenocarcinoma from extra-thoracic origin.

References

1. Lozano R, Naghavi M, Foreman K, et al. Global and regional mortality from 235 causes of death for 20 age groups in 1990 and 2010: a systematic analysis for the global burden of disease study 2010. Lancet. 2012;380:2095–128.
2. Zappa C, Mousa SA. Non-small cell lung cancer: current treatment and future advances. Transl Lung Cancer Res. 2016;5(3):288–300.
3. Travis WD, Brambilla E, Burke AP, Marx A, Nicholson AG, editors. WHO classification of Tumours of the lung, pleura, thymus and heart. Geneva: WHO Press; 2015.
4. Borczuk AC. Assessment of invasion in lung adenocarcinoma classification, including adenocarcinoma in situ and minimally invasive adenocarcinoma. Mod Pathol. 2012;25:S1–S10.
5. Suzuki K, Asamura H, Kusumoto M, et al. 'Early' peripheral lung cancer: prognostic significance of ground glass opacity on thin-section computed tomographic scan. Ann Thorac Surg. 2002;74:1635–9.
6. Travis WD, Brambilla E, Noduchi M, et al. International association for the study of lung cancer/american thoracic society/european

respiratory society international multidisciplinary classification of lung adenocarcinoma. J Thorac Oncol. 2011;6:244–85.
7. Nakamura S, Fukui T, Taniguchi T, et al. Prognostic impact of tumor size eliminating the ground glass opacity component: modified clinical T descriptors of the tumor, node, metastasis classification of lung cancer. J Thorac Oncol. 2013;8:1551–7.
8. Russell PA, Barnett SA, Walkiewicz M, et al. Correlation of mutation status and survival with predominant histologic subtype according to the new IASLC/ATS/ERS lung adenocarcinoma classification in stage III (N2) patients. J Thorac Oncol. 2013;8:461–8.
9. Russell PA, Wainer Z, Wright GM, et al. Does lung adenocarcinoma subtype predict patient survival? A clinicopathologic study based on the new International Association for the Study of Lung Cancer/American Thoracic Society/European Respiratory Society international multidisciplinary lung adenocarcinoma classification. J Thorac Oncol. 2011;9:1496–504.
10. Kadota K, Yeh Y, Sima C, et al. The cribriform pattern identifies a subset of acinar predominant tumors with poor prognosis in patients with stage I lung adenocarcinoma: a conceptual proposal to classify cribriform predominant tumors as a distinct histologic subtype. Mod Pathol. 2014;27(5):690–700. https://doi.org/10.1038/modpathol.2013.188.
11. Kamiya K, Hayashi Y, Douguchi K, et al. Histopathological features and prognostic significance of the micropapillary pattern in lung adenocarcinoma. Mod Pathol. 2008;8:992–1001.
12. Yoshizawa A, Motoi N, Riely GJ, et al. Impact of proposed IASLC/ATS/ERS classification of lung adenocarcinoma: prognostic subgroups and implications for further revision of staging based on analysis of 514 stage I cases. Mod Pathol. 2011;24:653–64.
13. Stenhouse G, Fyfe N, King G, et al. Thyroid transcription factor 1 in pulmonary adenocarcinoma. J Clin Pathol. 2004;57:383–7.
14. Lindeman NI, Cagle PT, Beasley MB, et al. Molecular testing guideline for selection of lung cancer patients for EGFR and ALK tyrosine kinase inhibitors: guideline from the College of American Pathologists, International Association for the Study of Lung Cancer, and Association for Molecular Pathology. J Thorac Oncol. 2013;8(7):823–59.
15. Paez JG, Janne PA, Lee JC, et al. EGFR mutations in lung cancer: correlation with clinical response to gefitinib therapy. Science. 2004;5676:1497–500.
16. Pao W, Miller V, Zakowski M, et al. EGF receptor gene mutations are common in lung cancers from ‘never smokers’ and are associated with sensitivity of tumors to gefitinib and erlotinib. Proc Natl Acad Sci U S A. 2004;101:13306–11.
17. Thunnissen E, Beasley MB, Borczuk AC, et al. Reproducibility of histopathological subtypes and invasion in pulmonary adenocarcinoma. An international interobserver study. Mod Pathol. 2012;25:1574–83.
18. Maeyashiki T, Suzuki K, Hattori A, et al. The size of consolidation on thin-section computed tomography is a better predictor of survival than the maximum tumour dimension in resectable lung cancer. Eur J Cardiothorac Surg. 2013;43(5):915–8.
19. Tsutani Y, Miyata Y, Nakayama H, et al. Prognostic significance of using solid versus whole tumor size on high-resolution computed tomography for predicting pathologic malignant grade tumors in clinical stage IA lung adenocarcinoma: a multicenter study. J Thorac Cardiovasc Surg. 2012;143(3):607–12.
20. Amin MB, Edge SB, Greene FL, et al., editors. AJCC cancer staging manual. 8th ed. New York, NY: Springer; 2017.
21. Jones KD. Whence *Lepidic*?: the history of a Canadian neologism. Arch Pathol Lab Med. 2013;12:1822–4.
22. Chung J, Chloe G, Jheon S, et al. Epidermal growth factor receptor mutation and pathologic-radiologic correlation between multiple lung nodules with ground-glass opacity differentiates multicentric origin from intrapulmonary spread. J Thorac Oncol. 2009;4:1490–5.
23. Detterbeck FC, Marom EM, Arenberg DA, et al. The IASLC lung cancer staging project: background data and proposals for the application of TNM staging rules to lung cancer presenting as multiple nodules with ground glass or lepidic features or a pneumonic type of involvement in the forthcoming eighth edition of the TNM classification. J Thorac Oncol. 2015;11(5):666–80.
24. Takamochi K, Oh S, Matsuoka J, Suzuki K. Clonality status of multifocal lung adenocarcinomas based on the mutation patterns of EGFR and K-ras. Lung Cancer. 2012;75:313–720.

7 Solid Pulmonary Adenocarcinoma Versus Large-Cell Undifferentiated Carcinoma

Jared Cobb and Chen Zhang

Case Presentation

A 51-year-old female smoker presents with longstanding dry cough for several months, which was initially thought to be due to bronchitis. Over the next month, the patient continues to show worsening of symptoms and develops new-onset hemoptysis, 10-pound weight loss, shortness of breath with exertion, increasing fatigue, and loss of appetite. Her chest computed tomography (CT) is remarkable for a 4.0 cm right lower lobe mass along the posterior lateral segment, with fluorine 18 fluorodeoxyglucose (FDG) avidity on positron-emission tomography (PET)/CT. These findings raise the concern for malignancy, without evidence of mediastinal or distant metastases. Subsequently, a CT-guided biopsy reveals a poorly differentiated non-small-cell carcinoma (NSCLC) without apparent squamous or glandular elements. The patient's past medical history, family history, and social history are otherwise noncontributory. Shortly thereafter, the patient proceeds to right lower lobectomy with mediastinal lymph node dissection via video-assisted thoracoscopic surgery (VATS).

Gross examination reveals a subpleural, gray-white, and well-circumscribed 4.4 cm mass. Histologic sections reveal a high-grade infiltrative malignant neoplasm composed of nests and sheets of polygonal cells lacking discernable acini, tubules, or papillae (Fig. 7.1a). Immunohistochemical analysis reveals the cells of interest to stain positively for cytokeratin AE1/AE3 (not shown) and TTF-1 (Fig. 7.1b) and negatively for p40 (Fig. 7.1c). A mucicarmine stain highlights abundant intracytoplasmic mucin (Fig. 7.1d). Programmed death-ligand 1 (PD-L1) immunohistochemical stain exhibits a tumor proportion score (TPS) of 70%, and the patient is subsequently treated with pembrolizumab.

J. Cobb
Department of Pathology and Laboratory Medicine, Indiana University School of Medicine, Indianapolis, IN, USA

C. Zhang (✉)
Weill Cornell Medicine, Department of Pathology and Laboratory Medicine, New York, NY, USA
e-mail: fjr9007@med.cornell.edu

H. Xu et al. (eds.), *Practical Lung Pathology*, Practical Anatomic Pathology, https://doi.org/10.1007/978-3-031-14402-8_7

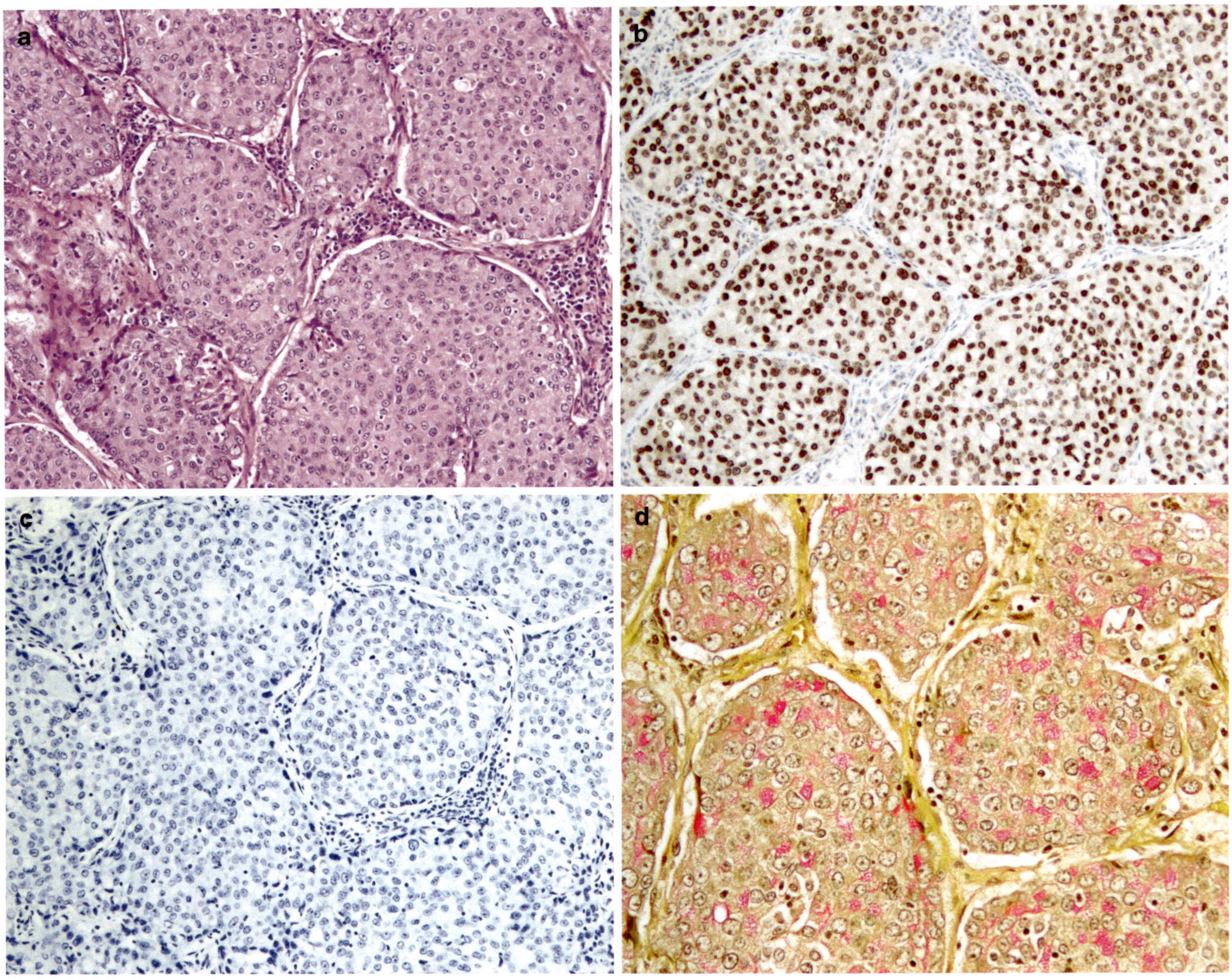

Fig. 7.1 Histologic features of solid pulmonary adenocarcinoma (SPA). (**a**) The tumor consists of nests and sheets of polygonal epithelial cells with round-to-oval nuclei and abundant eosinophilic cytoplasm. The nuclei are moderately atypical with inconspicuous nucleoli. No keratinization, glandular formation, or mucin production is seen. H&E, 100×. (**b**) Tumor cells show strong and diffuse nuclear positivity on TTF-1 immunohistochemical stain. (**c**) Tumor cells are negative for squamous marker p40. (**d**) Mucicarmine stain demonstrates abundant intracytoplasmic mucin vacuoles that are difficult to appreciate on H&E stain. 200×

Final Diagnosis: Solid-Type Pulmonary Adenocarcinoma

What Are the Clinical and Prognostic Features of Solid-Type Pulmonary Adenocarcinoma (SPA), and How Do They Differ from Large-Cell Undifferentiated Carcinoma (LCUC)?

SPA and LCUC typically present in a similar fashion with shortness of breath, cough, and pneumonia. Primary lung adenocarcinomas are more common in smokers and more frequently identified incidentally, compared to LCUC [1–3]. Additionally, paraneoplastic syndromes, although common in primary lung carcinomas, are less frequently observed in adenocarcinoma compared to other histologic types [3]. Prognostically, SPA and LCUC are not different from other types of NSCLC, with the main prognostic indicators being performance status at diagnosis and tumor node metastasis (TNM) stage [3]. From the histologic standpoint, poor prognostic indicators for both entities include a high histologic grade, extensive tumor necrosis, increased mitotic figures, few tumor-infiltrating lymphocytes, and vascular invasion. Genetically, for both SPA and LCUC, *KRAS* activation is associated with a poor prognosis as well as *p53* mutation and overexpression of c-erbB2 [4–6]. As molecular studies in these tumors advance, studies may continue to identify prognostically significant subsets of NSCLCs.

Can Radiologic Studies Be Used to Distinguish SPA from LCUC?

SPA and primary lung adenocarcinomas in general are frequently found in the peripheral lung and under 4.0 cm in size unlike LCUC which more commonly presents centrally with associated mediastinal lymphadenopathy and at a size larger than 4.0 cm [3]. Additionally, LCUC may present with involvement of the large bronchi, visceral pleura, or chest wall [7]. However, SPA only presents with pleura and chest wall involvement in approximately 15% of cases [3, 8]. By CT scan both pure SPA and LCUC are likely to present as a densely solid mass [9–12]. However, in mixed adenocarcinoma with a solid-predominant pattern, additional features may be identified such as a ground-glass periphery indicating a potential mixed bronchoalveolar pattern [13]. At the time of gross evaluation, a ground-glass component may be difficult to discern in an otherwise solid-appearing mass. Thus, comparing the radiologic impression to the tissue submitted for histologic evaluation can be helpful in difficult cases.

What Are the Pathologic Features of SPA and LCUC? How Can Special Stains Be Used to Distinguish These Two Entities?

Both SPA and LCUC are poorly differentiated non-squamous epithelial neoplasm that lack acini, tubules, and papillae. SPA is defined by the presence of cytoplasmic mucin in at least five tumor cells in two high-power fields. Diffuse and strong positivity on immunohistochemical stains of TTF-1 and/or napsin A also confirms the diagnosis. Compared with SPA, LCUC commonly demonstrates a higher degree of cytologic atypia, with large polygonal tumor cells, vesicular nuclei, prominent nucleoli, and moderate amounts of eosinophilic or clear cytoplasm (Fig. 7.2a–d). By definition, LCUC is a diagnosis of exclusion after ruling out any component of squamous cell carcinoma, adenocarcinoma, or small-cell carcinoma by morphology and immunohistochemical and/or mucin stains. In contrast to SPA which may be diagnosed on small biopsies with positive TTF-1 and/or mucin staining, LCUC can only be diagnosed on resection specimens after adequate sampling and examination of the entire tumor.

Other diagnostic considerations include poorly differentiated squamous cell carcinoma and mixed-type adenocarcinoma [1]. The mixed subtype comprises approximately 80% of resected pulmonary adenocarcinomas, and careful sampling is required to exclude the presence of different architectural patterns such as papillary, acinar, and lepidic patterns [14]. With a majority solid component, in the presence of additional architectural patterns, the diagnosis becomes solid-predominant pulmonary adenocarcinoma. Poorly differentiated squamous cell carcinoma is effectively excluded by the lack of p40 immunohistochemical staining.

Ultimately, LCUC is primarily a diagnosis of exclusion. Although rare cells in LCUC may contain intracellular mucin, most tumors lack significant mucicarmine staining and are negative for TTF-1, p40, and neuroendocrine markers [15, 16]. Additionally, extensive sampling will fail to reveal typical patterns of pulmonary adenocarcinoma. If these are present, other diagnosis should be considered, including the possibility of a collision tumor.

Are Genetic/Molecular Findings Useful in the Diagnosis and Treatment of SPA and LCUC?

The molecular findings for SPA and LCUC are largely similar, including point mutations in oncogenes such as *KRAS* and tumor suppressor genes such as *p53* and *Rb/p16Ink4* being the most common [17–19]. *KRAS* mutations typically occur at codon 12 from cancers arising in smokers and may be present in up to 30% of SPAs but are less common in other types of lung cancer including LCUC [20]. Furthermore, *KRAS* mutations correlate with poor survival and render *EGFR* inhibitors ineffective [4]. Later developments in the carcinogenesis pathway include loss of heterozygosity in multiple chromosomes including 2q, 9q, 18q, and 22q [21]. In addition to *EGFR* inhibitors, FDA-approved therapies targeting PD-1-, *BRAF*-, *ROS1*-, and *ALK*-positive NSCLCs are currently in use.

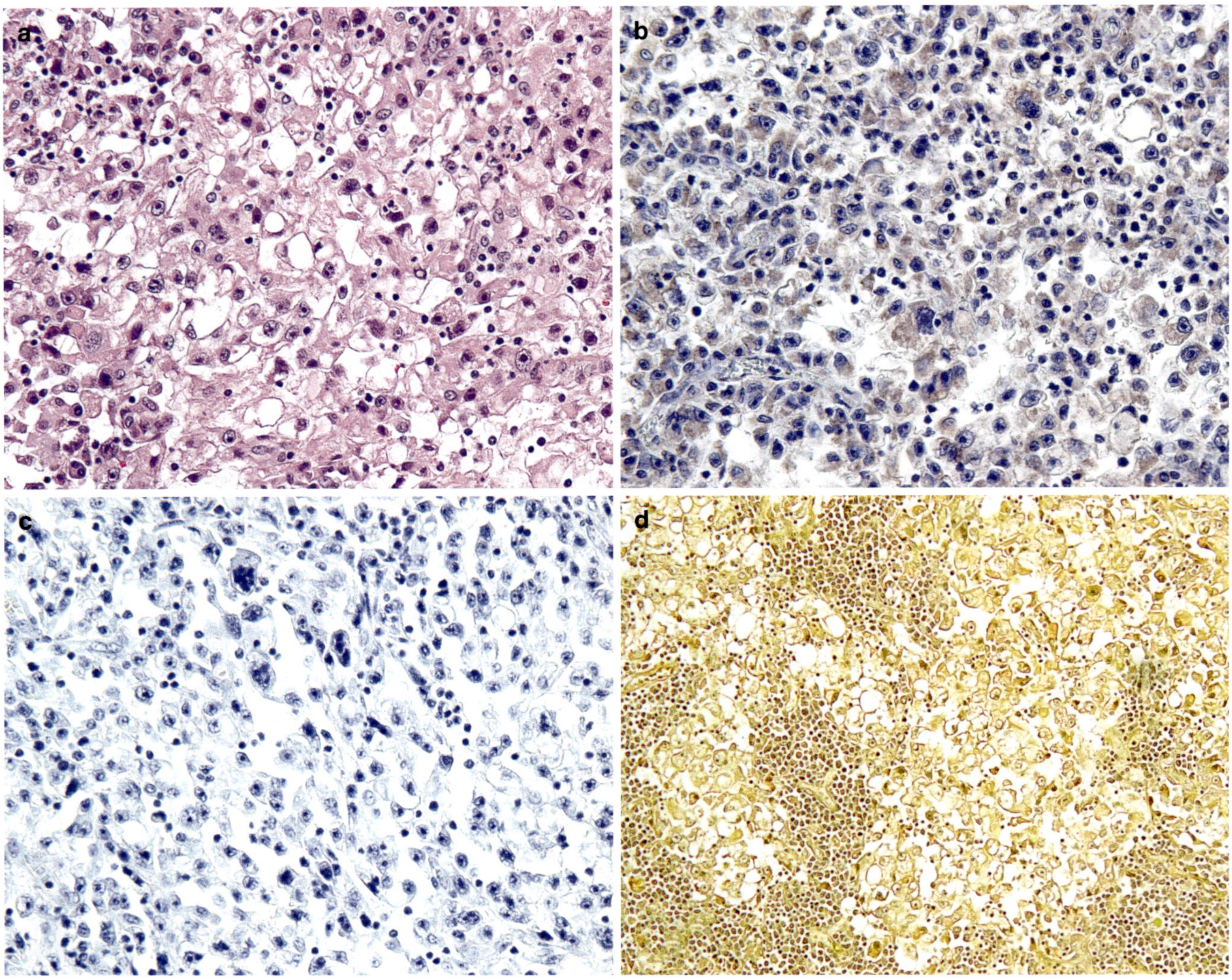

Fig. 7.2 Histologic features of large-cell undifferentiated carcinoma (LCUC). (**a**) The tumor consists of sheets of large polygonal pleomorphic cells with vesicular nuclei, prominent nucleoli, and moderate amount of eosinophilic and clear cytoplasm. No keratinization, glandular formation, or mucin production is seen. H&E, 200×. (**b–d**) The tumor cells stain negative for TTF-1 (**b**), p40 (**c**), and mucicarmine (**d**)

References

1. Travis W, Brambilla E, Burke A, Marx A, Nicholson A. WHO classification of tumors of the lung, pleura, thymus and heart. 4th ed. Lyon: International Agency for Research on Cancer (IARC); 2015.
2. Anon. Pretreatment evaluation of non-small-cell lung cancer. The American Thoracic Society and The European Respiratory Society. Am J Respir Crit Care Med. 1997;156:320–32.
3. Colby TV, Koss M, Travis WD. Tumors of the lower respiratory tract. 3rd ed. Washington, DC: Armed Forces Institute of Pathology; 1995.
4. Rodenhuis S, Slebos RJ, Boot AJ, Evers SG, Mooi WJ, Wagenaar SS, et al. Incidence and possible clinical significance of K-ras oncogene activation in adenocarcinoma of the human lung. Cancer Res. 1988;48:5738–41.
5. Mitsudomi T, Hamajima N, Ogawa M, Takahashi T. Prognostic significance of p53 alterations in patients with nonsmall cell lung cancer: a meta-analysis. Clin Cancer Res. 2000;6:4055–63.
6. Nemunaitis J, Klemow S, Tong A, Courtney A, Johnston W, Mack M, et al. Prognostic value of K-ras mutations, ras oncoprotein, and c-erb B-2 oncoprotein expression in adenocarcinoma of the lung. Am J Clin Oncol. 1998;21:155–60.
7. Brambilla E, Moro D, Veale D, Brichon PY, Stoebner P, Paramelle B, Brambilla C. Basal cell (basaloid) carcinoma of the lung: a new morphologic and phenotypic entity with separate prognostic significance. Hum Pathol. 1992;23:993–1003.
8. Fraser RS, Müller NL, Colman N, Pare PD. Pulmonary carcinoma. In: Fraser RS, Müller NL, Colman N, Pare PD, editors. Fraser's and Pare's diagnosis of diseases of the chest. Philadelphia: Saunders; 1999. p. 1069–228.
9. Henschke CI. I-ELCAP protocol. International Collaboration to Screen for Lung Cancer. 2003. http://ICScreen.med.cornell.edu/.
10. Kondo T, Yamada K, Noda K, Nakayama H, Kameda Y. Radiologicprognostic correlation in patients with small pulmonary adenocarcinomas. Lung Cancer. 2002;36:49–57.
11. Nagao M, Murase K, Yasuhara Y, Ikezoe J, Eguchi K, Mogami H, et al. Measurement of localized ground-glass attenuation on thin-section computed tomography images: correlation with the progression of bronchioloalveolar carcinoma of the lung. Investig Radiol. 2002;37:692–7.

12. Takashima S, Maruyama Y, Hasegawa M, Yamanda T, Honda T, Kadoya M, Sone S. Prognostic significance of high-resolution CT findings in small peripheral adenocarcinoma of the lung: a retrospective study on 64 patients. Lung Cancer. 2002;36:289–95.
13. Kodama K, Higashiyama M, Yokouchi H, Takami K, Kuriyama K, Mano M, Nakayama T. Prognostic value of ground-glass opacity found in small lung adenocarcinoma on high-resolution CT scanning. Lung Cancer. 2001;33:17–25.
14. Teraski H, Niki T, Matsuno Y, Yamada T, Maeshima A, Asamura H, et al. Lung adenocarcinoma with mixed bronchiolo-alveolar and invasive components: clinicopathological features, subclassification by extent of invasive foci, and immunohistochemical characterization. Am J Surg Pathol. 2003;27:937–51.
15. Sturm N, Lantuejoul S, Laverriere MH, Papotti M, Brichon PY, Brambilla C, Brambilla E. Thyroid transcription factor 1 and cytokeratins 1, 5, 10, 14 (34betaE12) expression in basaloid and large-cell neuroendocrine carcinomas of the lung. Hum Pathol. 2001;32:918–25.
16. Sturm N, Rossi G, Lantuejoul S, Laverriere MH, Papotti M, Brichon PY, et al. Cytokeratins 1, 5, 10, 14 (34betaE12) expression along the whole specturm of neuroendocrine proliferations of the lung, from neuroendocrine cell hyperplasia to small cell carcinoma. Histopathology. 2002;41:1–11.
17. Takahashi T, Nau MM, Chiba I, Birrer MJ, Rosenberg RK, Vinocour M, et al. p53: a frequent target for genetic abnormalities in lung cancer. Science. 1989;246:491–4.
18. Brambilla E, Moro D, Gazzeri S, Brambilla C. Alterations of expression of Rb, p16(INK4A) and cyclin D1 in non-small cell lung carcinoma and their clinical significance. J Pathol. 1999;188:351–60.
19. Yokota J, Kohno T. Molecular footprints of human lung cancer progression. Cancer Sci. 2004;95:197–204.
20. Slebos RJ, Kibbelaar RE, Dalesio O, Kooistra A, Stam J, Meijer CJ, et al. Kras oncogene activation as a prognostic marker in adenocarcinoma of the lung. N Engl J Med. 1990;323:561–5.
21. Shiseki M, Kohno T, Adachi J, Okazaki T, Otsuka T, Mizoguchi H, Noguchi M, Hirohashi S, Yokota J. Comparative allelotype of early and advanced stage non-small cell lung carcinomas. Genes Chromosomes Cancer. 1996;17:71–7.

8 Large-Cell Neuroendocrine Carcinoma Versus Solid-Predominant Lung Adenocarcinoma

Sophia Shaddy and Eric C. Huang

Case Presentation

A 65-year-old man with a past medical history of smoking presents with persistent dyspnea and cough. His chest computed tomography (CT) scan shows a 3.7 cm right upper lobe lung mass. The core-needle biopsy demonstrates solid nests and rosette-like malignant cells with finely granular chromatin, moderate amount of eosinophilic cytoplasm, and brisk mitotic activity. Immunohistochemical stains are positive for TTF-1 and show focal positivity for synaptophysin, chromogranin, and CD56. The biopsy is diagnosed as poorly differentiated carcinoma favoring large-cell neuroendocrine carcinoma (LCNEC).

The subsequent lobectomy from the right upper lobe contains similar malignant cells with predominantly organoid architecture and notable necrosis (Fig. 8.1a). High-power examination shows a large cell size, fine chromatin, variably prominent nucleoli, scant-to-moderate amount of eosinophilic and granular cytoplasm, and numerous mitotic figures (Fig. 8.1b). Malignant cells are diffusely positive for TTF-1, synaptophysin, and CD56 with focal positivity for chromogranin. Ki-67 labeling index is estimated to be greater than 70%.

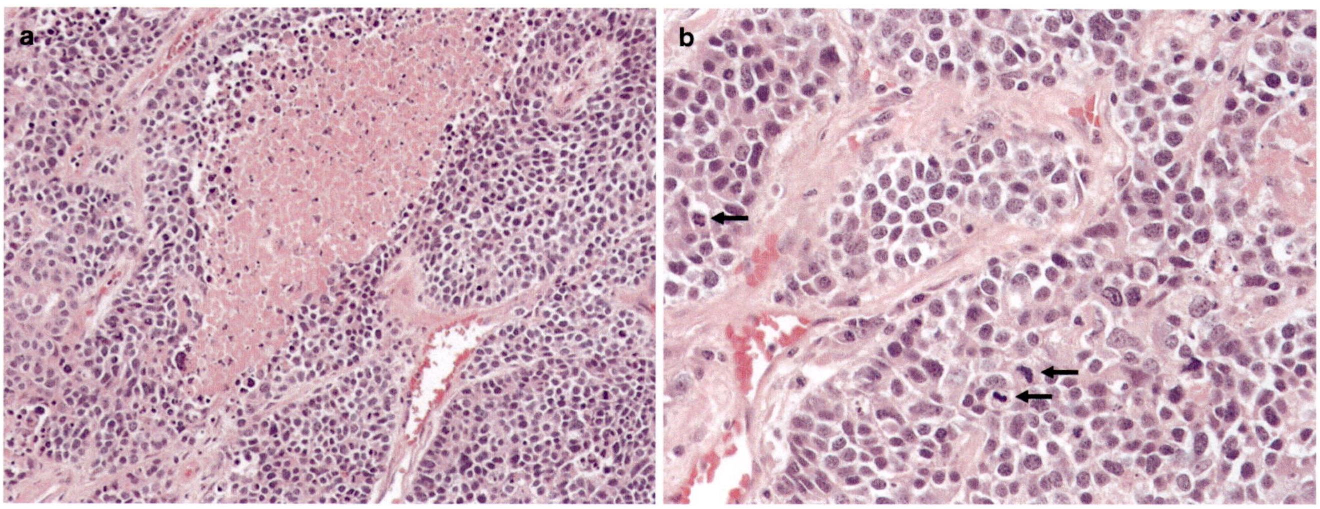

Fig. 8.1 (a) Low power showing organoid pattern with necrosis (H&E, 200×). (b) High power showing neuroendocrine nuclear features along with prominent nucleoli and numerous mitotic figures (arrows) (H&E, 400×)

S. Shaddy · E. C. Huang (✉)
Department of Laboratory Medicine and Pathology, University of Washington School of Medicine, Seattle, WA, USA
e-mail: ecchuang@uw.edu

H. Xu et al. (eds.), *Practical Lung Pathology*, Practical Anatomic Pathology, https://doi.org/10.1007/978-3-031-14402-8_8

Diagnosis: Large-Cell Neuroendocrine Carcinoma (LCNEC)

What Are the Key Clinicopathologic Findings of LCNEC and Solid Adenocarcinoma of the Lung?

LCNEC of the lung is a rare high-grade neuroendocrine malignancy that was previously classified as a variant of large-cell carcinoma [1–4]. Now classified with typical carcinoid (TC), atypical carcinoid (AC), and small-cell lung carcinoma (SCLC) as a subtype of neuroendocrine tumor, LCNEC accounts for approximately 3% of all lung tumors with a predisposition for older male smokers [3, 5–8]. Though LCNEC can be morphologically diverse, these tumors demonstrate a characteristic neuroendocrine appearance on histologic examination such as organoid, trabecular, or rosette-like architectural pattern, granular-to-coarse "salt-and-pepper" chromatin, and moderate amount of eosinophilic cytoplasm. Additionally, increased mitotic rate (>10 mitoses per 10 high-power fields) and necrosis are present [1, 2, 7, 8]. A large cell size (defined as greater than the diameter of three lymphocytes) and prominent nucleoli are distinct features of LCNEC not seen in other neuroendocrine tumors of the lung [1]. Neuroendocrine differentiation is confirmed by detection of dense-core granules by electron microscopy or more commonly, by immunohistochemical expression of synaptophysin, chromogranin, and/or CD56 [1, 9].

Solid-predominant adenocarcinoma is one of five architectural subtypes of invasive lung adenocarcinoma according to the 2015 WHO classification and is associated with older male nonsmokers [5, 10–12]. Malignant cells are arranged in sheets, and individual cells show vesicular nuclei, prominent nucleoli, and abundant cytoplasm (Fig. 8.2a, b) [13, 14]; intracellular mucin must be demonstrated with histochemical stains in five or more neoplastic cells in at least two high-power fields. Solid neoplastic cells lacking mucin but expressing pneumocyte markers (TTF-1 and/or napsin A) are also included in this category [14]. This subtype, as with micropapillary, is associated with a poor prognosis among the adenocarcinoma subtypes, and emerging studies identified a distinct molecular profile [11, 14–16].

Are There any Features on Radiologic Imaging that Would Help Diagnose and Differentiate LCNEC and Solid-Predominant Adenocarcinoma?

There are no clear radiologic features distinguishing LCNEC from solid adenocarcinoma and other non-small-cell carcinomas. However, certain radiologic findings may suggest the presence of either LCNEC or a solid component of adenocarcinoma. Knowledge of these parameters could help predict prognosis and would be beneficial in therapeutic planning, particularly for inoperable patients.

LCNEC is often peripherally located with a well-defined, lobular appearance on CT scans [17, 18]. In a large series of 38 cases by Oshiro et al., LCNEC was also found to lack air bronchograms and calcifications, and larger LCNEC showed inhomogeneous enhancement secondary to necrosis [17].

Few radiologic findings indicate the possibility of a solid component of adenocarcinoma, most notably a lack of ground-glass opacity, as compared to other subtypes of adenocarcinoma findings on imaging. Lung tumor CT findings of greater than stage I disease, size ≥2.5 cm, solid mass, and lack of ground-glass opacity are associated with solid or

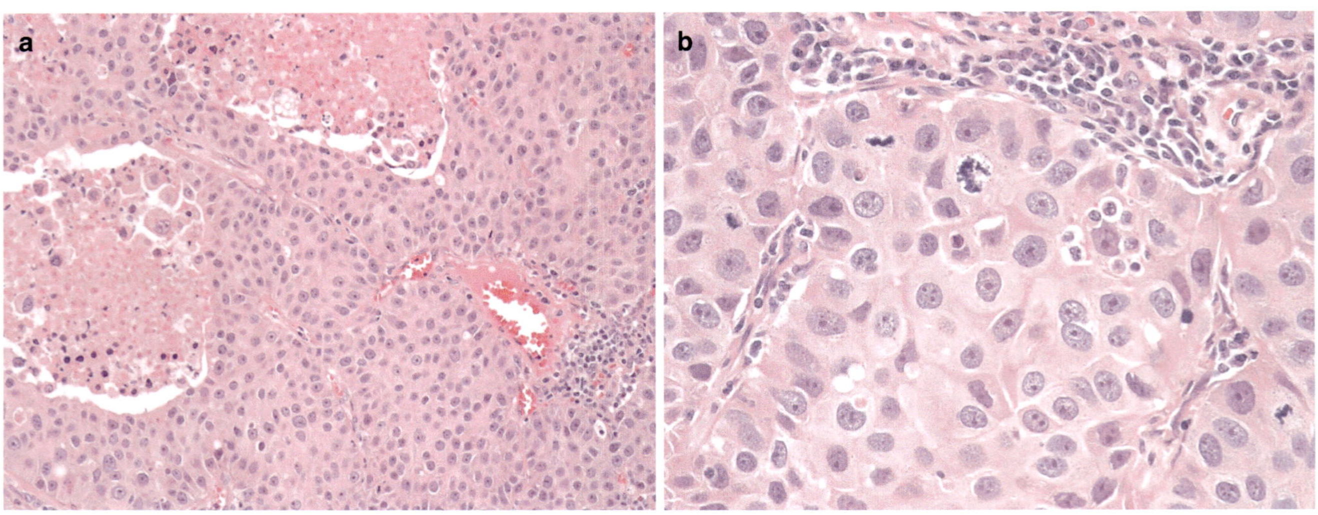

Fig. 8.2 (**a**) Solid predominant adenocarcinoma mimicking an organoid growth pattern with areas of necrosis (H&E, 200×). (**b**) Higher power, however, shows prominent nucleoli and abundant cytoplasm with lack of characteristic neuroendocrine nuclear features (H&E, 400×)

micropapillary subtype on histology. Additionally, positron-emission tomography (PET) standardized uptake value (SUV) maximum of ≥7 indicates a higher likelihood of either solid or micropapillary subtype [10].

What Immunohistochemical Stains Are Helpful for Diagnosing and Differentiating These Two Entities, Particularly on Small Biopsy/Cytology Specimens?

LCNEC and solid-predominant adenocarcinoma share morphologic features, such as enlarged nuclei and prominent nucleoli, which can make differentiating these two entities difficult on small core biopsy or cytology samples. If clear adenocarcinoma morphology is present on routine histologic evaluation, the diagnosis can be made by light microscopy alone, and the presence of a particular subtype should be mentioned when possible. For cases without definite adenocarcinoma morphology, the use of one adenocarcinoma marker such as TTF-1 and one squamous marker such as p40 is recommended as the minimal first round panel of stains in order to conserve tissue for potential molecular testing [19–21].

However, if neuroendocrine features are suggested on histologic evaluation, a larger panel of stains is necessary to distinguish LCNEC from solid-predominant adenocarcinoma. The addition of napsin A and neuroendocrine markers such as chromogranin, synaptophysin, and/or CD56 can help in this scenario as both entities are positive for TTF-1 (Fig. 8.3) [19, 21–23]. A staining pattern of TTF-1 and napsin A dual positivity supports the diagnosis of adenocarcinoma, while napsin A negativity and positivity of at least one neuroendocrine marker support the diagnosis of LCNEC (Table 8.1). In addition, histochemical stains such as mucicarmine are very helpful in diagnosis of solid adenocarcinoma if the neoplastic cells are negative for TTF-1 or napsin A; intracellular mucin must be demonstrated with histochemical stains in five or more solid adenocarcinoma cells in at least two high-power fields [14].

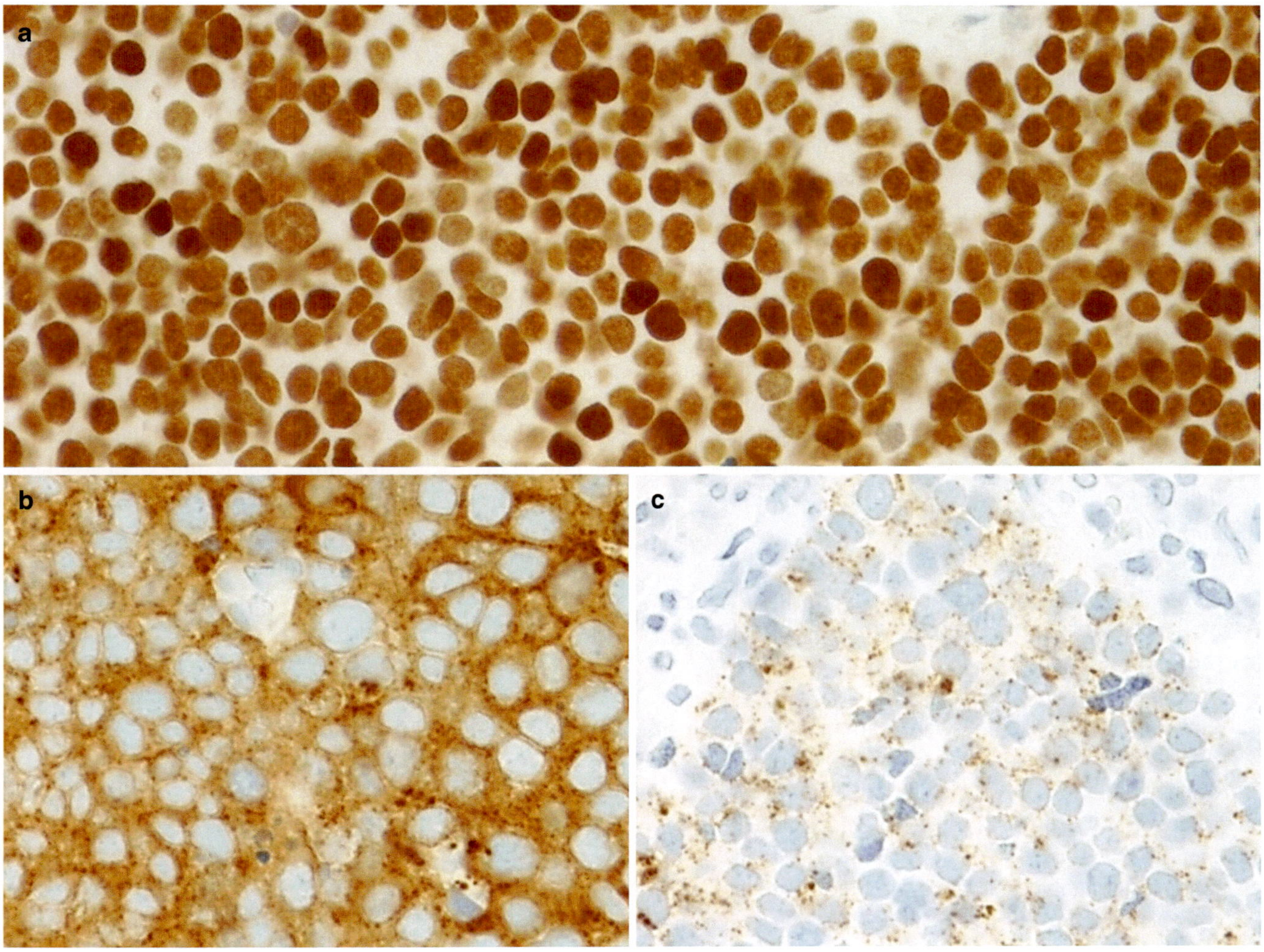

Fig. 8.3 LCNEC with TTF-1 (**a**), synaptophysin (**b**), and chromogranin (**c**) positivity (400×)

Table 8.1 Summary of helpful stains to differentiate LCNEC from primary lung adenocarcinoma

	LCNEC	Adenocarcinoma (lung primary)
TTF-1	+	+
Napsin A	–[a]	+
Neuroendocrine marker	+	–/+
(Synaptophysin, chromogranin, CD56)		

[a]Napsin A can be focal and weak or moderate staining in LCNEC [18]

Biopsy and cytology specimens are the mainstay of diagnosing lung cancer since most patients present in advanced, unrespectable stages. Given the increasing prevalence of targeted molecular therapy, pathologists must make prudent decisions during the diagnostic work-up in order to provide a specific classification while also preserving tissue for ancillary molecular testing [19, 21]. For these reasons, it is essential that morphologic findings dictate the appropriate panel of immunohistochemical stains [5, 12, 19].

Are There any Diagnostic Pitfalls with Immunohistochemistry to Be Aware of?

In general, the combination of positive TTF-1 and positive napsin A supports a diagnosis of adenocarcinoma when differentiating LCNEC from solid-predominant adenocarcinoma. However, a rare subset of LCNEC can express napsin A [22]. In comparison with adenocarcinoma, LCNEC has weaker and more focal napsin A staining which can alert pathologists to a potential pitfall. Weak napsin A staining with positive neuroendocrine markers in a tumor with neuroendocrine morphology would best be classified as LCNEC over adenocarcinoma [22].

It should also be noted that the routine use of neuroendocrine markers in the evaluation of poorly differentiated non-small-cell lung carcinoma (NSCLC) without definitive neuroendocrine morphology is not recommended due to lack of clinical relevance in these types of tumors with positive staining [24, 25].

What Are Genetic Differences, and Is There any Impact on Therapy?

Current targetable mutations are infrequently found in LCNEC [26]. However, few case reports of LCNEC with *EGFR/ALK* mutations have been described, suggesting routine screening for druggable mutations in LCNEC would be of benefit [27].

Although targetable mutations for therapy are lacking in LCNEC, genomic profiling of LCNEC demonstrates distinct genomic subsets that are also associated with differences in therapeutic outcomes. The most frequently described subtypes consist of SCLC- and NSCLC-like mutations due to overlapping molecular alterations with each respective group. LCNEC in the SCLC-like group show molecular alterations in RB1 and TP53, which are frequently associated with SCLC. Mutations typically associated with adenocarcinoma seen in the NSCLC-like subtype include *STK11*, *KRAS*, *and KEAP1-NFE2L2*. Interestingly, *STK11* and *KRAS* mutations were found to be mutually exclusive with *RB1* and *TP53* co-alterations [26, 28–30].

There is no consensus on whether SCLC or NSCLC treatments should be applied to metastatic cases, and both platinum-etoposide, a SCLC therapy, and NSCLC regimens are acceptable [30, 31]. However, recent studies show the NSCLC-like molecular subtype responds better to NSCLC treatments (gemcitabine/taxane) than to the SCLC platinum-etoposide regimen. Additionally, LCNEC with KRAS mutations (NSCLC-like molecular subtype) do not respond as well to platinum-etoposide regimens as SCLC [6, 22, 27, 30].

Molecular alterations in KRAS, ALK, ROS1, and RET have been associated with the solid-predominant subtype of adenocarcinoma [14, 15, 32, 33]. Most in keeping with previous studies that show a solid component has a negative association with *EGFR* mutations, the presence and amount of a solid morphology have been linked to increased frequency of *KRAS* mutations and decreased frequency of *EGFR* mutations [12, 15, 33]. Though solid-predominant lung adenocarcinoma is unlikely to benefit from *EGFR* targeted therapy, *ALK* inhibitors, such as crizotinib, may play an important therapeutic role in this subtype. Solid-predominant morphology is an independent predictor of the presence of *ALK* rearrangements in a multivariate analysis by Nishino et al. [34]. Additionally, Pan et al. found solid-predominant subtype to be enriched in *ALK* mutations, along with *ROS1* and *RET* [32]. The association and identification of a solid morphologic component with particular molecular alterations may help guide molecular testing when available material is from limited biopsy/cytology specimens.

Biopsy and cytology specimens are the primary diagnostic material in the majority of lung carcinoma cases. It is important to gain as much useful clinicopathologic information to aid in the diagnosis of LCNEC and solid-predominant adenocarcinoma especially if the small biopsy or cytology sample is all the material that is available for potential molecular testing.

References

1. Travis WD, Linnoila RI, Tsokos MG, Hitchcock CL, Cutler GB, Nieman L, et al. Neuroendocrine tumors of the lung with proposed criteria for large-cell neuroendocrine carcinoma. An ultrastructural, immunohistochemical, and flow cytometric study of 35 cases. Am J Surg Pathol. 1991;15(6):529–53.

2. Jiang SX, Kameya T, Shoji M, Dobashi Y, Shinada J, Yoshimura H. Large cell neuroendocrine carcinoma of the lung: a histologic and immunohistochemical study of 22 cases. Am J Surg Pathol. 1998;22(5):526–37.
3. Travis WD, Brambilla E, Nicholson AG, Yatabe Y, Austin JHM, Beasley MB, et al. The 2015 World Health Organization classification of lung tumors: impact of genetic, clinical and radiologic advances since the 2004 classification. J Thorac Oncol. 2015;10(9):1243–60.
4. Yang X, Lin D. Changes of 2015 WHO histological classification of lung cancer and the clinical significance. Zhongguo Fei Ai Za Zhi. 2016;19(6):332–6.
5. Travis WD, Brambilla E, Burke AP, Marx A, Nicholson AG. WHO classification of tumours of the lung, pleura, thymus and heart. Lyon: International Agency for Research on Cancer; 2015.
6. Naidoo J, Santos-Zabala ML, Iyriboz T, Woo KM, Sima CS, Fiore JJ, et al. Large cell neuroendocrine carcinoma of the lung: clinicopathologic features, treatment, and outcomes. Clin Lung Cancer. 2016;17(5):e121–e9.
7. Hung YP. Neuroendocrine tumors of the lung: updates and diagnostic pitfalls. Surg Pathol Clin. 2019;12(4):1055–71.
8. Fasano M, Della Corte CM, Papaccio F, Ciardiello F, Morgillo F. Pulmonary large-cell neuroendocrine carcinoma: from epidemiology to therapy. J Thorac Oncol. 2015;10(8):1133–41.
9. Derks JL, Dingemans AC, van Suylen RJ, den Bakker MA, Damhuis RAM, van den Broek EC, et al. Is the sum of positive neuroendocrine immunohistochemical stains useful for diagnosis of large cell neuroendocrine carcinoma (LCNEC) on biopsy specimens? Histopathology. 2019;74(4):555–66.
10. Cha MJ, Lee HY, Lee KS, Jeong JY, Han J, Shim YM, et al. Micropapillary and solid subtypes of invasive lung adenocarcinoma: clinical predictors of histopathology and outcome. J Thorac Cardiovasc Surg. 2014;147(3):921–8.e2.
11. Zhang Y, Li J, Wang R, Li Y, Pan Y, Cai D, et al. The prognostic and predictive value of solid subtype in invasive lung adenocarcinoma. Sci Rep. 2014;4:7163.
12. Travis WD, Brambilla E, Noguchi M, Nicholson AG, Geisinger KR, Yatabe Y, et al. International association for the study of lung cancer/american thoracic society/european respiratory society international multidisciplinary classification of lung adenocarcinoma. J Thorac Oncol. 2011;6(2):244–85.
13. Travis WD, Brambilla E, Riely GJ. New pathologic classification of lung cancer: relevance for clinical practice and clinical trials. J Clin Oncol. 2013;31(8):992–1001.
14. Truini A, Santos Pereira P, Cavazza A, Spagnolo P, Nosseir S, Longo L, et al. Classification of different patterns of pulmonary adenocarcinomas. Expert Rev Respir Med. 2015;9(5):571–86.
15. Morales-Oyarvide V, Mino-Kenudson M. High-grade lung adenocarcinomas with micropapillary and/or solid patterns: a review. Curr Opin Pulm Med. 2014;20(4):317–23.
16. Xu S, Xi J, Jiang W, Lu S, Wang Q. Solid component and tumor size correlate with prognosis of stage IB lung adenocarcinoma. Ann Thorac Surg. 2015;99(3):961–7.
17. Oshiro Y, Kusumoto M, Matsuno Y, Asamura H, Tsuchiya R, Terasaki H, et al. CT findings of surgically resected large cell neuroendocrine carcinoma of the lung in 38 patients. AJR Am J Roentgenol. 2004;182(1):87–91.
18. Shin AR, Shin BK, Choi JA, Oh YW, Kim HK, Kang EY. Large cell neuroendocrine carcinoma of the lung: radiologic and pathologic findings. J Comput Assist Tomogr. 2000;24(4):567–73.
19. Travis WD, Brambilla E, Noguchi M, Nicholson AG, Geisinger K, Yatabe Y, et al. Diagnosis of lung cancer in small biopsies and cytology: implications of the 2011 International Association for the Study of Lung Cancer/American Thoracic Society/European Respiratory Society classification. Arch Pathol Lab Med. 2013;137(5):668–84.
20. Mani H, Zander DS. Immunohistochemistry: applications to the evaluation of lung and pleural neoplasms: part 1. Chest. 2012;142(5):1316–23.
21. Inamura K. Update on immunohistochemistry for the diagnosis of lung cancer. Cancers (Basel). 2018;10(3):72.
22. Rekhtman N, Pietanza CM, Sabari J, Montecalvo J, Wang H, Habeeb O, et al. Pulmonary large cell neuroendocrine carcinoma with adenocarcinoma-like features: napsin a expression and genomic alterations. Mod Pathol. 2018;31(1):111–21.
23. Inage T, Nakajima T, Fujiwara T, Sakairi Y, Wada H, Suzuki H, et al. Pathological diagnosis of pulmonary large cell neuroendocrine carcinoma by endobronchial ultrasound-guided transbronchial needle aspiration. Thorac Cancer. 2018;9(2):273–7.
24. Travis WD, Brambilla E, Nicholson AG. Testing for neuroendocrine immunohistochemical markers should not be performed in poorly differentiated NSCCs in the absence of neuroendocrine morphologic features according to the 2015 WHO classification. J Thorac Oncol. 2016;11(2):e26–7.
25. Ionescu DN, Treaba D, Gilks CB, Leung S, Renouf D, Laskin J, et al. Nonsmall cell lung carcinoma with neuroendocrine differentiation--an entity of no clinical or prognostic significance. Am J Surg Pathol. 2007;31(1):26–32.
26. Rekhtman N, Pietanza MC, Hellmann MD, Naidoo J, Arora A, Won H, et al. Next-generation sequencing of pulmonary large cell neuroendocrine carcinoma reveals small cell carcinoma-like and non-small cell carcinoma-like subsets. Clin Cancer Res. 2016;22(14):3618–29.
27. Derks JL, Leblay N, Lantuejoul S, Dingemans AC, Speel EM, Fernandez-Cuesta L. New insights into the molecular characteristics of pulmonary carcinoids and large cell neuroendocrine carcinomas, and the impact on their clinical management. J Thorac Oncol. 2018;13(6):752–66.
28. Hiroshima K, Mino-Kenudson M. Update on large cell neuroendocrine carcinoma. Transl Lung Cancer Res. 2017;6(5):530–9.
29. George J, Walter V, Peifer M, Alexandrov LB, Seidel D, Leenders F, et al. Integrative genomic profiling of large-cell neuroendocrine carcinomas reveals distinct subtypes of high-grade neuroendocrine lung tumors. Nat Commun. 2018;9(1):1048.
30. Derks JL, Leblay N, Thunnissen E, van Suylen RJ, den Bakker M, Groen HJM, et al. Molecular subtypes of pulmonary large-cell neuroendocrine carcinoma predict chemotherapy treatment outcome. Clin Cancer Res. 2018;24(1):33–42.
31. Derks JL, van Suylen RJ, Thunnissen E, den Bakker MA, Groen HJ, Smit EF, et al. Chemotherapy for pulmonary large cell neuroendocrine carcinomas: does the regimen matter? Eur Respir J. 2017;49(6):1601838.
32. Pan Y, Zhang Y, Li Y, Hu H, Wang L, Li H, et al. ALK, ROS1 and RET fusions in 1139 lung adenocarcinomas: a comprehensive study of common and fusion pattern-specific clinicopathologic, histologic and cytologic features. Lung Cancer. 2014;84(2):121–6.
33. Rekhtman N, Ang DC, Riely GJ, Ladanyi M, Moreira AL. KRAS mutations are associated with solid growth pattern and tumor-infiltrating leukocytes in lung adenocarcinoma. Mod Pathol. 2013;26(10):1307–19.
34. Nishino M, Klepeis VE, Yeap BY, Bergethon K, Morales-Oyarvide V, Dias-Santagata D, et al. Histologic and cytomorphologic features of ALK-rearranged lung adenocarcinomas. Mod Pathol. 2012;25(11):1462–72.

Poorly Differentiated Squamous Cell Carcinoma Versus Solid Pattern Adenocarcinoma

9

Anshu Bandhlish and Haodong Xu

Case Presentation

A 67-year-old man was a former smoker with a 30 pack-year history of smoking and end-stage liver disease due to hepatitis C with cirrhosis and hepatocellular carcinoma. He denied any respiratory symptoms. When evaluated for a liver transplant, chest computerized tomography (CT) demonstrated a 1.5 cm peripheral nodule with cavitation involving the right lower lobe and associated with mild atelectasis in the lung bases and small right pleural effusion (Fig. 9.1). He had a CT-guided biopsy which demonstrated a poorly differentiated carcinoma with abundant eosinophilic cytoplasm. No obvious keratinization, intercellular bridges, or intra-cytoplasmic mucin was identified to suggest squamous cell carcinoma or adenocarcinoma (Fig. 9.2a). Immunohistochemical stains demonstrate that the neoplastic cells are diffusely and strongly positive for p40 (Fig. 9.2b) while being negative for TTF-1 (Fig. 9.2c).

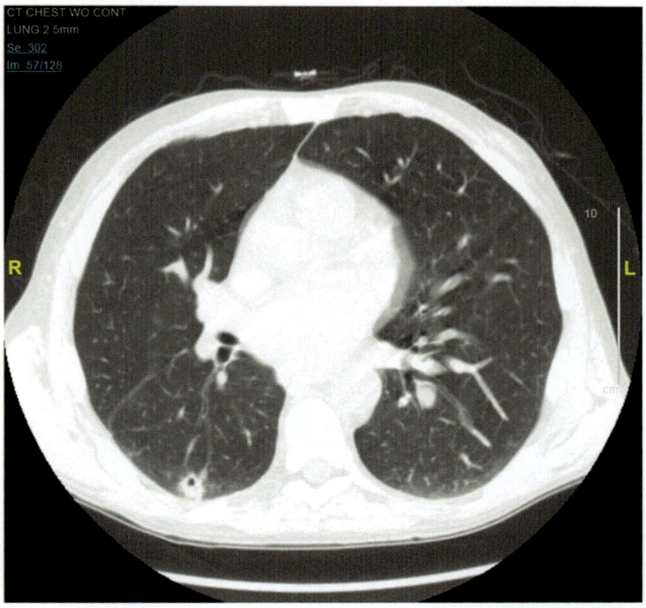

Fig. 9.1 Chest CT showed a 1.5 cm peripheral nodule with cavitation in the right lower lobe with mild atelectasis in the lung bases

A. Bandhlish (✉) · H. Xu
Department of Laboratory Medicine and Pathology, University of Washington Medical Center, Seattle, WA, USA
e-mail: anshuba@uw.edu

H. Xu et al. (eds.), *Practical Lung Pathology*, Practical Anatomic Pathology, https://doi.org/10.1007/978-3-031-14402-8_9

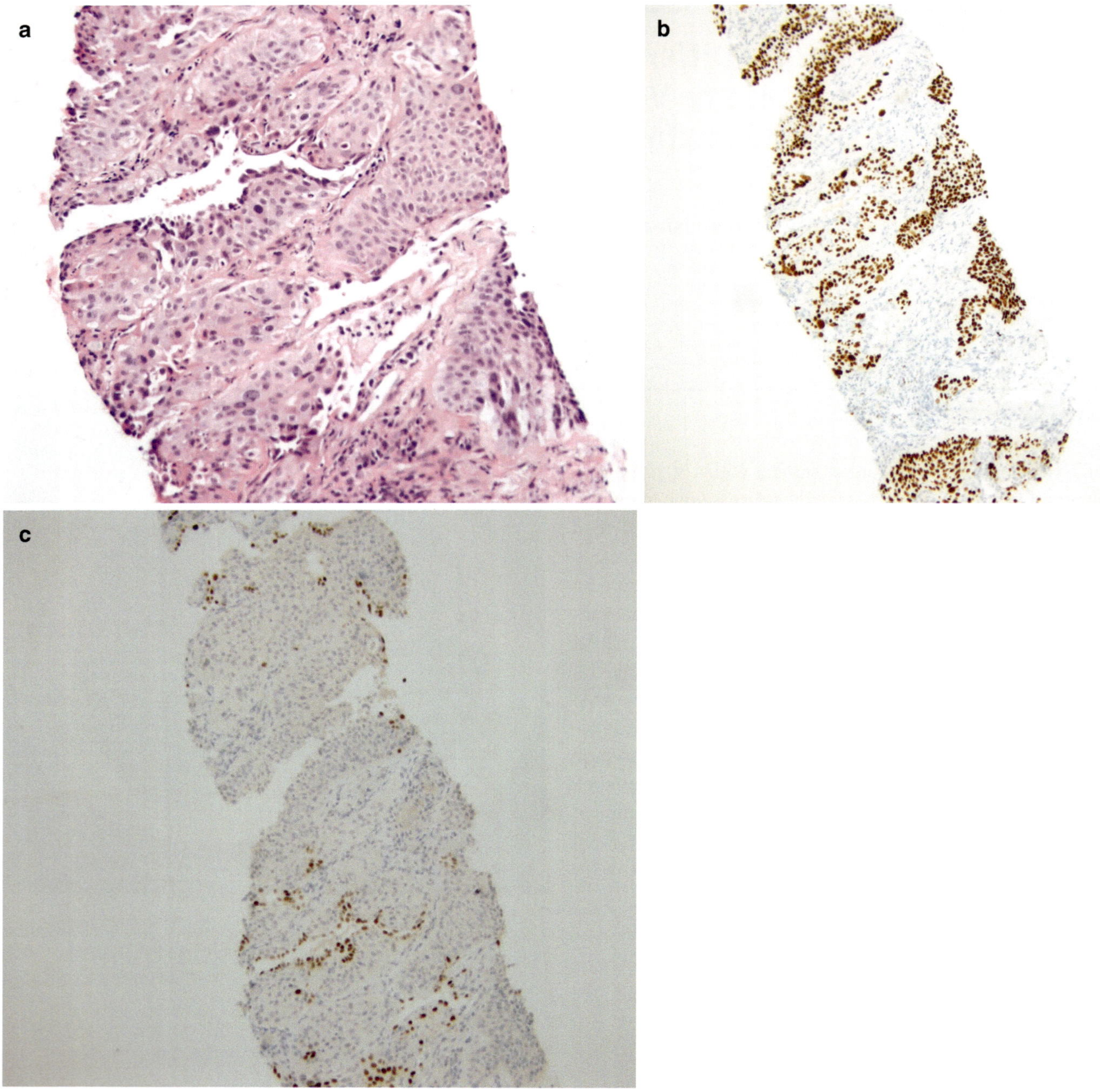

Fig. 9.2 Poorly differentiated squamous cell carcinoma. Histological section shows nests of a large cohesive malignant cell proliferation with abundant eosinophilic cytoplasm (**a**, 400×). Immunohistochemical stains show the neoplastic cells are diffusely and strongly positive for p40 (**b**, 100×), and they are negative for TTF-1; TTF-1 highlights the reactive type II pneumocytes (**c**, 100×)

Pathologic Diagnosis: Poorly Differentiated Squamous Cell Carcinoma

What Are the Histopathologic Features of Lung Adenocarcinoma and Squamous Cell Carcinoma?

Squamous cell carcinoma is characterized by neoplastic cells with abundant eosinophilic cytoplasm, sharp cell borders, intercellular bridges, and keratinization, whereas adenocarcinoma is characterized by the presence of malignant glands and/or the presence of intracytoplasmic mucin [1].

Classification of invasive lung adenocarcinoma is based on semiquantitative assessment of histologic patterns (in 5% increments) with the goal of choosing a single, predominant pattern as per the International Association for the study of Lung Cancer, American Thoracic Society, and European Respiratory Society, and it is classified as lepidic, acinar, papillary, micropapillary, and solid predominant adenocarcinoma [2–5]. Non-keratinizing squamous cell carcinomas can be difficult to distinguish from poorly differentiated solid adenocarcinomas which are composed of solid sheets of polygonal tumor cells without glandular differentiation and/or intracytoplasmic mucin.

What Are the Immunohistochemical Stains Often Utilized to Differentiate Poorly Differentiated Lung Squamous Cell Carcinoma from Solid Adenocarcinoma?

The inherent challenge in accurately classifying poorly differentiated lung carcinomas has paved way for a wide use of immunohistochemistry to evaluate non-small-cell lung carcinomas (NSCLC) that are difficult to classify on routine hematoxylin and eosin (H&E) stains. In most biopsies, a limited panel of p40 and TTF-1 immunostains is sufficient for accurate classification, and additional squamous markers such as p63 and CK5/6 and glandular markers such as napsin-A and CK7 can be utilized in cases with an unusual morphology [6]. A panel comprising of TTF-1 and p40 immunohistochemical stains, accompanied sometimes by a mucicarmine stain. Awareness of sensitivity and specificity of the various immunohistochemical stains is important during routine diagnostic evaluation. p40 has been shown to have greater specificity than p63 for squamous cell carcinoma, although the sensitivity of both stains is equal [7–9]. Our case showed diffuse strong positivity for p40 (Fig. 9.2b) rather than scattered and weak staining sometimes seen in the solid adenocarcinomas and TTF-1 (8G7G3/1) negativity (Fig. 9.2c). Immunohistochemical markers to routinely identify squamous lineage are CK5/6, p40, and p63. The *P63* gene is a member of the p53/p63/p73 family of transcription factors and plays a critical role in the development and homeostasis of squamous epithelium [8, 10]. Studies using antibodies against p63 have demonstrated positive results in a small percentage of lung adenocarcinomas [6, 8]. Unlike one of the p63 isoforms, ΔNp63, detected by antibody p40, is highly specific for squamous and basal cells and is overexpressed in squamous cell carcinoma in multiple organs [8–11].

TTF-1 antibody, used for the diagnosis of lung adenocarcinoma, is homeodomain-containing transcription factor that is predominantly found in normal type II alveolar pneumocytes [7]. TTF-1 antibodies for tissue diagnosis have been developed in three major clones: SPT24, SP141, and 8G7G3/1. In a study evaluating the utility of these three different antibody clones using tissue microarrays from 665 cases of resected lung cancer and 428 pulmonary metastases, positive immunoreactivity was seen in 89%, 93%, and 93% of lung ADC and 0%, 6%, and 8% of SCC, using the TTF-1 clones 8G7G3/1, SPT24, and SP141, respectively. These findings indicate that clone 8G7G3/1 is more specific but less sensitive compared to SPT24 and SP14 [12]. For clones SPT24 or SP141, a cutoff of 10% positive tumor cells is reported more useful than 1% to help overcome the problem of low specificity [12]. Another study using tissue microarrays of 480 resection specimens of poorly differentiated squamous cell carcinoma showed that all cases of both keratinizing and non-keratinizing squamous cell carcinomas were diffusely positive for p40 (99% and 98%, respectively) and negative for TTF-1 (8G7G3/1). Clone SPT24 exhibited focal and weak reactivity in 6% of pulmonary SCC. This study also confirmed the higher specificity for TTF-1 8G7G3/1 clone than SPT24 clone for differentiating lung ADC from SCC. Basaloid squamous cell carcinoma showed diffuse expression of p40 in 80% of cases [13].

These immunohistochemical stains should be interpreted with caution given the presence of occasional pitfalls, such as positivity for p63 and TTF-1 (SPT24 clone) in a small percentage of lung adenocarcinomas and squamous cell carcinomas, respectively [13]. p63 positivity in scattered cells is not entirely specific and does not help us further classify these tumors [7]. Benign TTF-1 and napsin A-positive entrapped and reactive pneumocytes and associated napsin A-positive macrophages should not be misinterpreted as carcinoma cells [1].

Mucin stains, such as mucicarmine, periodic acid-Schiff with diastase (PASD), and Alcian Blue-periodic acid-Schiff (ABPAS), can be utilized in poorly differentiated carcinomas although the sensitivity is low [7, 14]. Careful interpretation of mucin stains should be performed so as not to interpret apoptotic or necrotic tumor cells, macrophages, trapped benign epithelium, glycogen, or stromal mucin as cytoplasmic mucin [14]. Squamous cell carcinomas and large-cell carcinomas of the lung may show rare cells with intracytoplasmic mucin and are not indicative of solid pattern adenocarcinoma. Intracellular mucin should be present in at least five tumor cells in two high-power fields, for classification as solid adenocarcinoma with mucin [15].

What Are the Differences in the Prognosis and Molecular Findings between Lung Squamous Cell Carcinoma and Adenocarcinoma?

The emergence of targeted therapies for NSCLC has increased the demands for accurate histologic classification of NSCLC. The widespread use of next-generation sequencing (NGS) has facilitated access to vast amount of data regarding the molecular profiles of lung cancer. Among the various patterns of invasive adenocarcinoma, solid subtype correlates with poor prognosis. Disease-free survival at 5 years is 70% for solid adenocarcinoma, compared to 100% for low-grade and 83–90% for intermediate-grade tumors

[16]. Accurate diagnosis of the poor prognostic group of lung adenocarcinoma, including solid adenocarcinoma, is important, as these patients may be candidates for adjuvant therapy. The importance of immunohistochemistry in the accurate diagnosis of lung carcinoma must be emphasized, given that targeted therapy varies, since molecular alterations are different between adenocarcinoma and squamous cell carcinoma. *EGFR* mutations are the most common targeted driver mutation in lung adenocarcinoma (more commonly seen in micropapillary and lepidic pattern); these are more often identified in female and East Asian patients with a non−/light smoking history [1, 17]. *ALK* rearrangements are seen in approximately 4–5% of adenocarcinomas, more typically with acinar pattern, non-/light smoking history, and onset of disease at younger age. Various clinical trials have demonstrated the efficacy of tyrosine kinase inhibitors (TKI) or *ALK* inhibitors in patients with *ALK* gene rearranged NSCLC. *ROS1* and *RET* rearrangements are described in approximately 1% of cases. *RET* fusions are usually seen in poorly differentiated adenocarcinoma [17].

Squamous cell carcinoma, on the other hand, has significant mutations in genes such as *TP53*, *CDKN2A*, *PTEN*, *PIC3CA*, *KEAP1*, *MLL2*, *HLA-A*, *NFE2L2*, *NOTCH1*, *RB1*, and *PDYN*, with up to 90% harboring *TP53* mutations [17]. Two recent genetic alterations with potential for targeted therapy have been identified in a small percentage of pulmonary squamous cell carcinomas: these include mutations in *DDR2* (discoidin domain receptor tyrosine kinase 2) and FGFR1 (fibroblast growth factor 1) amplification [18].

References

1. Inamura K. Update on immunohistochemistry for the diagnosis of lung cancer. Cancers (Basel). 2018;10(3):72. https://doi.org/10.3390/cancers10030072.
2. Kuhn E, Morbini P, Cancellieri A, Damiani S, Cavazza A, Comin CE. Adenocarcinoma classification: patterns and prognosis. Pathologica. 2018;110(1):5–11.
3. Russell PA, Wainer Z, Wright GM, Daniels M, Conron M, Williams RA. Does lung adenocarcinoma subtype predict patient survival? A clinicopathologic study based on the new International Association for the Study of Lung Cancer/American Thoracic Society/European Respiratory Society international multidisciplinary lung adenocarcinoma classification. J Thorac Oncol. 2011;6(9):1496–504. https://doi.org/10.1097/JTO.0b013e318221f701.
4. Travis WD, Brambilla E, Noguchi M, et al. International association for the study of lung cancer/american thoracic society/european respiratory society international multidisciplinary classification of lung adenocarcinoma. J Thorac Oncol. 2011;6(2):244–85. https://doi.org/10.1097/JTO.0b013e318206a221.
5. Travis WD, Brambilla E, Noguchi M, et al. Diagnosis of lung adenocarcinoma in resected specimens: implications of the 2011 International Association for the Study of Lung Cancer/American Thoracic Society/European Respiratory Society classification. Arch Pathol Lab Med. 2013;137(5):685–705. https://doi.org/10.5858/arpa.2012-0264-RA.
6. Tacha D, Yu C, Bremer R, Qi W, Haas T. A 6-antibody panel for the classification of lung adenocarcinoma versus squamous cell carcinoma. Appl Immunohistochem Mol Morphol. 2012;20(3):201–7. https://doi.org/10.1097/PAI.0b013e31823d7f0e.
7. Woo JS, Reddy OL, Koo M, Xiong Y, Li F, Xu H. Application of immunohistochemistry in the diagnosis of pulmonary and pleural neoplasms. Arch Pathol Lab Med. 2017;141(9):1195–213. https://doi.org/10.5858/arpa.2016-0550-RA.
8. Nonaka D. A study of ΔNp63 expression in lung non-small cell carcinomas. Am J Surg Pathol. 2012;36(6):895–9. https://doi.org/10.1097/PAS.0b013e3182498f2b.
9. Bishop JA, Teruya-Feldstein J, Westra WH, Pelosi G, Travis WD, Rekhtman N. p40 (ΔNp63) is superior to p63 for the diagnosis of pulmonary squamous cell carcinoma. Mod Pathol. 2012;25(3):405–15. https://doi.org/10.1038/modpathol.2011.173.
10. Nobre AR, Albergaria A, Schmitt F. p40: a p63 isoform useful for lung cancer diagnosis - a review of the physiological and pathological role of p63. Acta Cytol. 2013;57(1):1–8. https://doi.org/10.1159/000345245.
11. Moses MA, George AL, Sakakibara N, et al. Molecular mechanisms of p63-mediated squamous cancer pathogenesis. Int J Mol Sci. 2019;20(14):3590. https://doi.org/10.3390/ijms20143590.
12. Vidarsdottir H, Tran L, Nodin B, et al. Comparison of three different TTF-1 clones in resected primary lung cancer and epithelial pulmonary metastases. Am J Clin Pathol. 2018;150(6):533–44. https://doi.org/10.1093/ajcp/aqy083.
13. Kadota K, Nitadori J, Rekhtman N, Jones DR, Adusumilli PS, Travis WD. Reevaluation and reclassification of resected lung carcinomas originally diagnosed as squamous cell carcinoma using immunohistochemical analysis. Am J Surg Pathol. 2015;39(9):1170–80. https://doi.org/10.1097/pas.0000000000000439.
14. Micke P, Botling J, Mattsson JSM, et al. Mucin staining is of limited value in addition to basic immunohistochemical analyses in the diagnostics of non-small cell lung cancer. Sci Rep. 2019;9(1):1319. https://doi.org/10.1038/s41598-018-37722-0.
15. Travis WD, Brambilla E, Nicholson AG, et al. The 2015 World Health Organization classification of lung tumors: impact of genetic, clinical and radiologic advances since the 2004 classification. J Thorac Oncol. 2015;10(9):1243–60. https://doi.org/10.1097/JTO.0000000000000630.
16. Yoshizawa A, Motoi N, Riely GJ, et al. Impact of proposed IASLC/ATS/ERS classification of lung adenocarcinoma: prognostic subgroups and implications for further revision of staging based on analysis of 514 stage I cases. Mod Pathol. 2011;24(5):653–64. https://doi.org/10.1038/modpathol.2010.232.
17. Kashima J, Kitadai R, Okuma Y. Molecular and morphological profiling of lung cancer: a foundation for "next-generation" pathologists and oncologists. Cancers (Basel). 2019;11(5):599. https://doi.org/10.3390/cancers11050599.
18. Popper HH, Ryska A, Tímár J, Olszewski W. Molecular testing in lung cancer in the era of precision medicine. Transl Lung Cancer Res. 2014;3(5):291–300. https://doi.org/10.3978/j.issn.2218-6751.2014.10.01.

Invasive Mucinous Adenocarcinoma Versus Ciliated Muconodular Papillary Tumor

10

Yu Yang and Chen Zhang

Case Presentation

A 45-year-old female patient presents with a productive cough which has persisted for 7 months. She has no history of cigarette smoking or other significant past medical history. A chest computed tomography (CT) scan demonstrates airspace consolidation within the left upper lobe with air bronchograms, suggesting of pneumonia. A bronchoalveolar lavage (BAL) specimen is obtained, and the BAL specimen is sent for culture and cytologic examination. The culture is negative. The cytological examination reveals abundant mucin but no atypical cells. She undergoes antibiotic treatment for a month without improvement of her symptoms. A CT scan is repeated and shows a rapid increase in the size of the parenchymal opacity in the left upper lobe (Fig. 10.1). A decision is made to do a video-assisted thoracoscopic surgery (VATS) wedge biopsy.

Grossly, the lung wedge biopsy specimen shows an intact, smooth pleural surface. The cut surface is diffusely consolidated with a gelatinous appearance.

The hematoxylin and eosin (H&E)-stained sections prepared from the wedge biopsy show a mucinous epithelial neoplasm growing along the pre-existing, unaltered alveolar septa. The underlying alveolar structure is preserved, but the alveolar spaces are filled with mucin and abundant alveolar macrophages (Fig. 10.2a). The neoplastic cells are tall and columnar with abundant intracytoplasmic mucin and basally located nuclei showing mild cytologic atypia (Fig. 10.2b). The majority of the tumor cells grow in a lepidic pattern; in some areas, the tumor cells form papillary or micropapillary structures, without a desmoplastic reaction or destruction of the alveolar structure (Fig. 10.2c).

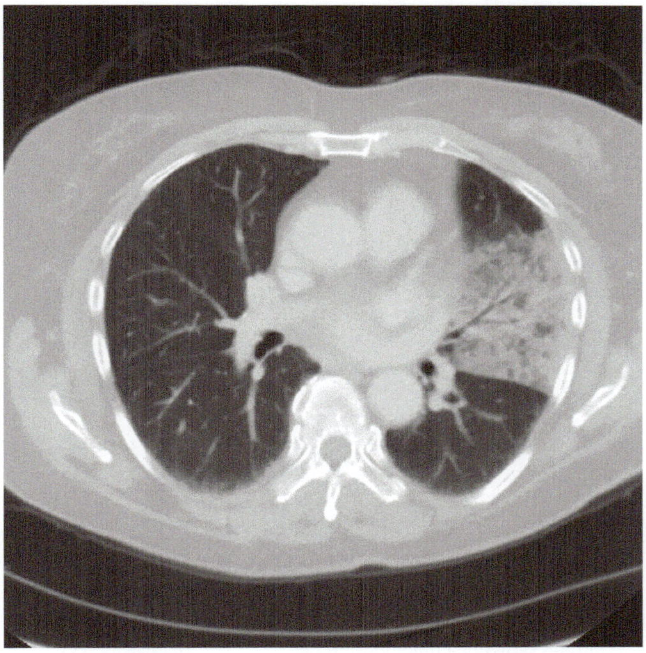

Fig. 10.1 Imaging features of invasive mucinous adenocarcinoma (IMA) of the lung. Chest CT image shows airspace consolidation within the left upper lobe with air bronchograms

By immunohistochemistry, the tumor cells are positive for CK7 and negative for CK20, CDX2, napsin A, and TTF-1.

KRAS gene mutation is detected by direct sequencing of codons 12 and 13 in exon 2 and codon 61 in exon 3. *EGFR* gene mutation is not detected by real-time polymerase chain reaction or direct sequencing of exons 18, 19, 20, and 21. Fluorescence in situ hybridization (FISH) studies show no evidence of *ALK* or *ROS-1* gene rearrangements.

Y. Yang
Department of Pathology and Laboratory Medicine, Indiana University School of Medicine, Indianapolis, IN, USA

C. Zhang (✉)
Weill Cornell Medicine, Department of Pathology and Laboratory Medicine, New York, NY, USA
e-mail: fjr9007@med.cornell.edu

H. Xu et al. (eds.), *Practical Lung Pathology*, Practical Anatomic Pathology, https://doi.org/10.1007/978-3-031-14402-8_10

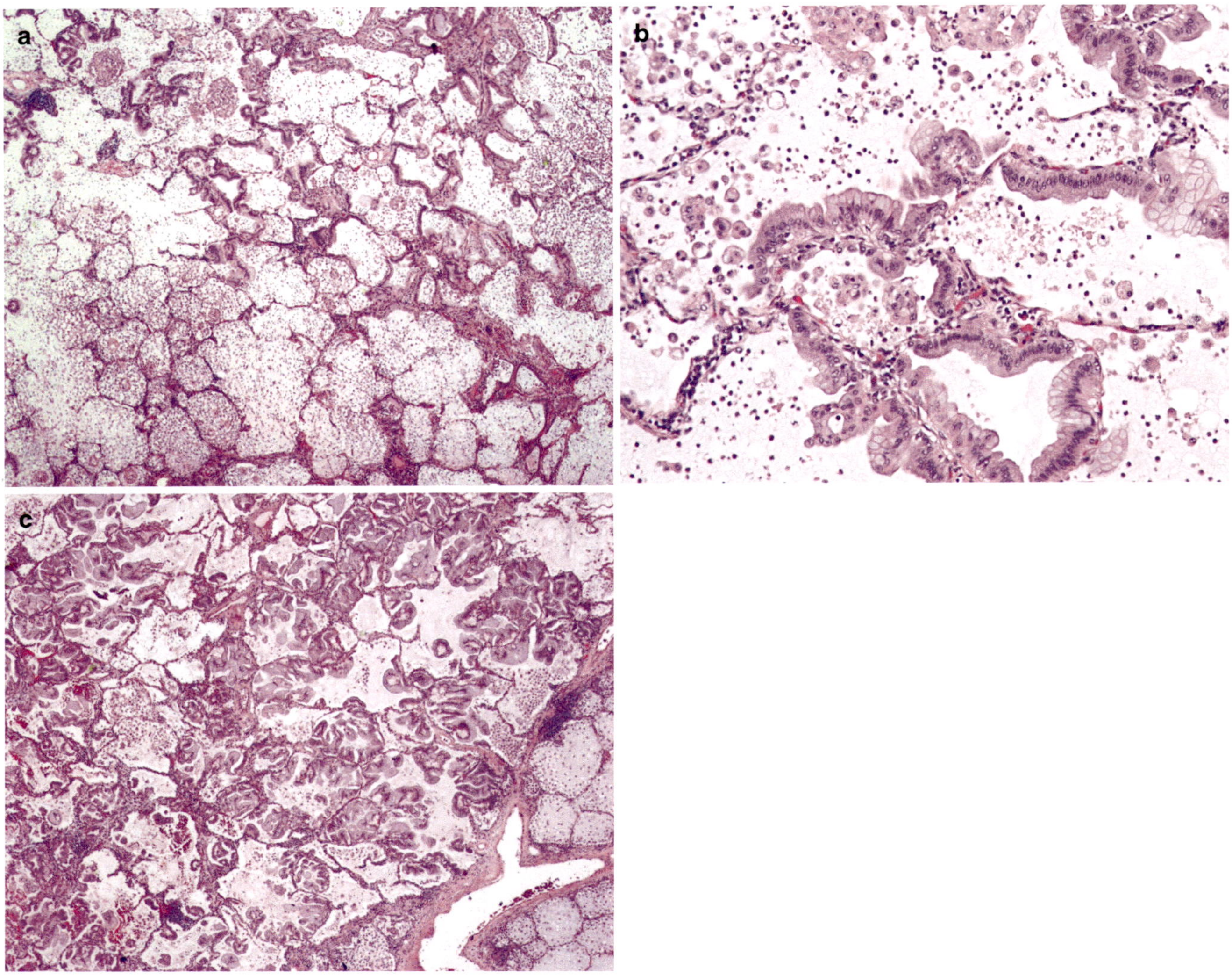

Fig. 10.2 Histologic features of IMA. (**a**) A low-magnification photomicrograph showing a mucinous epithelial neoplasm growing along the unaltered alveolar septa (lepidic growth pattern). The alveolar spaces are filled with mucin and macrophages. H&E, 20×. (**b**) A higher-magnification view of the neoplastic epithelium consisting of columnar cells with abundant apical intracellular mucin and basally located oval nuclei. There is minimal cytological atypia. H&E, 100×. (**c**) Another low-magnification microscopic field of the same tumor showing a mixture of lepidic, papillary, and micropapillary growth patterns. H&E, 20×

Final Diagnosis: Invasive Mucinous Adenocarcinoma (IMA) of the Lung

What Are the Clinical and Prognostic Features of IMA, and how Do they Differ from Ciliated Muconodular Papillary Tumor (CMPT)?

In 2015, the World Health Organization (WHO) announced a new classification of lung tumors in which mucinous bronchioloalveolar adenocarcinomas were reclassified as IMA, a variant of pulmonary adenocarcinoma [1]. The incidence of IMA among patients with a primary resected lung adenocarcinoma is about 1.5% [2]. The clinical presentation of this neoplasm varies considerably. Although some patients present incidentally with a solitary mass on imaging, most present with cough and other respiratory symptoms mimicking pneumonia. A significant proportion of patients present with mucinous bronchorrhea. Compared to other primary lung adenocarcinomas, IMAs show greater tendency to be multicentric, multilobar, or bilateral. The multifocality in IMA is thought to be the result of tumor spread through airspaces rather than metastasis via lymphatics and blood vessels within the lungs. After matching by clinical stage, the lung-cancer-specific mortality of IMA is not significantly different from those of other histologic types of lung adenocarcinoma. However, due to the greater tendency for multifocality of IMA, patients with IMA tend to present at higher clinical stages, hence with poorer prognosis [1–3].

CMPT of the lung is a newly recognized and extremely rare entity within the spectrum of mucinous tumors of the peripheral lung. Prior to the first report of this tumor in 2002, examples of this neoplasm were most likely diagnosed as a well-differentiated ciliated papillary adenocarcinoma, low-grade adenocarcinoma, glandular papilloma, or glandular metaplasia with mucinous features [4]. CMPTs are peripherally located small tumors that do not cause significant symptoms. Most of the cases reported to date are incidentally detected by CT-based screening for lung cancer. CPMT is considered benign. To date, no reported cases of CMPT have developed recurrence or metastases during follow-up ranging from 2 to120 months after resection [5–7].

How Can Radiologic Studies Be Used to Distinguish IMA from CMPT?

On chest CT scan, IMA is usually described as ground-glass opacities with or without consolidation, occupying the majority or the entire lobe of the lung. Multifocal, multilobar, and bilateral distributions are common. The radiological findings often mimic multifocal pneumonia.

On the other hand, CMPT is radiologically recognized as solitary, small, peripheral, solid, or partially solid nodules measuring 1 cm in average diameter with irregular contours. These lesions are commonly misinterpreted as early-stage adenocarcinoma on chest CT scan.

What Are the Pathologic Features of IMA and CPMT? How Can Immunohistochemistry Be Used to Distinguish these Two Entities?

Histologically, IMA consists of tall columnar non-ciliated epithelial cells with abundant intracytoplasmic mucin and basally located nuclei with minimal cytologic atypia (Fig. 10.2a–c). These cells line the alveolar septa in a lepidic manner but may show a mixture of acinar, papillary, and/or micropapillary growth patterns. The alveolar spaces are often filled with mucin and abundant alveolar macrophages. The immunophenotype of IMA resembles mucinous adenocarcinoma of the upper gastrointestinal and pancreaticobiliary tract, with frequent expression of CK7 and variable expressivity of CK20 and CDX2, often without napsin A and TTF-1 expression.

CMPT is characterized by a glandular, papillary, or tubulopapillary growth pattern associated with chronic lymphoplasmacytic infiltrates and columnar ciliated cells and mucous cells with continuous basal cell layers with abundant extracellular mucin filling alveoli (Fig. 10.3a and b). No nuclear atypia, mitotic activity, and necrosis are present. Immunohistochemical staining with p63 highlights a continuous layer of basal cells at the periphery of the glandular and papillary structures (Fig. 10.3c). TTF-1 stains the basal cells, mucous cells, and ciliated cells (Fig. 10.3d).

The extreme rarity and lack of awareness of the morphologic appearance of CMPT may result in a misdiagnosis of IMA, especially on fine-needle aspirates, small biopsies, or frozen sections. Features shared between CMPT and IMA are the presence of columnar mucinous cells, abundant extracellular mucus, and a diverse growth pattern. However, the presence of a trilineage proliferation with basal, mucinous, and ciliated cells together with the lack of mitosis and/or atypia helps distinguish CMPT from IMA. The predominantly lepidic growth pattern of IMA, presence of other growth patterns, nuclear atypia, and lack of basal and ciliated cells also differ from CMPT. Immunohistochemically, IMA is often negative for TTF-1 and napsin A (Table 10.1).

Are Genetic/Molecular Findings Different Between IMA and CMPT?

Genetically, IMA is known to frequently harbor *KRAS* mutation and lack *EGFR* mutation [2, 3]. Frequent *BRAF*, *AKT1*, or *EGFR* mutations have been found in CMPT. Cases of CMPT with *KRAS* mutation and *ALK* rearrangement have also been reported [8, 9].

How to Differentiate IMA from Colloid Adenocarcinoma or Mucinous Adenocarcinoma Metastatic to the Lung?

The histologic features of colloid adenocarcinoma include excess extracellular mucin containing rare tumor epithelial cells. Some colloid adenocarcinomas were formerly referred to as "mucinous cystadenocarcinoma." Features common to both IMA and colloid adenocarcinoma are the presence of goblet cells and columnar mucinous epithelium. However, colloid adenocarcinoma typically contains abundant extracellular mucin in which clusters of mucin-producing epithelium float and pools of mucin efface the native alveolar architecture. In contrast, alveolar architecture is preserved in IMAs.

Metastatic mucinous adenocarcinoma from pancreatic and gastrointestinal tract or of ovarian origin may be similar in appearance to IMA and must be excluded clinically and radiologically. Immunohistochemistry may play a role in determining the site of tissue origin of metastatic mucinous adenocarcinoma. The vast majority of cases of colorectal origin are diffusely CK20+, MUC-2+, homogenous CDX-2+, and nuclear beta-catenin+. In addition, rectal/anal origin tumors may also be positive for CK7. Tumors of appendiceal origin are heterogeneously CDX-2+, positive for CK7, and negative for nuclear expression of beta-catenin. Mucinous adenocarcinoma of the pancreas, biliary tree, and stomach is usually positive for CK7, focally positive for CK20, and het-

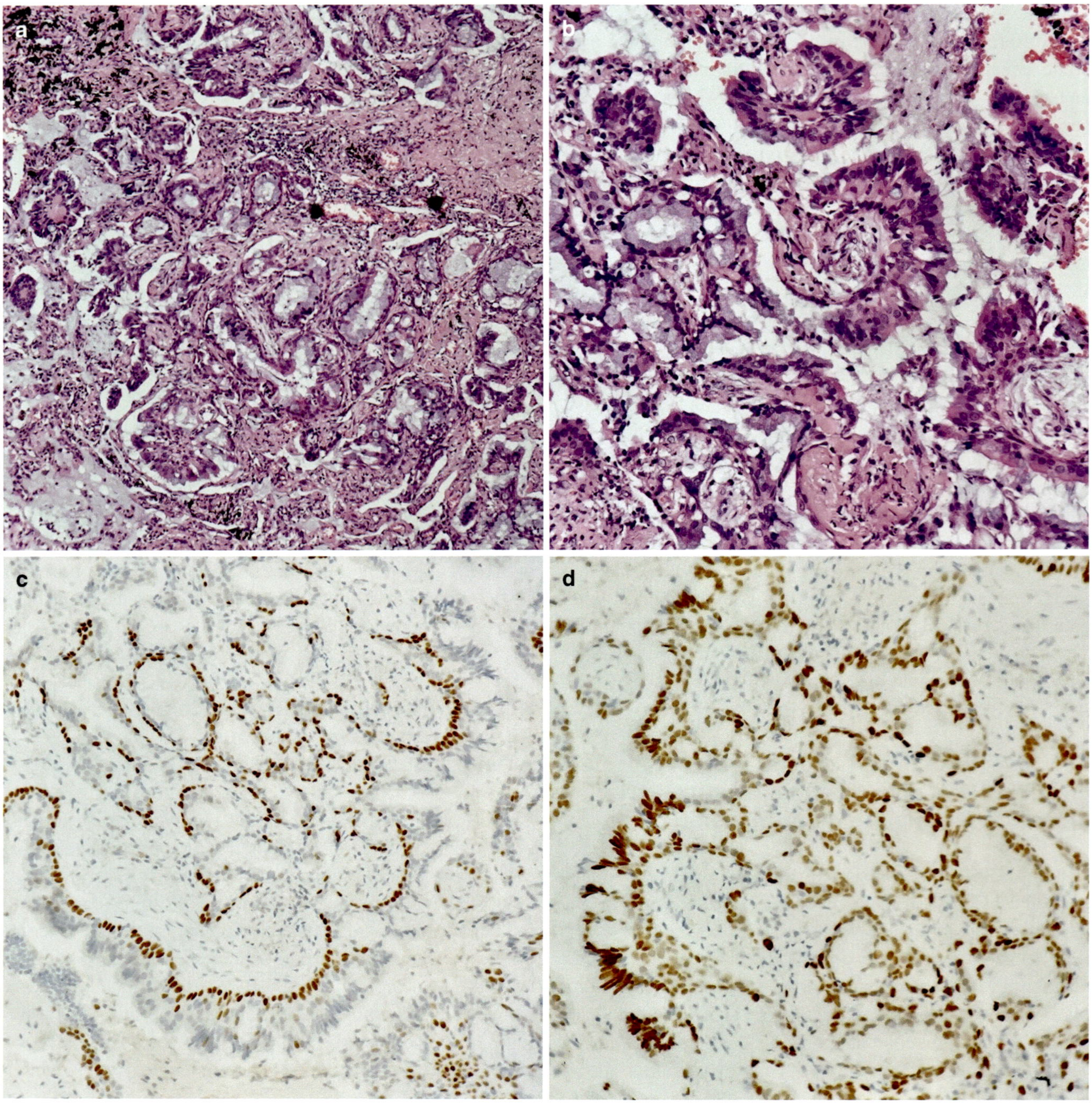

Fig. 10.3 Histological features of ciliated muconodular papillary tumor (CMPT) of the lung. Courtesy of Dr. Wenjuan Yu, Department of Pathology, Affiliated Hospital of Qingdao University, China. (**a**) The tumor exhibits tubulopapillary growth pattern associated with chronic lymphoplasmacytic infiltrates. H&E, 100×. (**b**) The tumor is composed of ciliated cells, mucous cells, and basal cells. H&E, 200×. (**c**) p63 is positive in the continuous layer of basal cells (100×). (**d**) TTF-1 highlights the basal cells, mucous cells, and ciliated cells (100×)

Table 10.1 Difference between invasive mucinous adenocarcinoma (IMA) and ciliated muconodular papillary tumor (CMPT)

	IMA	CMPT
Clinical presentation	Cough, mucous sputum	Asymptomatic
Incidence	Rare	Extremely rare
Radiology	Large areas of ground-glass opacity with or without consolidation; commonly multifocal	Solitary peripheral small lung nodule with an average diameter of 1 cm
Histology		
Growth pattern	Predominantly lepidic, mixed with papillary, micropapillary patterns	Glandular, papillary, tubulopapillary
Stromal invasion	+/−	−
Basal cells	No	Yes
Ciliated cells	No	Yes
Mucinous cells	Yes	Yes
Extracellular mucus	Present	Present
Atypia and mitoses	+/−	−
Phenotype	CK7+,CK20+(50%),TTF-1-	TTF-1+; p63+ in basal cells
Molecular	*KRAS* mutation	*BRAF*, *EGFR* mutations
Prognosis	Malignant	Benign

erogeneously positive for CDX-2. Mucinous adenocarcinomas of ovarian origin are positive for CK7, MUC-1, and PAX8 but are rarely positive for CK20, CDX2, and beta-catenin. Mucinous adenocarcinoma which originates in the breast is positive for CK7, ER, and WT-1 [10, 11].

How to Diagnose a Tumor with Mixed Morphologic Features of IMA and Invasive Nonmucinous Adenocarcinoma?

A mixture of mucinous and nonmucinous adenocarcinoma occurs occasionally. If the percentage of the IMA component is <10%, the diagnosis is based on the predominantly nonmucinous adenocarcinoma component. In such cases the percentage of IMA should be mentioned in a comment. If the percentage of invasive mucinous adenocarcinoma component is >90%, the diagnosis is IMA. If there is at least 10% of each component, the tumor should be classified as "mixed invasive mucinous/nonmucinous adenocarcinoma." The percentage and subtype of invasive nonmucinous adenocarcinoma should be mentioned in a comment. In addition, an invasive adenocarcinoma may produce mucin which can be identified by light microscopy or mucin stains, but the characteristic goblet cell or columnar cell morphology is lacking. Tumors of this type should be diagnosed as invasive adenocarcinoma with mucinous features [12, 13].

References

1. Travis WD, Brambilla E, Burke AP, Marx A, Nicholson AG. WHO classification of Tumours of the lung, pleura, thymus and heart. 4thed. ed. Lyon: International Agency for Research on Cancer (IARC); 2015.
2. Moon SW, Choi SY, Moon MH. Effect of invasive mucinous adenocarcinoma on lung cancer-specific survival after surgical resection: a population-based study. J Thorac Dis. 2018;10(6):3595–608.
3. Chinokawa H, Ishii G, Nagai K, Kawase A, Yoshida J, Nishimura M, et al. Distinct clinicopathologic characteristics of lung mucinous adenocarcinoma with KRAS mutation. Hum Pathol. 2013;44(12):2636–42.
4. Isaila B, Ananthanarayanan V, Pambuccian S. Ciliated Muconodular papillary tumor of the lung: a new entity formerly regarded as a well-differentiated adenocarcinoma. AJSP: Rev Rep. 2018;23(1):30–7.
5. Kamata T, Yoshida A, Kosuge T, Watanabe S, Asamura H, Tsuta K. Ciliated muconodular papillary tumors of the lung: a clinicopathologic analysis of 10 cases. Am J Surg Pathol. 2015;39(6):753–60.
6. Kon T, Baba Y, Fukai I, Watanabe G, Uchiyama T, Murata T. Ciliated muconodular papillary tumor of the lung: a report of five cases. Pathol Int. 2016;66(11):633–9.
7. Lu YW, Yeh YC. Ciliated muconodular papillary tumors of the lung. Arch Pathol Lab Med. 2019;143(1):135–9. https://doi.org/10.5858/arpa.2017-0275-RS.
8. Liu L, Aesif SW, Kipp BR, Voss JS, Daniel S, Aubry MC, et al. Ciliated Muconodular papillary tumors of the lung can occur in Western patients and show mutations in BRAF and AKT1. Am J Surg Pathol. 2016;40(12):1631–6.
9. Kamata T, Sunami K, Yoshida A, Shiraishi K, Furuta K, Shimada Y, et al. Frequent BRAF or EGFR mutations in ciliated Muconodular papillary tumors of the lung. J Thorac Oncol. 2016;11(2):261–5.
10. Heymann JJ, Hoda RS, Scognamiglio T. Polyclonal napsin a expression: a potential diagnostic pitfall in distinguishing primary from metastatic mucinous tumors in the lung. Arch Pathol Lab Med. 2014;138(8):1067–71.
11. Chu PG, Chung L, Weiss LM, Lau SK. Determining the site of origin of mucinous adenocarcinoma: an immunohistochemical study of 175 cases. Am J Surg Pathol. 2011;35(12):1830–6.
12. Travis WD, Brambilla E, Noguchi M, Nicholson AG, Geisinger KR, Yatabe Y, et al. International association for the study of lung cancer/American thoracic society/European respiratory society international multidisciplinary classification of lung adenocarcinoma. J Thorac Oncol. 2011;6(2):244–85.
13. Boland JM, Maleszewski JJ, Wampfler JA, Voss JS, Kipp BR, Yang P. Pulmonary invasive mucinous adenocarcinoma and mixed invasive mucinous/nonmucinous adenocarcinoma-a clinicopathological and molecular genetic study with survival analysis. Hum Pathol. 2018;71:8–19.

Mucoepidermoid Carcinoma Versus Adenosquamous Carcinoma

11

Jennifer J. Chia and Gregory A. Fishbein

Case Presentation

A 24-year-old female non-smoker presented with a 3-week history of fever, cough, and thick purulent sputum. A chest X-ray showed a right lower lobe consolidated mass. Sputum cultures grew *Streptococcus pneumoniae*. A diagnosis of community-acquired pneumonia was made. Antibiotics were prescribed, and the patient's symptoms resolved by the follow-up visit. Six months later, she presented with similar symptoms, this time including bouts of hemoptysis. High-resolution computed tomography (CT) demonstrated lobar consolidation in the right lower lobe and a 3.3 cm polypoid mass in the right mainstem bronchus. Bronchoscopy was performed confirming an obstructing right-mainstem endobronchial mass measuring approximately 3 cm. An endobronchial biopsy was performed and was nondiagnostic, showing almost exclusively acellular mucinous debris. Bronchioalveolar lavage demonstrated abundant mucin with rare, atypical cells, suspicious for adenocarcinoma. It was felt that excision would be both therapeutic and diagnostic; a right lower lobectomy with mediastinoscopic lymph node sampling was performed.

Pathologic examination of the right lower lobe showed grossly consolidated lung parenchyma with mucopurulent airway plugging. There was a 3-cm polypoid mass with smooth and glistening outer surface affixed to the lumen of the mainstem bronchus (Fig. 11.1).

Histologic sections showed an infiltrative mass within the bronchial submucosa with both solid and cystic components (Fig. 11.2).

Focally, vaguely squamoid nests were present, but frank keratinization was absent. Tumor cells were round to ovoid with eosinophilic to clear cytoplasm. Prominent mucocytes were scattered within tumor islands and lining the cystic components (Fig. 11.3).

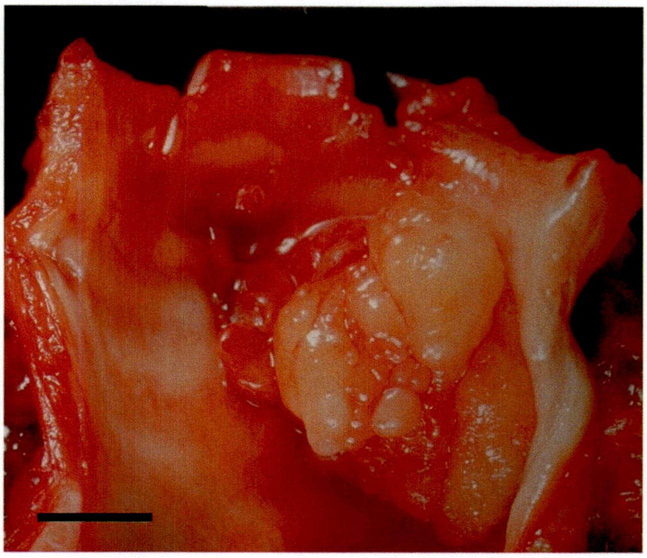

Fig. 11.1 Gross photograph demonstrating a polypoid exophytic endobronchial mass (scale bar = 1 cm)

Mitoses were inconspicuous, and necrosis was not identified. Immunohistochemistry for TTF-1 and napsin-A was negative in the tumor cells. Fluorescent in situ hybridization (FISH) studies were positive for rearrangement of the *MAML2* (11q21) gene. The background lung parenchyma showed post-obstructive pneumonia. Mediastinal lymph nodes were negative for metastases.

J. J. Chia · G. A. Fishbein (✉)
David Geffen School of Medicine at UCLA, Department of Pathology and Laboratory Medicine, Los Angeles, CA, USA
e-mail: gfishbein@mednet.ucla.edu

H. Xu et al. (eds.), *Practical Lung Pathology*, Practical Anatomic Pathology, https://doi.org/10.1007/978-3-031-14402-8_11

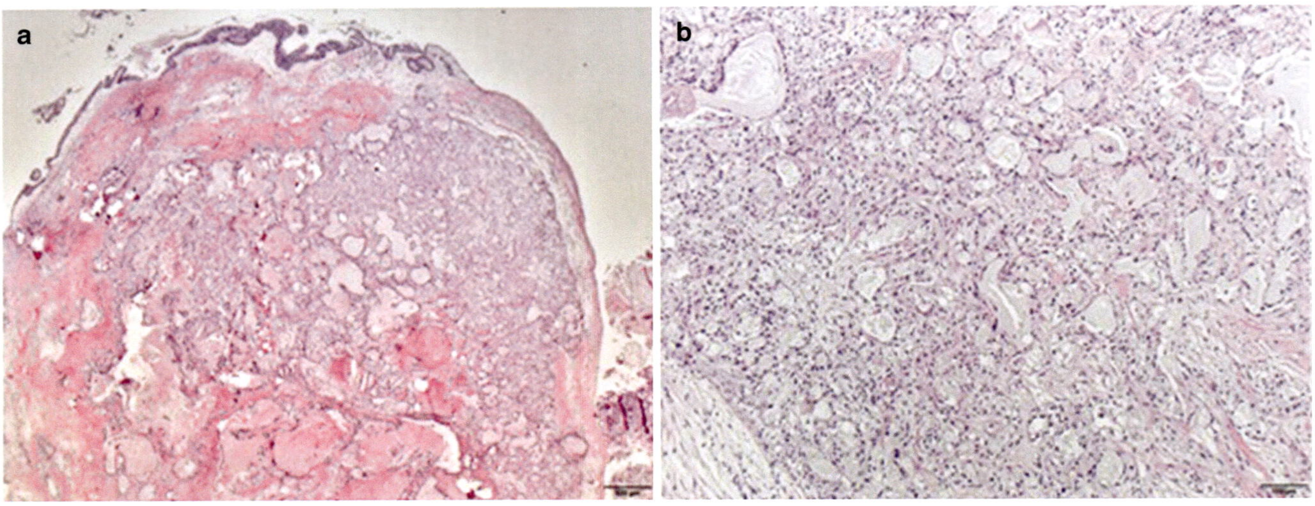

Fig. 11.2 Low- and mid-power photomicrographs of the endobronchial mass (H&E). Sections show an exophytic submucosal proliferation of tumor cells with infiltrative borders (**a**, 20×). The tumor has abundant mucin-filled cysts and an intervening solid component (**b**, 100×)

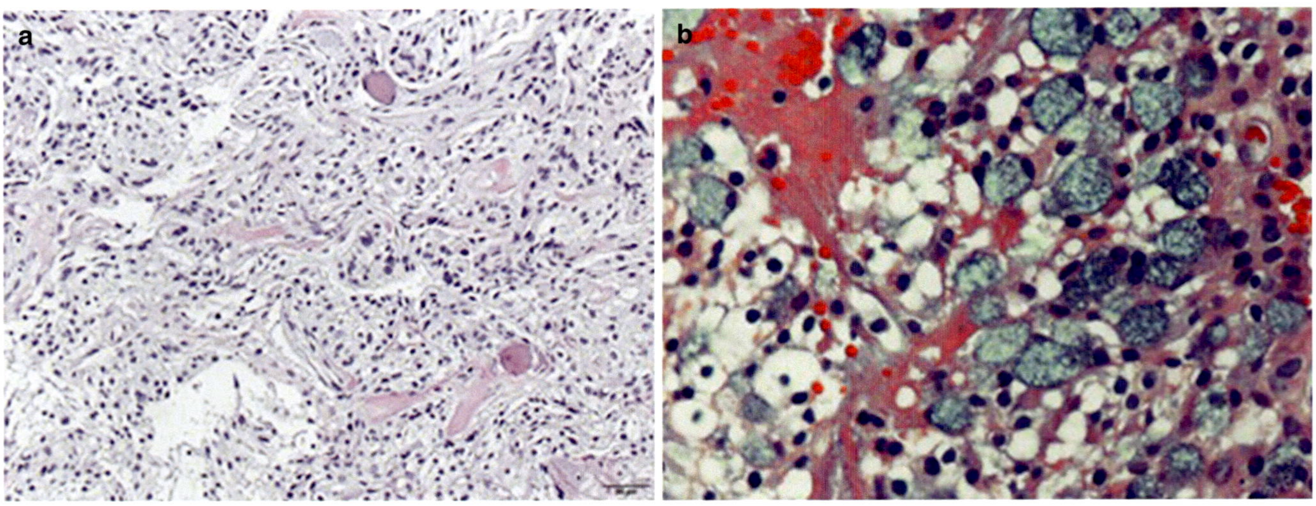

Fig. 11.3 High-magnification photomicrographs demonstrating multiple cell types (H&E). Cells are round to ovoid with eosinophilic to clear cytoplasm. Solid areas have a vaguely squamoid appearance (**a**, 200×). Mucin-secreting cells (mucocytes) with prominent intracytoplasmic mucin droplets can be seen at a high power (**b**, 600×)

Final Diagnosis: Mucoepidermoid Carcinoma, Low Grade

What Is Mucoepidermoid Carcinoma?

Mucoepidermoid carcinoma is a malignant salivary gland-type neoplasm most often occurring in the major salivary glands of the head and neck. Like any salivary gland-type tumor, they may rarely arise from the bronchial and bronchiolar submucosal seromucinous glands. Mucoepidermoid carcinomas characteristically are composed of three cell types: squamoid cells, mucin-secreting cells (a.k.a. mucocytes), and intermediate-type cells. While a subset of tumor cells is squamoid in appearance and immunophenotype, true keratinization is absent.

How Common Is Bronchopulmonary Mucoepidermoid Carcinoma?

Although mucoepidermoid carcinomas are the most common salivary-type malignancy in the lung, primary lung mucoepidermoid carcinomas are rare, accounting for less than 0.5% of lung cancers [1]. The incidence peaks in the fourth decade of life, but about half of cases occur in patients less than 30 years old [2]. Moreover, in children and adolescents, mucoepidermoid carcinoma is the third most common type of primary lung cancer [3].

How Do Patients with Bronchopulmonary Mucoepidermoid Carcinoma Present?

Bronchopulmonary mucoepidermoid carcinoma generally manifests as an endobronchial mass. Therefore, it is not surprising that patients with bronchopulmonary mucoepidermoid carcinoma tend to present with obstructive symptoms. These symptoms may include wheezing, cough, and hemoptysis. Younger patients may initially be misdiagnosed with asthma. Older patients may receive a diagnosis of chronic obstructive pulmonary disease (COPD). As in the case above, some patients may develop post-obstructive pneumonia and present with lobar consolidation secondary to infection.

When Should I Consider Mucoepidermoid Carcinoma in the Differential Diagnosis?

Mucoepidermoid carcinoma should always be considered in the differential diagnosis of an endobronchial mass. The radiographic appearance may be similar to a carcinoid tumor, which is more common in both the pediatric and adult populations. Mucinous adenocarcinoma is exceedingly rare in young people and non-smokers. Therefore, a mucinous endobronchial neoplasm in either of these groups is likely to be a mucoepidermoid carcinoma.

What Ancillary Studies Are Helpful to Establish a Diagnosis of Mucoepidermoid Carcinoma?

The diagnosis of mucoepidermoid carcinoma can be established on H&E sections by identifying the characteristic three cell types: squamoid cells, intermediate cells, and mucin-secreting cells. When tumors are solid and/or the squamoid and intermediate cells predominate, a mucicarmine stain can be very helpful to identify inconspicuous mucocytes. Immunohistochemistry is of limited utility. Squamoid cells expectedly stain with markers of squamous differentiation, such as CK5/6, p63, and p40. Similarly, mucocytes stain with markers of glandular differentiation, such as CEA and MUC5AC. CK7 tends to be positive in all cell types. Neuroendocrine and pneumocytic (e.g., TTF-1, napsin-A) markers are generally negative. It is now recognized that 80–100% of bronchopulmonary mucoepidermoid carcinomas harbor the fusion gene *CRTC1(MECT1)-MAML2* [4–6], an alteration considered specific to mucoepidermoid carcinoma. These include both high- and low-grade tumors. FISH using break-apart probes for the *MAML2* (11q21) gene is an important diagnostic tool. In the appropriate morphologic context, rearrangement of *MAML2* is diagnostic of mucoepidermoid carcinoma.

How Are Bronchopulmonary Mucoepidermoid Carcinomas Graded?

There are numerous systems for grading mucoepidermoid carcinoma. In general, they are three-tier systems, stratifying lesions into low (grade I), intermediate (grade II), and high (grade III) based on the degree of cystic component, cytologic atypia, necrosis, mitotic activity, vascular invasion, and perineural invasion [7, 8]. In the lung, however, mucoepidermoid carcinoma is usually subclassified as either low- or high-grade [2]. Low-grade tumors have more mucin-secreting cells and prominent cystic component with surrounding squamoid and intermediate cells. Low-grade tumors lack necrosis and perineural or lymphatic invasion. Cytologic atypia is minimal, and mitoses are generally <4/10 high-power fields. High-grade tumors are more solid. The squamoid and intermediate cells predominate; mucocytes may be difficult to identify. High-grade mucoepidermoid carcinomas demonstrate significant cytologic atypia, necrosis, and increased mitotic activity and may be accompanied by lymphovascular or perineural invasion.

How Do I Distinguish High-Grade Mucoepidermoid Carcinoma from Adenosquamous Carcinoma?

High-grade mucoepidermoid carcinoma can be difficult if not impossible to differentiate from adenosquamous carcinoma. Adenosquamous carcinoma is a non-small-cell lung cancer, usually poorly differentiated, with components of both squamous cell carcinoma and adenocarcinoma, each constituting greater than 10% of the entire tumor [9]. There is considerable morphologic and immunophenotypic overlap between these uncommon entities. Often the diagnosis of high-grade mucoepidermoid carcinoma is considered controversial and should be rendered only after careful evaluation. Features that argue against high-grade mucoepidermoid carcinoma include keratinization, mucosal squamous dysplasia and/or squamous cell carcinoma in situ, and TTF-1 and/or napsin-A positivity. High-grade mucoepidermoid carcinoma should be considered in cases with exophytic endobronchial growth and/or a transition from areas of conventional low-grade mucoepidermoid carcinoma. FISH analysis (or other molecular techniques) demonstrating rearrangement of the *MAML2* gene is diagnostic of mucoepidermoid carcinoma. Table 11.1 summarizes the above features.

Table 11.1 Features favoring a diagnosis of high-grade pulmonary mucoepidermoid carcinoma versus pulmonary adenosquamous carcinoma

High-grade mucoepidermoid carcinoma	Adenosquamous carcinoma
Exophytic endobronchial growth	Keratinization
Transition from low-grade MEC	Surface epithelial dysplasia/CIS
MAML2 gene rearrangement	TTF-1 and/or napsin-A positivity

MEC mucoepidermoid carcinoma, *CIS* carcinoma in situ

Do I Need to See Three Cell Populations to Suggest a Diagnosis of Mucoepidermoid Carcinoma?

Although the three cell types – squamous, intermediate, and mucin-secreting – are the definitional features of mucoepidermoid carcinoma, all three cell types may not be readily identified in practice. Particularly in small biopsies of low-grade tumors in which glandular elements predominate, definitive squamoid cells may either be unsampled or inconspicuous. Clinical context is paramount. The finding of a mucinous endobronchial lesion in a young person or non-smoker should raise suspicion for mucoepidermoid carcinoma, whether or not a squamoid component can be identified. In such cases, FISH for *MAML2* rearrangement should be performed. If positive, a diagnosis of bronchopulmonary mucoepidermoid carcinoma can be confidently rendered.

References

1. Turnbull AD, Huvos AG, Goodner JT, Foote FW. Mucoepidermoid tumors of bronchial glands. Cancer. 1971;28:539–44.
2. Ishikawa Y, Alvarez-Fernandez E, Aubry MC, Dacic S, Nicholson AG. Mucoepidermoid carcinoma. In: Travis W, Brambilla E, Burke A, Marx A, Nicholson A, editors. WHO Classif. Tumours lung, pleura, thymus hear. 4th ed. International Agency for Research on Cancer: Lyon; 2015. p. 99–100.
3. Welsh JH, Maxson T, Jaksic T, Shahab I, Hicks J. Tracheobronchial mucoepidermoid carcinoma in childhood and adolescence: case report and review of the literature. Int J Pediatr Otorhinolaryngol. 1998;45:265–73.
4. Huo Z, Wu H, Li J, Li S, Wu S, Liu Y, et al. Primary Pulmonary Mucoepidermoid Carcinoma: Histopathological and Moleculargenetic Studies of 26 Cases. PLoS One. 2015;10:e0143169.
5. Salem A, Bell D, Sepesi B, Papadimitrakopoulou V, El-Naggar A, Moran CA, et al. Clinicopathologic and genetic features of primary bronchopulmonary mucoepidermoid carcinoma: the MD Anderson Cancer Center experience and comprehensive review of the literature. Virchows Arch. 2017;470:619–26.
6. Roden AC, García JJ, Wehrs RN, Colby TV, Khoor A, Leslie KO, et al. Histopathologic, immunophenotypic and cytogenetic features of pulmonary mucoepidermoid carcinoma. Mod Pathol. 2014;27:1479–88.
7. Goode RK, Auclair PL, Ellis GL. Mucoepidermoid carcinoma of the major salivary glands: clinical and histopathologic analysis of 234 cases with evaluation of grading criteria. Cancer. 1998;82:1217–24.
8. Brandwein MS, Ivanov K, Wallace DI, Hille JJ, Wang B, Fahmy A, et al. Mucoepidermoid carcinoma: a clinicopathologic study of 80 patients with special reference to histological grading. Am J Surg Pathol. 2001;25:835–45.
9. Travis W, Brambilla E, Burke A, Marx A, Nicholson A. WHO classification of Tumours of the lung, pleura, thymus and heart. 4th ed. IARC: Lyon; 2015.

12 Large-Cell (Undifferentiated) Carcinoma (LCC) Versus Large-Cell Neuroendocrine Carcinoma (LCNEC)

Aimi T. Rothrock, Mufaddal Najmuddin, and Faqian Li

Case Presentation 1

A 71-year-old female with a long history of cigarette smoking presented initially with a right preauricular mass. A workup including a computed tomography (CT) of the neck revealed a 2 cm mass in the lower right parotid gland as well as an incidental finding of a 2 cm irregularly shaped cavitary mass in the left upper lung. A FNA of the preauricular mass was consistent with Warthin's tumor. PET scan showed a hypermetabolic nodule at the posterior aspect of the right upper lobe of the lung measuring 2.1 × 1.9 cm with a standardized uptake value (SUV) max 12.3, as well as a stable cavitary lesion at the left upper lobe (1.4 × 1.4 cm, SUV max 1.6). A right upper lobectomy revealed a solid 2.9 cm mass composed of large polygonal cells with abundant cytoplasm and nesting growth pattern (Fig. 12.1a, c, e). Nuclear chromatin was vesicular with prominent nucleoli. Immunohistochemical (IHC) stains showed that the tumor cells were diffusely positive for cytokeratin AE1/AE3, synaptophysin, chromogranin, and CD56 (Fig. 12.1b, d, f, respectively). There was focal TTF-1 and CK7 positivity, but cytokeratin 5/6 and p40 were negative in the tumor cells. The Ki-67 index was more than 60%. Based on the overall findings, a diagnosis of LCNEC was made. Resection margins were negative, and all lymph nodes were free of carcinoma; thus, the patient was staged as T2aN0M0.

A. T. Rothrock
Department of Pathology and Laboratory Medicine, University of Texas Health Science Center At San Antonio, San Antonio, TX, USA

Department of Pathology and Laboratory Medicine, Albany Medical College, Albany, NY, USA

M. Najmuddin · F. Li (✉)
Department of Pathology and Laboratory Medicine, University of Texas Health Science Center At San Antonio, San Antonio, TX, USA
e-mail: lif2@uthscsa.edu

H. Xu et al. (eds.), *Practical Lung Pathology*, Practical Anatomic Pathology, https://doi.org/10.1007/978-3-031-14402-8_12

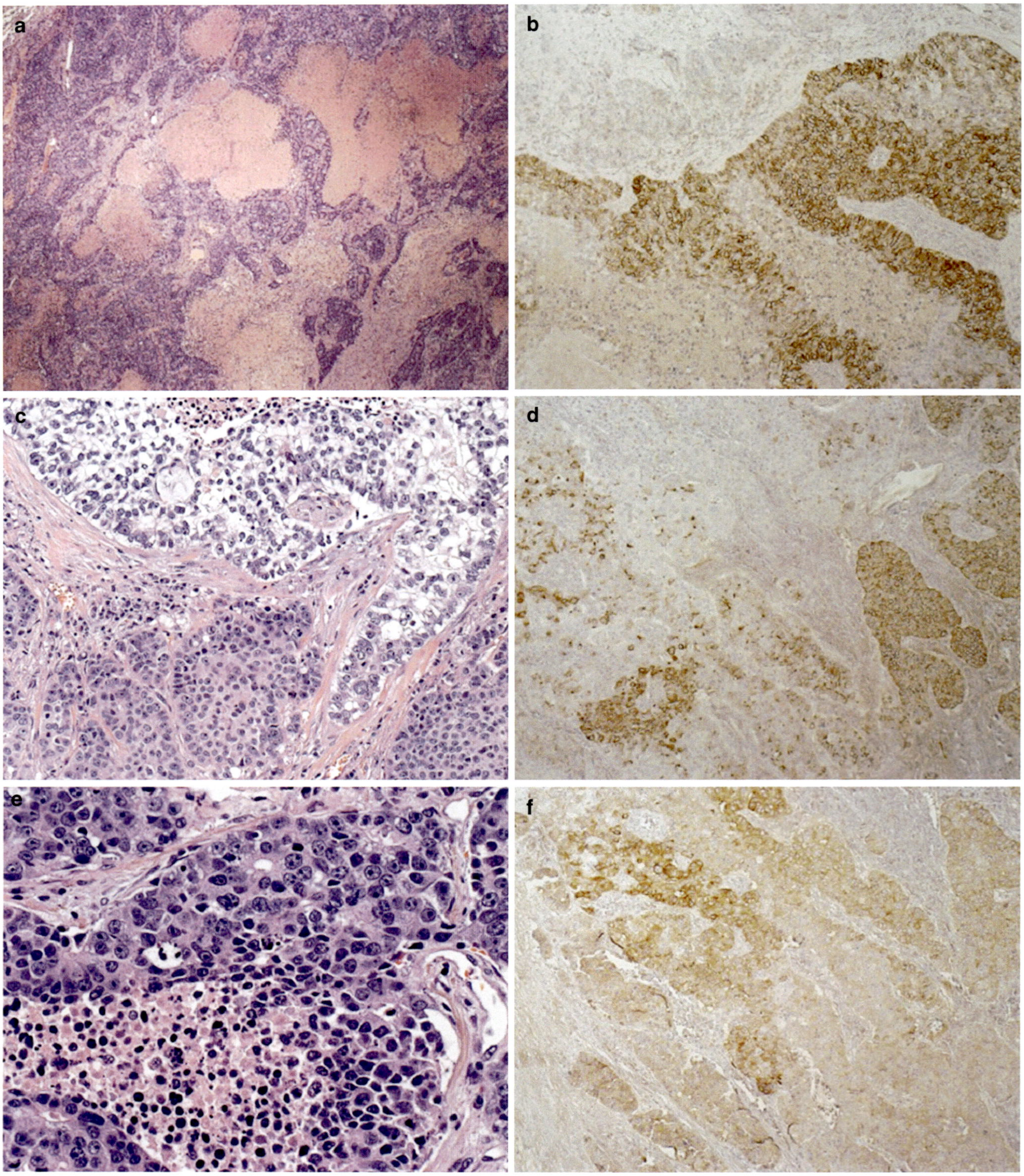

Fig. 12.1 Large-cell neuroendocrine carcinoma. (**a**) Large and small tumor nests with peripheral nuclear palisading and central comedo-like necrosis. H&E, 100×. (**c**) Focal areas of cytoplasmic clearing are seen. The nuclei of neoplastic cells in both areas have similar vesicular chromatin. H&E, 200×. (**d**) Tumor nests with rosette (arrow). H&E, 400×. Tumor positive for neuroendocrine markers CD56 (**b**), highlighting the cell membrane, chromogranin (**d**), and synaptophysin (**f**) in the cytoplasm. IHC 100×

Case Presentation 2

A 76-year-old male with a history of 40–50 pack-year cigarette smoking and follicular lymphoma, currently in remission, had been followed for multiple pulmonary nodules since 2004. In 2016, a CT revealed an irregular solid nodule at the anterolateral right upper lobe that measured 1.4 × 1.0 cm, which was larger than previous imaging studies. A wedge resection revealed a 1.1 × 0.6 cm yellow-tan nodule. Microscopically, there were sheets and clusters of large epithelial cells with abundant eosinophilic cytoplasm and focal clearing (Fig. 12.2). There was significant nuclear pleomorphism with vesicular chromatin, prominent nucleoli, and irregular nuclear contours. Mitotic figures were frequent, and multinucleated tumor giant cells comprised less than 10% of total tumor cells. IHC studies demonstrated that the lesional cells were positive for cytokeratin AE1/AE3 with variable intensity and negative for CK8/18, EMA, CK5/6, CK7, calretinin, desmin, CD45, ERG, melan-A, S-100, p40, TTF-1, and NE markers. Therefore, this tumor was best classified as LCC after extensive workup to rule out other concurrent malignancy and potential metastasis. Lymph nodes sampled for staging purposes were negative for metastasis.

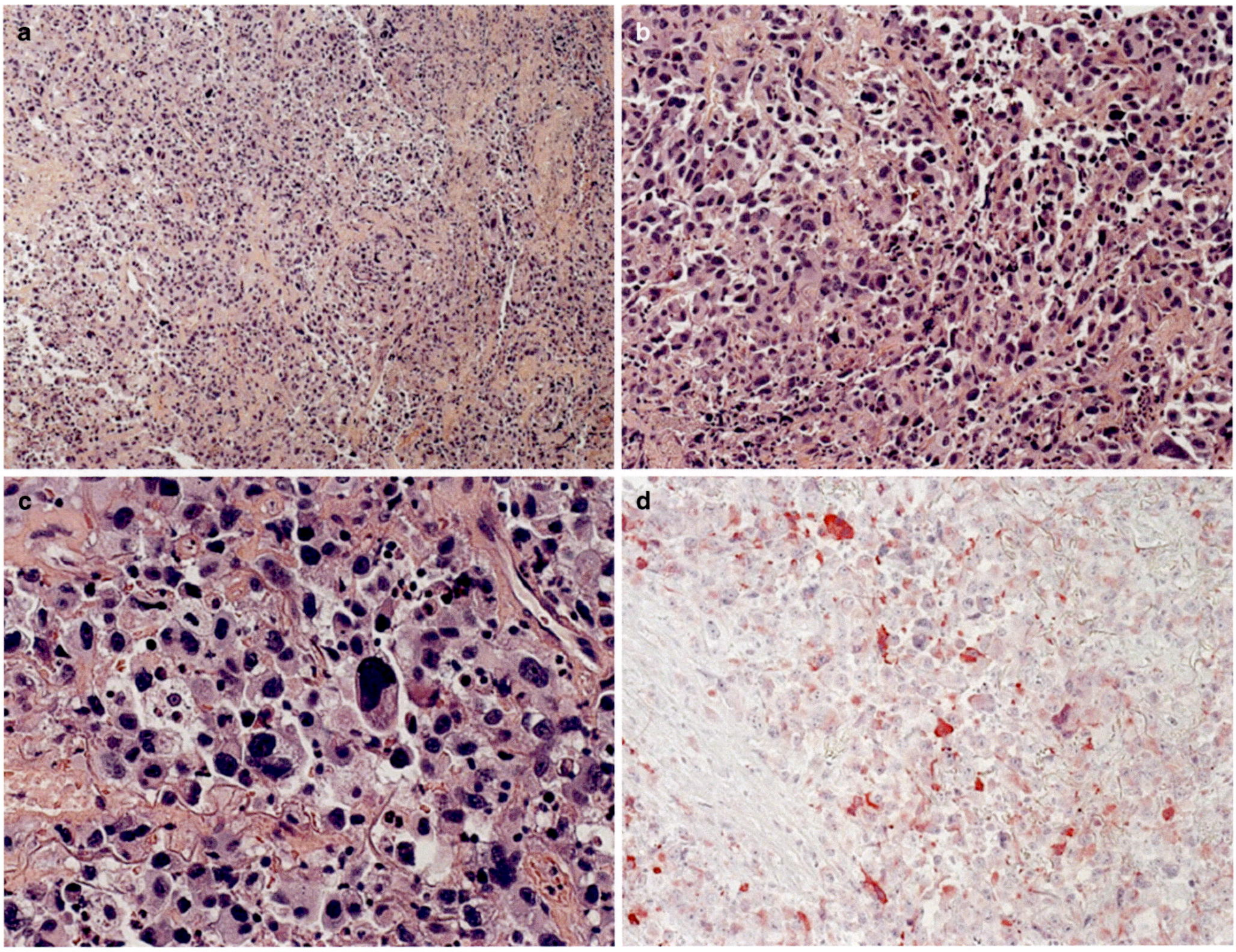

Fig. 12.2 Large-cell carcinoma. (**a**) Individual tumor cells contain abundant cytoplasm with marked nuclear pleomorphism and occasional tumor giant cells, with focal necrosis. H&E, 100×. (**b**) Focal areas contain rhabdoid cells and neutrophils. H&E, 200×. (**c**) Tumor cells have vesicular chromatin and prominent nucleoli. H&E, 400×. (**d**) Tumor cells are positive for cytokeratin AE1/AE3. IHC 200×

What Are the Diagnostic Definitions of LCC and LCNEC?

LCC: According to the 2015 WHO classification, "Large cell carcinoma is an undifferentiated non-small cell carcinoma (NSCC) that lacks the cytological, architectural, and immunohistochemical features of small cell carcinoma, adenocarcinoma or squamous cell carcinoma" [1]. In this definition, "small cell carcinoma" should be replaced with "neuroendocrine tumor or carcinoma" to better address additionally excluded entities such as well-differentiated carcinoids or LCNEC.

In resection specimens, diagnosis of LCC requires thorough sampling and IHC workup to exclude SCC, ADC, or NEC. When morphological features of SCC or ADC are present, IHC markers are not required to assess poorly differentiated areas for further classification. However, if NE morphology is present, NE markers are needed to exclude combined NEC with SCC and/or ADC. Solid pattern ADC can be diagnosed if there are five or more intracellular mucin droplets in each of two high-power fields, confirmed by histochemical stains for mucin. In patients with a history of carcinoma with clinical suspicion for metastasis, cell lineage markers can be performed to support the diagnosis. In a case without morphological features of SCC, ADC, or NEC, immunohistochemical markers to support SCC (p40, p63, and cytokeratin5/6) or ADC (TTF1 and napsin-A) are required for further classification. If a carcinoma is positive for p40, p63, or cytokeratin5/6 but negative for TTF1 and napsin-A, it can be diagnosed as nonkeratinizing SCC. On the other hand, a carcinoma can be classified as solid ADC if it is TTF1 and/or napsin-A positive. It is debatable how strong or what percentage of tumors should be positive for these markers. Generally, focal staining for p40, p63, and/or CK5/6 in scattered tumor cells is allowed in ADC with strong TTF1 and/or napsin-A positivity [2]. Adenosquamous cell carcinoma can be diagnosed when both SCC and ADC markers are distinctly positive in non-overlapping areas, each accounting for more than 10% of tumor cells. Lack of p40 staining strongly argues against SCC [3]. When a carcinoma shows weak and scattered positivity for both SCC and ADC markers in less than 10% of tumor cells, it is best diagnosed with "LCC with unclear immunohistochemical features." "LCC with null immunohistochemical features" is negative for both SCC and ADC markers. In practices without immunohistochemical and mucin stains performed, "LCC with no stains available" is a valid diagnosis.

LCC cannot be diagnosed in small biopsy or cytology specimens, but similar stepwise assessments by morphology, IHC, and mucin stains are still applied, as done for resection specimens [1]. NSCC NOS rather than LCC is used when no clear SCC, ADC, or NE morphology or IHC pattern is present.

LCNEC: According to the 2015 WHO classification, "Large cell neuroendocrine carcinoma is a non-small cell lung carcinoma (NSCLC) that shows histological features of neuroendocrine morphology (including rosettes and peripheral palisading) and expresses immunohistochemical markers of neuroendocrine differentiation" [4]. In resection specimens, diagnosis of LCNEC requires careful search for areas of NE morphology which can be subtle, as well as IHC stains for NE markers: chromogranin A, synaptophysin, and CD56. Chromogranin A and synaptophysin are less sensitive but more specific than CD56 [4, 5]. LCNEC is usually weaker for chromogranin A and synaptophysin than carcinoid tumor [6]. Clear-cut positivity for one of these three NE markers is sufficient to diagnose LCNEC when NE morphology is present. If there is no NE morphology, NE markers should not be assessed, as up to 36% of ADC or SCC can be positive for one of the three NE markers [5, 7, 8]. Newly described NE markers such as INSM1 [9] and hASH1 [6] are more specific but have not been included in the 2015 WHO classification. If NSCC shows NE morphology but is negative for NE, SCC, or ADC markers, it should be classified as LCC rather than LCC with NE morphology to avoid confusion. When LCNEC coexists with ADC or SCC, the diagnosis should be combined LCNEC and ADC or SCC. However, at least 10% of LCNEC is required to diagnose combined LCNEC and SCLC, ADC, or SCC.

LCNEC cannot be diagnosed in small biopsies or cytology specimens. In a case with both NE morphology and positive NE markers, "NSCC possible LCNEC" is a possible term to use. If a carcinoma has NE morphology but is negative for NE markers, a noncommittal diagnosis of "NSCC with NE morphology" is appropriate with a comment: "this is a NSCC where LCNEC is suspected, but stains failed to demonstrate NE differentiation."

What Are the Clinical and Prognostic Features of LCC, and How Do they Differ from LCNEC?

Both LCC and LCNEC are extremely aggressive with a poor prognosis. It is debatable whether LCNEC has worse prognosis than LCC or whether LCNEC benefits from SCLC treatment protocol, either as first-line therapy or in adjuvant settings. Given that these tumors accounts for only 1–3% of all lung carcinomas, no prospective or retrospective clinical studies with sufficient cases have been documented. In addition, a number of studies characterizing these tumors were conducted before IHC stains were commonly used for separating SCC, NEC, and ADC from LCC, as suggested in the 2015 WHO classification.

A prior review of The Surveillance, Epidemiology, and End Results (*SEER*) database from 2001 to 2007 revealed no statistically significant differences in prognosis between LCNEC and other LCC compared to SCLC [10]. In addition, it is not clear whether strict diagnostic criteria were uniformly applied to classify the tumors in this study.

In another single institution review of 28 LCC and 26 LCNEC treated with surgical resection, LCC showed better overall and disease-free survival than LCNEC [11]. In another study of 366 resected cases of lung NE tumors, including 141 LCNEC and 113 SCLC, the overall survival curves of LCNEC and SCLC superimpose each other, suggesting a similarly poor prognosis [12].

In a study with 27 patients, SCLC protocol with platinum-etoposide seems more effective to treat LCNEC than a combination of NSCLC regimens [13]. LCNEC may also benefit from SCLC treatment protocol after surgical resection [14]. However, another evaluation of 26 patients has shown a significantly worse overall survival of SCLC protocol for LCNEC relative to a combination of NSCLC therapies [15]. A detailed retrospective analysis has revealed that NSCLC drug combinations determine the treatment outcomes [16]. Platinum-based NSCLC chemotherapy with gemcitabine, docetaxel, paclitaxel, or vinorelbine is more effective for LCNEC than the NSCLC regimen with platinum-pemetrexed and the SCLC protocol with platinum-etoposide, while the platinum-pemetrexed combination has worse overall survival for LCNEC patients than platinum-etoposide therapy.

How Has Molecular Genetics Played a Role in Defining LCNEC and LCC?

The identification of specific gene mutations in molecular signaling pathways has led to the development of novel targeted therapies for lung cancer. Based on genetic profiling, LCC does not form a distinct group and instead shows genetic alterations similar to ADC; however, targetable molecular alterations typical of ADC such as *EGFR* mutations and translocation of *ALK* and *ROS1* are usually not identified in LCC [17, 18]. In cases when LCC shows *EGFR*, *ALK*, or *ROS-1* alteration, it is better classified as solid pattern ADC, even in the absence of TTF-1 or napsin-A immunoreactivity. This allows patients to receive appropriate targeted therapies. In light of these findings, it can be suggested that LCC be considered as a poorly differentiated form of ADC which lacks expression of its usual immunohistochemical markers [19]. Expression profiling also fails to identify a distinct LCC group, and cases of LCC are often clustered along with either SCC or ADC [18].

On the other hand, LCNEC forms three distinct genetic groups: (1) SCLC-like with p53 and Rb1 double inactivation, (2) NSCLC-like with a genetic profile often similar to ADC and occasionally SCC, and (3) carcinoid-like with mutations in *MEN-1* and low total mutation burden [20–22]. These three groups of LCNEC are also identified based on gene expression changes [18, 22]. In LCNEC, diagnostic morphological and immunophenotypic findings do not reflect their molecular alterations and gene expression profiles [23]. It is not surprising to see that LCNEC is a mixed group containing molecular features of SCLC, carcinoids, and NSCLC as LCNEC was subclassified from these different tumors. Further refinement of morphological and IHC criteria for LCNEC based on recent molecular studies will make the diagnosis of LCNEC more accurate and reflect its genetic basis.

Summary

When evaluating lung cancer, the first diagnostic step is to histologically assess whether SCC, ADC, or NE morphology is present. If SCC, ADC, or NEC morphological features are not obvious under the microscope, IHC stains for ADC and SCC markers are required. Negative staining patterns would render the diagnosis of LCC with null IHC features. If inconclusive, LCC with unclear IHC features can be reported. These two subtypes of LCC are not a molecularly defined entity based on recent molecular profiling and can show molecular features similar to ADC. In the future, LCC may be classified as ADC without ADC marker expression as long as SCC is carefully ruled out.

In contrast to LCC, LCNEC requires both NE morphology and positivity with NE markers by IHC. LCNEC has three distinct subtypes according to molecular alterations and unique expression profiles. The current diagnostic criteria for LCNEC based on both NE morphology and NE marker positivity require further refinement to reflect its genetic basis and potential therapeutic targets.

References

1. Nicholson AG, Beasley MB, Caporaso NE, Carvalho L, Dalurzo ML, Devesa SS, et al. Large cell carcinoma. In: Travis WDBE, Burke AP, Marx A, Nicholson AG, editors. WHO classification of Tumours of of the lung, pleura, thymus and heart. 4th ed. Lyon, France: International Agency for Research on Cancer (IARC); 2015. p. 80–5.
2. Rekhtman N, Ang DC, Sima CS, et al. Immunohistochemical algorithm for differentiation of lung adenocarcinoma and squamous cell carcinoma based on large series of whole-tissue sections with validation in small specimens. Mod Pathol. 2011;24:1348.
3. Pelosi G, Fabbri A, Papotti M, et al. Dissecting pulmonary large-cell carcinoma by targeted next generation sequencing of several cancer genes pushes genotypic-phenotypic correlations to emerge. J Thorac Oncol. 2015;10(11):1560–9.
4. Brambilla EBM, Chirieac LR, Austin JHM, Capelozzi VL, Devesa SS, Gazdar A, et al. Large cell neuroendocrine carcinoma. In: Travis WD, Brambilla E, Burke AP, Marx A, Nicholson AG, editors. WHO classification of Tumours of of the lung, pleura, thymus

and heart. 4th ed. Lyon, France: International Agency for Research on Cancer (IARC); 2015. p. 69–72.
5. Ionescu DN, Treaba D, Gilks CB, et al. Nonsmall cell lung carcinoma with neuroendocrine differentiation--an entity of no clinical or prognostic significance. Am J Surg Pathol. 2007;31(1):26–32.
6. Ye B, Cappel J, Findeis-Hosey J, et al. hASH1 is a specific immunohistochemical marker for lung neuroendocrine tumors. Human Pathol. 2016;48:142–7.
7. Howe MC, Chapman A, Kerr K, et al. Neuroendocrine differentiation in non-small cell lung cancer and its relation to prognosis and therapy. Histopathology. 2005;46(2):195–201.
8. Pelosi G, Pasini F, Sonzogni A, et al. Prognostic implications of neuroendocrine differentiation and hormone production in patients with stage I nonsmall cell lung carcinoma. Cancer. 2003;97(10):2487–97.
9. Mukhopadhyay S, Dermawan JK, Lanigan CP, et al. Insulinoma-associated protein 1 (INSM1) is a sensitive and highly specific marker of neuroendocrine differentiation in primary lung neoplasms: an immunohistochemical study of 345 cases, including 292 whole-tissue sections. Mod Pathol. 2019;32(1):100–9.
10. Varlotto JM, Medford-Davis LN, Recht A, et al. Should large cell neuroendocrine lung carcinoma be classified and treated as a small cell lung cancer or with other large cell carcinomas? J Thorac Oncol. 2011;6(6):1050–8.
11. Iyoda A, Hiroshima K, Toyozaki T, et al. Clinical characterization of pulmonary large cell neuroendocrine carcinoma and large cell carcinoma with neuroendocrine morphology. Cancer. 2001;91(11):1992–2000.
12. Asamura H, Kameya T, Matsuno Y, et al. Neuroendocrine neoplasms of the lung: a prognostic Spectrum. J Clin Oncol. 2006;24(1):70–6.
13. Rossi G, Cavazza A, Marchioni A, et al. Role of chemotherapy and the receptor tyrosine kinases KIT, PDGFRα, PDGFRβ, and met in large-cell neuroendocrine carcinoma of the lung. J Clin Oncol. 2005;23(34):8774–85.
14. Iyoda A, Hiroshima K, Moriya Y, et al. Prospective study of adjuvant chemotherapy for pulmonary large cell neuroendocrine carcinoma. Ann Thorac Surg. 2006;82(5):1802–7.
15. Naidoo J, Santos-Zabala ML, Iyriboz T, et al. Large cell neuroendocrine carcinoma of the lung: Clinico-pathologic features, treatment, and outcomes. Clin Lung Cancer. 2016;17(5):e121–9.
16. Derks JL, van Suylen RJ, Thunnissen E, et al. Chemotherapy for pulmonary large cell neuroendocrine carcinomas: does the regimen matter? Eur Resp J. 2017;49(6):1601838.
17. The clinical lung cancer genome project (CLCGP) and network genomic medicine (NGM). A genomics-based classification of human lung tumors. Sci Transl Med. 2013;5(209):209ra153.
18. Karlsson A, Brunnström H, Micke P, et al. Gene expression profiling of large cell lung cancer links transcriptional phenotypes to the new histological WHO 2015 classification. J Thorac Oncol. 2017;12(8):1257–67.
19. Driver BR, Portier BP, Mody DR, et al. Next-generation sequencing of a cohort of pulmonary large cell carcinomas reclassified by World Health Organization 2015 criteria. Arch Pathol Lab Med. 2016;140(4):312–7.
20. Miyoshi T, Umemura S, Matsumura Y, et al. Genomic profiling of large-cell neuroendocrine carcinoma of the lung. Clin Cancer Res. 2017;23(3):757–65.
21. Rekhtman N, Pietanza MC, Hellmann MD, et al. Next-generation sequencing of pulmonary large cell neuroendocrine carcinoma reveals small cell carcinoma-like and non-small cell carcinoma-like subsets. Clin Cancer Res. 2016;22(14):3618–29.
22. George J, Walter V, Peifer M, et al. Integrative genomic profiling of large-cell neuroendocrine carcinomas reveals distinct subtypes of high-grade neuroendocrine lung tumors. Nat Commun. 2018;9(1):1048.
23. Travis WD, Brambilla E, Burke AP, Marx A, Nicholson AG. WHO classification of Tumours of of the lung, pleura, thymus and heart. Lyon, France: International Agency for Research on Cancer (IARC); 2015.

Large-Cell Neuroendocrine Carcinoma Versus Small-Cell Carcinoma of the Lung

13

Rebecca Baldassarri, Stephen Baldassarri, and Guoping Cai

Case Presentation

A 60-year-old woman with a history of chronic obstructive pulmonary disease (COPD), hypertension, and anxiety presented to her primary care physician for routine follow-up care. She felt reasonably well and denied symptoms of cough, shortness of breath, hemoptysis, or chest discomfort. She took a daily long-acting bronchodilator for COPD, which controlled her respiratory symptoms adequately. Her social history was notable for a prior heavy cigarette smoking (40 pack-years). She quit cigarette smoking 5 years prior to her visit.

Since she met the US Preventive Services Task Force (USPSTF) criteria for lung cancer screening, a shared decision-making discussion was held with her physician, and a decision was made to proceed with a low-dose chest computed tomography (CT) scan. Her CT scan showed a well-circumscribed 2 cm × 2 cm pulmonary nodule located peripherally in the right upper lobe. A follow-up positron-emission tomography (PET) scan showed that the nodule was highly PET avid (SUV = 10). There was neither hilar nor mediastinal lymphadenopathy. The patient subsequently underwent video-assisted thoracoscopic surgery. Intraoperative biopsy with frozen section revealed non-small-cell carcinoma. A right upper lobe lobectomy was subsequently performed. Pathologic review of the specimen revealed a peripherally located, irregularly shaped, firm mass. Histologically, the tumor was compromised of large polygonal cells with prominent nucleoli arranged in nests and cords. Immunohistochemically, the tumor was positive for thyroid transcription factor 1 (TTF-1), synaptophysin, and insulinoma-associated protein 1 (INSM1) while negative for p40. The combined morphologic and immunohistochemical findings were consistent with large-cell neuroendocrine carcinoma (LCNEC).

Final Pathologic Diagnosis: Large-Cell Neuroendocrine Carcinoma

How Do LCNEC Present Clinically? What Are the Imaging Findings?

LCNEC is a rare, highly aggressive neoplasm of the lung. Together with SCLC, LCNEC is considered a high-grade neuroendocrine carcinoma, with clinicopathologic features distinct from low-grade typical carcinoid and intermediate-grade atypical carcinoid. Like SCLC, LCNEC disproportionately affects older male smokers and presents at an advanced stage with poor prognosis [1].

The reported incidence of LCNEC in surgically resected specimens is approximately 2–3%. This is likely an underestimate of the true incidence, given that many patients are inoperable at the time of diagnosis and a confident diagnosis of LCNEC is difficult on small biopsies and cytologic specimens alone [1, 2]. Given the rarity of LCNEC, standardized treatment has not been established. Treatment approaches may be slightly different from those used in SCLC. Patients with limited stage disease are generally treated with surgery and chemotherapy and/or radiation therapy, while those with advanced stage disease receive etoposide or platinum-based therapies [1]. Overall survival is poor regardless of stage, with an overall 5-year survival rate of 35.3% [3].

LCNEC appears as peripherally located, expansile, and irregularly shaped mass on high-resolution computed tomography (HRCT). Calcification is variable, and bulky lymphadenopathy is typically absent. The imaging findings of

R. Baldassarri (✉)
Department of Pathology, Yale University School of Medicine, New Haven, CT, USA
e-mail: rebecca.baldassarri@yale.edu

S. Baldassarri · G. Cai
Division of Pulmonary and Critical Care, Department of Internal Medicine, Yale University School of Medicine, New Haven, CT, USA
e-mail: stephen.baldassarri@yale.edu; guoping.cai@yale.edu

H. Xu et al. (eds.), *Practical Lung Pathology*, Practical Anatomic Pathology, https://doi.org/10.1007/978-3-031-14402-8_13

LCNEC are nonspecific, without reliable features that distinguish it from other non-small-cell carcinomas [1, 2, 4]. As LCNEC tends to be peripherally located, symptoms commonly associated with centrally located lesions (cough, hemoptysis, and post-obstructive pneumonia) are less common. Rather, patients tend to be asymptomatic or exhibit nonspecific flu-like symptoms, dyspnea, or night sweats [2].

What Are the Key Pathologic Features of LCNEC?

Gross examination of LCNEC typically reveals a peripherally located, bulky circumscribed mass with a tan-yellow cut surface. The gross features of LCNEC are indistinguishable from other NSCLC [5]. Histologic features of LCNEC include neuroendocrine-type morphology (organoid, trabecular, or rosette pattern) with nuclear palisading, large nuclear size (greater than three times that of a mature lymphocyte), prominent nucleoli, relatively low nuclear/cytoplasmic (N/C) ratios, abundant necrosis, and high mitotic rate (>10 mitoses per 10 high-power fields) (Fig. 13.1) [1, 6].

Diagnosis of LCNEC is typically made retrospectively on resection specimens, as the recognition of salient features may be difficult on small pre-surgical specimens. Due to overlapping morphologic features, many LCNEC are diagnosed preoperatively as poorly differentiated non-small-cell carcinoma (NSCLC), atypical carcinoid (AC), SCLC, or high-grade neuroendocrine carcinoma, NOS [6].

Immunohistochemical staining of LCNEC is necessary to confirm neuroendocrine differentiation. The tumor cells exhibit variable reactivity for neuroendocrine markers such as chromogranin A, synaptophysin, CD56, and neuron-specific enolase (NSE) [1, 6, 7]. Positivity for CD56 or NSE should be interpreted carefully, as isolated positivity is not specific for neuroendocrine differentiation [6, 7]. Insulinoma-associated protein 1 (INSM1) is a new, highly specific marker of neuroendocrine differentiation that has been found to stain 75% of LCNEC (Fig. 13.2) [8].

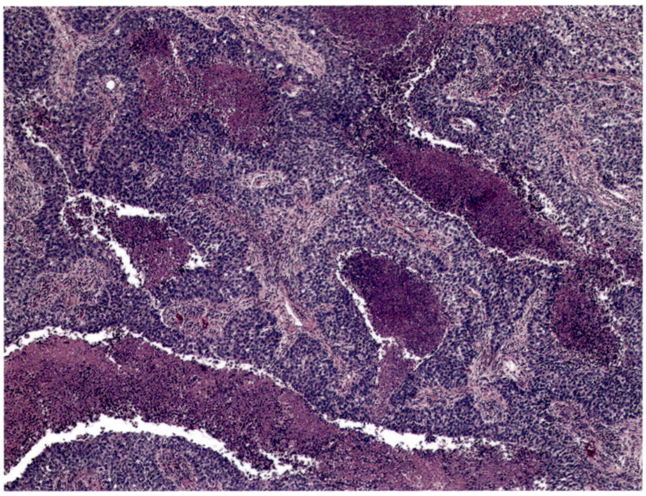

Fig. 13.1 Large-cell neuroendocrine carcinoma of the lung. Histologic section of the tumor shows neuroendocrine-type morphology, including nests and cords of malignant cells with necrosis. H&E 40× magnification

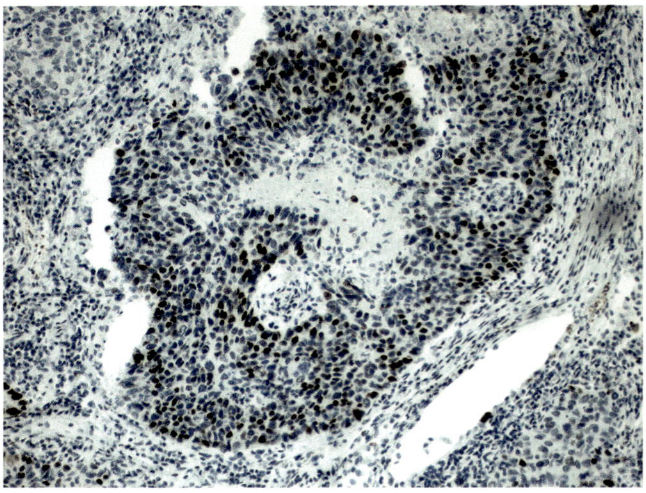

Fig. 13.2 LCNEC showing diffuse nuclear positivity for INSM1. IHC 100× magnification

What Are the Molecular Features of LCNEC?

Recent studies have shown that LCNEC segregates into distinct molecular subsets, including a SCLC-like group (harboring TP53/RB1 co-mutations and other SCLC-type alterations, such as *MYC* amplification) and a non-small-cell carcinoma (NSCLC)-like group that harbors mutations more commonly seen in adenocarcinomas, such as *STK11*, *KRAS*, and/or *KEAP*. The morphologic features of these LCNEC subsets parallel their molecular similarities, with the SCLC-like LCNEC group showing morphologic overlap with SCLC and the NSCLC-like LCNEC group displaying NSCLC-like morphologic features [7]. George et al. have analyzed LCNEC on a genomic and transcriptomic level, finding that LCNEC falls into two molecular subtypes: "type I LCNEC" (harboring bi-allelic *TP53* and *STK11/KEAP1* alterations) and "type II LCNEC" (with bi-allelic *TP53* and *RB1* inactivation). However, despite the genomic similarity to SCLC, type II LCNEC differs on a transcriptomic level from SCLC, with reduced expression of neuroendocrine markers [9].

What Are the Key Points in Differentiating LCNEC from SCLC?

What Are the Clinical and Radiographic Characteristics that Distinguish LCNEC from SCLC?

LCNEC and SCLC affect a similar cohort of patients—older men with a heavy smoking history. The imaging characteristics of LCNEC and SCLC are typically dissimilar. LCNEC tends to present as a peripheral mass without bulky lymphadenopathy, while SCLC typically presents as a centrally located lung mass with bulky mediastinal or hilar lymphadenopathy. However, a minority of SCLC (5%) can present as peripherally located lesions, and LCNEC can occasionally present in a central location [4, 10].

What Are the Architectural Features that Suggest LCNEC over SCLC?

There can be substantial overlap between LCNEC and SCLC on a morphologic basis, particularly in small biopsy or cytology samples. In general, architecture that favors SCLC includes a diffuse sheetlike growth, while "classic" neuroendocrine architectures are more commonly seen in LCNEC, including nesting, organoid, or trabecular growth patterns. LCNEC often shows nuclear palisading along the peripheral of tumor nests.

What Are the Cytologic Features that Suggest LCNEC over SCLC?

LCNEC and SCLC are usually morphologically distinct. As suggested by the names of the entities, tumor nuclear size is one distinguishing factor between LCENC and SCLC. However, while the nuclei of LCNEC are typically described as greater than three times the size of a mature lymphocyte, and the nuclei of SCLC are smaller than three times the size of a mature lymphocyte, in practice, there is significant overlap in nuclear size between LCNEC and SCLC, and distinction solely based on cell size is discouraged [7, 11]. Rather, a constellation of cytologic features points towards LCNEC. LCNEC has a lower N/C ratio than SCLC, with polygonal tumor cells and distinct cell borders, as opposed to fusiform cells of SCLC (Figs. 13.3 and 13.4) [11]. Examination of nuclear features reveals that LCNEC has coarse, vesicular chromatin with conspicuous nucleoli, while SCLC has absent or inconspicuous nucleoli, with more characteristic "salt and pepper" chromatin [7]. In addition, basophilic crusting of blood vessels (the Azzopardi phenomenon) is less pronounced in LCNEC compared to SCLC [1]. Features shared by both LCNEC and SCLC include a high mitotic rate and abundant necrosis [1].

In classic cases, the distinction between LCNEC and SCLC is straightforward; however, there exist borderline cases of high-grade neuroendocrine carcinomas that fall between LCNEC and SCLC. These borderline cases exhibit overlapping morphologic features, including nuclear size; it is these borderline cases that contribute to the low reproducibility rate in diagnosis of LCNEC [6, 11].

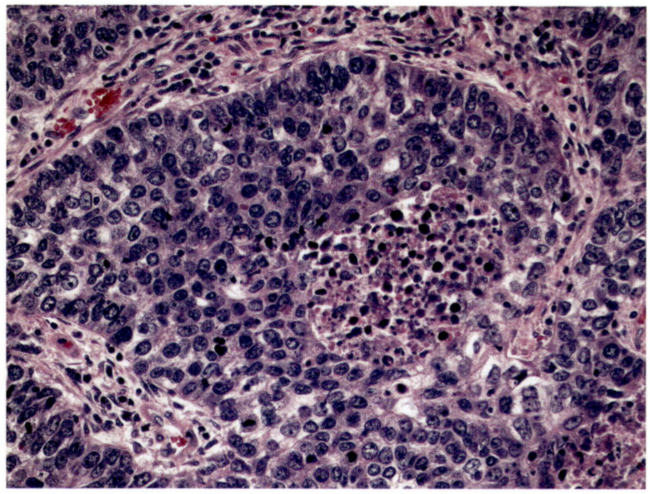

Fig. 13.3 Large-cell neuroendocrine carcinoma of the lung. Histological sections show that the tumor cells are polygonal with a moderate amount of cytoplasm. Tumor nuclei are greater than three times the size of a mature lymphocyte. Nuclei have coarse chromatin with conspicuous nucleoli. H&E 200× magnification

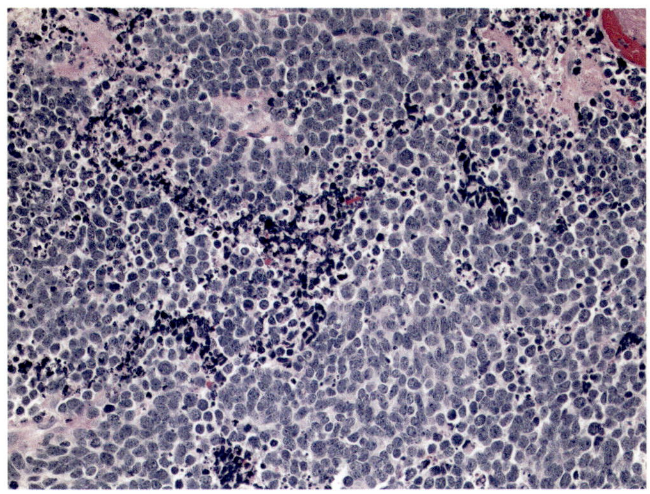

Fig. 13.4 Small-cell carcinoma of the lung. Histological section shows that the tumor cells have a high nuclear/cytoplasmic ratio with fusiform-shaped nuclei and nuclear molding. Tumor cells are less than three times the size of a mature lymphocyte. Chromatin is evenly distributed without prominent nucleoli. H&E 200× magnification

What Are the Immunohistochemical Differences Between LCNEC and SCLC?

LCNEC and SCLC can both show weak punctate "dot-like" reactivity for cytokeratins such as AE1/AE3. Both LCNEC and SCLC should be negative for high-molecular weight keratins such as CK903; if there is diffuse positivity for

CK903 with a SCLC-like morphology, one should consider the diagnosis of basaloid squamous cell carcinoma [11]. Most SCLC (90%) are positive for TTF1, while it is expressed in only 50% of LCNEC [12]. SCLC and LCNEC show variable positivity with neuroendocrine markers; however, positivity with at least one neuroendocrine marker is required to diagnose LCNEC. Most (70%) LCNEC co-express synaptophysin and chromogranin. Up to 25% of SCLC can be negative for synaptophysin and chromogranin; however, these cases are often positive for CD56. Still, about 10% of SCLC can be negative for all three (synaptophysin, chromogranin, and CD56) commonly used neuroendocrine markers [11]. INSM1, a new neuroendocrine marker, is highly sensitive for SCLC (98%), similar to synaptophysin (100%) and CD56 (95%). In contrast, the sensitivity of CD56 (92%) and synaptophysin (88%) surpassed that of INSM1 (75%) for the diagnosis of LCNEC [8].

References

1. Fasano M, Della Corte CM, Papaccio F, Ciardiello F, Morgillo F. Pulmonary large-cell neuroendocrine carcinoma: from epidemiology to therapy. J Thorac Oncol. 2015;10(8):1133–41.
2. Fernandez FG, Battafarano RJ. Large-cell neuroendocrine carcinoma of the lung: an aggressive neuroendocrine lung cancer. Semin Thorac Cardiovasc Surg. 2006;18(3):206–10.
3. Iyoda A, Jiang SX, Travis WD, Kurouzu N, Ogawa F, Amano H, et al. Clinicopathological features and the impact of the new TNM classification of malignant tumors in patients with pulmonary large cell neuroendocrine carcinoma. Mol Clin Oncol. 2013;1(3):437–43.
4. Akata S, Okada S, Maeda J, Park J, Yoshimura M, Saito K, et al. Computed tomographic findings of large cell neuroendocrine carcinoma of the lung. Clin Imaging. 2007;31(6):379–84.
5. Franks TJ, Galvin JR. Lung tumors with neuroendocrine morphology: essential radiologic and pathologic features. Arch Pathol Lab Med. 2008;132(7):1055–61. https://doi.org/10.1043/1543-2165(2008)132[1055:LTWNME]2.0.CO;2.
6. Iyoda A, Hiroshima K, Nakatani Y, Fujisawa T. Pulmonary large cell neuroendocrine carcinoma: its place in the spectrum of pulmonary carcinoma. Ann Thorac Surg. 2007;84(2):702–7.
7. Hiroshima K, Mino-Kenudson M. Update on large cell neuroendocrine carcinoma. Transl Lung Cancer Res. 2017;6(5):530–9.
8. Mukhopadhyay S, Dermawan JK, Lanigan CP, Farver CF. Insulinoma-associated protein 1 (INSM1) is a sensitive and highly specific marker of neuroendocrine differentiation in primary lung neoplasms: an immunohistochemical study of 345 cases, including 292 whole-tissue sections. Mod Pathol. 2019;32(1):100–9.
9. George J, Walter V, Peifer M, Alexandrov LB, Seidel D, Leenders F, et al. Integrative genomic profiling of large-cell neuroendocrine carcinomas reveals distinct subtypes of high-grade neuroendocrine lung tumors. Nat Commun. 2018;9(1):1048.
10. Carter BW, Glisson BS, Truong MT, Erasmus JJ. Small cell lung carcinoma: staging, imaging, and treatment considerations. Radiographics. 2014;34(6):1707–21.
11. Rekhtman N. Neuroendocrine tumors of the lung: an update. Arch Pathol Lab Med. 2010;134(11):1628–38.
12. Thunnissen E, Borczuk AC, Flieder DB, Witte B, Beasley MB, Chung JH, et al. The use of immunohistochemistry improves the diagnosis of small cell lung cancer and its differential diagnosis. An international reproducibility study in a demanding set of cases. J Thorac Oncol. 2017;12(2):334–46.

Atypical Carcinoid Tumor Versus Large-Cell Neuroendocrine Carcinoma

14

Esther C. Yoon and Guoping Cai

Case Presentation

A 66-year-old female never-smoker was referred to the Thoracic Oncology Program Clinic for a mass in the right lower lobe of the lung. She was recently hospitalized for recurrent bronchitis after 2 weeks of progressively worsening cough and wheezing. She denied nausea, emesis, fever, chills, weight loss, or hemoptysis. On physical examination, she appeared well developed and well nourished. Her pulmonary examination was unremarkable, and she had no lymphadenopathy in the cervical or supraclavicular regions.

She was managed with a course of antibiotics and steroids with improvement. During her hospitalization, computed tomography (CT) imaging revealed a 4.7 × 4.7 × 3.4 cm well-circumscribed mass in the base of the right lower lobe with increased attenuation of the dependent portion of the mass and focal atelectasis (Fig. 14.1). No pleural effusion, edema, or pneumothorax was identified. The mass has a standardized uptake value (SUV) maximum of 7.3 on positron-emission tomography (PET) scan. No hypermetabolic hilar or mediastinal lymphadenopathy was identified. The patient underwent lobectomy and mediastinal lymph node biopsy staging.

Grossly, a bulging peripheral mass was palpated. The overlying pleura was glistening and tan-pink without areas of puckering. Sectioning revealed a 4.5 × 4.5 × 3.5 cm well-circumscribed, spherical mass which abutted the pleura. The mass consisted of a firm, almost cartilaginous, eccentric area surrounded by a peripheral hemorrhagic gelatinous area (Fig. 14.2). The mass was well demarcated

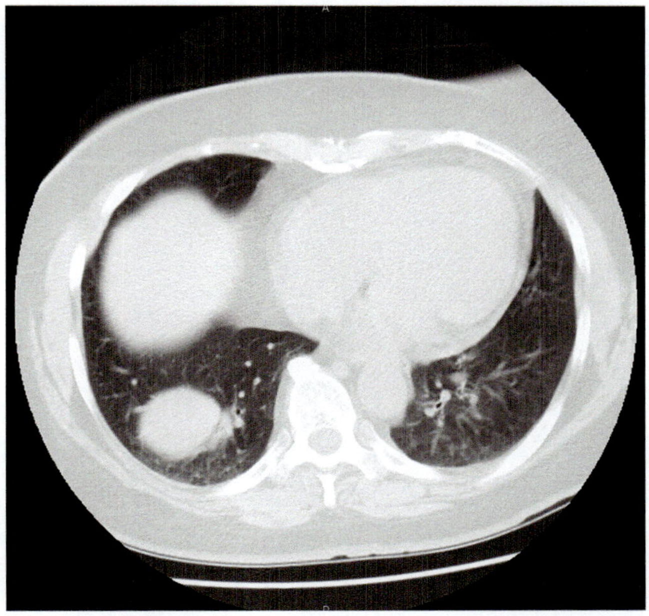

Fig. 14.1 CT image of atypical carcinoid. A well-circumscribed mass is shown in the right middle lobe near the base

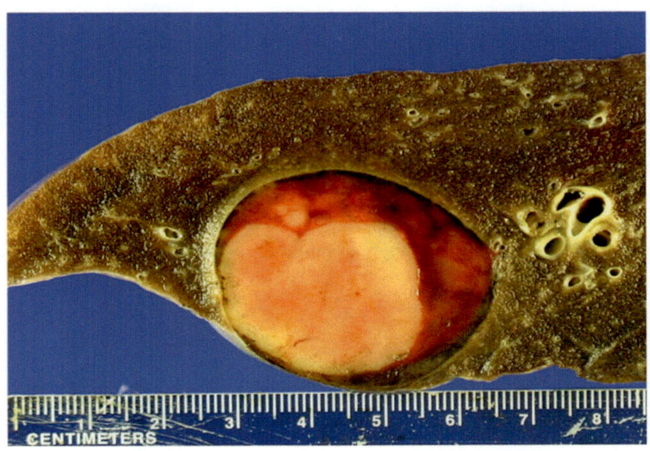

Fig. 14.2 Gross image of atypical carcinoid. The tumor is a well-circumscribed mass with an eccentric tan-white slightly lobulated firm area surrounded by hemorrhagic gelatinous area

E. C. Yoon
Department of Pathology, The University of Texas MD Anderson Cancer Center, Houston, TX, USA

G. Cai (✉)
Department of Pathology, Yale University School of Medicine, New Haven, CT, USA
e-mail: guoping.cai@yale.edu

H. Xu et al. (eds.), *Practical Lung Pathology*, Practical Anatomic Pathology, https://doi.org/10.1007/978-3-031-14402-8_14

from the surrounding pink spongy lung parenchyma. Lobar, segmental, and mediastinal lymph nodes were grossly unremarkable.

Microscopically, the tumor showed organoid growth pattern with prominent vascularity. There was focal necrosis. The neoplastic cells were polygonal and had moderate eosinophilic cytoplasm and oval-to-round nuclei with smooth nuclear membrane, finely granular chromatin, and inconspicuous nucleoli (Fig. 14.3). Focal areas showed cytological atypia including nuclear enlargement, nuclear polymorphism, and multinucleation. Mitotic figure count was four mitoses per 2 mm^2. The tumor cells are positive for chromogranin, synaptophysin, and CD56 with a Ki-67 proliferation index focally up to 5% (Fig. 14.4).

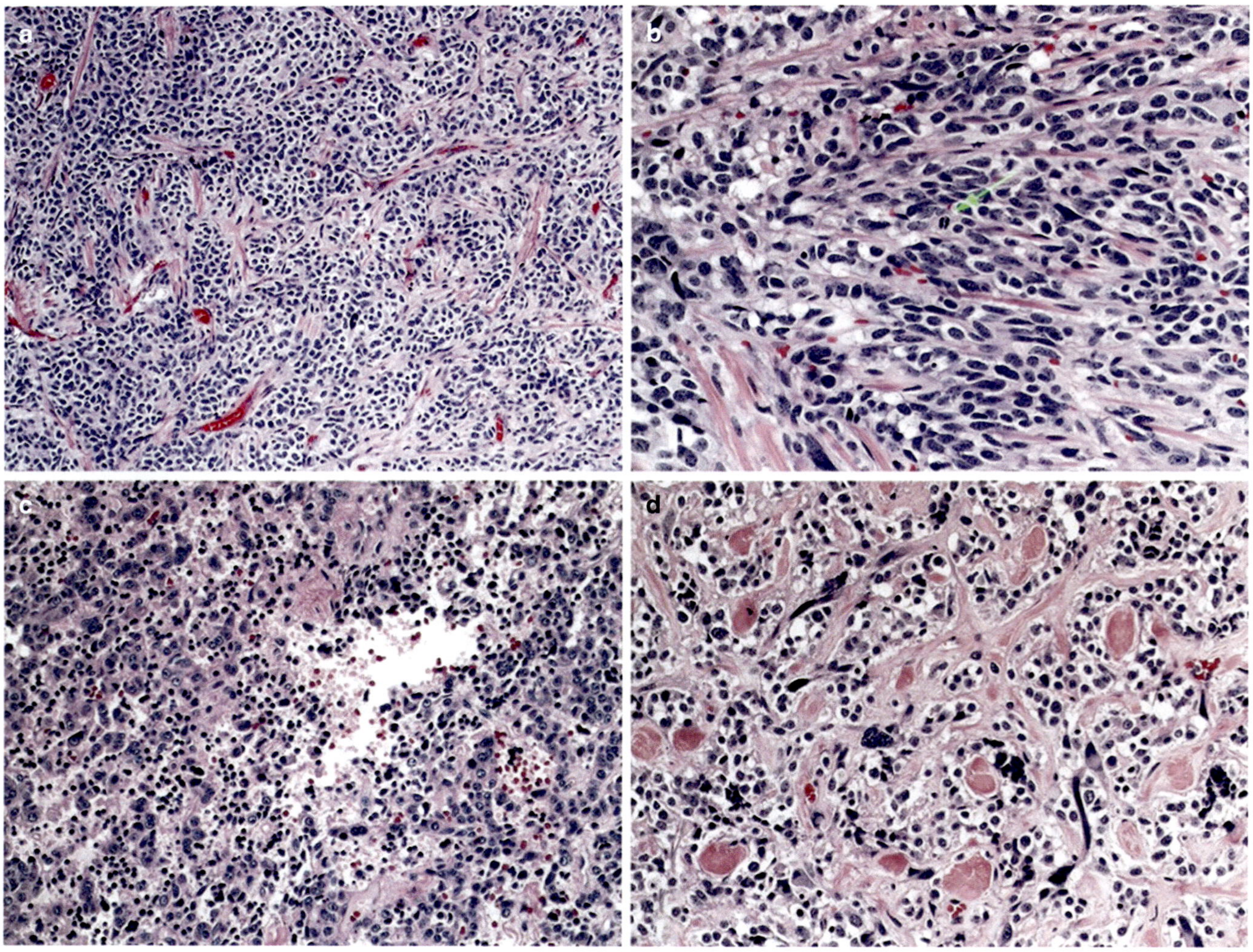

Fig. 14.3 Morphologic features of atypical carcinoid. The tumor has organoid and trabecular growth patterns with relative uniform cells (**a**). The tumor cells have moderate amount of eosinophilic cytoplasm and round-to-oval nuclei with finely granular chromatin and inconspicuous nucleoli. Mitotic rate is about four mitoses per 2 mm^2 (**b**). Focal necrosis (**c**) and nuclear atypia (**d**) are identified. H&E 100× magnification (**a**, **c**) and 200× magnification (**b**, **d**)

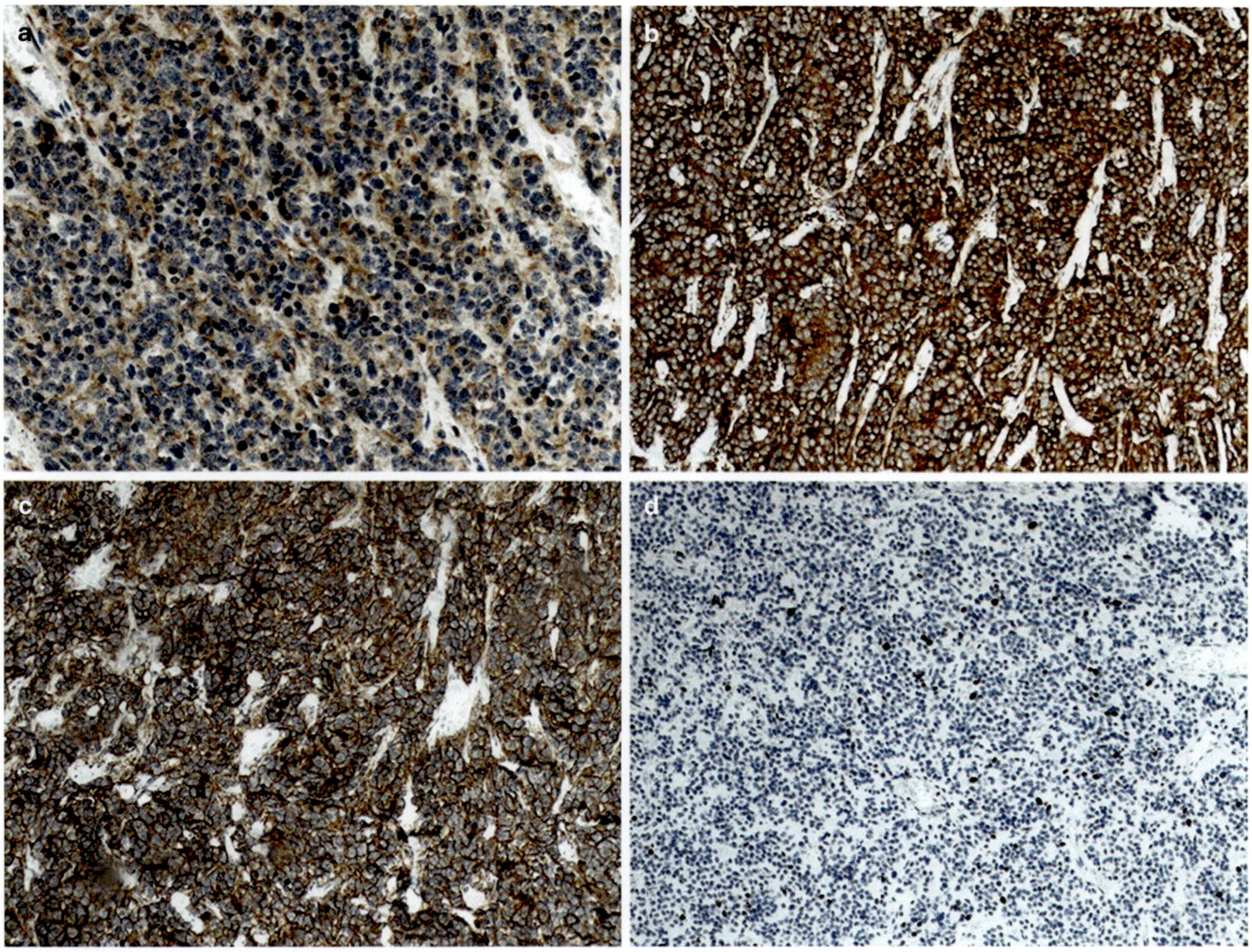

Fig. 14.4 Immunohistochemical profile of atypical carcinoid tumor. The tumor cells are positive for chromogranin (**a**), synaptophysin (**b**), and CD56 (**c**) with a Ki-67 proliferation index focally up to 5% (**d**). IHC 100× magnification (**a–d**)

Final Pathologic Diagnosis: Atypical Carcinoid

What Is the Definition of Atypical Carcinoid?

Atypical carcinoid tumor (AC) is an intermediate-grade neuroendocrine tumor with characteristic neuroendocrine histologic features (organoid, trabecular, insular, palisading, ribbon, rosette-like arrangements). The tumor is composed of uniform cells with low-to-moderate amount of eosinophilic, finely granular cytoplasm. Nuclei are round to oval with salt-and-pepper chromatin and inconspicuous nucleoli. Focal cytological atypia may or may not be present. ACs have an increased mitotic rate (2–10 per 2 mm^2) and/or presence of necrosis [1]. Necrosis is usually punctate, although larger zones of necrosis may be seen. By definition, carcinoid tumors are more than 0.5 cm in size.

What Are the Clinical Features of Atypical Carcinoid?

Carcinoid tumors are uncommon, accounting for 0.5–5% of all lung cancers [2]. Typical carcinoids (TC) comprise about 90% of all pulmonary carcinoid tumors, while the remaining 10% are AC [2]. Patients with carcinoid tumors are usually in the fourth to sixth decade of life, with a younger age for TCs than ACs. Although carcinoid tumors are not usually associated with smoking or any known environmental factor, more AC patients are current or former smokers [3]. Up to half of carcinoid tumors are asymptomatic and found incidentally on imaging studies; however, symptoms may manifest when large airways become irritated or obstructed. These symptoms include coughing, wheezing, hemoptysis, atelectasis, and pneumonia [2]. Paraneoplastic syndromes are rare [4]. The majority of carcinoid tumors are sporadic, but approximately 5% of tumors arise in the setting of MEN1 syndrome [3, 5].

Complete surgical excision is the treatment of choice for carcinoid tumors. ACs have a worse prognosis than TCs with 5-year overall survival of around 60% [2, 6]. Approximately 57% and 21% of AC patients have lymph node metastases and distant metastases [4], and the lymph node metastasis is associated with a high likelihood of developing recurrent disease [7]. Stage is the most important prognostic factor in carcinoid tumors [8].

What Are the Radiographic Features of Atypical Carcinoid?

ACs and TCs share similar imaging features. At the time of diagnosis, about 41% of ACs are confined to the lung [9]. The carcinoid tumors can occur at the central or peripheral lung regions, and when centrally located, the tumors often demonstrate evidence of an endobronchial luminal component [10]. On imaging, carcinoid tumors are highly vascular, well-defined round-to-ovoid lesions with smooth or lobulated margins [10]. Associated calcification, atelectasis, or bronchiectasis can also be present.

What Are the Pathologic Features of Atypical Carcinoid?

Macroscopically, ACs are firm, well-demarcated masses with tan to yellow cut surfaces. Focal hemorrhage and necrosis may be present. When ACs are associated with bronchi, the tumors typically protrude into the bronchial lumen, and the overlying bronchial epithelium may be intact or ulcerated. Occasionally, patients might have multiple tumors or tumorlets surrounding a main lesion. Microscopically, carcinoid tumors may exhibit a variety of growth patterns; but organoid/nested and trabecular growths are the most common patterns. Other growth patterns include solid, pseudoglandular, spindle, rosette, papillary, and follicular [1, 11]. Carcinoid tumors often show fibrovascular stroma with a high vascularity. The associated stroma can also be hyalinized, calcified, or ossified [11, 12]. Tumor cells are uniform and polygonal with scant-to-moderate eosinophilic cytoplasm. Additional cytologic features include round-to-ovoid nuclei, finely stippled chromatin imparting a characteristic "salt-and-pepper" pattern, and inconspicuous nucleoli. In some instances, nuclear atypia and pleomorphism can be marked, and as such these features themselves should not be used to diagnose more aggressive tumors such as atypical carcinoid tumor [8]. By definition, ACs have an intermediate mitotic activity (2–10 mitoses per $2mm^2$) and/or focal necrosis [1]. The immunohistochemical profile of carcinoid tumors is characteristic, including strong staining for classic neuroendocrine markers such as chromogranin, synaptophysin, and CD56. Carcinoid tumors usually stain positive for cytokeratins, but up to 20% of tumors can be cytokeratin negative [11].

Is there a Precursor Lesion to Atypical Carcinoid?

There are preexisting neuroendocrine cells in the normal airway. Various stimuli such as infection, bronchiectasis, persistent high altitude, and various smoking-associated conditions can induce bronchiolar neuroendocrine cell hyperplasia (NEH). Frequently, NEH is present in the background of resected carcinoid tumor lung specimens [13]. Recently, diffuse idiopathic pulmonary neuroendocrine cell hyperplasia (DIPNECH) is recognized to be a precursor lesion for carcinoid tumors [1, 14].

What Are the Genetic and Molecular Alterations Seen in Atypical Carcinoid?

The most frequent gene alterations found in carcinoid tumors are *MEN1*, *PSIP1*, *ARID1A*, and *EIF1AX* [15]. TCs and also ACs demonstrate allelic imbalance in the 11q13 region of *MEN1* gene [16]. *MEN1* gene mutations and loss of expression are almost exclusively seen in carcinoid tumors and extremely rare in high-grade neuroendocrine carcinomas [17], whereas *TP53* and *RB1* mutations are extremely rare in carcinoid tumors but highly frequent in high-grade neuroendocrine carcinomas [15].

What Is the Differential Diagnosis for Atypical Carcinoid?

A definite diagnosis of AC is relied on through pathologic examination of a resected tumor. In small biopsy specimens, other neuroendocrine tumors (TC, SCLC, and LCNEC) should be included in the differential. The wide variety of growth patterns can resemble adenocarcinoma, mucoepidermoid carcinoma, adenoid cystic carcinoma, and metastatic tumors such as metastatic neuroendocrine tumor of gastrointestinal origin.

What Are the Pathologic Features to Differentiate Large-Cell Neuroendocrine Carcinomas from Atypical Carcinoid?

LCNEC is an undifferentiated, non-small-cell carcinoma that shows neuroendocrine morphology and neuroendocrine differentiation confirmed by immunohistochemistry with positivity of at least one neuroendocrine maker and/or by electron microscopy [1]. Grossly, they are lobulated with relatively smooth edges and yellow-tan to red on cut section with areas of necrosis. Microscopically, LCNECs have organoid nesting, trabecular growth, peripheral palisading, and rosette-like growth patterns (Fig. 14.5). The tumor cells are large and polygonal with ample pink cytoplasm, thus having lower nuclear-to-cytoplasmic ratios. The tumor cells have irregular nuclear contour and coarse chromatin with prominent nucleoli. There are large areas of necrosis and a very high mitotic count (typically more than 10 mitoses per 2 mm^2 with an average of 75 mitoses per 2 mm^2) [1]. LCNECs stain for at least one neuroendocrine marker (chromogranin, synaptophysin, or CD56), and around 50% of LCNECs express TTF-1 and have a high Ki-67 proliferation index, ranging 50–100% (Fig. 14.6) [11]. Rarely, a tumor a mitotic rate of greater than ten mitoses per 2 mm^2 can show a carcinoid-like morphology, which should be classified as LCNEC according to the current WHO guidelines [1]. However, the carcinoid tumors with an increased mitotic rate have been recently documented [18, 19].

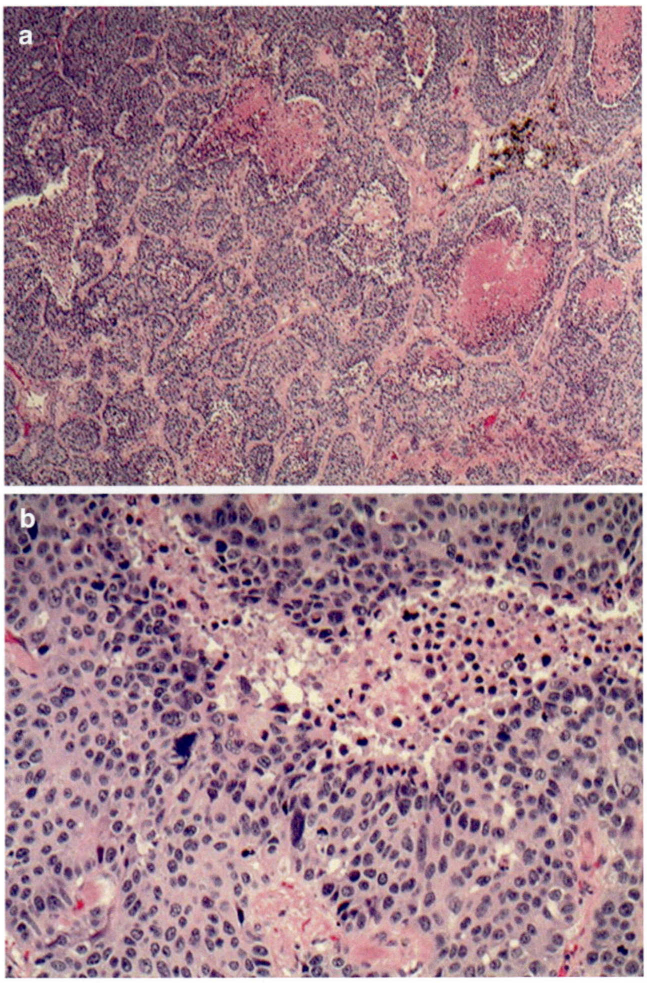

Fig. 14.5 Morphologic features of large-cell neuroendocrine carcinoma. The tumor cells are arranged in organoid nesting growth pattern, and there are large areas of necrosis (**a**). The tumor cells are large and polygonal with eosinophilic cytoplasm (**b**). The nuclei have irregular nuclear contour and coarse chromatin with prominent nucleoli. A high mitotic rate is noted. H&E 40× magnification (**a**) and 200× magnification (**b**)

At the genetic and molecular levels, LCNECs are distinct from ACs and more closely related to small-cell carcinomas of the lung (SCLCs) or other non-small-cell lung carcinomas (NSCLCs). Like SCLCs, LCNECs may have *P53* and *RB* mutations [1]. Higher occurrences of *MYCL*, *SOX2*, and *FGFR1* amplifications have also been reported, as well as *PTEN* mutation or loss [17, 20, 21]. Abnormal expression or loss of heterozygosity (LOH) for 3p, 5q, 11q, 13q, and 5p gain is common in both LCNEC and SCLC [22]. Interestingly, a distinct second set of LCNECs has no *RB1* or *TP53* alterations, instead harboring mutations of *STK11*, *KRAS*, or *KEAP1* mutations, similar to NSCLCs [20, 21].

How Does Large-Cell Neuroendocrine Carcinoma Differ Clinically from Atypical Carcinoid?

LCNECs comprise approximately 2–3% of lung carcinomas, and the vast majority of afflicted patients are smokers [23]. There is male predominance, and the average age of occurrence is between ages 60 and 70 [24, 25]. Patients typically present with cough, chest pain, dyspnea, or weight loss; however, since LCNECs are often peripheral tumors, patients can be asymptomatic with LCNECs found only incidentally on imaging study. Radiologically, LCNECs appear as nodules or masses with irregular borders, averaging 3.0–4.0 cm in size [26, 27]. At the time of diagnosis, 40% of patients have distant metastasis, and 60–80% have lymph node metastasis [28]. The prognosis of LCNEC is worse with 5-year overall survival rate of <50% [25]. The optimal treatment for LCNECs has not been established, but for early-stage disease, surgery is preferred with patients typically receiving multimodality therapies including adjuvant chemotherapy [29].

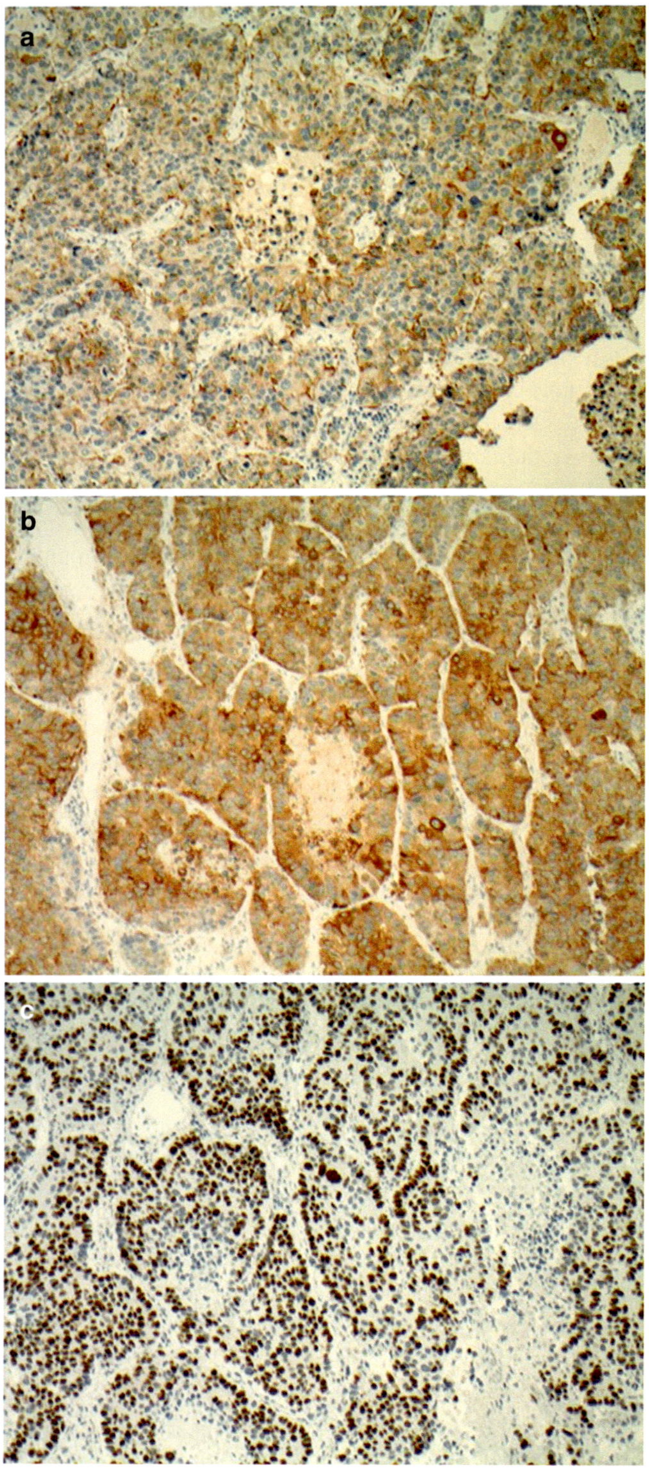

Fig. 14.6 Immunohistochemical profile of large-cell neuroendocrine carcinoma. The tumor cells are positive for chromogranin (**a**) and synaptophysin (**b**) with a high Ki-67 proliferation index (>50%) (**c**). IHC 100× magnification (**a**–**c**)

References

1. Travis WD, Brambilla E, Burke AP, Marx A, Nicholson AG. WHO classification of tumors of the lung, pleura, thymus, and heart. Geneva, Switzerland: IARC Press; 2015.
2. Herde RF, Kokeny KE, Reddy CB, Akerley WL, Hu N, Boltax JP, et al. Primary pulmonary carcinoid tumor: a long-term single institution experience. Am J Clin Oncol. 2018;41(1):24–9.
3. Caplin ME, Baudin E, Ferolla P, Filosso P, Garcia-Yuste M, Lim E, et al. Pulmonary neuroendocrine (carcinoid) tumors: European neuroendocrine tumor society expert consensus and recommendations for best practice for typical and atypical pulmonary carcinoids. Ann Oncol. 2015;26(8):1604–20.
4. Fink G, Krelbaum T, Yellin A, Bendayan D, Saute M, Glazer M, et al. Pulmonary carcinoid: presentation, diagnosis, and outcome in 142 cases in Israel and review of 640 cases from the literature. Chest. 2001;119(6):1647–51.
5. Sachithanandan N, Harle RA, Burgess JR. Bronchopulmonary carcinoid in multiple endocrine neoplasia type 1. Cancer. 2005;103(3):509–15.
6. Ha SY, Lee JJ, Cho J, Hyeon J, Han J, Kim HK. Lung parenchymal invasion in pulmonary carcinoid tumor: an important histologic feature suggesting the diagnosis of atypical carcinoid and poor prognosis. Lung Cancer. 2013;80(2):146–52.
7. Thomas CF Jr, Tazelaar HD, Jett JR. Typical and atypical pulmonary carcinoids : outcome in patients presenting with regional lymph node involvement. Chest. 2001;119(4):1143–50.
8. Travis WD, Rush W, Flieder DB, Falk R, Fleming MV, Gal AA, et al. Survival analysis of 200 pulmonary neuroendocrine tumors with clarification of criteria for atypical carcinoid and its separation from typical carcinoid. Am J Surg Pathol. 1998;22(8):934–44.
9. Skuladottir H, Hirsch FR, Hansen HH, Olsen JH. Pulmonary neuroendocrine tumors: incidence and prognosis of histological subtypes. A population-based study in Denmark. Lung Cancer. 2002;37(2):127–35.
10. Rosado de Christenson ML, Abbott GF, Kirejczyk WM, Galvin JR, Travis WD. Thoracic carcinoids: radiologic-pathologic correlation. Radiographics. 1999;19(3):707–36.
11. Travis WD. Pathology and diagnosis of neuroendocrine tumors: lung neuroendocrine. Thorac Surg Clin. 2014;24(3):257–66.
12. Borczuk AC. Neuroendocrine neoplasms of the lung. In: Kennedy JF, editor. Practical pulmonary pathology a diagnostic approach. 3rd ed. Philadelphia, PA: Elsevier; 2018. p. 439–66.
13. Miller RR, Muller NL. Neuroendocrine cell hyperplasia and obliterative bronchiolitis in patients with peripheral carcinoid tumors. Am J Surg Pathol. 1995;19(6):653–8.
14. Aguayo SM, Miller YE, Waldron JA Jr, Bogin RM, Sunday ME, Staton GW Jr, et al. Brief report: idiopathic diffuse hyperplasia of pulmonary neuroendocrine cells and airways disease. N Engl J Med. 1992;327(18):1285–8.
15. Fernandez-Cuesta L, Peifer M, Lu X, Sun R, Ozretic L, Seidal D, et al. Frequent mutations in chromatin-remodelling genes in pulmonary carcinoids. Nat Commun. 2014;5:3518.
16. Debelenko LV, Brambilla E, Agarwal SK, Swalwell JI, Kester MB, Lubensky IA, et al. Identification of MEN1 gene mutations in sporadic carcinoid tumors of the lung. Hum Mol Genet. 1997;6(13):2285–90.
17. Rossi G, Bertero L, Marchio C, Papotti M. Molecular alterations of neuroendocrine tumours of the lung. Histopathology. 2018;72(1):142–52.

18. Onuki N, Wistuba II, Travis WD, Virmani AK, Yashima K, Brambilla E, et al. Genetic changes in the spectrum of neuroendocrine lung tumors. Cancer. 1999;85(3):600–7.
19. Quinn AM, Chaturvedi A, Nonaka D. High-grade neuroendocrine carcinoma of the lung with carcinoid morphology: a study of 12 cases. Am J Surg Pathol. 2017;41(2):263–70.
20. Rekhtman N, Desmeules P, Litvak AM, Pietanza MC, Santos-Zabala ML, Ni A, et al. Stage IV lung carcinoids: spectrum and evolution of proliferation rate, focusing on variants with elevated proliferation indices. Mod Pathol. 2019;32(8):1106–22.
21. Rekhtman N, Pietanza MC, Hellmann MD, Naidoo J, Arora A, Won H, et al. Next-generation sequencing of pulmonary large cell neuroendocrine carcinoma reveals small cell carcinoma-like and non-small cell carcinoma-like subsets. Clin Cancer Res. 2016;22(14):3618–29.
22. Takeuchi T, Minami Y, Iijima T, Kameya T, Asamura H, Noguchi M. Characteristics of loss of heterozygosity in large cell neuroendocrine carcinomas of the lung and small cell lung carcinomas. Pathol Int. 2006;56(8):434–9.
23. Paci M, Cavazza A, Annessi V, Putrino I, Ferrari G, De Franco S, et al. Large cell neuroendocrine carcinoma of the lung: a 10-year clinicopathologic retrospective study. Ann Thorac Surg. 2004;77(4):1163–7.
24. Takei H, Asamura H, Maeshima A, Suzuki K, Kondo H, Niki T, et al. Large cell neuroendocrine carcinoma of the lung: a clinicopathologic study of eighty-seven cases. J Thorac Cardiovasc Surg. 2002;124(2):285–92.
25. Veronesi G, Morandi U, Alloisio M, Terzi A, Cardillo G, Filosso P, et al. Large cell neuroendocrine carcinoma of the lung: a retrospective analysis of 144 surgical cases. Lung Cancer. 2006;53(1):111–5.
26. Jung KJ, Lee KS, Han J, Kwon OJ, Kim J, Shim YM, et al. Large cell neuroendocrine carcinoma of the lung: clinical, CT, and pathologic findings in 11 patients. J Thorac Imaging. 2001;16(3):156–62.
27. Iyoda A, Hiroshima K, Toyozaki T, Haga Y, Fujisawa T, Ohwada H. Clinical characterization of pulmonary large cell neuroendocrine carcinoma and large cell carcinoma with neuroendocrine morphology. Cancer. 2001;91(11):1992–2000.
28. Gridelli C, Rossi A, Airoma G, Bianco R, Costanzo R, Daniele B, et al. Treatment of pulmonary neuroendocrine tumours: state of the art and future developments. Cancer Treat Rev. 2013;39(5):466–72.
29. Iyoda A, Makino T, Koezuka S, Otsuka H, Hata Y. Treatment options for patients with large cell neuroendocrine carcinoma of the lung. Gen Thorac Cardiovasc Surg. 2014;62(6):351–6.

Small-Cell Carcinoma Versus Atypical Carcinoid Tumor

15

Esther C. Yoon, Xuchen Zhang, and Guoping Cai

Case Presentation

A 57-year-old male with a history of smoking (45 pack-years until the last 5 months) presented to an outpatient clinic with a chief complaint of persistent cough for two and half months. In the preceding days, he reported a small amount of hemoptysis. He worked in an industrial environment and reported exposure to various chemicals, heavy metals, and asbestos throughout his adult life. Computed tomography (CT) revealed a 2.5 cm mass in the left suprahilar region with suspicion for an endobronchial involvement (Fig. 15.1). There was no evidence of pleural effusion. The patient eventually underwent a left upper lobectomy.

Gross examination of lobectomy specimen showed that the pleura is glistening and tan-pink with minimal anthracosis and no areas of puckering. On sectioning, a 2.5 cm tan-white to white-gray well-circumscribed mass was identified. The mass was medially abutting but not grossly invading the bronchi and vasculature. The remaining parenchyma was pink-red, spongy, and unremarkable. There were multiple palpable peribronchial lymph nodes.

Microscopically, the tumor cells are arranged haphazardly in sheets without a discernible architectural pattern and vaguely separated by thin fibrous septa (Fig. 15.2). The neoplastic cells are small with scant cytoplasm and a high nuclear-to-cytoplasmic ratio. The tumor nuclei have "salt-and-pepper" chromatin with no distinct nucleoli. Nuclear molding and extensive necrosis are seen. Immunohistochemically, the tumor cells are positive for insulinoma-associated protein 1 (INSM1) (Fig. 15.3a), chromogranin, synaptophysin (Fig. 15.3b), and CD56 (Fig. 15.3c) while negative for TTF1 and napsin A. The tumor has a Ki-67 index up to 70% (Fig. 15.3d).

E. C. Yoon
Department of Pathology, The University of Texas MD Anderson Cancer Center, Houston, TX, USA

X. Zhang · G. Cai (✉)
Department of Pathology, Yale University School of Medicine, New Haven, CT, USA
e-mail: guoping.cai@yale.edu

H. Xu et al. (eds.), *Practical Lung Pathology*, Practical Anatomic Pathology, https://doi.org/10.1007/978-3-031-14402-8_15

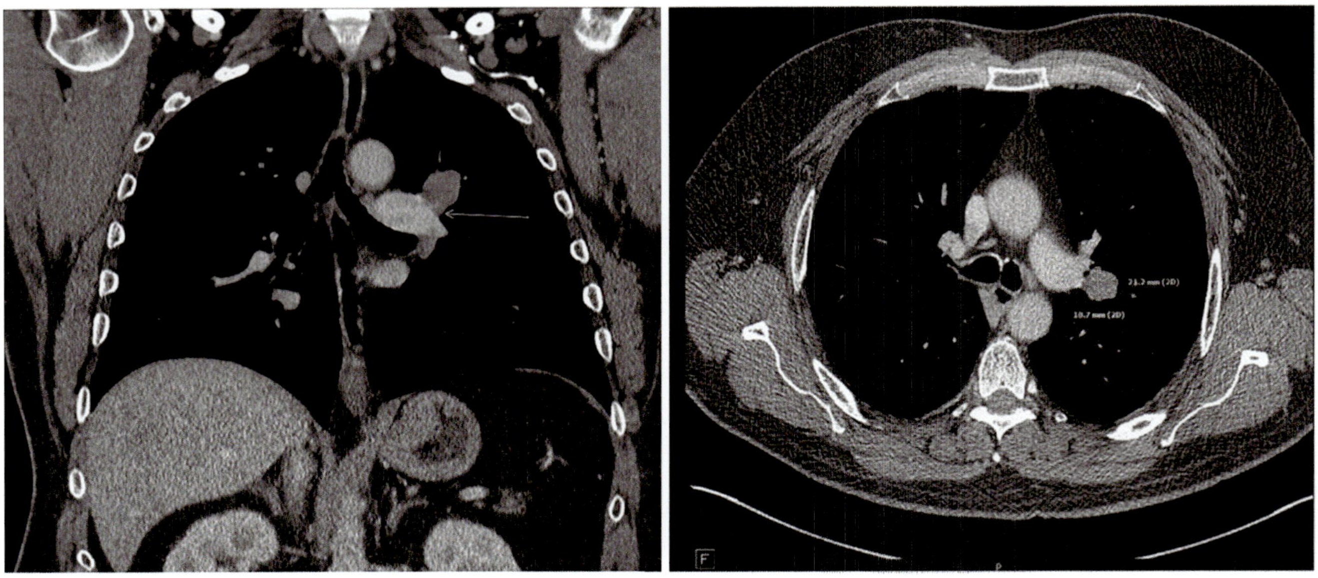

Fig. 15.1 CT scan image of small-cell carcinoma. A well-circumscribed mass is shown in the left suprahilar region with suspicion for endobronchial involvement

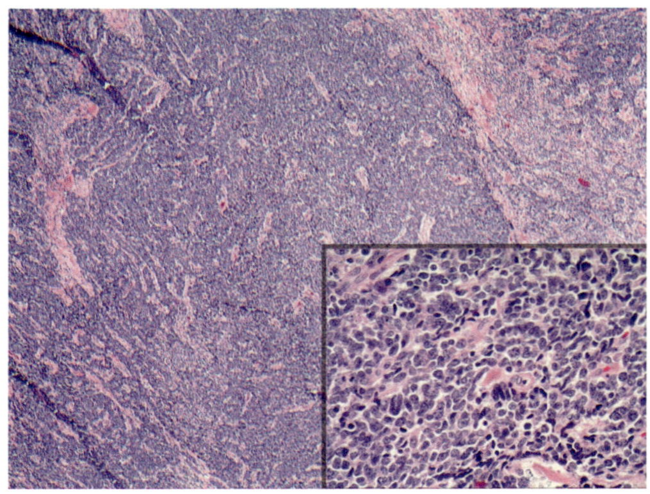

Fig. 15.2 Morphologic features of small-cell carcinoma. The tumor is composed of sheets of small cells with scant cytoplasm, high nuclear-to-cytoplasmic ratio, and speckled chromatin. Mitosis is frequently seen. H&E: 40× magnification with insert 400× magnification

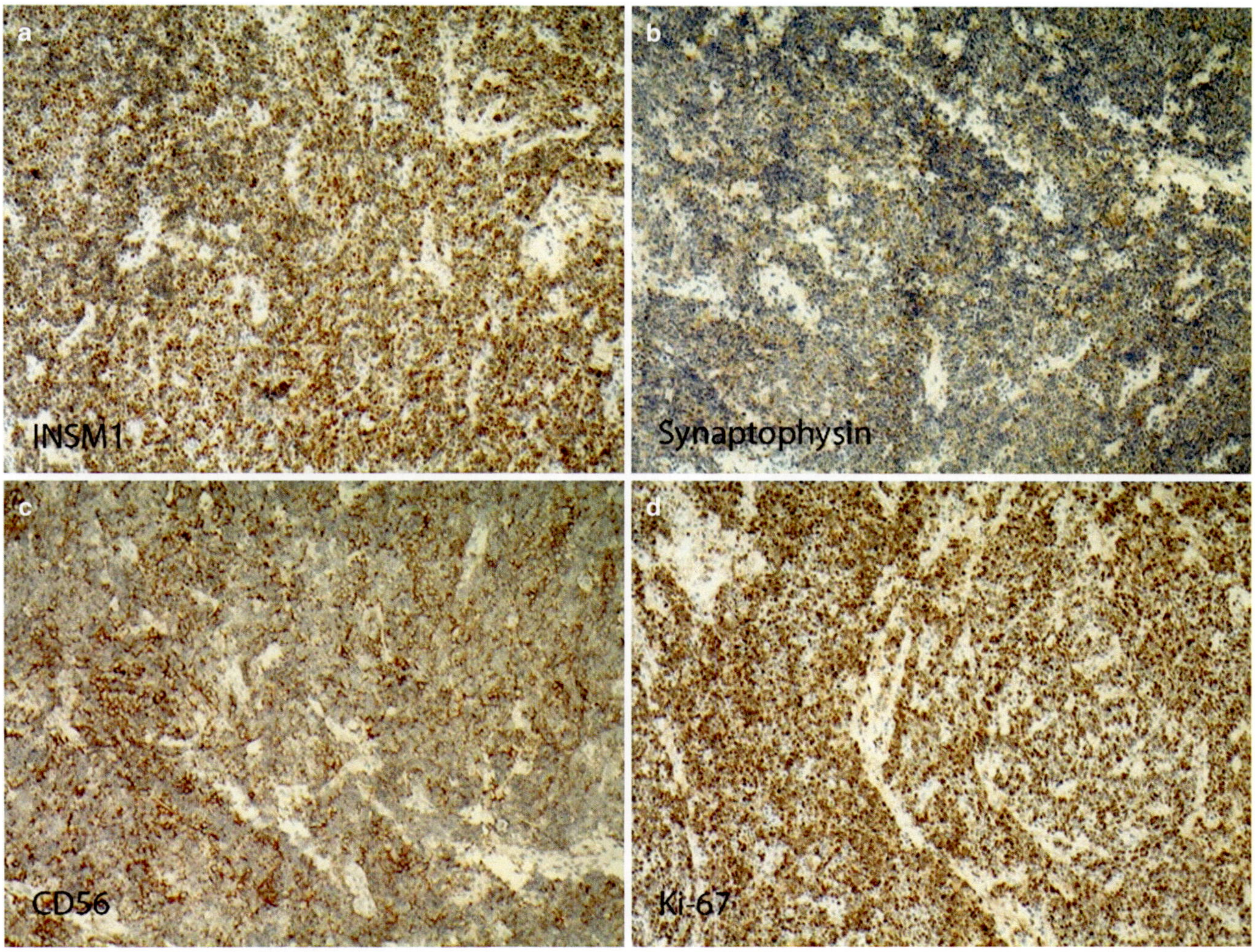

Fig. 15.3 Immunohistochemical profile of small-cell carcinoma. The tumor cells are positive for INSM1 (**a**), synaptophysin (**b**), and CD56 (**c**) with a Ki-67 index close to 70% (**d**). IHC: **a**–**d**, 100× magnification

Pathologic Diagnosis: Small-Cell Carcinoma of the Lung (SCLC)

What Is the Definition of SCLC of the Lung?

Small-cell carcinoma of the lung (SCLC) is an aggressive, high-grade malignant epithelial tumor with characteristic histomorphologic features, including scant cytoplasm, finely granular nuclear chromatin, and absent/inconspicuous nucleoli. Nuclear molding is prominent, and tumors invariably have extensive necrosis with high mitotic counts.

What Are the Clinical and Prognostic Features of SCLC?

SCLC is the most common type of pulmonary neuroendocrine tumor [1], comprising about 15% of all lung cancers [2, 3]. SCLC usually occurs in patients of 63–70 years of age [4, 5] and has a strong association with smoking. Most patients are diagnosed at advanced stage with only 14% of SCLCs being confined to the lung at the time of diagnosis [5]. SCLC is a high-grade malignancy with 5- and 10-year survival rates of only 2–5% and 1–2%, respectively [2, 5, 6]. The median survival is 16–22 months for limited disease and 8–13 months for advanced-stage disease [7, 8]. The recommended treatment for SCLC is chemotherapy, chemoradiation, or chemotherapy followed by radiation [9].

What Are the Typical Symptoms of Patients with SCLC?

Patients can present with symptoms related to central and mediastinal tumor mass effect, including chest pain, hemoptysis, and hoarseness. Those with advanced disease may also have constitutional symptoms such as malaise, anorexia, and weight loss. Up to 3–5% of SCLC patients can present with paraneoplastic syndromes, such as syndrome of inappropriate antidiuretic hormone secretion, Lambert-Eaton myasthenic syndrome, sensory neuropathy, limbic encephalitis, and cancer-associated retinopathy [10–12].

What Are the Radiographic Features of SCLC?

Most of SCLCs are located centrally and typically manifest as a mediastinal or hilar mass with associated lymphadenopathy, which may displace or narrow the tracheobronchial tree and/or major vessels [13, 14]. Other findings include atelectasis, noncontiguous parenchymal mass, and pleural effusion. Only 5–10% of SCLCs manifest as peripheral nodule without associated lymphadenopathy [15, 16].

What Are the Pathologic Features of SCLC?

Grossly, SCLCs are bulky tumors with tan-white cut surface and extensive necrosis. The tumor cells are typically small (<3 times the diameter of mature lymphocytes) with scant cytoplasm (high nuclear-to-cytoplasmic ratio), round-to-fusiform-shaped nuclei, speckled "salt-and-pepper" pattern chromatin, and absent or inconspicuous nucleoli [17]. Nuclear molding is frequent, and cellular fragility can cause "crush artifact" where nuclear chromatin streaks, particularly in small biopsies. The tumor cells can sometimes be large with more cytoplasm and show scattered pleomorphic giant tumor cells; however, these should not represent more than 10% of neoplastic cells [18]. SCLCs have large areas of geographic necrosis and a high mitotic rate (average 60–80 mitoses per 2 mm^2) [17]. The tumor cells are often arranged in sheets without the typical architectural patterns seen in other neuroendocrine tumors; however, various classic growth patterns such as nested/organoid, peripheral palisading, trabecular, and rosettes have been described [17, 18].

Immunohistochemistry may not be necessary, since the characteristic morphologic features can be sufficient for diagnosis on good-quality H&E sections. However, SCLCs express at least one of the several neuroendocrine markers (chromogranin, synaptophysin, and N-CAM (CD56)) [18]. A recently described neuroendocrine marker, INSM1, has been shown to have a high sensitivity and specificity for diagnosis of lung neuroendocrine neoplasms [19, 20]. Since it is a nuclear stain, INSM1 may be particularly helpful in tumors with severe crush artifact. Up to 90% of SCLCs are also positive for TTF-1 [21, 22]. Cytokeratin stains are weak with a perinuclear dot-like staining pattern [23]. The proliferation index by Ki-67 (MIB-1) is high, usually ranging from 80 to 100% of tumor nuclei [24]. High Ki-67 index can efficiently separate low and intermediate neuroendocrine carcinomas from high-grade neuroendocrine carcinomas, even in the presence of well-differentiated morphology [25].

What Are the Genetic and Molecular Alterations Seen in SCLC?

More than 90% of SCLCs have mutations or deletions in *TP53* and *RB1* [26–28]. Other genetic alterations are inactivating mutations of genes in the *NOTCH* family [28] and multiple deletions in chromosomes 3p, 4q, 5q, 10q, 13q, and 17p, as well as gains in 3q and 5p [26]. Amplification of *MYC* [29] and methylation of caspase-8 [30], key anti-apoptotic genes, are reportedly characteristic of SCLCs. Mutations in *EGFR* and translocation in the *ALK* are not typical features of SCLCs [31].

What Is the Differential Diagnosis of SCLC?

The differential diagnosis includes other neuroendocrine tumors, particularly atypical carcinoid tumor (ACs), lymphoma, and other "small round blue cell tumors" (SRBCT).

How Does One Differentiate SCLC from Atypical Carcinoid (AC)?

Atypical carcinoids (ACs) are intermediate-grade neuroendocrine tumors characterized by classic "neuroendocrine" growth patterns. Grossly, ACs are firm, highly vascularized, and well-demarcated masses with tan cut surfaces and occasional hemorrhage [17, 31]. The tumor cells are classically uniform and polygonal, with scant-to-moderate eosinophilic cytoplasm, round-to-oval nuclei with salt-and-pepper chromatin, and inconspicuous nucleoli (Fig. 15.4). Necrosis is usually focal, and mitotic rate ranges from 2 to 10 per 2 mm^2 [17]. A variety of growth patterns can occur in ACs, but organoid and trabecular growth patterns are most frequently seen [17]. In ACs, the tumor cells have fair amount of cytoplasm, necrosis is focal, and Ki-67 index is less than 20%.

Similar to SCLC, ACs also express neuroendocrine markers (chromogranin, synaptophysin, CD56) (Fig. 15.5) and INSM1 [20]. TTF-1 expression is variable, and cytokeratin stains are usually positive; however, up to 20% of the tumor cells can lack keratin expression [24]. The Ki-67 proliferation index is low to moderate (5–20%) [32]. 50–70% of ACs

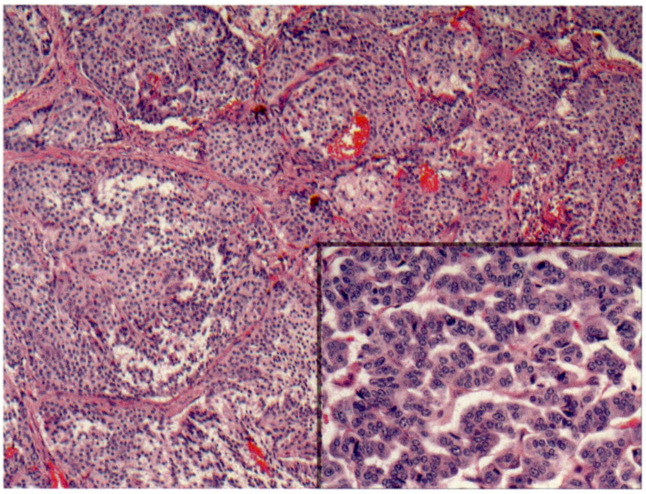

Fig. 15.4 Morphologic features of atypical carcinoid (AC). AC of the lung is composed of uniform tumor cells with a moderate amount of eosinophilic cytoplasm, oval-to-round nuclei, and increased mitotic figures. H&E: 100× magnification with insert 400× magnification

have *MEN1* mutations and loss of 11q [17]. Other molecular alterations described include mutations in *PSIP1*, *ARID1A*, and *EIF1AX*. In contrast to SCLC, *TP53* and *RB1* gene mutations are rare in AC [27].

How Does AC Differ Clinically from SCLC?

ACs are much rarer and comprise less than 1% of all lung cancer cases. The patients are usually in their fifth to sixth decade of life [4]. Approximately 70–75% of ACs are centrally located and involve the major bronchi, and up to 90% of patients with a central tumor present with obstructive symptoms such as cough, dyspnea, hemoptysis, and post-obstructive pneumonia [33]. Peripherally located tumors tend to be asymptomatic and discovered incidentally. Paraneoplastic syndromes are rare but can include carcinoid syndrome, Cushing syndrome, and ectopic secretion of growth hormone-releasing hormone.

At the time of diagnosis, 40–50% of ACs have metastasized to the lymph nodes, and approximately 20% of ACs have distant metastasis [17]. The 5-year and 10-year overall survival ranges from 56 to 79% and 35 to 56%, respectively [34, 35]. Currently, surgical resection with nodal staging is recommended when feasible.

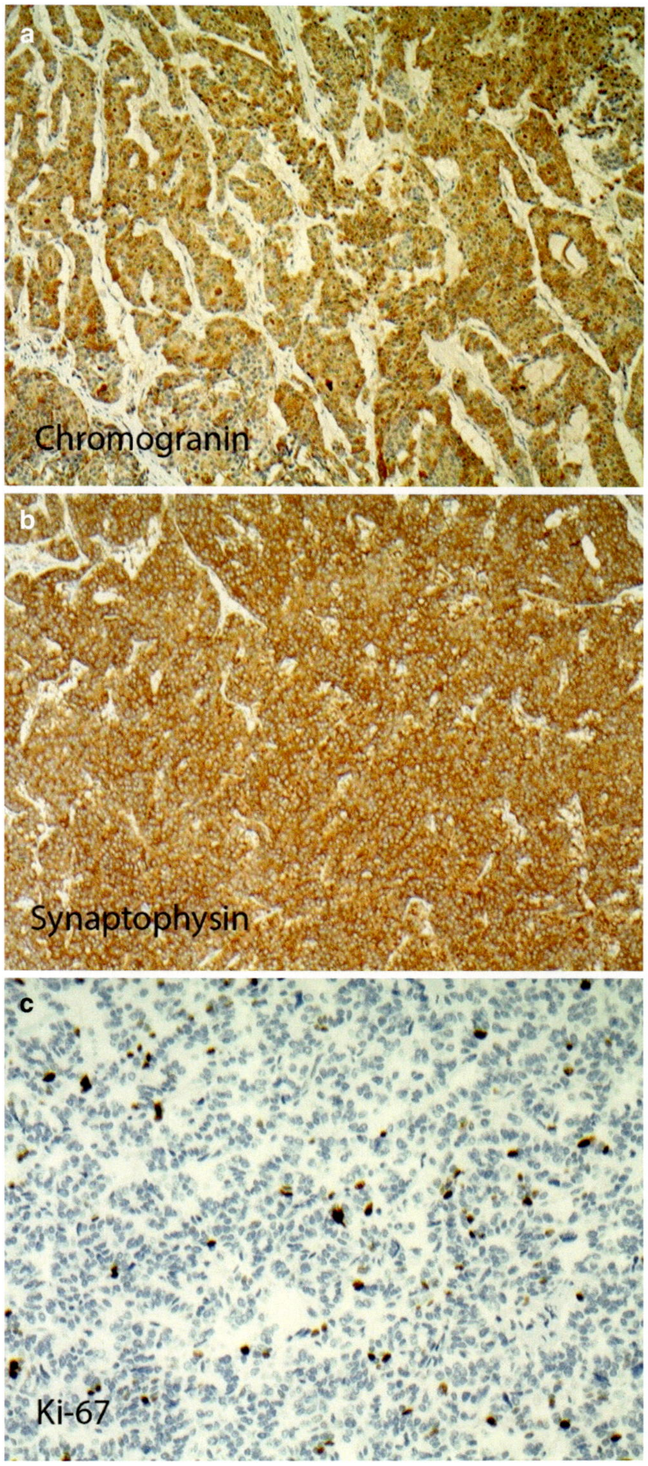

Fig. 15.5 Immunohistochemical profile of atypical carcinoid tumor. The tumor cells are positive for chromogranin (**a**) and synaptophysin (**b**). Ki-67 proliferation index is ~5% (**c**). IHC: **a**–**c**, 100× magnification

References

1. Siegel R, Ma J, Zou Z, Jemal A. Cancer statistics, 2014. CA Cancer J Clin. 2014;64(1):9–29.
2. Govindan R, Page N, Morgensztern D, Read W, Tierney R, Vlahiotis A, et al. Changing epidemiology of small-cell lung cancer in the United States over the last 30 years: analysis of the surveillance, epidemiologic, and end results database. J Clin Oncol. 2006;24(28):4539–44.
3. Travis WD. Update on small cell carcinoma and its differentiation from squamous cell carcinoma and other non-small cell carcinomas. Mod Pathol. 2012;25(Suppl 1):S18–30.
4. Litzky LA. Pulmonary neuroendocrine tumors. Surg Pathol Clin. 2010;3(1):27–59.
5. Skuladottir H, Hirsch FR, Hansen HH, Olsen JH. Pulmonary neuroendocrine tumors: incidence and prognosis of histological subtypes. A population-based study in Denmark. Lung Cancer. 2002;37(2):127–35.
6. Paci M, Cavazza A, Annessi V, Putrino I, Ferrari G, De Franco S, et al. Large cell neuroendocrine carcinoma of the lung: a 10-year clinicopathologic retrospective study. Ann Thorac Surg. 2004;77(4):1163–7.
7. Lally BE, Urbanic JJ, Blackstock AW, Miller AA, Perry MC. Small cell lung cancer: have we made any progress over the last 25 years? Oncologist. 2007;12(9):1096–104.
8. Simon GR, Turrisi A. American College of Chest P. management of small cell lung cancer: ACCP evidence-based clinical practice guidelines (2nd edition). Chest. 2007;132(3 Suppl):324S–39S.
9. De Ruysscher D, Pijls-Johannesma M, Vansteenkiste J, Kester A, Rutten I, Lambin P. Systematic review and meta-analysis of randomised, controlled trials of the timing of chest radiotherapy in patients with limited-stage, small-cell lung cancer. Ann Oncol. 2006;17(4):543–52.
10. Gandhi L, Johnson BE. Paraneoplastic syndromes associated with small cell lung cancer. J Natl Compr Cancer Netw. 2006;4(6):631–8.
11. Elrington GM, Murray NM, Spiro SG, Newsom-Davis J. Neurological paraneoplastic syndromes in patients with small cell lung cancer. A prospective survey of 150 patients. J Neurol Neurosurg Psychiatry. 1991;54(9):764–7.
12. Dalmau J, Rosenfeld MR. Paraneoplastic syndromes of the CNS. Lancet Neurol. 2008;7(4):327–40.
13. Rosado de Christenson ML, Abbott GF, Kirejczyk WM, Galvin JR, Travis WD. Thoracic carcinoids: radiologic-pathologic correlation. Radiographics. 1999;19(3):707–36.
14. Chong S, Lee KS, Chung MJ, Han J, Kwon OJ, Kim TS. Neuroendocrine tumors of the lung: clinical, pathologic, and imaging findings. Radiographics. 2006;26(1):41–57; discussion -8
15. Quoix E, Fraser R, Wolkove N, Finkelstein H, Kreisman H. Small cell lung cancer presenting as a solitary pulmonary nodule. Cancer. 1990;66(3):577–82.
16. Yabuuchi H, Murayama S, Sakai S, Hashiguchi N, Murakami J, Muranaka T, et al. Resected peripheral small cell carcinoma of the lung: computed tomographic-histologic correlation. J Thorac Imaging. 1999;14(2):105–8.
17. Travis WD, Brambilla E, Burke AP, Marx A, Nicholson AG. WHO classification of tumors of the lung, pleura, thymus, and heart. Geneva, Switzerland: IARC Press; 2015.
18. Nicholson SA, Beasley MB, Brambilla E, Hasleton PS, Colby TV, Sheppard MN, et al. Small cell lung carcinoma (SCLC): a clinicopathologic study of 100 cases with surgical specimens. Am J Surg Pathol. 2002;26(9):1184–97.
19. Fujino K, Motooka Y, Hassan WA, Ali Abdalla MO, Sato Y, Kudoh S, et al. Insulinoma-associated protein 1 is a crucial regulator of neuroendocrine differentiation in lung cancer. Am J Pathol. 2015;185(12):3164–77.
20. Mukhopadhyay S, Dermawan JK, Lanigan CP, Farver CF. Insulinoma-associated protein 1 (INSM1) is a sensitive and highly specific marker of neuroendocrine differentiation in primary lung neoplasms: an immunohistochemical study of 345 cases, including 292 whole-tissue sections. Mod Pathol. 2019;32(1):100–9.
21. Folpe AL, Gown AM, Lamps LW, Garcia R, Dail DH, Zarbo RJ, et al. Thyroid transcription factor-1: immunohistochemical evaluation in pulmonary neuroendocrine tumors. Mod Pathol. 1999;12(1):5–8.
22. Kaufmann O, Dietel M. Expression of thyroid transcription factor-1 in pulmonary and extrapulmonary small cell carcinomas and other neuroendocrine carcinomas of various primary sites. Histopathology. 2000;36(5):415–20.
23. Marchevsky AM, Wick MR. Diagnostic difficulties with the diagnosis of small cell carcinoma of the lung. Semin Diagn Pathol. 2015;32(6):480–8.
24. Pelosi G, Rodriguez J, Viale G, Rosai J. Typical and atypical pulmonary carcinoid tumor overdiagnosed as small-cell carcinoma on biopsy specimens: a major pitfall in the management of lung cancer patients. Am J Surg Pathol. 2005;29(2):179–87.
25. Rindi G, Klersy C, Inzani F, Fellegara G, Ampollini L, Ardizzoni A, et al. Grading the neuroendocrine tumors of the lung: an evidence-based proposal. Endocr Relat Cancer. 2014;21(1):1–16.
26. Swarts DR, Ramaekers FC, Speel EJ. Molecular and cellular biology of neuroendocrine lung tumors: evidence for separate biological entities. Biochim Biophys Acta. 2012;1826(2):255–71.
27. Rossi G, Bertero L, Marchio C, Papotti M. Molecular alterations of neuroendocrine tumours of the lung. Histopathology. 2018;72(1):142–52.
28. George J, Lim JS, Jang SJ, Cun Y, Ozretic L, Kong G, et al. Comprehensive genomic profiles of small cell lung cancer. Nature. 2015;524(7563):47–53.
29. Johnson BE, Russell E, Simmons AM, Phelps R, Steinberg SM, Ihde DC, et al. MYC family DNA amplification in 126 tumor cell lines from patients with small cell lung cancer. J Cell Biochem Suppl. 1996;24:210–7.
30. Shivapurkar N, Toyooka S, Eby MT, Huang CX, Sathyanarayana UG, Cunningham HT, et al. Differential inactivation of caspase-8 in lung cancers. Cancer Biol Ther. 2002;1(1):65–9.
31. Borczuk AC. Neuroendocrine neoplasms of the lung. In: Kennedy JF, editor. Practical pulmonary pathology a diagnostic approach. 3rd ed. Philadelphia, PA: Elsevier; 2018. p. 439–66.
32. Travis WD. Pathology and diagnosis of neuroendocrine tumors: lung neuroendocrine. Thorac Surg Clin. 2014;24(3):257–66.
33. Wolin EM. Challenges in the diagnosis and Management of Well-Differentiated Neuroendocrine Tumors of the lung (typical and atypical carcinoid): current status and future considerations. Oncologist. 2015;20(10):1123–31.
34. Fink G, Krelbaum T, Yellin A, Bendayan D, Saute M, Glazer M, et al. Pulmonary carcinoid: presentation, diagnosis, and outcome in 142 cases in Israel and review of 640 cases from the literature. Chest. 2001;119(6):1647–51.
35. Travis WD, Rush W, Flieder DB, Falk R, Fleming MV, Gal AA, et al. Survival analysis of 200 pulmonary neuroendocrine tumors with clarification of criteria for atypical carcinoid and its separation from typical carcinoid. Am J Surg Pathol. 1998;22(8):934–44.

Typical Versus Atypical Carcinoid and Diffuse Idiopathic Neuroendocrine Cell Hyperplasia Versus Carcinoid Tumorlets

16

Ryan J. Morse and Haodong Xu

Case Presentation

A 63-year-old woman presented to the emergency room with a few months of weight loss and progressive hoarseness, with new-onset dyspnea and cough. Over the past few days, she had noted chills, rigors, and fever. A chest computed tomography (CT) showed a 2.8 cm mass adjacent to the left upper lobe mainstem bronchus, with impingement of the airway and atelectasis distally (Fig. 16.1).

Bronchoscopy performed at an outside hospital showed a speckled pink-white endobronchial mass which almost completely occluded the bronchial lumen. A biopsy demonstrated oval-shaped to spindled cells with occasional large, pleomorphic nuclei (Fig. 16.2). Immunohistochemistry showed that the neoplastic cells were negative for TTF-1 and p40. A diagnosis of non-small-cell carcinoma was rendered. The patient was referred to our institution for resection; on review of the biopsy slides, carcinoid tumor was suspected. Additional immunohistochemical stains were then performed which showed that the neoplastic cells were diffusely positive for Cam5.2, synaptophysin, and chromogranin with Ki-67 reactivity in 1% of the tumor cells (Fig. 16.3). These findings support the diagnosis of carcinoid tumor.

After the revised diagnosis, the patient underwent a lobectomy of the left upper lobe. Gross examination identified a circumscribed, tan-pink mass with focal hemorrhage arising from the mainstem bronchus wall with protrusion into the bronchial lumen. There was consolidation distal to the mass, consistent with recurrent post-obstructive pneumonia (Fig. 16.4). Histologic examination was again notable for organoid nests of oval-shaped to spindled cells with occasional pleomorphic nuclei (Fig. 16.5). No mitotic figures or necrosis was identified.

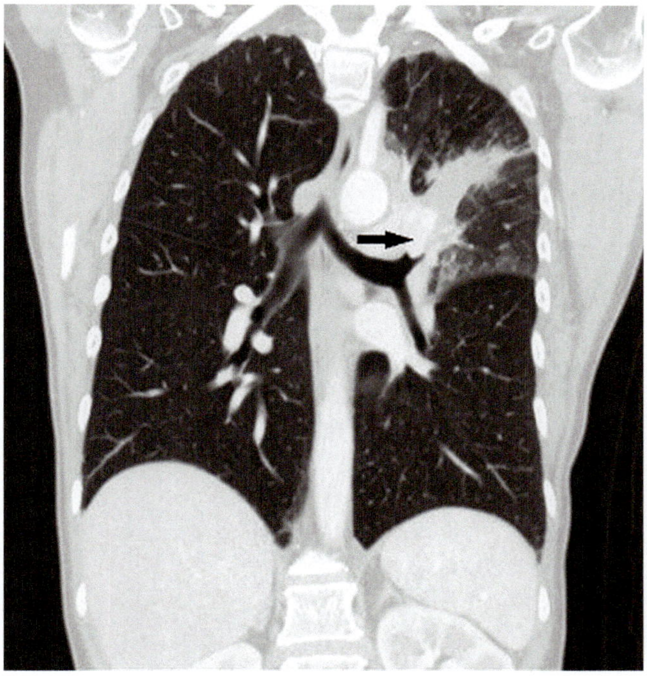

Fig. 16.1 Features of carcinoid tumor in the coronal CT. Coronal CT shows a mass (*arrow*) intimately associated with bronchus, post-obstructive atelectasis, and pneumonia distal to the mass

R. J. Morse · H. Xu (✉)
Department of Laboratory Medicine and Pathology, University of Washington Medical Center, Seattle, WA, USA
e-mail: xuh8@uw.edu

H. Xu et al. (eds.), *Practical Lung Pathology*, Practical Anatomic Pathology, https://doi.org/10.1007/978-3-031-14402-8_16

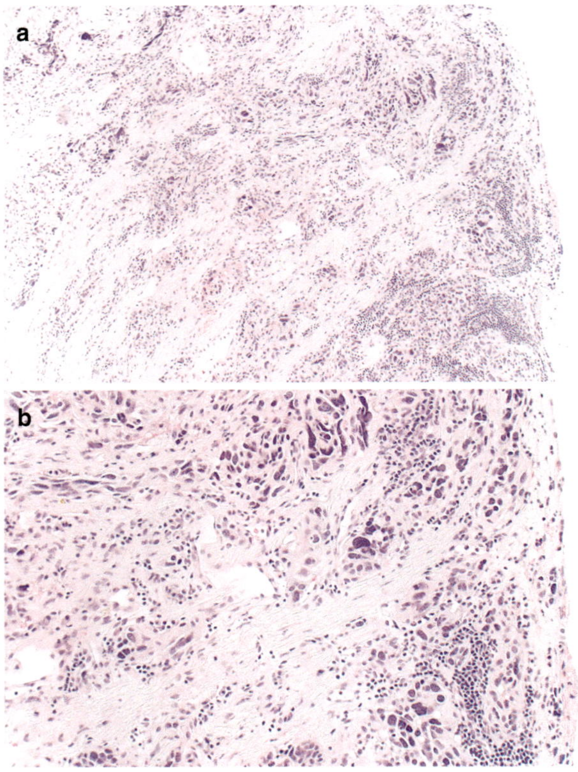

Fig. 16.2 Histologic sections of the endobronchial biopsy demonstrated the oval-shaped to spindled cells with occasional large, pleomorphic nuclei (**a**, H&E: 100× and **b**, H&E: 200×)

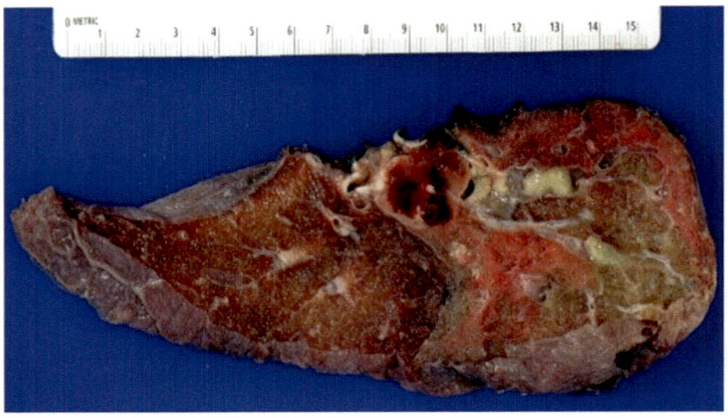

Fig. 16.4 Gross pathologic appearance of a carcinoid tumor. The mass protruded into the bronchial lumen with infiltration into the wall. There are mucus plugs in the distal bronchus; the areas of the lung parenchyma show congestion

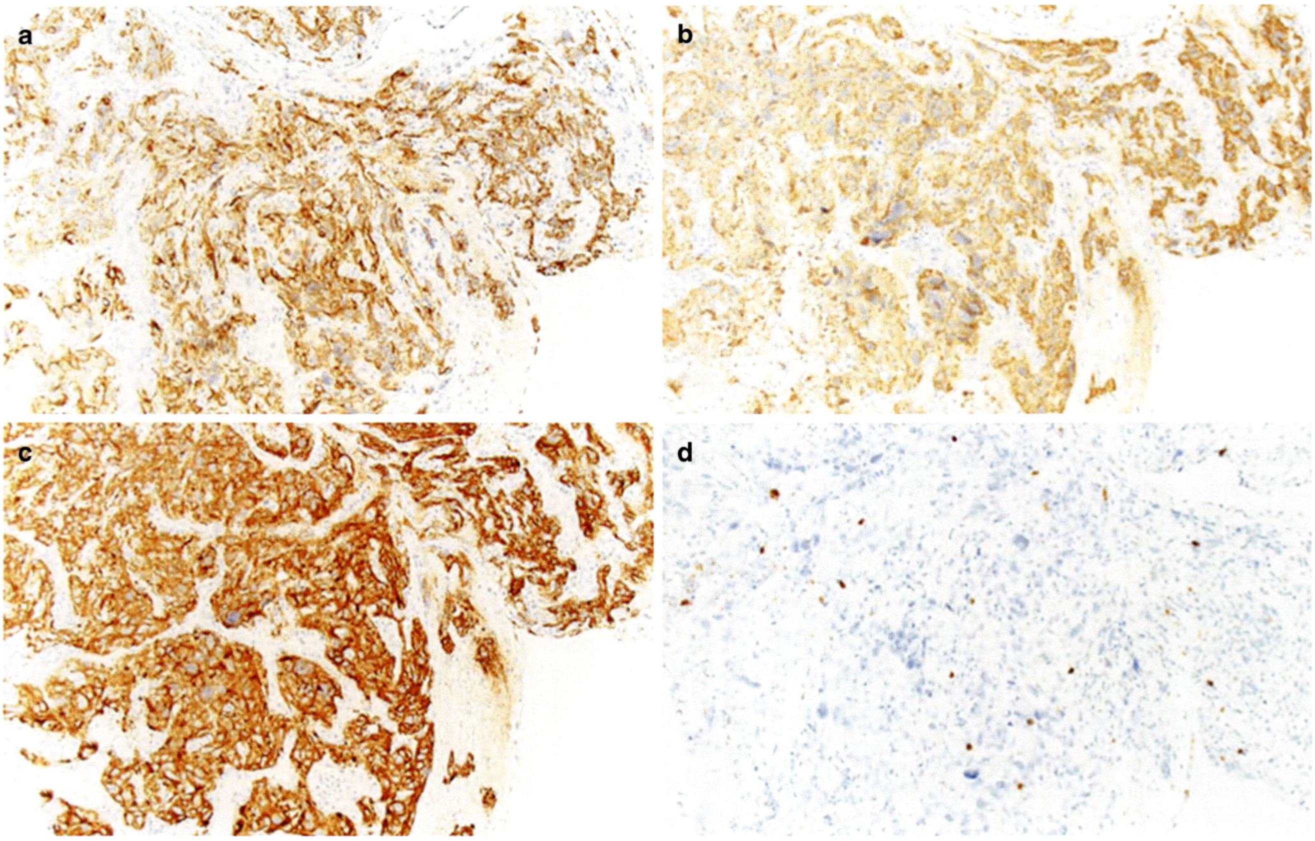

Fig. 16.3 Immunohistochemical (IHC) stains show that the neoplastic cells are diffusely positive for Cam5.2 (**a**), chromogranin (**b**), synaptophysin (**c**), and Ki67 (**d**). IHC: 200×

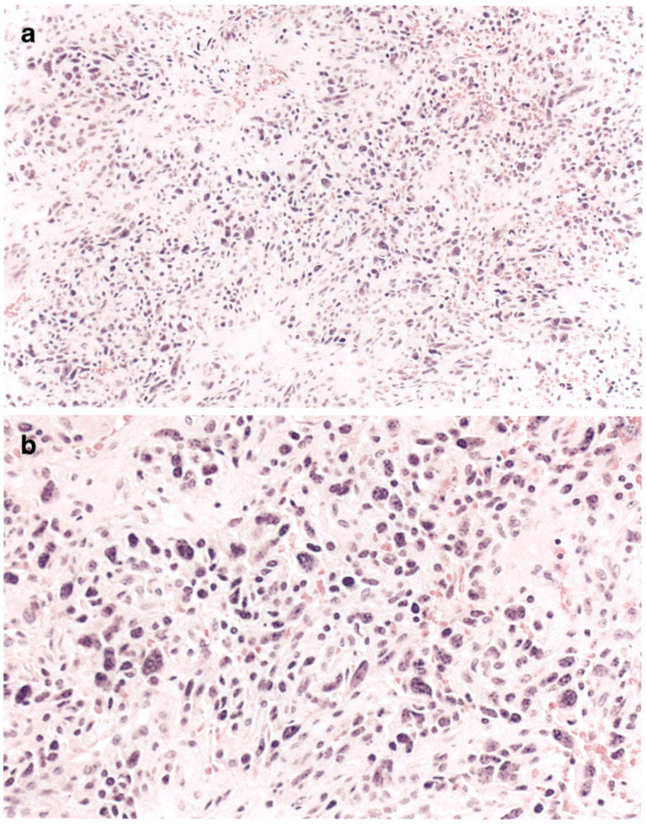

Fig. 16.5 Histologic sections of the tumor demonstrated the sheet of oval-shaped to spindled cells with occasional large, pleomorphic nuclei (**a**, H&E: 200× and **b**, H&E: 400×)

Final Pathologic Diagnosis: Typical Carcinoid

Where Are Pulmonary Neuroendocrine Cells Found, and What Is Neuroendocrine Hyperplasia?

Neuroendocrine cell rests are a normal component of the lung, present as scattered, in apparent neuroepithelial cells (called Kulchitsky cells) within the bronchial and bronchiolar epithelium [1]. Neuroendocrine cell hyperplasia (NECH) is defined as increased numbers of these neuroendocrine cells forming aggregates/clusters which remain confined to the basement membrane (Fig. 16.6). NECH can be seen as a reactive process associated with a number of inflammatory and neoplastic conditions and is commonly highlighted by immunohistochemical stains for synaptophysin and chromogranin performed for other reasons [2, 3].

What Is Pulmonary Carcinoid Tumor, and What Are its Clinical Features?

Carcinoid tumors are uncommon primary neuroendocrine neoplasms arising from the neuroendocrine cell rests or from pluripotent epithelial stem cells located in the bronchial and bronchiolar epithelium. Pulmonary carcinoid tumors are thus intimately associated with the airways [2, 4, 5].

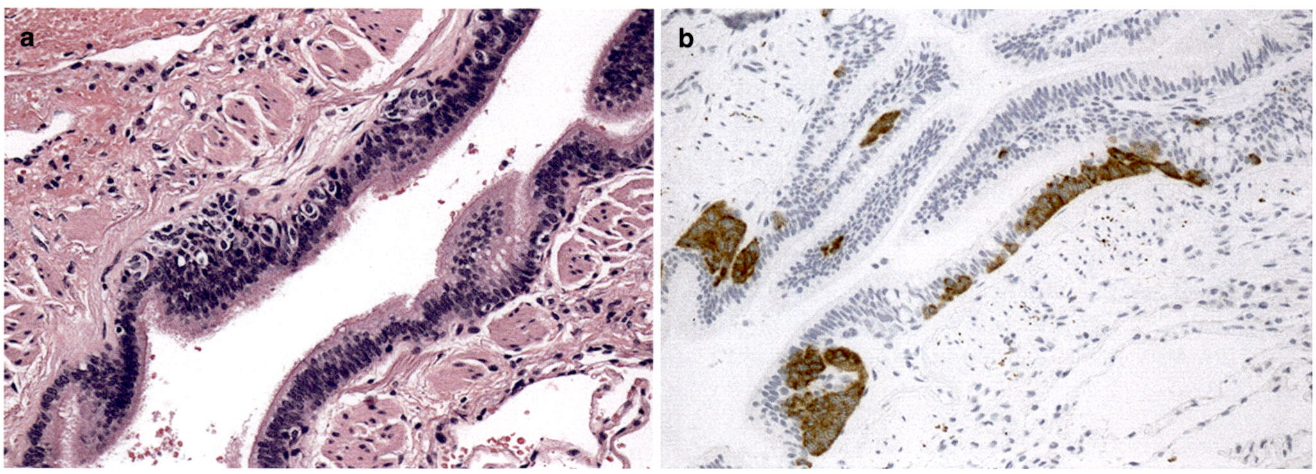

Fig. 16.6 Neuroendocrine cells are usually unapparent, and the histologic findings of neuroendocrine cell hyperplasia (NECH) can be subtle (**a**, H&E: 200×), but can be highlighted with synaptophysin (**b**, IHC: 200×) above the basement membrane

Similar to carcinoids of other sites, bronchopulmonary carcinoids predominantly affect middle-aged adults and are classified as TC and AC. Overall, these tumors occur earlier than most other primary pulmonary malignancies. TC generally occurs in the 40s to 50s, with AC occurring slightly later in the 50s to 60s. TC affects males and females approximately equally, with a slight female predominance for AC in some series [2, 6].

As a mass-forming bronchopulmonary lesion, the most common presenting symptoms are persistent cough and hemoptysis, although up to a quarter of cases are detected incidentally. Post-obstructive pneumonia is not an uncommon complication [6, 7]. As they are of neuroendocrine origin, ACTH production and the carcinoid syndrome can occur; however, these phenomena are rare and more often seen in carcinoids of other primary sites [2].

What Are the Characteristic Histopathologic and Immunohistochemical Features?

Pulmonary carcinoid tumors are characterized by polygonal to spindled epithelioid cells with a moderate amount of finely granular eosinophilic cytoplasm. "Organoid" nests or trabeculae are the most common architectural patterns, and prominent vascularity is typical (Fig. 16.7). They will be well circumscribed from the surrounding pulmonary parenchyma, although entrapped portions of bronchial wall and cartilage may be present [2, 4, 7].

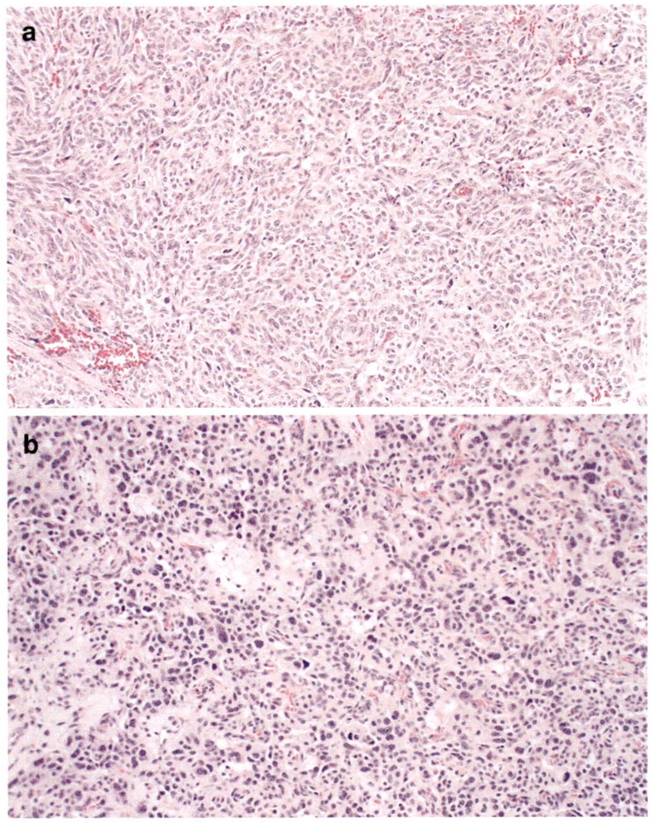

Fig. 16.7 Histologic features of typical carcinoids. Classically composed of epithelioid to spindled cells with moderate amounts of eosinophilic cytoplasm in organoid nests (**a**, H&E: 200×). The nuclei are generally banal; however, large, heterochromatic, and pleomorphic nuclei similar to the degenerative "ancient change" seen in other neuroendocrine neoplasms can be present (**b**, H&E: 200×)

The nuclei of most carcinoid tumors are bland, with smooth nuclear contours and granular, speckled, or "salt-and-pepper" chromatin [2]. As demonstrated above, unusual cases will demonstrate severe pleomorphism, with bizarre hyperchromatic nuclei. While potentially alarming, and possibly contributing to misdiagnosis, this morphology does not portend aggressive behavior and is not used in the consideration of atypical carcinoids [8].

Immunohistochemically, the majority of carcinoid tumors will strongly express neuroendocrine markers such as CD56 (76%), synaptophysin (90%), and chromogranin (92%). Up to 80% will stain positive with cytokeratins. Staining for TTF-1 is more variable, with positivity in only 20–50% of cases [2, 3, 6].

What Is an Atypical Carcinoid, and What Features Distinguish them from Typical Carcinoid?

AC is an intermediate-grade neuroendocrine neoplasm with more aggressive clinical behavior and the primary diagnostic consideration when evaluating bronchopulmonary carcinoids. While not diagnostic, nuclear pleomorphism, patchy loss of staining with neuroendocrine markers, and a Ki-67 proliferation index >2% are suggestive of AC, warranting close evaluation [2, 9, 10].

There are two histologic features which define AC. The first is necrosis, with a single focus being sufficient for the diagnosis of AC. The other is an increased mitotic rate of two to ten mitoses per 2 mm^2 (Fig. 16.8) [2, 4]. Both of these features may be focal, and, as such, the exclusion of AC requires thorough evaluation of resection specimens.

Are there any Features Which Have Prognostic Significance?

The main prognostic feature is the presence of atypical features, with AC having a 5-year survival rate of approximately 60%, as compared to >90% for TC [2, 5]. The presence of an elevated Ki-67 proliferation index has been shown to be an independent factor predicting worse overall survival [10], as has the presence of lymph node metastases [11].

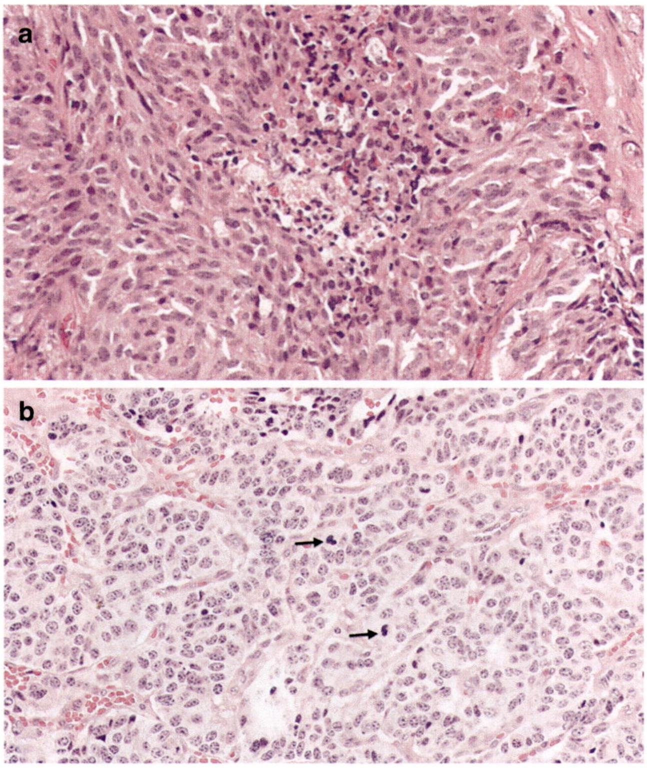

Fig. 16.8 Atypical carcinoid with focal necrosis (**a**, H&E: 400×) and/or increased mitotic activity with >2 mitoses/2 mm^2 (**b**, H&E: 400×, arrows)

How Do I Differentiate Pulmonary Carcinoid from Other Primary Pulmonary Malignancies?

While carcinoids are typically apparent on resection specimens, crush artifact, poor sampling, and presence of neoplastic cells with bizarre nuclei in biopsy specimens can obscure the characteristic cytologic and architectural features. In these instances, immunohistochemical stains for p40 or p63, as well as neuroendocrine markers, can be helpful in the differentiation of carcinoid tumors from poorly differentiated squamous cell carcinoma. Poorly differentiated adenocarcinoma will express TTF-1 with less common expression neuroendocrine markers [4].

Tumors with morphologic features of carcinoid tumor and > 10 mitoses per 2 mm^2 warrant classification as large-cell neuroendocrine carcinoma, given their greater likelihood to have aggressive behavior [4].

How Is Primary Pulmonary Carcinoid Differentiated from Metastasis?

Primary pulmonary carcinoid is usually unifocal. The presence of multifocal lesions, or a history of carcinoid tumors elsewhere, should prompt investigation for possible metastatic disease. Immunoreactivity for TTF-1 may help suggest primary pulmonary carcinoid. If negative, additional stains more specific to a presumed originating site are warranted. As an example, gastrointestinal carcinoid tumors metastatic to the lung will be TTF-1 negative but retain CDX2 expression [6].

What Is DIPNECH, and how Is it Differentiated from NECH?

Diffuse idiopathic pulmonary neuroendocrine cell hyperplasia (DIPNECH) is a rare entity in which multiple foci of neuroendocrine cell proliferation are seen in the bilateral lungs in the absence of an underlying pulmonary process. The majority of patients diagnosed with DIPNECH are nonsmokers in the sixth to seventh decade of life, with a 4:1 female predominance [3, 6, 7, 12–14]. The prevalence has increased in recent years, possibly due to increased recognition as a disease entity, and as such the exact incidence is uncertain [3, 12]. If symptomatic, the most common presenting symptoms are persistent cough and dyspnea/wheezing. Many cases are detected incidentally on imaging, which is characterized by numerous reticulonodular bronchial/bronchiolar nodules bilaterally (Fig. 16.9a). Bronchial wall thickening and mosaic air trapping are seen in some cases. Pulmonary function tests will show an obstructive or mixed obstructive and restrictive pattern. The majority of cases will remain relatively stable, with a small subset progressing to end-stage lung disease requiring transplantation due to bronchiolar obstruction and obliteration. The mechanism underlying this process is unclear [3, 7, 12, 13].

DIPNECH is a defined entity within the WHO classification, although the criteria for it are somewhat vague and nonspecific. More definitive criteria for the histologic diagnosis of DIPNECH have been proposed by multiple authors. One such example from Marchesky et al. is the presence of five or more neuroendocrine cells, either singly or in clusters, located within the basement membrane of the bronchiolar epithelium of at least three bronchioles in the setting of three or more carcinoid tumorlets [15]. However, there is no current consensus regarding any of the proposed criteria in the literature [3, 12]. Overall, while an important diagnostic consideration whenever NECH is identified, DIPNECH is, in some respects, predominantly a clinical diagnosis and requires clinical and radiographic correlation.

What Are Carcinoid Tumorlets, and how Are they Distinguished from NECH and DIPNECH?

Carcinoid tumorlets, on the other hand, are localized neuroendocrine cell proliferations which are typically seen in association with underlying primary lung disease, such as long-standing bronchiectasis or pulmonary fibrosis. They are also not infrequently seen adjacent to carcinoid tumors. Affected patients tend to be older, in their seventh to eighth decade of life, but otherwise share a similar female predominance to DIPNECH [6, 7, 16]. Clinically asymptomatic, they are typically incidental findings on radiographic studies (Fig. 16.9b) or examination of pulmonary resection specimens [16, 17].

Generally, these tumorlets are thought to develop in response to localized hypoxia or inflammation [17]. Although considered to be benign lesions, their recognition and consideration are important as their presence is associated with an increased risk of development of carcinoid tumors, both typical and atypical. As such, careful gross and microscopic examination of pulmonary specimens for their presence is warranted [7, 16].

Carcinoid tumorlets are differentiated from NECH by infiltration beyond the bronchial or bronchiolar basement membrane (Fig. 16.10).

By definition, they are 5 mm or less in size but are otherwise histologically and immunophenotypically identical to typical carcinoid tumors. Rare cases with atypia and lymph node metastases have been reported [7]. If necrosis and/or increased mitotic activity are present, these should be treated and staged as atypical carcinoids.

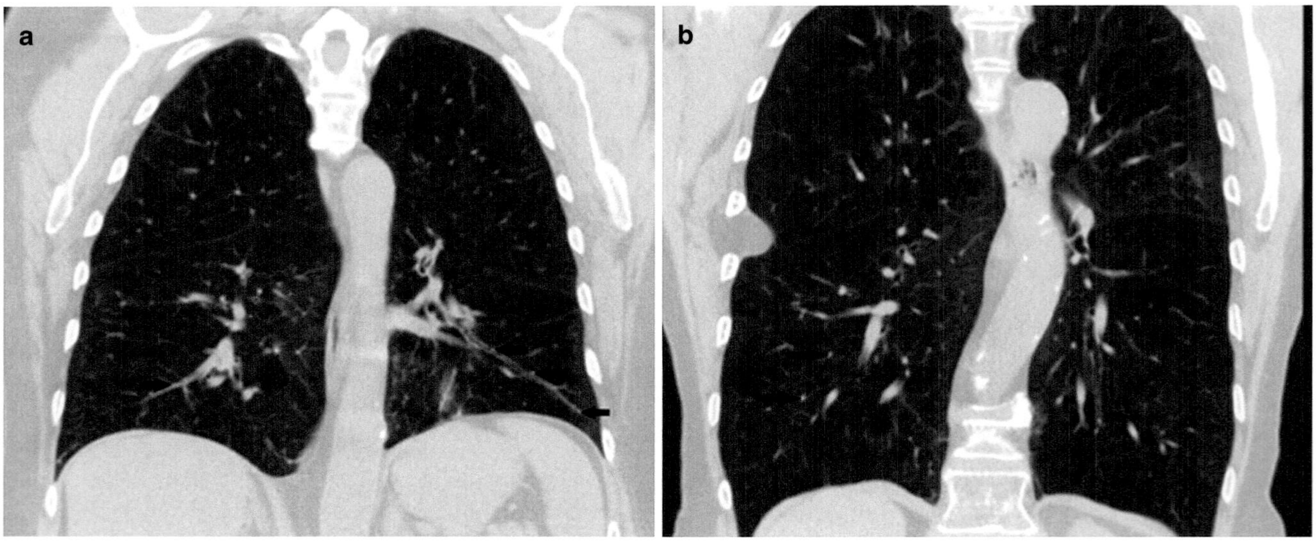

Fig. 16.9 CT findings in DIPNECH and carcinoid tumorlets. The presence of multiple nodules arranged linearly along the walls of bronchi and bronchioles bilaterally is characteristic of DIPNECH (**a**). Carcinoid tumorlets, on the other hand, are typically more localized, with presence of interstitial lung disease in the background (**b**)

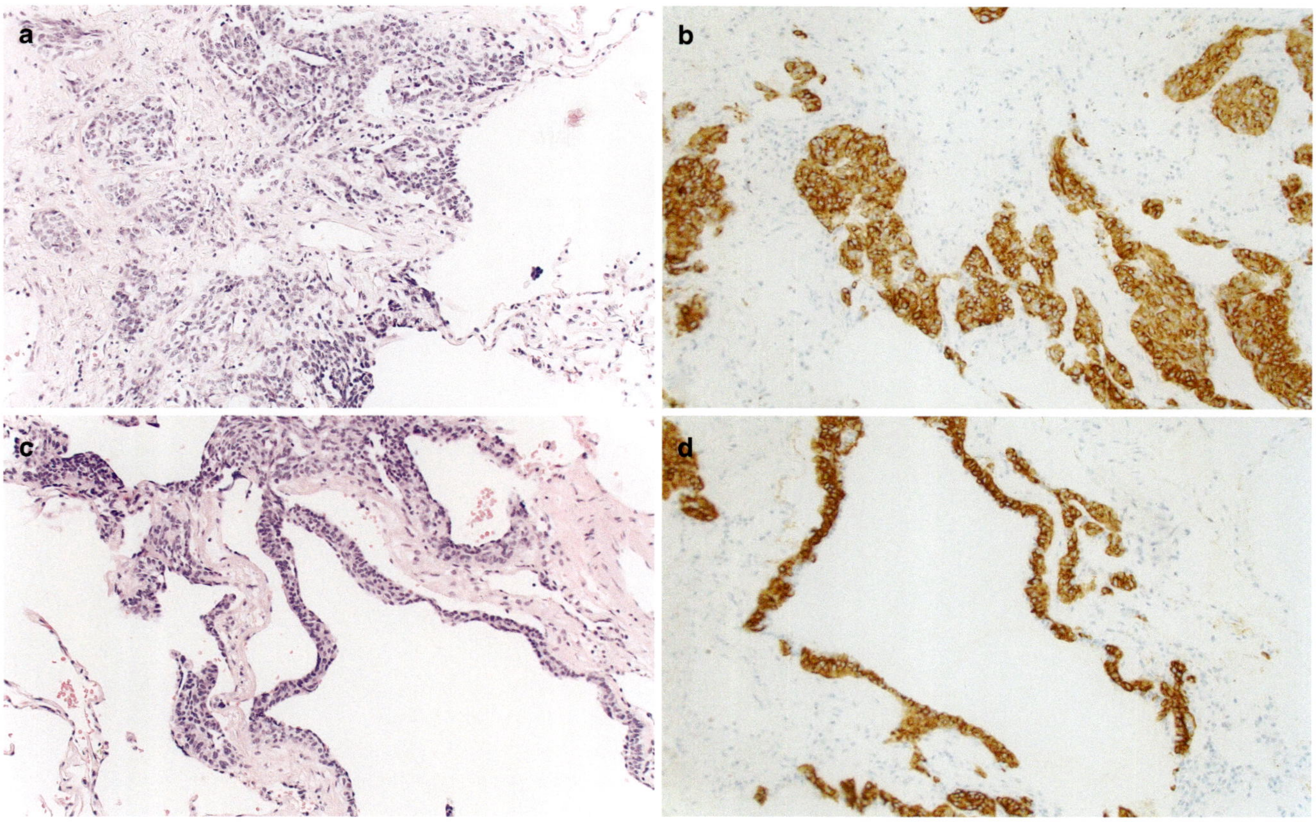

Fig. 16.10 Histologic difference between tumorlet and DIPNECH of the lung. Histologic section demonstrated tumorlet with nests of oval-shaped neuroendocrine cell infiltrates beyond the basement membrane of the bronchiole with stromal fibrosis (**a**), while DIPNECH exhibited an oval-shaped neuroendocrine cell proliferation intact basement membrane (**c**). There are adjacent emphysematous changes. H&E, (**a** and **c**): 200×. Immunohistochemical stain showed the neuroendocrine cells were positive for synaptophysin (**b** and **d**). IHC, (**b** and **d**): 200×

References

1. Linnoila RI. Functional facets of the pulmonary neuroendocrine system. Lab Investig. 2006;86(5):425–44.
2. Rekhtman N. Neuroendocrine tumors of the lung: an update. Arch Pathol Lab Med. 2010;134(11):1628–38.
3. Mengoli MC, Rossi G, Cavazza A, Franco R, Marino FZ, Migaldi M, et al. Diffuse idiopathic pulmonary neuroendocrine cell hyperplasia (DIPNECH) syndrome and carcinoid tumors with/without NECH: a clinicopathologic, radiologic, and Immunomolecular comparison study. Am J Surg Pathol. 2018;42(5):646–55.
4. Travis WD, Brambilla E, Nicholson AG, Yatabe Y, Austin JHM, Beasley MB, et al. The 2015 World Health Organization classification of lung tumors: impact of genetic, clinical and radiologic advances since the 2004 classification. J Thorac Oncol. 2015;10(9):1243–60.
5. Pinchot SN, Holen K, Sippel RS, Chen H. Carcinoid tumors. Oncologist. 2008;13(12):1255–69.
6. Koo CW, Baliff JP, Torigian DA, Litzky LA, Gefter WB, Akers SR. Spectrum of pulmonary neuroendocrine cell proliferation: diffuse idiopathic pulmonary neuroendocrine cell hyperplasia, tumorlet, and carcinoids. AJR Am J Roentgenol. 2010;195(3):661–8.
7. Dincer HE, Podgaetz E, Andrade RS. Pulmonary neuroendocrine tumors: Part I. Spectrum and characteristics of tumors. J Bronchology Interv Pulmonol. 2015;22:267–73.
8. Sheppard MN. Nuclear pleomorphism in typical carcinoid tumours of the lung: problems in frozen section interpretation. Histopathology. 1997;30(5):478–80.
9. Marchevsky AM, Hendifar A, Walts AE. The use of Ki-67 labeling index to grade pulmonary well-differentiated neuroendocrine neoplasms: current best evidence. Mod Pathol. 2018;31(10):1523–31.
10. Pelosi G, Rindi G, Travis WD, Papotti M. Ki-67 antigen in lung neuroendocrine tumors: unraveling a role in clinical practice. J Thorac Oncol. 2014;9(3):273–84.
11. García-Yuste M, Matilla JM. The significance of histology: typical and atypical bronchial carcinoids. Thorac Surg Clin. 2014;24(3):293–7.
12. Rossi G, Cavazza A, Spagnolo P, Sverzellati N, Longo L, Jukna A, et al. Diffuse idiopathic pulmonary neuroendocrine cell hyperplasia syndrome. Eur Respir J. 2016;47(6):1829–41.
13. Davies SJ, Gosney JR, Hansell DM, Wells AU, du Bois RM, Burke MM, et al. Diffuse idiopathic pulmonary neuroendocrine cell hyperplasia: an under-recognised spectrum of disease. Thorax. 2007;62(3):248–52.
14. Gorshtein A, Gross DJ, Barak D, Strenov Y, Refaeli Y, Shimon I, et al. Diffuse idiopathic pulmonary neuroendocrine cell hyperplasia and the associated lung neuroendocrine tumors. Cancer. 2012;118(3):612–9.
15. Marchevsky AM, Wirtschafter E, Walts AE. The spectrum of changes in adults with multifocal pulmonary neuroendocrine proliferations: what is the minimum set of pathologic criteria to diagnose DIPNECH? Human Patholol. 2015;46(2):176–81.
16. Ginsberg MS, Akin O, Berger DM, Zakowski MF, Panicek DM. Pulmonary Tumorlets: CT findings. Am J Roentgenol. 2004;183(2):293–6.
17. Kallianos A, Velentza L, Zarogoulidis P, Baka S, Kosmidis C, Labaki S, et al. Progressive dyspnea due to pulmonary carcinoid tumorlets. Respir Med Case Rep. 2017;6(21):84–5.

Minute Meningothelial-Like Nodules Versus Tumorlet

17

Sophia Shaddy and Eric C. Huang

Case Presentation

Computed tomography (CT) from a 65-year-old female shows a suspicious 2.0 cm right upper lobe lung mass and multiple sub-centimeter randomly distributed nodules within the same lobe. Biopsy of the mass is interpreted as lung adenocarcinoma, and the decision is made to pursue a right upper lobe lobectomy. On gross examination of the lobectomy specimen, the small nodules are tan and well circumscribed and range in size from 2 to 4 mm. Microscopic examination shows whorled nests of bland ovoid nuclei with finely granular chromatin and eosinophilic cytoplasm. Immunohistochemical study on the small nodules is negative for cytokeratin and neuroendocrine markers. Based on these findings, the diagnosis of minute pulmonary meningothelial-like nodules (MPMNs) is rendered (Fig. 17.1).

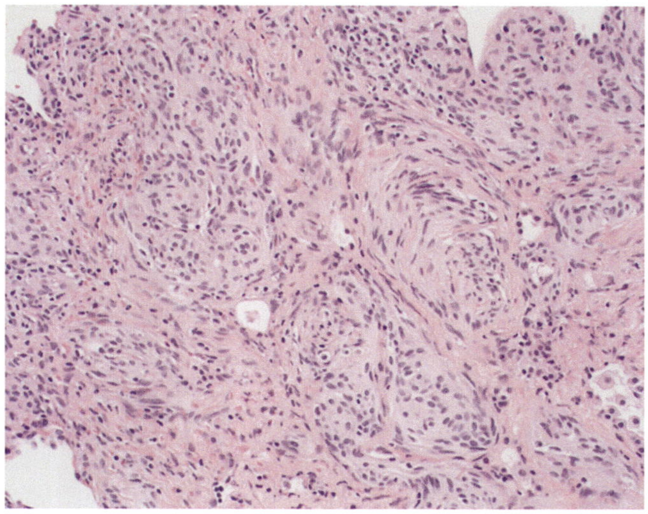

Fig. 17.1 Tissue section of MPMN showing whorled clusters of bland cells with ovoid nuclei and eosinophilic cytoplasm (H&E 200×)

S. Shaddy · E. C. Huang (✉)
Department of Laboratory Medicine and Pathology, University of Washington School of Medicine, Seattle, WA, USA
e-mail: ecchuang@uw.edu

H. Xu et al. (eds.), *Practical Lung Pathology*, Practical Anatomic Pathology, https://doi.org/10.1007/978-3-031-14402-8_17

Pathologic Diagnosis: Minute Pulmonary Meningothelial-Like Nodules (MPMNs)

What Are MPMNs and its Main Differential on Microscopic Evaluation?

MPMNs are benign proliferations of cells with bland, oval-to-spindled nuclei, finely granular chromatin, and granular, eosinophilic cytoplasm arranged in nests or whorls that involve the alveolar septa [1, 2] (Fig. 17.2). MPMNs are more commonly found in women in the sixth decade and have been associated with underlying chronic lung disease, chronic ischemic heart disease, and primary pulmonary malignancy elsewhere in the lungs [3–7]. They are usually asymptomatic, found incidentally, are less than 5 mm in size, and occur as single or multiple nodules randomly distributed throughout the lung lobes [4, 8, 9]. Diffuse pulmonary meningotheliomatosis is a rare condition with disseminated bilateral pulmonary involvement by MPMNs and restrictive pulmonary disease-like symptoms [3, 10].

MPMNs can mimic metastatic malignancy on imaging [9]; however, on microscopy MPMNs are readily classified as benign. The main differential is another benign, small lung lesion called pulmonary tumorlet, especially on low-power scanning (Fig. 17.3a). Pulmonary tumorlets are neuroendocrine cell proliferations and appear as well-circumscribed nodules on imaging [11–14]. Morphologically,

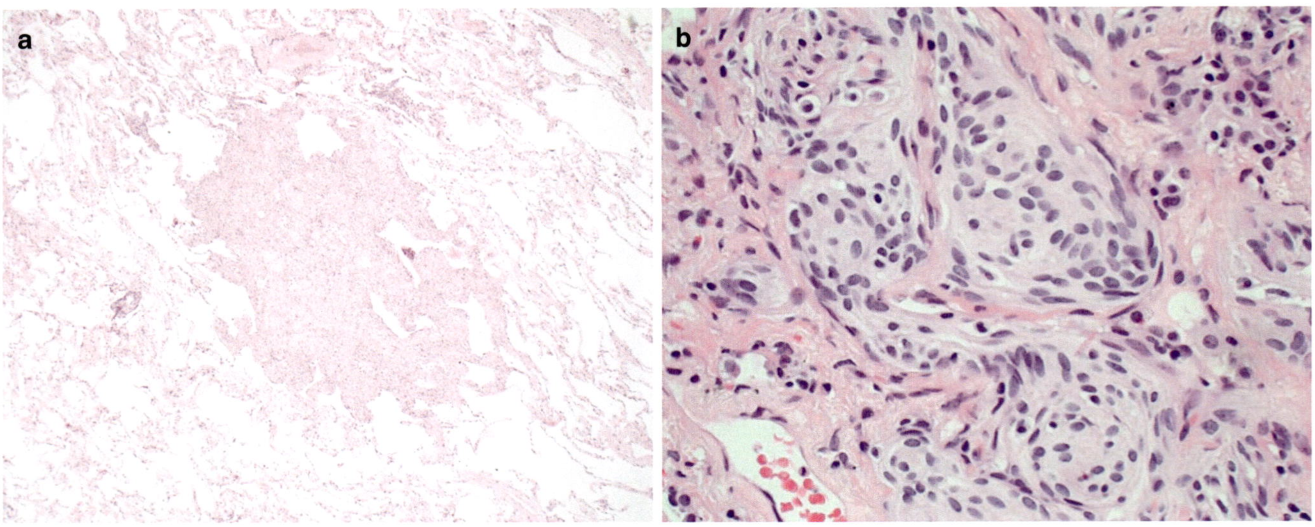

Fig. 17.2 (**a**) Low-power view of MPMN showing a well-circumscribed nodule (H&E 40×). (**b**) High power shows whorled nests of cells with bland nuclei and eosinophilic cytoplasm (H&E 400×)

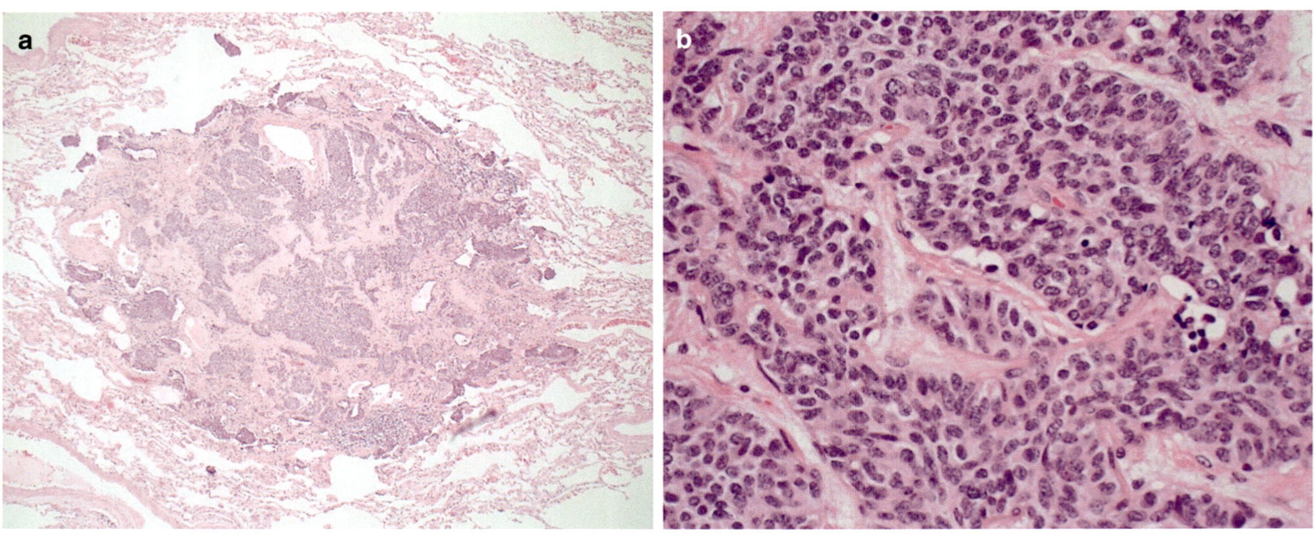

Fig. 17.3 Tumorlet histology. (**a**) Low power shows a well-circumscribed nodule of nested cells measuring less than 5 mm (H&E 40×). (**b**) High-power magnification shows typical neuroendocrine features such as finely stippled chromatin and scant cytoplasm. This lesion also lacks mitotic figures and necrosis (H&E 400×)

tumorlets are identical to typical carcinoid tumors of the lung, showing organoid growth pattern, fine nuclear chromatin, scant pink cytoplasm, and a low mitotic rate, but are less than 5 mm in size (Fig. 17.3b). The presumed normal counterpart of tumorlets is the Kulchitsky cell, and early electron microscopy studies show tumorlets contain neurosecretory granules, indicating neuroendocrine cell origin [13, 15]. Like MPMNs, tumorlets also occur more frequently in women in the sixth decade, are often incidentally found, and are associated with areas of chronic lung injury [13, 14]).

Are MPMNs Related to Central Nervous System Meningiomas and/or Primary Pulmonary Meningiomas?

Originally, MPMNs were thought to arise from chemoreceptor cell precursors when described by Korn et al. in 1960, hence the original name "chemodectoma" [16]. However, ultrastructural and immunohistochemical findings show these lesions more closely resemble meningothelial cells [1]. Though MPMNs are linked to meningothelial cell origin, there is no significant association with central nervous system meningiomas or primary pulmonary meningiomas [1, 3, 6]. The exact pathogenesis of MPMNs remains unclear; however, most studies conclude it is likely a reactive process [4, 8, 17].

What Immunohistochemical Findings Can Help Differentiate MPMNs from Pulmonary Tumorlets?

Tumorlets have a neuroendocrine immunohistochemical profile (with expression of synaptophysin and chromogranin) (Fig. 17.4a and b) and are positive for cytokeratins (Table 17.1). Additionally, tumorlets can be positive for TTF-1 [11]. MPMNs are negative for keratin, synaptophysin, and chromogranin (Fig. 17.5c and d) but have been shown to express patchy CD56 [4]. MPMNs have a similar immunohistochemical profile to central nervous system meningiomas and are positive for EMA (Fig. 17.5a), vimentin (Fig. 17.5b), and PR (variably) [9].

Why Is it Important for Pathologists to Be Aware of MPMNs and Pulmonary Tumorlets?

Both MPMNs and tumorlets are considered benign lesions. However, they can mimic malignancy on imaging studies [6, 11, 12] and may be sampled for diagnostic or staging purposes. It is important to be aware of these entities to avoid misdiagnosis as malignancy or metastatic disease in order to ensure appropriate patient care and management.

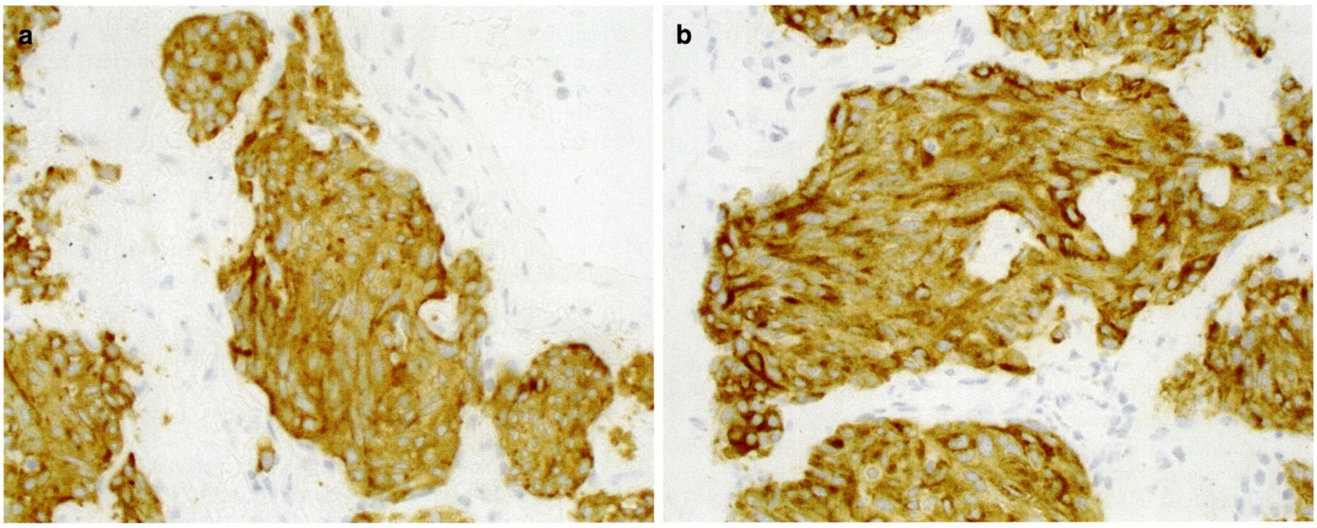

Fig. 17.4 Tumorlet showing strong positivity for neuroendocrine markers (**a**) synaptophysin and (**b**) chromogranin (400×)

Table 17.1 Summary of stains differentiating MPMN from tumorlet

	MPMN	Tumorlet
Synaptophysin, chromogranin	–	+
Keratin	–	+
TTF1	–	+/–

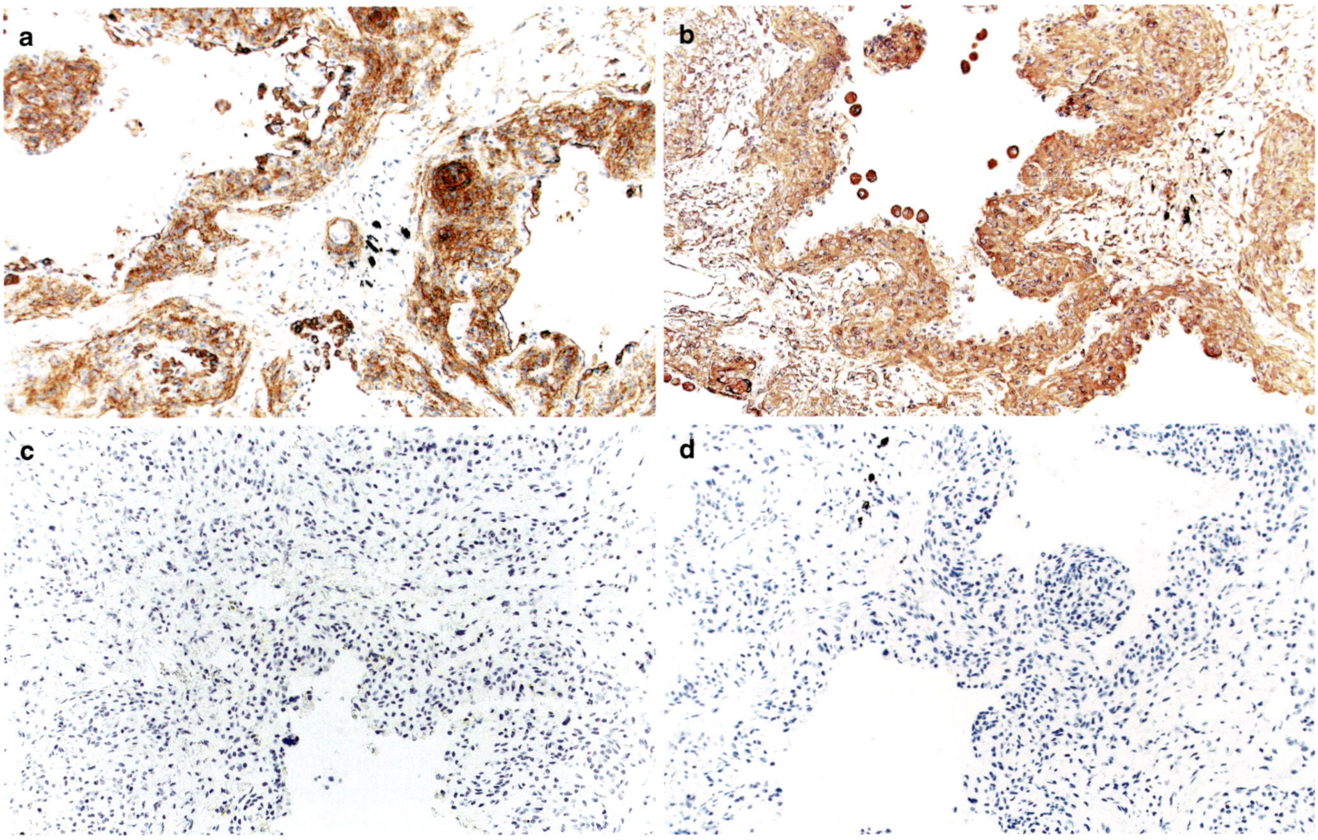

Fig. 17.5 MPMN showing positivity for (**a**) EMA and (**b**) vimentin and negativity for (**c**) synaptophysin and (**d**) chromogranin (200×). (Figure courtesy of Haodong Xu, MD, PhD, University of Washington Medical Center, Department of Laboratory Medicine and Pathology, Seattle, WA)

References

1. Gaffey MJ, Mills SE, Askin FB. Minute pulmonary meningothelial-like nodules. A clinicopathologic study of so-called minute pulmonary chemodectoma. Am J Surg Pathol. 1988;12(3):167–75.
2. Ionescu DN, Sasatomi E, Aldeeb D, Omalu BI, Finkelstein SD, Swalsky PA, et al. Pulmonary meningothelial-like nodules: a genotypic comparison with meningiomas. Am J Surg Pathol. 2004;28(2):207–14.
3. Suster S, Moran CA. Diffuse pulmonary meningotheliomatosis. Am J Surg Pathol. 2007;31(4):624–31.
4. Mukhopadhyay S, El-Zammar OA, Katzenstein AL. Pulmonary meningothelial-like nodules: new insights into a common but poorly understood entity. Am J Surg Pathol. 2009;33(4):487–95.
5. Mizutani E, Tsuta K, Maeshima AM, Asamura H, Matsuno Y. Minute pulmonary meningothelial-like nodules: clinicopathologic analysis of 121 patients. Hum Pathol. 2009;40(5):678–82.
6. Asakawa A, Horio H, Hishima T, Yamamichi T, Okui M, Harada M. Clinicopathologic features of minute pulmonary meningothelial-like nodules. Asian Cardiovasc Thorac Ann. 2017;25(7–8):509–12.
7. Tao L, Chen Y, Huang Q, Yong J, Yan S, Huang Y. Constant expression of somatostatin receptor 2a in minute pulmonary meningothelial-like nodules. J Clin Pathol. 2019;72(8):525–8.
8. Sellami D, Gotway MB, Hanks DK, Webb WR. Minute pulmonary meningothelial-like nodules: thin-section CT appearance. J Comput Assist Tomogr. 2001;25(2):311–3.
9. Peng XX, Yan LX, Liu C, Wang SY, Li WF, Gao X, et al. Benign disease prone to be misdiagnosed as malignant pulmonary nodules: minute meningothelioid nodules. Thorac Cancer. 2019;10(5):1182–7.
10. Huang EC, Zhang Y, Bishop JW, Gandour-Edwards RF, Afify AM. Diffuse pulmonary meningotheliomatosis: a diagnostically challenging entity on fine-needle aspiration cytology. Diagn Cytopathol. 2015;43(9):727–30.
11. Aubry MC, Thomas CF, Jett JR, Swensen SJ, Myers JL. Significance of multiple carcinoid tumors and tumorlets in surgical lung specimens: analysis of 28 patients. Chest. 2007;131(6):1635–43.
12. Ginsberg MS, Akin O, Berger DM, Zakowski MF, Panicek DM. Pulmonary tumorlets: CT findings. AJR Am J Roentgenol. 2004;183(2):293–6.
13. Churg A, Warnock ML. Pulmonary tumorlet. A form of peripheral carcinoid. Cancer. 1976;37(3):1469–77.
14. Travis WD. Pathology and diagnosis of neuroendocrine tumors: lung neuroendocrine. Thorac Surg Clin. 2014;24(3):257–66.
15. Ranchod M. The histogenesis and development of pulmonary tumorlets. Cancer. 1977;39(3):1135–45.
16. Korn D, Bensch K, Liebow AA, Castleman B. Multiple minute pulmonary tumors resembling chemodectomas. Am J Pathol. 1960;37(6):641–72.
17. Niho S, Yokose T, Nishiwaki Y, Mukai K. Immunohistochemical and clonal analysis of minute pulmonary meningothelial-like nodules. Hum Pathol. 1999;30(4):425–9.

Primary Lung Versus Metastatic Adenocarcinoma

18

Rouba Hadi and Haodong Xu

Case Presentation

A 62-year-old female, never-smoker, with a history of ovarian cancer years ago for which she underwent surgical resection with four cycles of chemotherapy, presented to the thoracic clinic with a persistent non-productive cough. A computed tomography (CT) of the chest was performed and showed a 6 cm mass in the right lower lobe of the lung posterior to the hilum and extending to the pleura. A biopsy was performed and reported as adenocarcinoma of likely lung origin, given the immunohistochemical reactivity of the neoplastic cells forTTF-1, PAX-8, napsin-A, CK7, and ER. Positron-emission tomography-CT (PET-CT) performed one month later demonstrated that there were two hypermetabolic masses, 6.0 cm in the right lower lobe and 2.4 cm in the right hilum, respectively (Fig. 18.1a, b). There was no evidence of other organ involvement. The patient was transferred to a tertiary center for surgical intervention and further management. Upon re-review of her lung biopsy, the material from the patient's right salpingo-oophorectomy in March 2008 was requested for comparison. A similar endometrioid morphology in both cases was noted, as shown in Fig. 18.2, which was taken from the lung biopsy, leading to additional immunohistochemical studies. It was noticed that the ovarian mass also expressed PAX8, TTF-1, and napsin-A. A right upper and lower bilobectomy and excision of the hilar mass, as well as biopsies of lymph nodes from different mediastinal levels, were performed. Histological sections of the lung and hilar masses show morphologic features of endometrioid adenocarcinoma (Fig. 18.3a, b). The neoplastic cells are strongly positive for TTF-1 (Fig. 18.3c) and PAX8 (Fig. 18.3d). In light of these overall findings, the patient's current lung mass and hilar lymph node metastasis were consistent with metastatic ovarian endometrioid adenocarcinoma. After surgery was completed, the patient was referred to gynecological oncology for further management.

R. Hadi · H. Xu (✉)
Department of Laboratory Medicine and Pathology, University of Washington Medical Center, Seattle, WA, USA
e-mail: xuh8@uw.edu

H. Xu et al. (eds.), *Practical Lung Pathology*, Practical Anatomic Pathology, https://doi.org/10.1007/978-3-031-14402-8_18

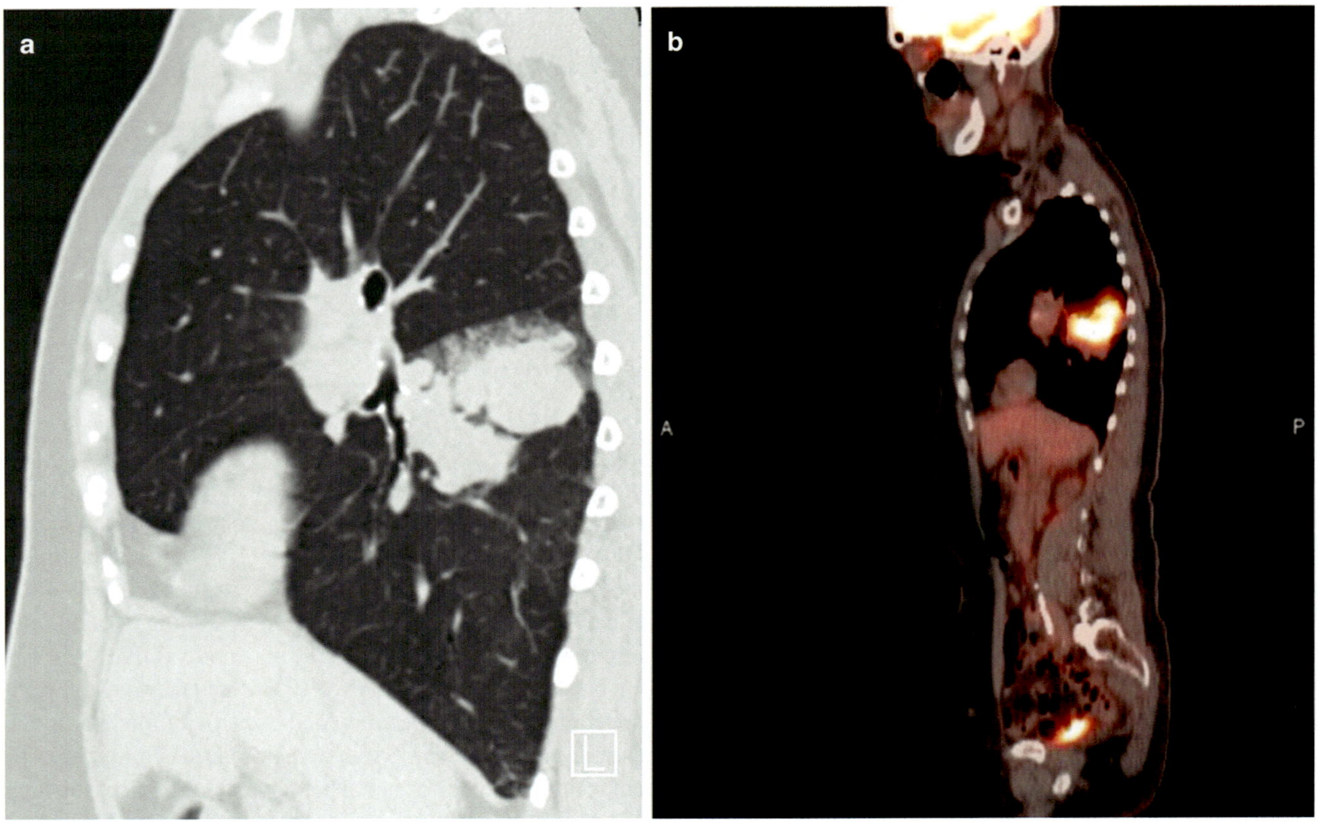

Fig. 18.1 Chest CT image shows a mass in the right lower lobe and a mass in the right hilum (**a**), which are hypermetabolic in PET scan (**b**)

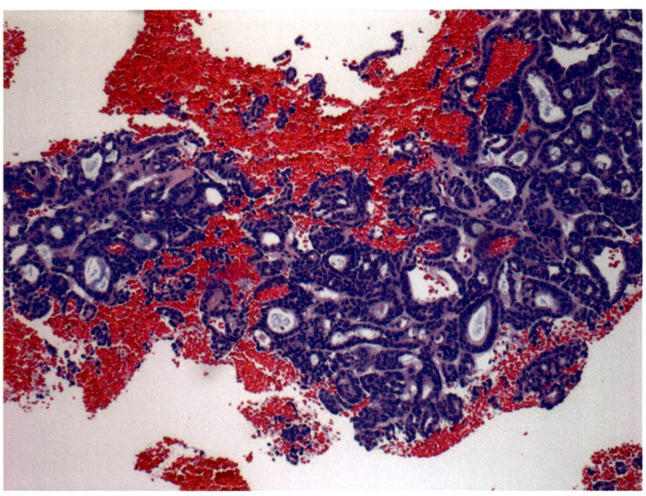

Fig. 18.2 H&E-stained slide of the patient's right lung mass biopsy shows a malignant gland proliferation with the unique endometrioid-like morphology, which is not a common feature of typical primary lung adenocarcinoma, acinar pattern. H&E: 200×. The salpingo-oophorectomy resection specimen dating back ten years to the current presentation had a similar morphology

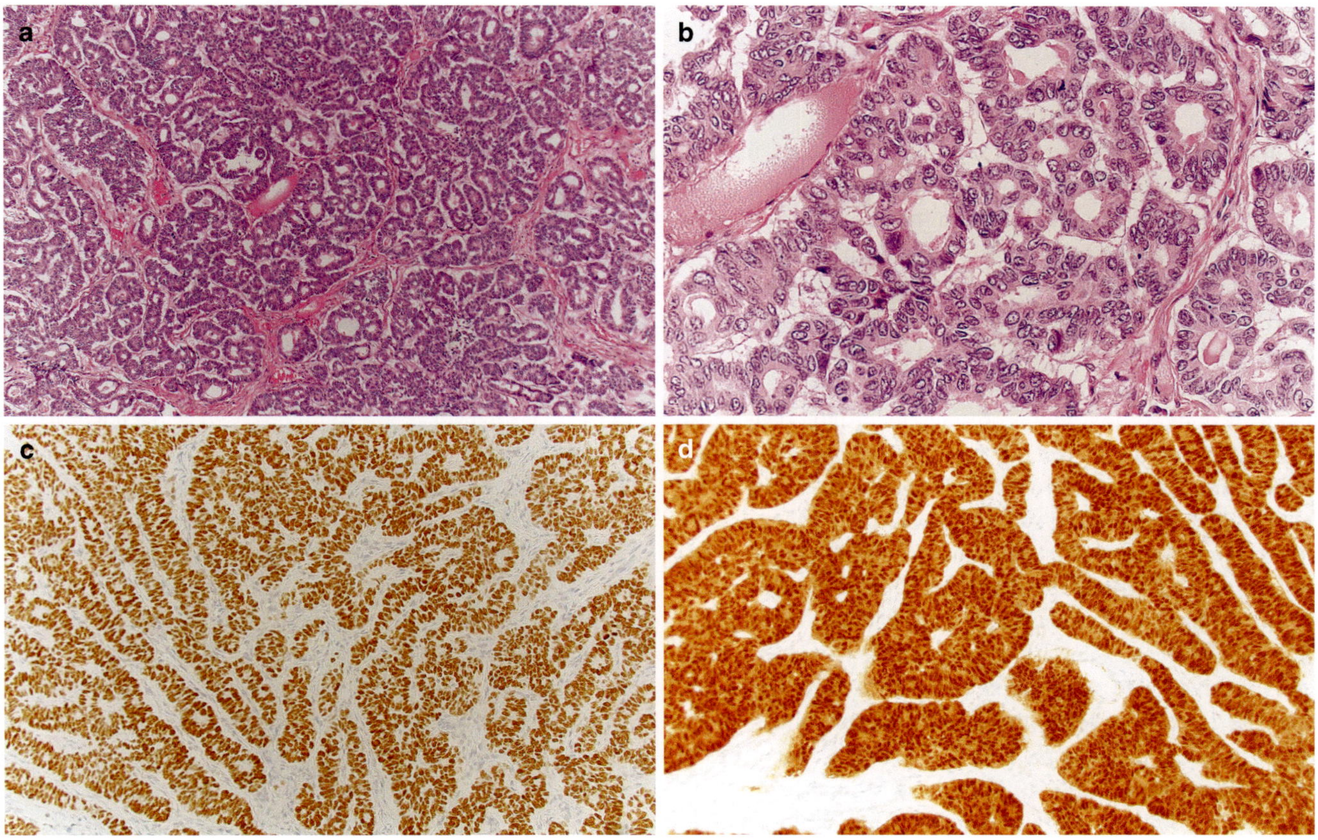

Fig. 18.3 H&E-stained slides of the patient's lung resection specimen show that a gland-forming neoplasm is present making nests and cords, with fairly uniform cells that are frequently polarized with more abundant cytoplasm adjacent to the lumens. The overall features are those of endometrioid carcinoma. H&E: 100× (**a**) and 400× (**b**). Immunohistochemical stains show that the neoplastic cells are positive for TTF-1 (**c**) and PAX8 (**d**). IHC: 200×

Pathologic Diagnosis: Lung, Right Upper and Lower Lobes. Bilobectomy: Adenocarcinoma, Consistent with Metastasis from Ovarian Endometrioid Carcinoma

What Is the Clinical Relevance of Distinguishing Metastasis from Primary Lung Adenocarcinoma, and Will it Change Prognosis?

Establishing a diagnosis that favors metastatic adenocarcinoma involving the lung versus a primary lung adenocarcinoma carries a significant impact on future therapeutic interventions. Even in a setting of known adenocarcinoma of lung origin, it is necessary to report intrapulmonary metastasis from multiple synchronous primaries as this will change staging and therapeutic interventions [1]. Knowing this, the distinction between primary lung adenocarcinoma and metastatic adenocarcinoma of extrapulmonary origin becomes even more important. A patient with an isolated lung lesion, if truly of lung origin, will usually only require surgical management, in the form of a lobectomy and possibly mediastinal lymph node staging. However, in the case of extrapulmonary metastasis, treatment will almost always involve some form of chemotherapy (usually with radiation). Prognosis also becomes significantly different. With colorectal adenocarcinomas, which can metastasize to the lung in up to 20% of patients, rare cases have been reported where patients developed synchronous lung and colorectal adenocarcinomas. In these patients, surgical resection and chemotherapy regimens are drastically different. Synchronous curative resection of the two lesions is the primary management step, and adjuvant chemotherapy for colorectal cancer should not be given. In cases where the synchronous primaries were missed and the patients given adjuvant chemotherapy for presumed metastasis, there were severely unfavorable outcomes reported [2]. Of note, patients with synchronous primaries have been found to have a better prognosis than those with metastatic colorectal carcinoma alone [2].

What Imaging Findings Are Helpful in Distinguishing Metastasis from Primary Lung Adenocarcinoma?

Radiographic imaging plays a big role in the assessment of lung lesions. CT imaging of the chest allows radiologists to evaluate some characteristics of a lung mass such as its location and size, as well as more detailed features such as a lepidic-growth pattern versus invasion, mucinous versus solid components, and even the presence of lymphovascular space invasion [3]. When imaging detects multiple lung nodules in a patient with a history of an extrapulmonary malignancy, it is likely that this represents metastatic disease [4, 5]. In addition to the presence multiple pulmonary nodules, another key feature that would favor metastasis is cavitation/necrosis [5]. Still, in the setting of an isolated lung lesion, determining metastasis from primary lung cancer on imaging remains a challenge. Furthermore, the odds of a patient having primary lung cancer when there has been an extrapulmonary malignancy are not as low as one would expect. A study reviewing 800 cases of patients with extrathoracic cancer who later presented with a solitary pulmonary lesion found that 500 of these patients had primary cancer of the lung. Approximately 200 (40%) of these patients had solitary metastasis from their extrathoracic primary [4]. Other studies have reported that for patients with a history of an extrapulmonary malignancy, the ones most likely to present with a metastatic nodule in the lung are those with a history of melanoma, sarcoma, or testicular carcinoma [6]. In these cases, the size of the nodule and distance from the pleura were found to be statically significant in the prediction of malignancy. Nodules greater than 10 mm in size and measuring more than 10 mm away from the pleura were most likely to be malignant [6]. All in all, although some features are helpful in the radiologic assessment of lung nodules, imaging modalities alone are not enough for definitive diagnosis.

What Histopathologic Features Are Helpful in Distinguishing Metastasis from Primary Lung Adenocarcinoma, and how Is Immunohistochemistry Contributory?

The histologic subtypes of lung adenocarcinoma are many and include lepidic, acinar, papillary, micropapillary, solid, invasive mucinous (including mixed invasive mucinous and non-mucinous), colloid, fetal, enteric, and minimally invasive adenocarcinoma [7]. Given this wide variation in morphologic patterns, to assess whether an adenocarcinoma in the lung is a primary versus a metastasis using histopathology alone is extremely challenging. While the presence of atypical adenomatous hyperplasia (AAH) and/or adenocarcinoma in situ (AIS) can allow one to be confident in diagnosing primary lung adenocarcinoma, particularly in the presence of peripheral lepidic pattern of growth (given the appropriate clinical and radiographic context), the real dilemma happens when these preinvasive lesions are inconspicuous or absent, and the tumor lacks lepidic component. Furthermore, both metastatic pancreatic and breast adenocarcinomas have been known to have a lepidic pattern of growth, mimicking primary lung adenocarcinoma with a lepidic pattern and complicating the diagnosis [8].

Immunohistochemistry has been historically useful when favoring primary lung adenocarcinoma over metastasis from an extrapulmonary malignancy. Thyroid transcription factor 1 (TTF-1) and napsin-A are routinely used and known to be strongly positive in most primary lung adenocarcinomas, staining up to 72% and 80% of cases, respectively [9]. Positivity with these markers however is not restricted to lung adenocarcinoma, as TTF-1 is also typically expressed in thyroid carcinoma (including those metastasizing to the lung) and small-cell carcinoma originating from organs such as the bladder, prostate, and esophagus [9]. More recent studies have even shown rare TTF-1 expression in endometrioid carcinoma and ovarian epithelial neoplasms including serous and endometrioid adenocarcinomas [10]. Although rarely described, napsin-A can be positive in thyroid carcinoma, renal cell carcinoma, and ovarian clear cell carcinoma [9].

It is also important to note that while these markers are sensitive, certain histologic subtypes, specifically enteric and mucinous adenocarcinomas of the lung, may not show expression of either TTF-1 or napsin-A. Enteric-type lung adenocarcinoma may instead express CDX2, villin, and SATB2, known markers of enteric differentiation [9]. One study evaluated the immunohistochemical profile of seven different primary adenocarcinomas (lung, colorectal, gastric, pancreatic, bile duct, breast, and ovarian) and specifically looked at the expression of common site-specific markers such as CDX-2, CK7, CK20, TTF-1, CEA, SMAD4, and GCDFP-15, among others. In the conclusion, it was noted that in this specific study, no single markers other than TTF-1 and GCDFP-15 were entirely specific for a given site [11]. Overall, while immunohistochemistry may help support a diagnosis, it has its limitations and is alone insufficient to make a definitive diagnosis.

References

1. Girard N, Deshpande C, Lau C, Finley D, Rusch V, Pao W, et al. Comprehensive histologic assessment helps to differentiate multiple lung primary nonsmall cell carcinomas from metastases. Am J Surg Pathol. 2009;33:1752–64.
2. Peng YF, Gu J. Synchronous colorectal and lung cancer: report of three cases. World J Gastroenterol. 2008;14:969–73.
3. Tang ER, Schreiner AM, Pua BB. Advances in lung adenocarcinoma classification: a summary of the new international multidis-

ciplinary classification system (IASLC/ATS/ERS). J Thorac Dis. 2014;6(Suppl 5):S489–501.
4. Cahan WG, Shah JP, Castro EB. Benign solitary lung lesions in patients with cancer. Ann Surg. 1978;187(3):241–4.
5. Caparica R, Mak MP, Rocha CH, Velho PHI, Viana P, Moura MRL, et al. Pulmonary nodules in patients with nonpulmonary cancer: not always metastases. J Glob Oncol. 2016;2:138–44.
6. Hanamiya M, Aoki T, Yamashita Y, Kawanami S, Korogi Y. Frequency and significance of pulmonary nodules on thin-section CT in patients with extrapulmonary malignant neoplasms. Eur J Radiol. 2012;81:152–7.
7. Travis WD, Brambilla E, Nicholson AG, Yatabe Y, Austin JHM, Beasley MB, et al. The 2015 World Health Organization classification of lung tumors: impact of genetic, clinical and radiologic advances since the 2004 classification. J Thorac Oncol. 2015;10(9):1243–60.
8. Chauhan A, Monterroso C, Geradi D. A diagnostic dilemma: metastatic pancreatic adenocarcinoma mimicking organizing pneumonia. Am J Resp Crit Care Med. 2017;195:A6578.
9. Jagirdar J. Application of immunohistochemistry to the diagnosis of primary and metastatic carcinoma to the lung. Arch Pathol Lab Med. 2008;132(3):384–96.
10. Kubba LA, McCluggage WG, Liu J, Malpica A, Euscher ED, Silva EG, et al. Thyroid transcription factor-1 expression in ovarian epithelial neoplasms. Mod Pathol. 2008;21:485–90.
11. Park SY, Kim BH, Kim JH, Lee S, Kang GH. Panels of immunohistochemical markers help determine primary sites of metastatic adenocarcinoma. Arch Pathol Lab Med. 2007;131:1561–7.

19 Metastatic Urothelial Carcinoma Versus Squamous Cell Carcinoma

L. Angelica Lerma, Christopher M. Chandler, and Haodong Xu

Case Presentation

A 70-year-old man is a former smoker (1 pack-year) with a history of chemotherapy and radiation for left tonsillar squamous cell carcinoma 10 years ago, as well as for T2N0M0 high-grade urothelial carcinoma, diagnosed 2 years ago. Recent follow-up chest computed tomography (CT) showed a right apical spiculated, subpleural, solid pulmonary nodule (Fig. 19.1a). A positron-emission tomography (PET) scan showed an abnormal fluorodeoxyglucose (FDG) uptake (SUV max 3.19) corresponding to the nodule (Fig. 19.1b). The imaging findings were interpreted as most consistent with a new primary early stage lung cancer. Therefore, the patient was brought to the operating room for diagnostic and therapeutic wedge resection. Histologic sections of the 1.4 cm lung nodule showed a high-grade carcinoma with nested pattern of growth (Fig. 19.2). No glands, squamous differentiation, or neuroendocrine morphology was present. The major differential diagnosis includes primary poorly differentiated squamous cell carcinoma, metastatic urothelial carcinoma, and metastatic tonsillar squamous cell carci-

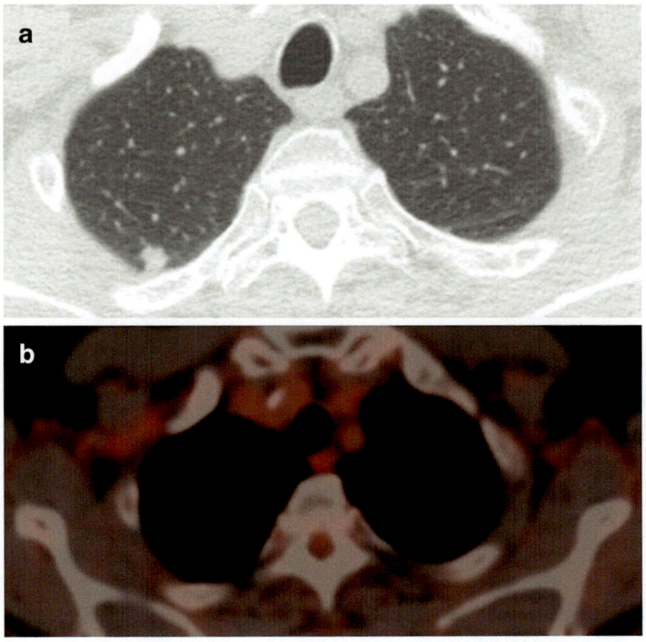

Fig. 19.1 Chest CT showing a subpleural spiculated nodule (**a**) with hypermetabolism on PET (**b**) in the right upper lobe

L. A. Lerma · C. M. Chandler · H. Xu (✉)
Department of Laboratory Medicine and Pathology, University of Washington Medical Center, Seattle, WA, USA
e-mail: xuh8@uw.edu

H. Xu et al. (eds.), *Practical Lung Pathology*, Practical Anatomic Pathology, https://doi.org/10.1007/978-3-031-14402-8_19

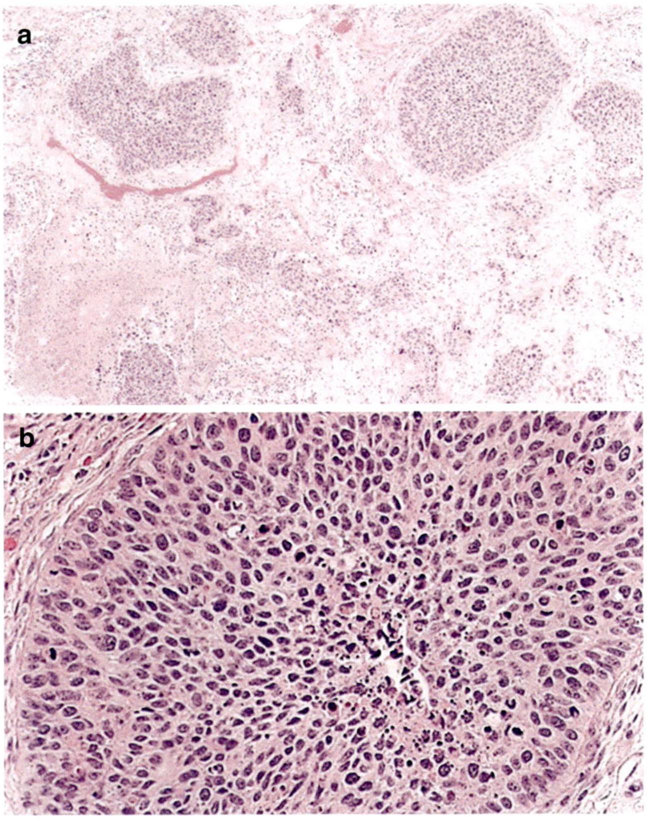

Fig. 19.2 Metastatic high-grade urothelial carcinoma. Histologic sections show a high-grade carcinoma with a nested pattern of growth (H&E, (**a**) 100× and (**b**) 400×)

noma. Slides from the two prior carcinomas were not available for comparison. Immunohistochemical stains showed that the neoplastic cells are positive for p40, GATA3, and uroplakin II (Fig. 19.3), but negative for p16. Based on the clinical history, histologic features, and immunohistochemical staining pattern, the diagnosis of metastatic high-grade urothelial carcinoma was rendered.

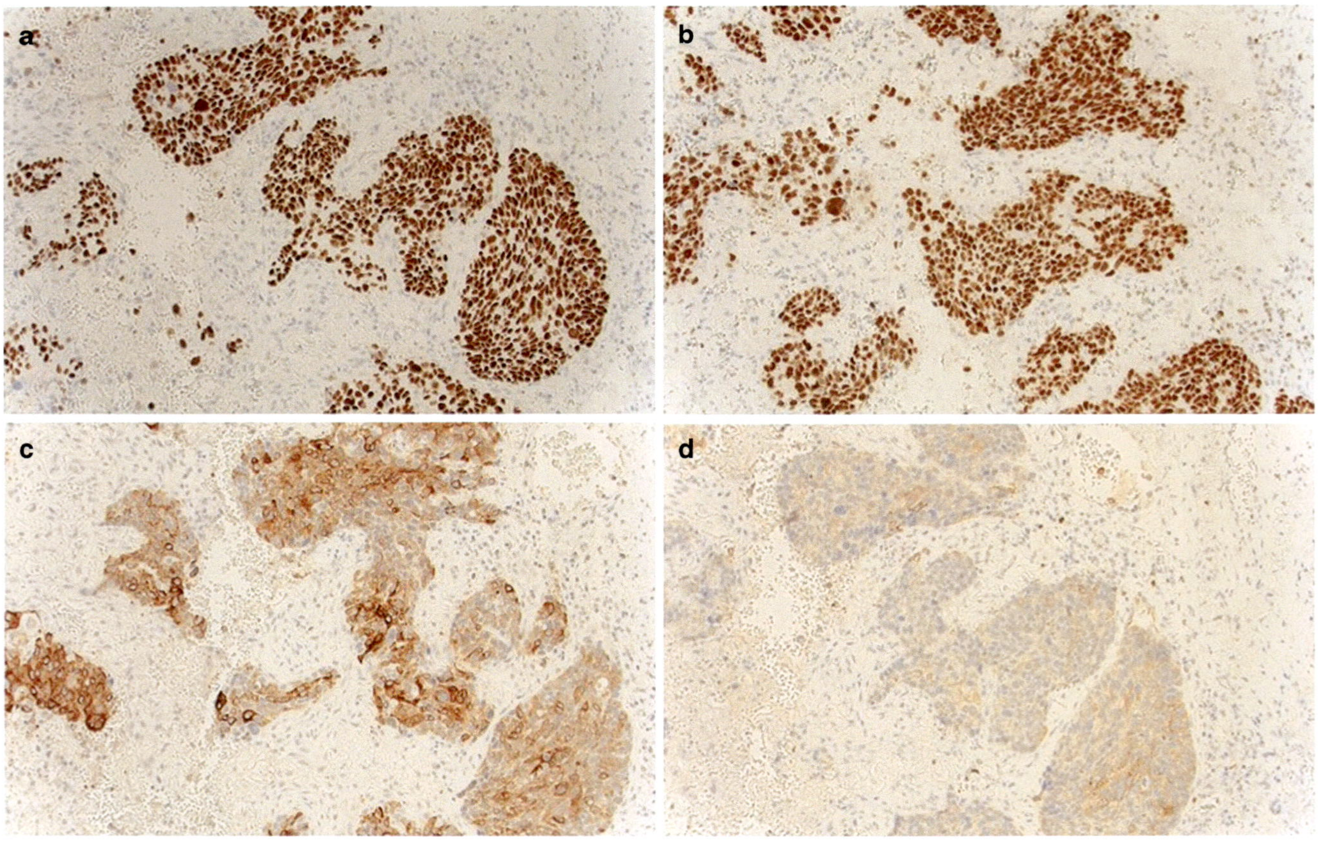

Fig. 19.3 Metastatic urothelial carcinoma with a characteristic immunohistochemical staining pattern. The neoplastic cells are positive for p40, GATA3, and uroplakin II (**a**, **b**, and **c** IHC 200×), and they are negative for p16 (**d** IHC, 200×)

Final Pathologic Diagnosis: Metastatic High-Grade Urothelial Carcinoma

What Are the Clinical, Radiologic, and Prognostic Features of Primary Squamous Cell Carcinoma of the Lung?

Lung cancer is the second most common cancer in women and men, of which squamous cell carcinoma comprises 30% of all cases [1, 2]. Pulmonary squamous cell carcinoma (pSCC) causes approximately 400,000 deaths annually around the world and is strongly associated with cigarette smoking (98% of patients) [3]. The risk of pSCC increases 10% per year of smoking and decreases at a rate of 11% per year upon cessation [4]. Clinical symptoms may include shortness of breath and chest pain [2].

The classic radiologic finding of pSCC is a centrally located, spiculated mass with or without cavitation involving lobar or segmental bronchi [2]. However, central lesions account for 43–65% of cases, and therefore pSCC should be considered in the differential of peripheral lesions [5, 6]. Koenigkam et al. describe lobulated margins as the predominant feature in the plurality of pSCCs [5]. Wang et al. reported the presence of mediastinal and ipsilateral hilar lymphadenopathy in 65% and 50% of central SCCs of the lung, in a series of 95 cases [7]. On the other hand, contralateral lung metastasis, contralateral hilar lymphadenopathy, and pleural nodules were fairly uncommon occurrences (6%, 3%, and 5%, respectively) [7].

The most important prognostic marker in pSCC is the pathologic stage. 5-year overall survival of all non-small-cell carcinomas is >77% for clinical stage IA disease, while it is <10% in patients with clinical stage IV disease [8]. Performance status at diagnosis is also correlated with overall survival [9]. Although only between 9% and 25% of tumors display cavitation on CT, it is a negative predictor of survival, independent of the TNM stage [5, 7, 10].

Patients with Muir-Torre, von Hippel-Lindau, and dysplastic nevus syndrome have an increased incidence of pSCC [6].

What Are the Clinical, Radiologic, and Prognostic Features of Metastatic Urothelial Carcinoma?

At the time of diagnosis, urothelial carcinoma (UC) patients are men in their seventh and eighth decade of life who present with painless hematuria as a first symptom of localized disease; however, 3.1% of patients are younger than 44 years of age at the time of diagnosis [11]. Overall, approximately 20% of cases have metastatic disease at the time of presentation, most commonly to regional lymph nodes [12, 13]. Distant metastases most frequently involve the lymph nodes, lung, liver, and bone [11, 14]. Rarely, patients with metastatic UC present with hemoptysis, dyspnea, and cough as a consequence of endobronchial metastases, cavitary metastases, or pulmonary tumor emboli [15, 16]. Stowell et al. reported a case of metastatic UC presenting as pleuritic chest pain as a result of a pneumothorax secondary to a cavitary metastasis [14].

Typically, lung involvement is identified by radiologic staging. In the lung parenchyma, metastatic UC may present as interstitial micronodules, multifocal nodules, or a single lesion, which may have cavitation in up to 4% of cases [15, 17]. Pleural metastases are present in 11% of cases [15].

Cisplatinum-based chemotherapy is the mainstay of treatment for metastatic disease, which is given to approximately half of patients [12, 13]. Approximately one quarter of patients with metastatic bladder cancer receive radiation treatment [13]. Even with current treatment options, the overall 5-year survival of patients with metastatic urothelial carcinoma is only 9.5% in the United States [13]. Luzzi et al. describe a series of 69 patients who underwent lung lobectomy with curative intent. In this study, patients with metastases of less than 3 cm had a 5-year survival of 59% vs. 33% for those patients with larger tumors [18].

What Are the Gross Examination Features of Lung SCC?

The tumors are gray-white, friable masses, frequently growing along the wall of the bronchus or into the lumen. Sectioning can range from firm to central necrosis with or without cavitation [2, 6].

What Are the Histologic Features of Lung SCC?

Squamous cell carcinomas resemble architecturally disorganized squamous epithelium. Tumor cells variably lack maturation, although most tumors can have areas of differentiation, in which keratinization is a prominent feature. Cytologically, an increased nuclear-to-cytoplasmic ratio, hyperchromatic nuclei, and atypical mitotic figures are readily apparent. SCC stains for p40, p63, CK5/6, EMA, and CEA by immunohistochemistry. Negative immunohistochemical stains include TTF-1 and napsin-A. Chu et al. report that 23% of pSCC can be positive for CK7. Of these, staining with p40 is more specific than p63 [19].

What Are the Gross Examination Features of Metastatic UC?

Of bladder cancers with metastasis, between 37% and 45% involve the lungs [20, 21]. The pattern of metastatic disease varies but is classically multiple nodules of varying sizes involving the bilateral lungs (Fig. 19.4). However, a single site of metastasis is not uncommon [6], as seen in our case.

What Are the Histologic Features of Metastatic UC?

Urothelial carcinoma has many different morphologies, although 90% of tumors are predominantly transitional cell carcinoma with areas of divergent differentiation [13, 15]. Classic UC is composed of pleomorphic cells and significant nuclear atypia [22]. The architecture can vary greatly, including nests, solid growth, and papillary architecture (Fig. 19.4). However, a subset of cells with squamous differentiation can be seen in up to 60% of UCs [23, 24].

How Does One Differentiate Between Metastatic UC and SCC?

Histologically, the features of metastatic UC and SCC often overlap. As mentioned, up to 60% of UCs can have squamous differentiation [23–25]. However, identification of squamous cell carcinoma in situ reliably indicates primary lung origin (Fig. 19.5). On fine-needle aspiration, cercariform cells (racket-form cells with eccentric nuclei, intranuclear inclusions, and small vacuoles in the cytoplasmic extensions) are encountered in UC and rarely in SCC [26]. Waxy metaplastic cytoplasm, dark pyknotic nuclei, and spindle cells on cytological preparations favor SCC [27].

Gruver et al. proposed a panel consisting of CK7, CK20, GATA3, uroplakin III, CK14, and desmoglein-3. Of these, uroplakin III demonstrated no staining in lung SCC; however, only 25% of UC metastases in the lung were positive for this marker [25]. Uroplakins are relatively specific immunohistochemical markers of urothelial differentiation but have recently been described as cross-reacting in breast carcinomas with apocrine differentiation and ovarian Brenner tumors [25, 28–30]. Uroplakin II has a sensitivity of approximately 53% and 73% in invasive and metastatic UC, respectively [31, 32]. Uroplakin III is less sensitive (25–36% metastatic UC) [25, 32].

Although the sensitivity of GATA3 in urothelial carcinoma is between 67 and 91%, there are some reports of reactivity in up to 23% of lung squamous cell carcinomas [22, 25, 33]. Of note, CK20 is rarely expressed in lung SCC (0–3%) and frequently found in pulmonary metastasis of UC (40–62%) [19, 25, 34]. CK7 has a similar profile, ranging from 0% to 7% in pSCC and from 88% to 100% in UC metastases [19, 25, 30, 35].

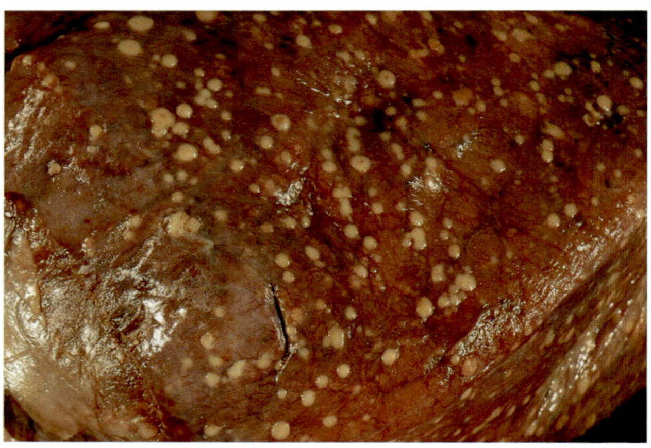

Fig. 19.4 Micronodules of metastatic urothelial carcinoma. Gross photograph of the pleural surface of a lung collected at the time of autopsy with innumerable micronodules of metastatic urothelial carcinoma

What Is the Prognosis of Metastatic Urothelial Cell Carcinoma and Primary Lung Squamous Cell Carcinoma?

UC at an advanced stage (including metastatic disease) has a median overall survival of 7.3 months with multiagent chemotherapy and 10.1 months with the use of checkpoint blockade agents [36]. The prognosis for squamous cell carcinoma of the lung varies greatly depending on stage; the American Cancer Society reports greater than 45% five-year survival for stage I disease and <1% in stage IV disease [1].

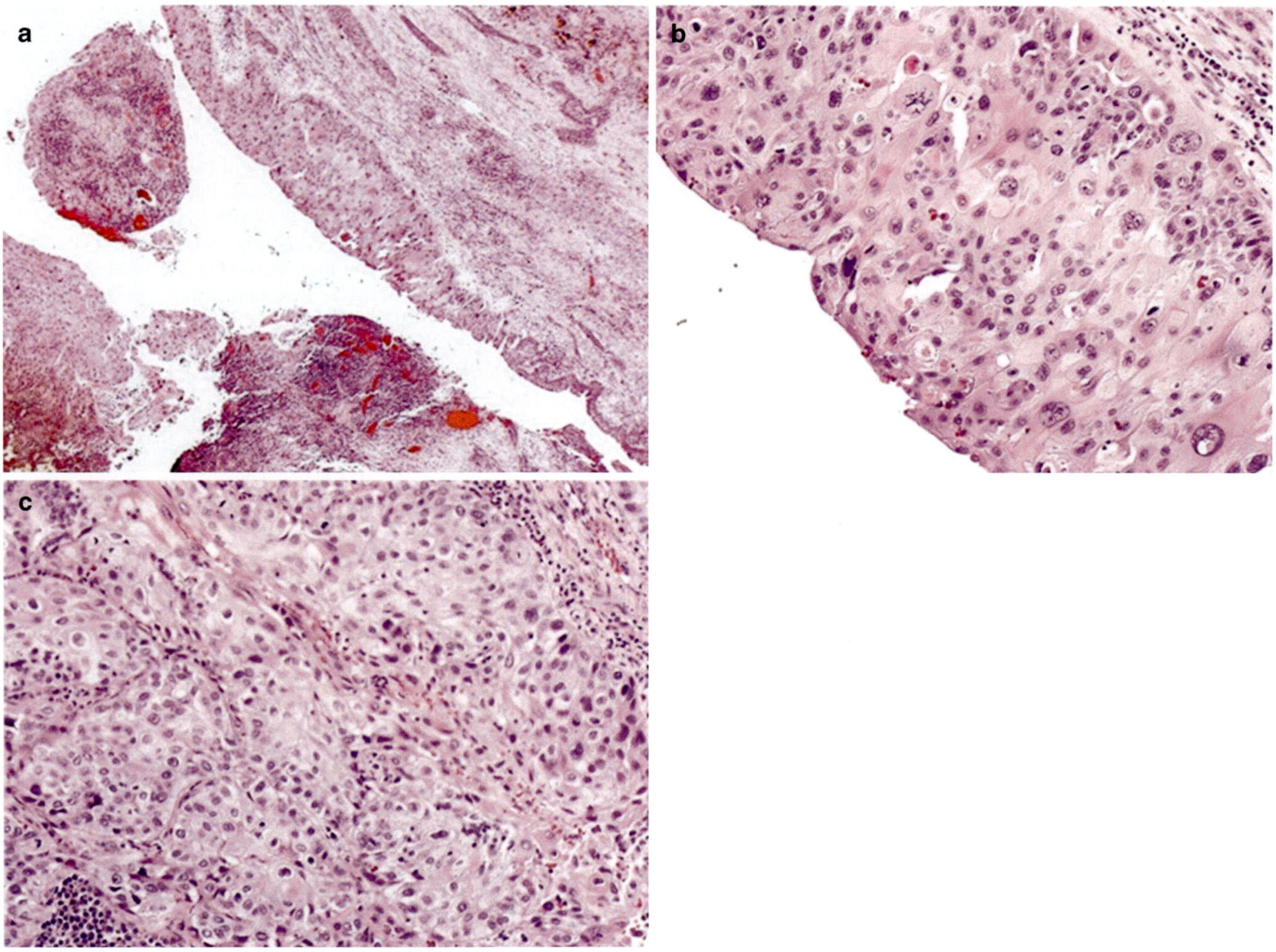

Fig. 19.5 Invasive squamous cell carcinoma of the lung is associated with carcinoma in situ. (**a**) Squamous cell carcinoma in situ in a bronchiole characterized by thickened, stratified squamous epithelium with disorganized, crowded, and atypical cells. (**b**) Squamous cell carcinoma in situ with pleomorphic squamous cells with increased nuclear-to-cytoplasmic ratios and mitotic figure. (**c**) Nearby invasive squamous cell carcinoma. H&E, (**a**) 100×; (**b**) 400×; (**c**) 200×

References

1. Siegel RL, Miller KD, Jemal A. Cancer statistics, 2019. CA Cancer J Clin. 2019;69(1):7–34. Available from: https://onlinelibrary.wiley.com/doi/abs/10.3322/caac.21551
2. Zander DS, Farver CF, editors. Pulmonary pathology. Philadelphia, PA: Elsevier; 2018. p. 759. (Foundations in diagnostic pathology)
3. Cancer Genome Atlas Network. Comprehensive genomic characterization of squamous cell lung cancers. Nature. 2012;489(7417):519–25.
4. Kenfield SA, Wei EK, Stampfer MJ, Rosner BA, Colditz GA. Comparison of aspects of smoking among four histologic types of lung cancer. Tob Control. 2008;17(3):198–204.
5. Koenigkam Santos M, Muley T, Warth A, de Paula WD, Lederlin M, Schnabel PA, et al. Morphological computed tomography features of surgically resectable pulmonary squamous cell carcinomas: impact on prognosis and comparison with adenocarcinomas. Eur J Radiol. 2014;83(7):1275–81.
6. Leslie KO, Wick MR. Practical Pulmonary Pathology E-Book: a Diagnostic Approach. London: Churchill Livingstone; 2011.
7. Wang Z, Li M, Huang Y, Ma L, Zhu H, Kong L, et al. Clinical and radiological characteristics of central pulmonary adenocarcinoma: a comparison with central squamous cell carcinoma and small cell lung cancer and the impact on treatment response. Onco Targets Ther. 2018;11:2509–17.
8. Goldstraw P, Chansky K, Crowley J, Rami-Porta R, Asamura H, Eberhardt WEE, et al. The IASLC lung cancer staging project: proposals for revision of the TNM stage groupings in the forthcoming (eighth) edition of the TNM classification for lung cancer. J Thorac Oncol. 2016;11(1):39–51.
9. Travis WD. Weltgesundheitsorganisation. In: International Agency for Research on Cancer, editor. WHO classification of tumours of lung, pleura, thymus and heart: ... reflects the views of a working group that convened for a consensus and editorial meeting at the International Agency for Research on Cancer, Lyon, April 24–26, 2014. 4. Lyon: International Agency for Research on Cancer; 2015. p. 412. (World Health Organization Classification of tumours).

10. Kolodziejski LS, Dyczek S, Duda K, Góralczyk J, Wysocki WM, Lobaziewicz W. Cavitated tumor as a clinical subentity in squamous cell lung cancer patients. Neoplasma. 2003;50(1):66–73.
11. Wong-You-Cheong JJ, Woodward PJ, Manning MA, Sesterhenn IA. From the archives of the AFIP: neoplasms of the urinary bladder: radiologic-pathologic correlation. Radiographics. 2006;26(2):553–80.
12. Svatek RS, Siefker-Radtke A, Dinney CP. Management of metastatic urothelial cancer: the role of surgery as an adjunct to chemotherapy. Can Urol Assoc J. 2009;3(6 Suppl 4):S228–31.
13. Royce TJ, Lin CC, Gray PJ, Shipley WU, Jemal A, Efstathiou JA. Clinical characteristics and outcomes of nonurothelial cell carcinoma of the bladder: results from the National Cancer Data Base. Urol Oncol. 2018;36(2):78.e1–78.e12.
14. Stowell JT, Betancourt-Cuellar SL, Carter BW, Wu CC, Walker CM. Thoracic manifestations of genitourinary neoplasms and treatment-related complications. J Thorac Imaging. 2019;34(3):W36–48.
15. Agrawal A, Sahni S, Vulisha AK, Gumpeni R, Shah R, Talwar A. Pulmonary manifestations of urothelial carcinoma of the bladder. Respir Med. 2017;128:65–9.
16. Rovirosa A, Salud A, Felip E, Capdevila F, Giralt J, Bellmunt J. Cavitary pulmonary metastases in transitional cell carcinoma of the urinary bladder. Urol Int. 1992;48(1):102–4.
17. Babaian RJ, Johnson DE, Llamas L, Ayala AG. Metastases from transitional cell carcinoma of urinary bladder. Urology. 1980;16(2):142–4.
18. Luzzi L, Marulli G, Solli P, Cardillo G, Ghisalberti M, Mammana M, et al. Long-term results and prognostic factors of pulmonary Metastasectomy in patients with metastatic transitional cell carcinoma. Thorac Cardiovasc Surg. 2017;65(7):567–71.
19. Chu P, Wu E, Weiss LM. Cytokeratin 7 and cytokeratin 20 expression in epithelial neoplasms: a survey of 435 cases. Mod Pathol. 2000;13(9):962–72.
20. Shinagare AB, Ramaiya NH, Jagannathan JP, Fennessy FM, Taplin M-E, Van den Abbeele AD. Metastatic pattern of bladder cancer: correlation with the characteristics of the primary tumor. Am J Roentgenol. 2011;196(1):117–22. Available from: http://www.ajronline.org/doi/10.2214/AJR.10.5036
21. Wallmeroth A, Wagner U, Moch H, Gasser TC, Sauter G, Mihatsch MJ. Patterns of metastasis in muscle-invasive bladder cancer (pT2–4): an autopsy study on 367 patients. Urol Int. 1999;62(2):69–75.
22. Chang A, Amin A, Gabrielson E, Illei P, Roden RB, Sharma R, et al. Utility of GATA3 immunohistochemistry in differentiating urothelial carcinoma from prostate adenocarcinoma and squamous cell carcinomas of the uterine cervix, anus, and lung. Am J Surg Pathol. 2012;36(10):1472–6.
23. Lagwinski N, Thomas A, Stephenson A, Campbell S, Hoschar A, El-Gabry E, et al. Squamous cell carcinoma of the bladder: a clinicopathologic analysis of 45 cases. Am J Surg Path. 2007;31(12):1777–87.
24. Izard JP, Siemens DR, Mackillop WJ, Wei X, Leveridge MJ, Berman DM, et al. Outcomes of squamous histology in bladder cancer: a population-based study. Urol Oncol. 2015;33(10):425.e7–13.
25. Gruver AM, Amin MB, Luthringer DJ, Westfall D, Arora K, Farver CF, et al. Selective immunohistochemical markers to distinguish between metastatic high-grade urothelial carcinoma and primary poorly differentiated invasive squamous cell carcinoma of the lung. Arch Pathol Lab Med. 2012;136(11):1339–46.
26. Vural Ç, Yildiz K, Çabuk D, Akgül A. Transthoracic fine-needle aspiration cytology of non-invasive, low-grade urothelial carcinoma with lung metastasis: a case report with review of the literature. J Cytol. 2015;32(2):132–5.
27. Kaur G, Bakshi P, Verma K. Fine needle aspiration cytology of metastatic urothelial carcinoma: study of seven cases with review of literature. J Cytol. 2012;29(2):116–20.
28. Yatabe Y, Dacic S, Borczuk AC, Warth A, Russell PA, Lantuejoul S, et al. Best practices recommendations for diagnostic immunohistochemistry in lung cancer. J Thorac Oncol. 2019;14(3):377–407.
29. Tajima S, Koda K. Uroplakin II expression in breast carcinomas showing apocrine differentiation: putting some emphasis on invasive pleomorphic lobular carcinoma as a potential mimic of urothelial carcinoma at metastatic sites. Dis Markers. 2016;2016:2940496.
30. Logani S, Oliva E, Amin MB, Folpe AL, Cohen C, Young RH. Immunoprofile of ovarian tumors with putative transitional cell (urothelial) differentiation using novel urothelial markers: histogenetic and diagnostic implications. Am J Surg Pathol. 2003;27(11):1434–41.
31. Tian W, Guner G, Miyamoto H, Cimino-Mathews A, Gonzalez-Roibon N, Argani P, et al. Utility of uroplakin II expression as a marker of urothelial carcinoma. Hum Pathol. 2015;46(1):58–64.
32. Smith SC, Mohanty SK, Kunju LP, Chang E, Chung F, Carvalho JC, et al. Uroplakin II outperforms uroplakin III in diagnostically challenging settings. Histopathology. 2014;65(1):132–8.
33. Miettinen M, McCue PA, Sarlomo-Rikala M, Rys J, Czapiewski P, Wazny K, et al. GATA3: a multispecific but potentially useful marker in surgical pathology: a systematic analysis of 2500 epithelial and nonepithelial tumors. Am J Surg Pathol. 2014;38(1):13–22.
34. Parker D, Folpe A, Bell J, Oliva E, Young R, Cohen C, et al. Potential utility of uroplakin III, thrombomodulin, high molecular weight cytokeratin, and cytokeratin 20 in noninvasive, invasive, and metastatic urothelial (transitional cell) carcinomas. Am J Surg Pathol. 2003;27(1):1–10.
35. Jiang J, Ulbright TM, Younger C, Sanchez K, Bostwick DG, Koch MO, et al. Cytokeratin 7 and cytokeratin 20 in primary urinary bladder carcinoma and matched lymph node metastasis. Arch Pathol Lab Med. 2001;125(7):921–3.
36. Teo MY, Iyer G. The landscape of immunotherapy in metastatic urothelial carcinoma. Curr Opin Urol. 2019;29(6):643–8.

Thymic Carcinoma Versus Lung Squamous Cell Carcinoma

20

Jennifer J. Chia and Gregory A. Fishbein

Case Presentation

A 55-year-old male non-smoker presented with 15-pound weight loss and 3 months of progressive mild chest pressure, shortness of breath, and dry cough. He also endorsed intermittent fevers over the last 2 weeks. Physical examination showed no cervical or axillary lymphadenopathy. A chest X-ray showed a large mediastinal mass. Chest computed tomography (CT) demonstrated a mass located in the anterior mediastinum with extension to the right lung (Fig. 20.1). An initial biopsy was interpreted as poorly differentiated squamous cell carcinoma, which could represent thymic squamous cell carcinoma invading the lung or pulmonary squamous cell carcinoma invading the anterior mediastinum. A thymectomy with pulmonary segmentectomy was performed.

The resection specimen contained a red-tan, smooth, firm mass measuring 6.3 cm in greatest dimension (Fig. 20.2) and directly underlying an attached portion of the lung. Cut surfaces showed a white-tan, friable mass with central hemorrhage and necrosis (not pictured).

Histologic examination of the mass demonstrated an infiltrative epithelial neoplasm with subtle squamous features including focal dyskeratotic cells, intercellular bridges, and focal keratinization (Fig. 20.3). Immunohistochemical stains (Fig. 20.4) were strongly positive for p40 and PAX8, supporting thymic origin. CD117 and CD5 were also positive. These findings were ultimately classified as thymic carcinoma.

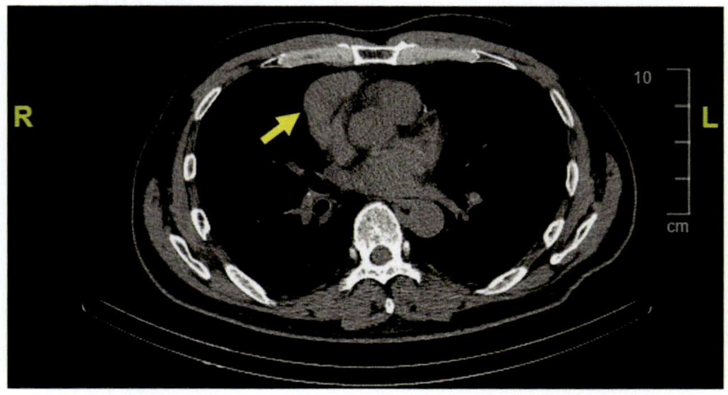

Fig. 20.1 CT without contrast showing a solid anterior mediastinal mass with extension to the right lung (arrow)

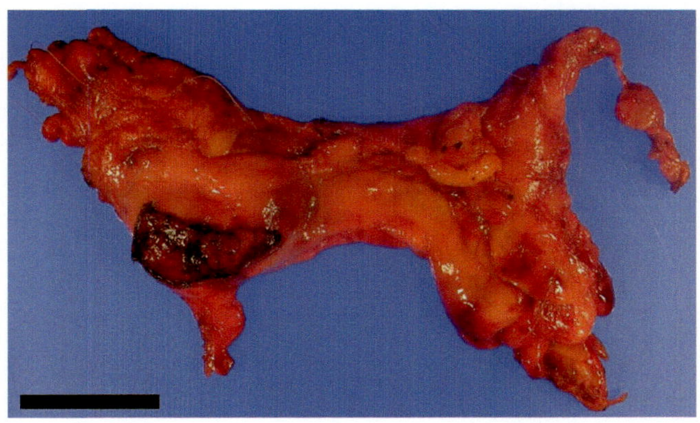

Fig. 20.2 Gross photograph demonstrating the anterior mediastinal resection with mass underlying the adherent portion of the lung. Scale bar represents 4 cm

J. J. Chia · G. A. Fishbein (✉)
Department of Pathology and Laboratory Medicine, David Geffen School of Medicine at UCLA, Los Angeles, CA, USA
e-mail: gfishbein@mednet.ucla.edu

H. Xu et al. (eds.), *Practical Lung Pathology*, Practical Anatomic Pathology, https://doi.org/10.1007/978-3-031-14402-8_20

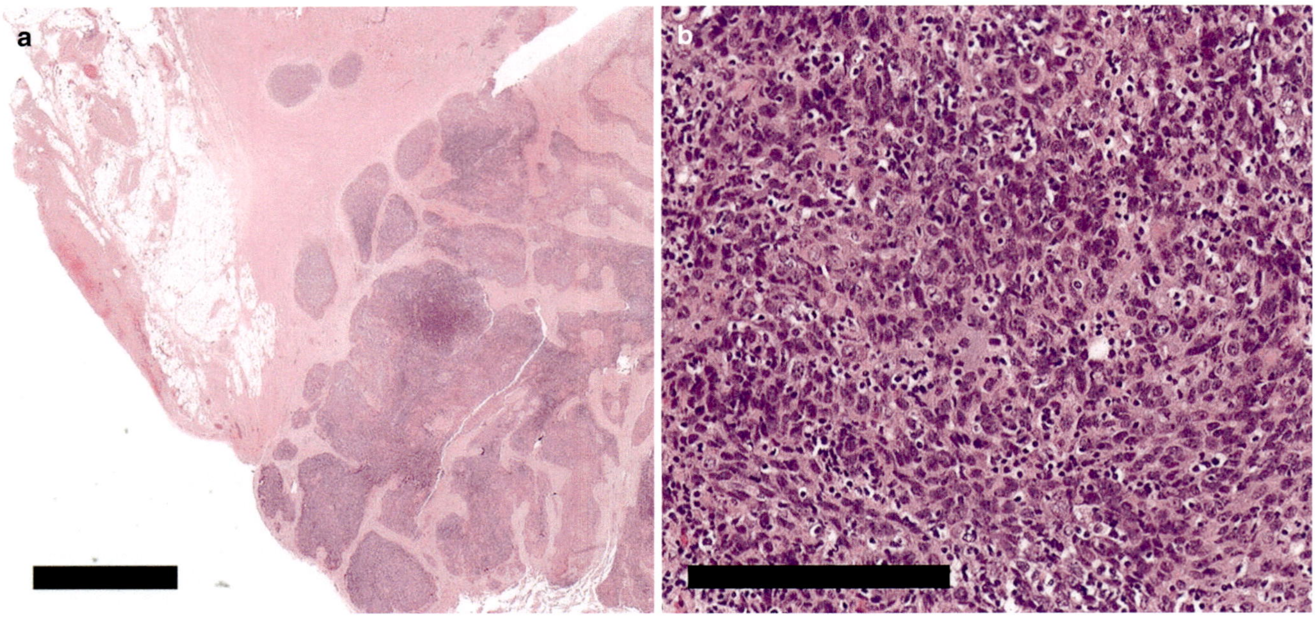

Fig. 20.3 Histologic evaluation of the thymic mass. (**a**) At low power, the normal thymic architecture is replaced by cohesive sheets and islands of tumor cells with predominantly smooth contours infiltrating into the surrounding soft tissue. Scale bar represents 2 mm. (**b**) At medium power, the tumor cells are moderately pleomorphic with dense eosinophilic cytoplasm and subtle keratinization. There are scattered admixed lymphocytes. Scale bar represents 200 μm

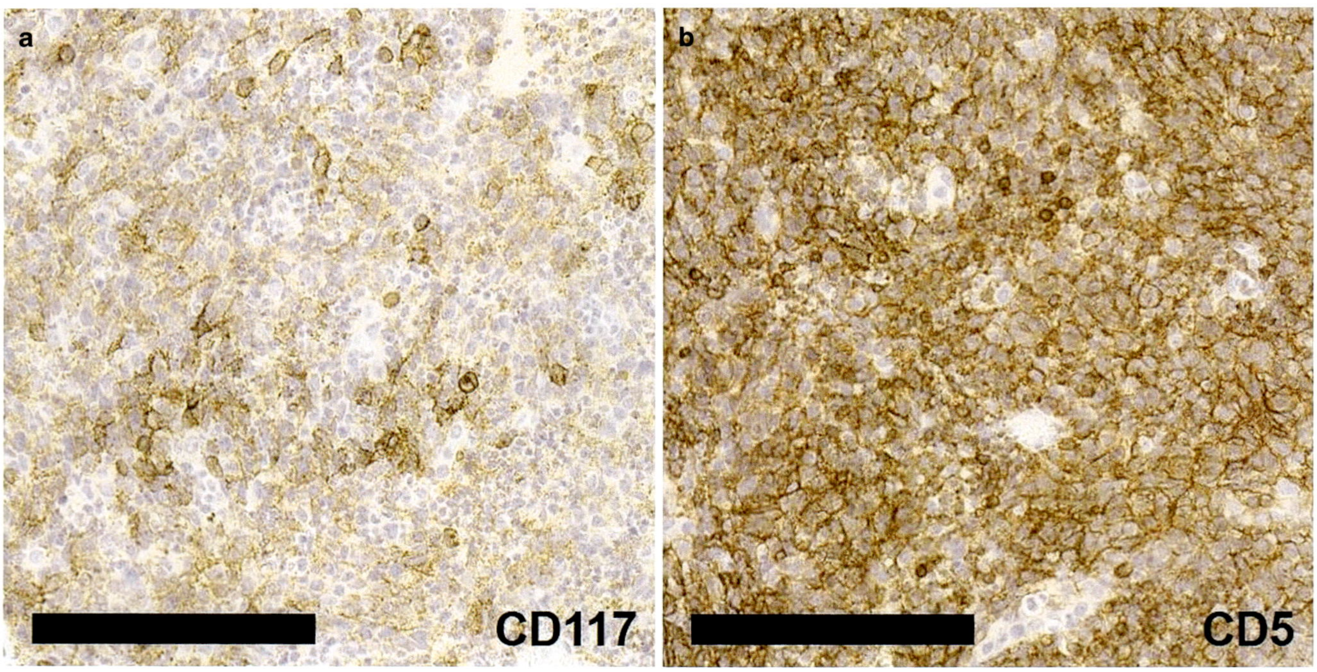

Fig. 20.4 Immunohistologic evaluation of the thymic mass. (**a**) CD117 (cKit) demonstrates patchy membrane staining. (**b**) CD5 demonstrates diffuse membrane staining. (**c**) PAX8 demonstrates diffuse nuclear staining, consistent with thymic origin. (**d**) p40 demonstrates diffuse nuclear staining, consistent with squamous differentiation. Scale bar represents 200 μm

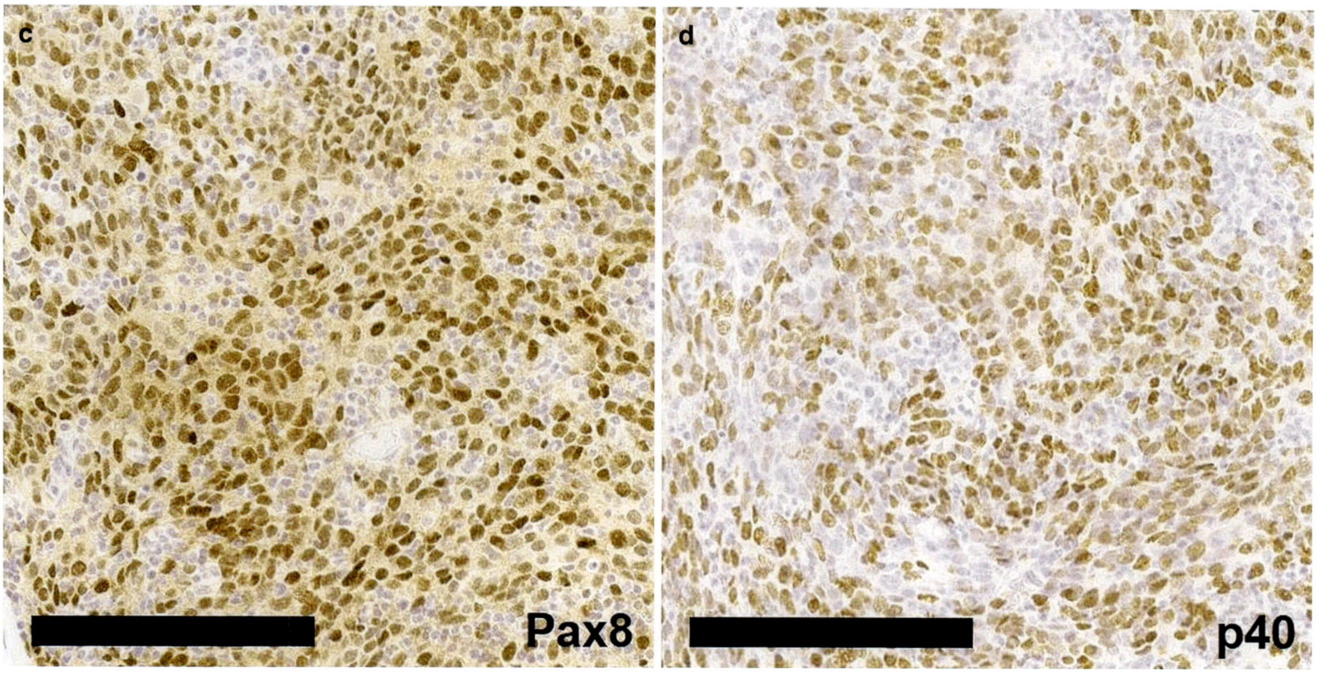

Fig. 20.4 (continued)

Final Diagnosis: Thymic Squamous Cell Carcinoma

Key Points for Differentiating Thymic Carcinoma Versus Lung Squamous Cell Carcinoma

How Do the Clinical Presentations of Patients with Thymic Carcinoma and Lung Squamous Cell Carcinoma Differ?

Patients with thymic carcinoma may be of any age, and there is no association with environmental risk factors (Table 20.1). In contrast, patients with squamous cell carcinoma of the lung tend to be older (>65 years) and are almost always smokers. The symptoms of thymic carcinoma are not specific but are usually related to compression of adjacent mediastinal structures by mass effect.

Are Imaging Features, Including Localization, Helpful in Determining the Origin of the Tumor?

Yes. The radiographic localization can be helpful, especially when an endobronchial component is identified. The presence of an endobronchial component strongly supports a primary lung squamous cell carcinoma (Figs. 20.5 and 20.6).

Table 20.1 Comparison of clinical features of thymic carcinoma and lung squamous cell carcinomas [1, 2]

Clinical features	Thymic carcinoma	Lung SCC
Age at presentation	Any, sixth decade most common	Predominantly >65 years
Signs and symptoms	Asymptomatic or mediastinal compression: Chest pain, cough, shortness of breath	Variable: May include progressive shortness of breath, cough, chest pain/pressure, hoarseness, hemoptysis; occasionally asymptomatic
Environmental factors	No association with tobacco smoke or other environmental factors	Tobacco smoke

SCC squamous cell carcinoma

Does Histology Alone Distinguish Between Thymic and Lung Squamous Cell Carcinoma?

No. Histology alone does not reliably distinguish these two entities. Thymic carcinoma can have a variety of histologic phenotypes, although 70% exhibits squamous differentiation [1]. Invasive squamous cell carcinoma of the lung will often have a moderately differentiated appearance, while those originating in the thymus tend to be more poorly differenti-

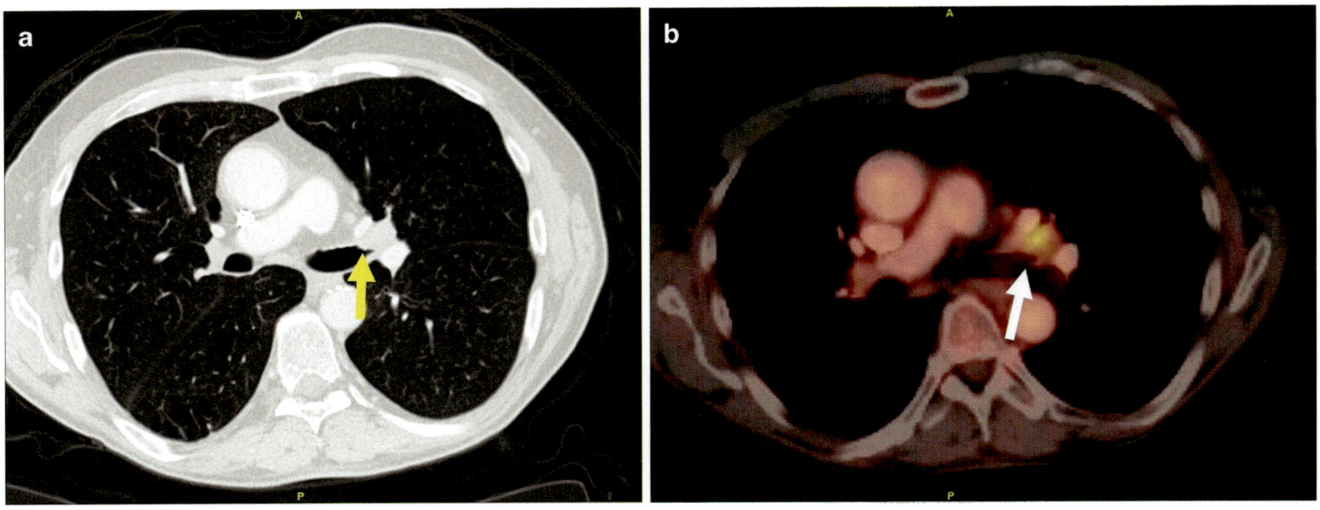

Fig. 20.5 Radiologic findings in lung squamous cell carcinoma. (**a**) CT with contrast demonstrated an enhancing, endobronchial mass (arrow). (**b**) PET-CT demonstrating FDG-avidity of the endobronchial mass (arrow)

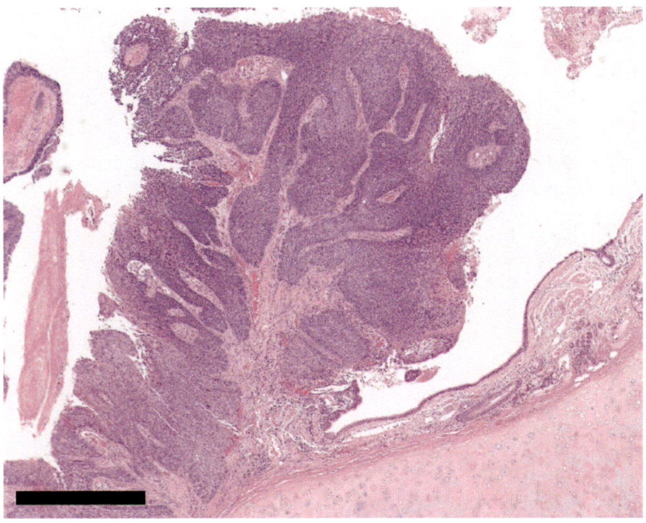

Fig. 20.6 Endobronchial component of lung squamous cell carcinoma. Scale bars represent 800 μm

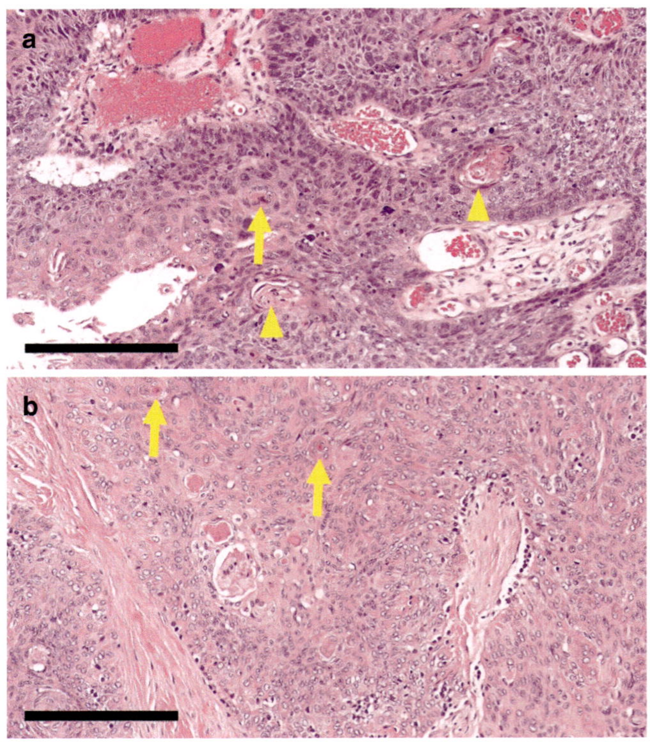

Fig. 20.7 Histologic comparison of lung squamous cell carcinoma and thymic carcinoma at medium power. (**a**) Lung squamous cell carcinoma with dyskeratotic cells (arrow), keratin pearls (arrow heads), and necrosis. (**b**) Thymic carcinoma invading the lung with abrupt keratinization (arrows). Scale bars represent 200 μm

ated with only focal keratinization and vague intercellular bridges (Fig. 20.7).

Extensive necrosis can be seen in both entities. The invasive, pushing borders of thymic carcinoma may be more rounded than in lung squamous cell carcinoma. However, this is not a reliable feature for diagnosis.

Can Immunohistochemistry Distinguish Between Thymic and Lung SCC?

Yes. In general, there are no immunohistochemical markers that can distinguish squamous carcinoma of the lung from squamous cell carcinoma originating from a distant site. The exception is the thymus. Squamous cell carcinoma from any site will usually be immunoreactive to high-molecular-weight cytokeratins (e.g., CK5/6), p63, and p40. However, the majority of thymic epithelial neoplasms, including thymic squamous cell carcinoma, also express PAX8. In addition, thymic squamous cell carcinoma tends to express CD5 and CD117. These markers can help distinguish thymic squamous cell carcinoma from squamous cell carcinoma of lung origin (Table 20.2). That said, the importance of radiographic localization cannot be overstated. The mass location, extent of invasion, and other radiographic features should also be taken into consideration. (Table 20.3) Both thymic carcinoma and lung squamous cell carcinoma have a propensity for local invasion; thus, a scenario in which squamous cell carcinoma is present in adjacent lung and thymic tissue is possible, as in the case presented above. When imaging and gross localization is equivocal, immunohistochemistry can be helpful to determine the primary site.

Does Molecular Testing Help to Distinguish Thymic Carcinoma and Lung SCC?

The pattern of molecular and cytogenetic alterations has been show to differ between thymic carcinoma and lung SCC; however, this has not been widely used diagnostically as the range of possible mutational changes in each of these malignancies is wide and shows some overlap [10]. Frequent chromosomal aberrations found in thymic carcinoma include loss of 16q, 6, 3p, and 17p and gain of 1q, 17q, and 18 [11]. This pattern is different than seen in lung carcinomas, which more frequently demonstrate loss of 3q, 11q, and 8q and gain of 3p, 5q, 9p, and 13q [11]. Thymic carcinomas may demonstrate mutations in *TP53* (20–40%), *KIT* (10%), *EGFR* (2.5%), and *KRAS* (6%); *Her2* gene amplification is relatively rare, found in 0–4% of cases [11–13]. *TP53* is also frequently mutated in lung SCC (>50%). Other common gene mutations found in lung SCC involve *CDK2A*, *PTEN*, *PIK3CA*, *KEAP1*, *MLL2*, *HLA-A*, *NFE2L2*, *NOTCH1*, and *RB1* [14]. Due to the mutagenic effects of cigarette smoke, lung SCC demonstrates a very high tumor mutational burden that is enriched in C>A single-nucleotide substitutions compared to other cancer mutational signatures [15]. While the detection of a tobacco smoking-associated mutational signature by genome or exome sequencing may favor lung origin, these molecular techniques are not typically used to distinguish between thymic carcinoma and lung SSC.

Table 20.2 Comparison of immunophenotype of thymic carcinoma and lung squamous cell carcinoma [1–4]

Immunohistochemistry	Thymic carcinoma	Lung SCC
PAX8	Positive (75%)	Negative
CD5	Positive (74%)	Negative
CD117	Positive (84%)	Negative
p63	Positive	Positive
p40	Positive	Positive
CK5/6	Positive	Positive

SCC squamous cell carcinoma

Table 20.3 Comparison of imaging features of thymic carcinoma and lung squamous cell carcinomas [5–9]

Imaging features	Thymic carcinoma	Lung SCC
Mass location	Anterior mediastinum	Main/lobar bronchus or peripheral
Imaging features	Solid mass with irregular thymic borders; may have necrotic or cystic areas	Solid mass; may have necrotic areas
Local invasion	May invade other mediastinal structures, including the lung	Invasion of bronchi and pleura most common; may extend to mediastinum

SCC squamous cell carcinoma

Squamous Cell Carcinoma Is Present in the Thymus. Could this Be a Metastasis of Primary Lung Squamous Cell Carcinoma?

Metastasis of primary lung SCC to the thymus has not been described, though metastasis of lung *adenocarcinoma* to the thymus has been reported [16]. In this unlikely scenario, immunohistochemistry may be helpful.

Does the Presence of Extra-Thoracic Metastasis Favor SCC of Lung Origin?

No. Thymic SCC can also lead to lymph node and distant metastases. The sites of metastases are similar: the bone, liver, lung, adrenal gland, and brain [2, 17].

Does Thymic SCC Arise from a Pre-existing Thymoma?

Only rarely. Most cases of thymic carcinoma arise without a thymoma component [2, 18]. Similarly, myasthenia gravis is only associated with thymic carcinoma when a thymoma component is present in the tumor [18].

References

1. Zhao Y, Zhao H, Hu D, Fan L, Shi J, Fang W. Surgical treatment and prognosis of thymic squamous cell carcinoma: a retrospective analysis of 105 cases. Ann Thorac Surg. 2013;96:1019–24.
2. Weissferdt A, Moran CA. Thymic carcinoma, part 1: a clinicopathologic and immunohistochemical study of 65 cases. Am J Clin Pathol. 2012;138:103–14.
3. Weissferdt A, Moran CA. Thymic carcinoma associated with multilocular thymic cyst. Am J Surg Pathol. 2011;35:1074–9.
4. Funai K, Yokose T, Ishii G, Araki K, Yoshida J, Nishimura M, et al. Clinicopathologic characteristics of peripheral squamous cell carcinoma of the lung. Am J Surg Pathol. 2003;27:978–84.
5. Hishima T, Fukayama M, Fujisawa M, Hayashi Y, Arai K, Funata N, et al. CD5 expression in thymic carcinoma. Am J Pathol. 1994;145:268–75.
6. Pan C-C, Chen PC-H, Chiang H. KIT(CD117) is frequently overexpressed in thymic carcinomas but is absent in thymomas. J Pathol. 2004;202:375–81.
7. Weissferdt A, Moran CA. Pax8 expression in thymic epithelial neoplasms. Am J Surg Pathol. 2011;35:1305–10.
8. Asirvatham JR, Esposito MJ, Bhuiya TA. Role of PAX-8, CD5, and CD117 in distinguishing thymic carcinoma from poorly differentiated lung carcinoma. Appl Immunohistochem Mol Morphol. 2014;22:372–6.

9. Kriegsmann M, Muley T, Harms A, Tavernar L, Goldmann T, Dienemann H, et al. Differential diagnostic value of CD5 and CD117 expression in thoracic tumors: a large scale study of 1465 non-small cell lung cancer cases. Diagn Pathol. 2015;10:210.
10. Girard N, Shen R, Guo T, Zakowski MF, Heguy A, Riely GJ, et al. Comprehensive genomic analysis reveals clinically relevant molecular distinctions between thymic carcinomas and thymomas. Clin Cancer Res. 2009;15:6790–9.
11. Travis W, Brambilla E, Burke A, Marx A, Nicholson A. WHO classification of Tumours of the lung, pleura, thymus and heart. 4th ed. IARC: Lyon; 2015.
12. Weissferdt A, Wistuba II, Moran CA. Molecular aspects of thymic carcinoma. Lung Cancer. 2012;78:127–32.
13. Perez-Moreno P, Brambilla E, Thomas R, Soria JC. Squamous cell carcinoma of the lung: molecular subtypes and therapeutic opportunities. Clin Cancer Res. 2012;18:2443–51.
14. Cancer Genome Atlas Research Network. Comprehensive genomic characterization of squamous cell lung cancers. Nature. 2012;489:519–25. Available from: http://www.ncbi.nlm.nih.gov/pubmed/22960745
15. Alexandrov LB, Kim J, Haradhvala NJ, Huang MN, Tian Ng AW, Wu Y, et al. The repertoire of mutational signatures in human cancer. Nature. 2020;578:94–101.
16. Demondion P, Validire P, Tredaniel J, Gossot D. Thymic metastasis from lung carcinoma. Interact Cardiovasc Thorac Surg. 2011;12:848–9.
17. Vladislav T, Jain RK, Alvarez R, Mehta RJ, Gökmen-Polar Y, Kesler KA, et al. Extrathoracic metastases of thymic origin: a review of 35 cases. Mod Pathol. 2012;25:370–7.
18. Suster S, Moran CA. Primary thymic epithelial neoplasms showing combined features of thymoma and thymic carcinoma. A clinicopathologic study of 22 cases. Am J Surg Pathol. 1996;20:1469–80.

Pulmonary Epithelioid Hemangioendothelioma Versus Carcinoma and Other Epithelioid Neoplasms

21

John M. Gross and Robert W. Ricciotti

Case Presentation

A healthy 35-year-old nonsmoking female underwent a routine chest radiograph prior to surgery for an elective cholecystectomy. Routine preoperative CBC, BMP, and urinalysis were all within normal limits. A physical examination was unremarkable, and neither family history nor occupational exposures were of any clinical significance. The chest radiograph showed a diffuse bilateral micronodular pulmonary infiltrate. A high-resolution CT scan showed multiple, bilateral small pulmonary nodules. The nodules were present in all lobes and adjacent to bronchioles and medium-sized vessels without associated hilar lymphadenopathy. Surgical lung biopsy revealed epithelioid cells with ample eosinophilic cytoplasm and intracytoplasmic vacuolization in a myxohyaline stroma (Figs. 21.1 and 21.2a,b). Immunohistochemistry revealed strong nuclear reactivity with CAMTA1 (Fig. 21.2c, d) as well as expression of CD34 and ERG (not shown), whereas TTF1, AE1/AE3, and p40 were negative.

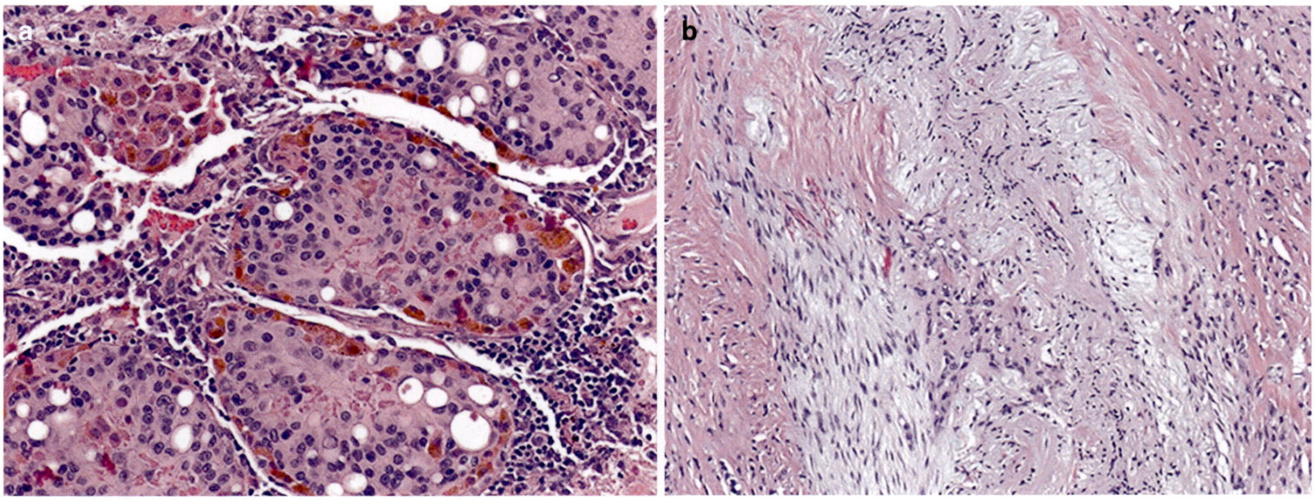

Fig. 21.1 (**a**) Histologic evaluation shows epithelioid cells growing in clusters in an alveolar filling pattern. (**b**) Other areas assume a more spindled pattern in a background myxoid stroma. (**c**) Tumor cells with ample eosinophilic cytoplasm growing in cords and clusters. (**d**) Many cells contain intracytoplasmic vacuoles/lumina with erythrocytes

J. M. Gross
Division of Anatomic Pathology, The Johns Hopkins Medical Institute, Baltimore, MD, USA

R. W. Ricciotti (✉)
Department of Laboratory Medicine and Pathology, University of Washington Medical Center, Seattle, WA, USA
e-mail: ricciott@uw.edu

H. Xu et al. (eds.), *Practical Lung Pathology*, Practical Anatomic Pathology, https://doi.org/10.1007/978-3-031-14402-8_21

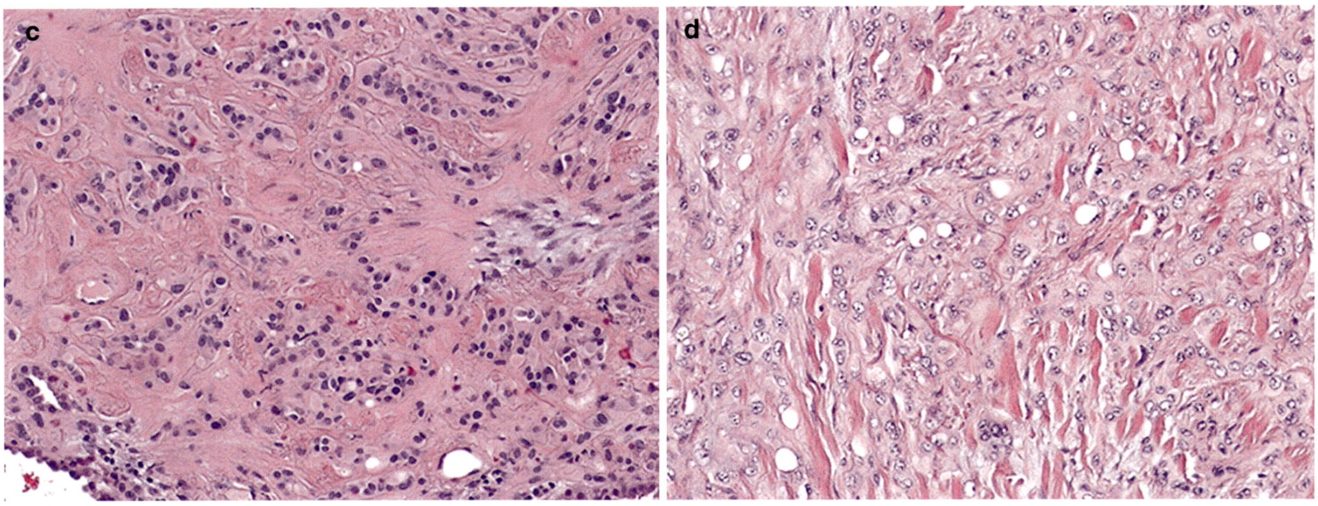

Fig. 21.1 (continued)

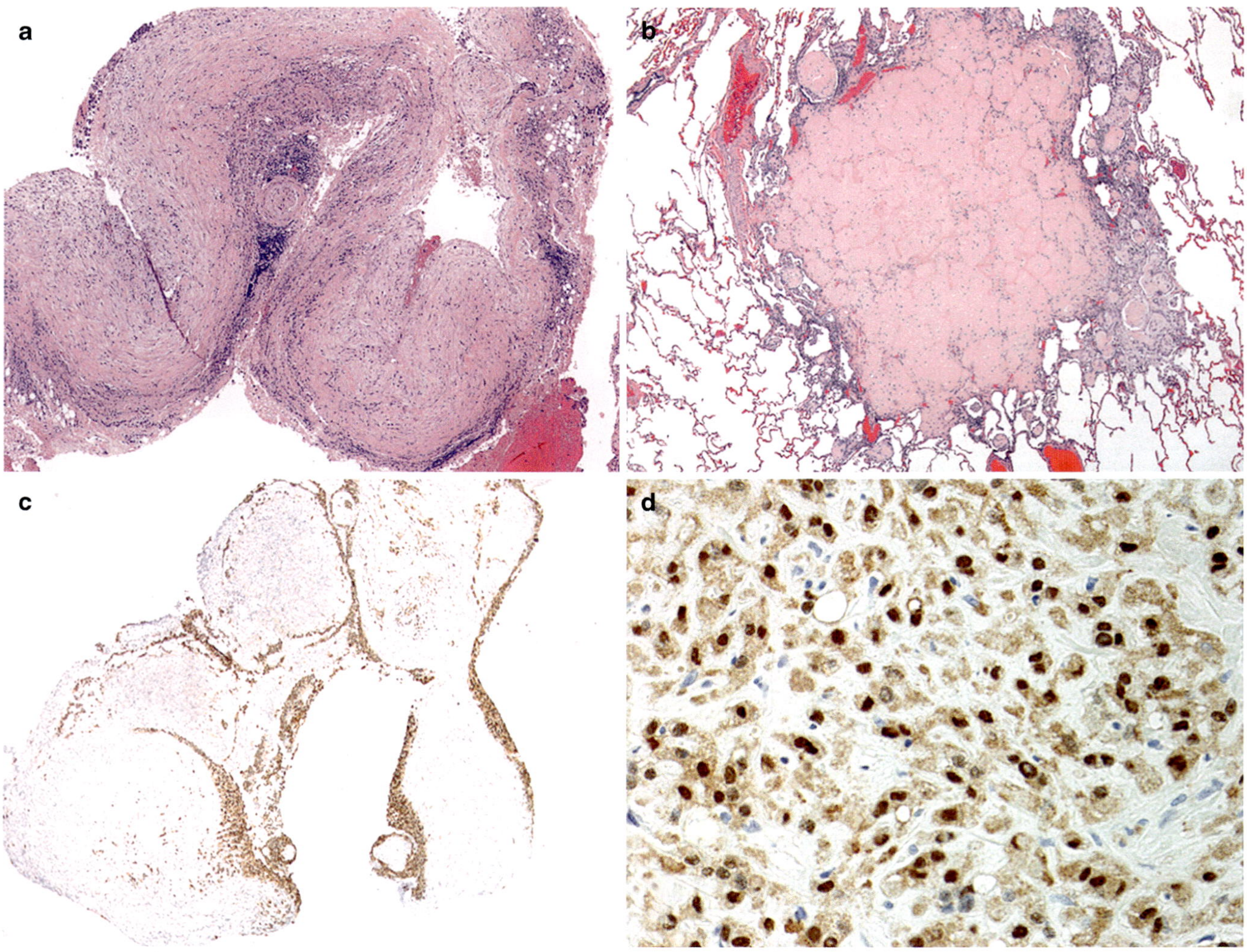

Fig. 21.2 (**a**) Tumor is present along the pleural surface and (**b**) as hyalinized, eosinophilic nodules within the lung parenchyma. (**c**) Immunohistochemistry for CAMTA1 is diffusely positive along the pleural surface. (**d**) Higher power shows the strong nuclear CAMTA1 expression

Final Diagnosis: Pulmonary Epithelioid Hemangioendothelioma

What Is the Definition of Epithelioid Hemangioendothelioma?

EHE is a malignant vascular neoplasm composed of epithelioid endothelial cells in a distinct myxohyaline stroma [1–3]. This neoplasm is characterized by a *WWTR1-CAMTA1* gene fusion [4–7] in >90% of cases and, less commonly, *YAP1-TFE3* fusions [8].

What Are the Epidemiologic Factors?

EHE affects patients of all ages but is most common after the second decade of life with a median age of onset at 38 years. It is especially rare in childhood. For unknown reasons, 60–80% of cases occur in women [1–3].

What Are the Clinical and Radiologic Considerations of Pulmonary Epithelioid Hemangioendothelioma?

EHE most often occurs as a soft tissue or bone tumor; however, primary visceral sites are not uncommon including the liver, lung, and pleura [1–3]. PEHE, including those of pleural origin, account for approximately 20% of cases. Most patients (50–70%) are symptomatic at presentation, with pain being the most common complaint followed by cough, dyspnea, hemoptysis, pleural effusion, and nonspecific systemic symptoms. Radiologic studies most often show multiple bilateral perivascular nodules (less than 2 cm) with either well or poorly defined borders. These findings are commonly misinterpreted as representing metastatic carcinoma or granulomas. A minority of patients present with a solitary lung nodule (<5 cm) or nodular/diffuse pleural involvement mimicking mesothelioma [9–12].

What Are the Macroscopic Features of Epithelioid Hemangioendothelioma?

EHE typically presents with multiple circumscribed nodules with a firm, gray-white cut surface. Tumors extending to the pleura show diffuse pleural thickening mimicking the gross appearance of malignant mesothelioma (Fig. 21.3a–c) [9–12].

What Are the Histologic and Immunophenotypic Features of Epithelioid Hemangioendothelioma?

The histologic and immunophenotypic features of PEHE are shown in Figs. 21.4, 21.5, 21.6, and 21.7. These tumors are often associated with arterioles, venules, or lymphatic vessels. At low power, PEHE most often forms rounded nodules with increased cellularity at the periphery and a hypocellular, sclerotic center. The tumor is composed of strands and nests of epithelioid cells often with intracytoplasmic lumina containing fragmented erythrocytes, so-called blister cells. The cells are embedded in a sclerotic myxohyaline stroma. At the periphery, PEHE often shows "micropolypoid" protrusions with tumor filling alveolar spaces (Figs. 21.1, 21.2, and 21.3) [9]. Significant pleomorphism is rare, and mitotic activity is generally low (<5/10 HPF) [1–3]. Rare calcification and ossification may occur [1].

EHE expresses an endothelial immunophenotype with positive CD31, CD34, FLI1, and ERG; however, the intensity of staining may vary. Epithelial-type antigens are expressed in 25–50% of tumors including CK7, CK8, CK18, AE1/AE3, and EMA [1–3]. Nuclear staining for CAMTA1, the surrogate antibody for the *WWTR1-CAMTA1* fusion, is useful to separate EHE from its mimics [13]. Nuclear TFE3 expression is seen in a subset of cases with *YAP1-TFE3* fusion (Figs. 21.6 and 21.7) [8].

What Are the Genetics of Epithelioid Hemangioendothelioma?

Epithelioid hemangioendothelioma harbors a unique translocation t(1;3)(p36;q23–25) resulting in a *WWTR1-CAMTA1* fusion. Three fusion-transcript variants have been described: exon 3 or 4 of *WWTR1* fused to either exon 8 or exon 9 of *CAMTA1*. The fusion gene encodes a putative transcription factor which places *CAMTA1* under the control of the *WWTR1* promoter resulting in overexpression of the C-terminus of *CAMTA1* culminating in dysregulation of downstream events [4–7]. A subset of cases, often associated with vasoformation and younger age at presentation, harbors *YAP1-TFE3* gene fusion. This variant fusion results in overexpression of the TFE3 protein, which can be detected by nuclear immunoreactivity with TFE3 antibodies [8].

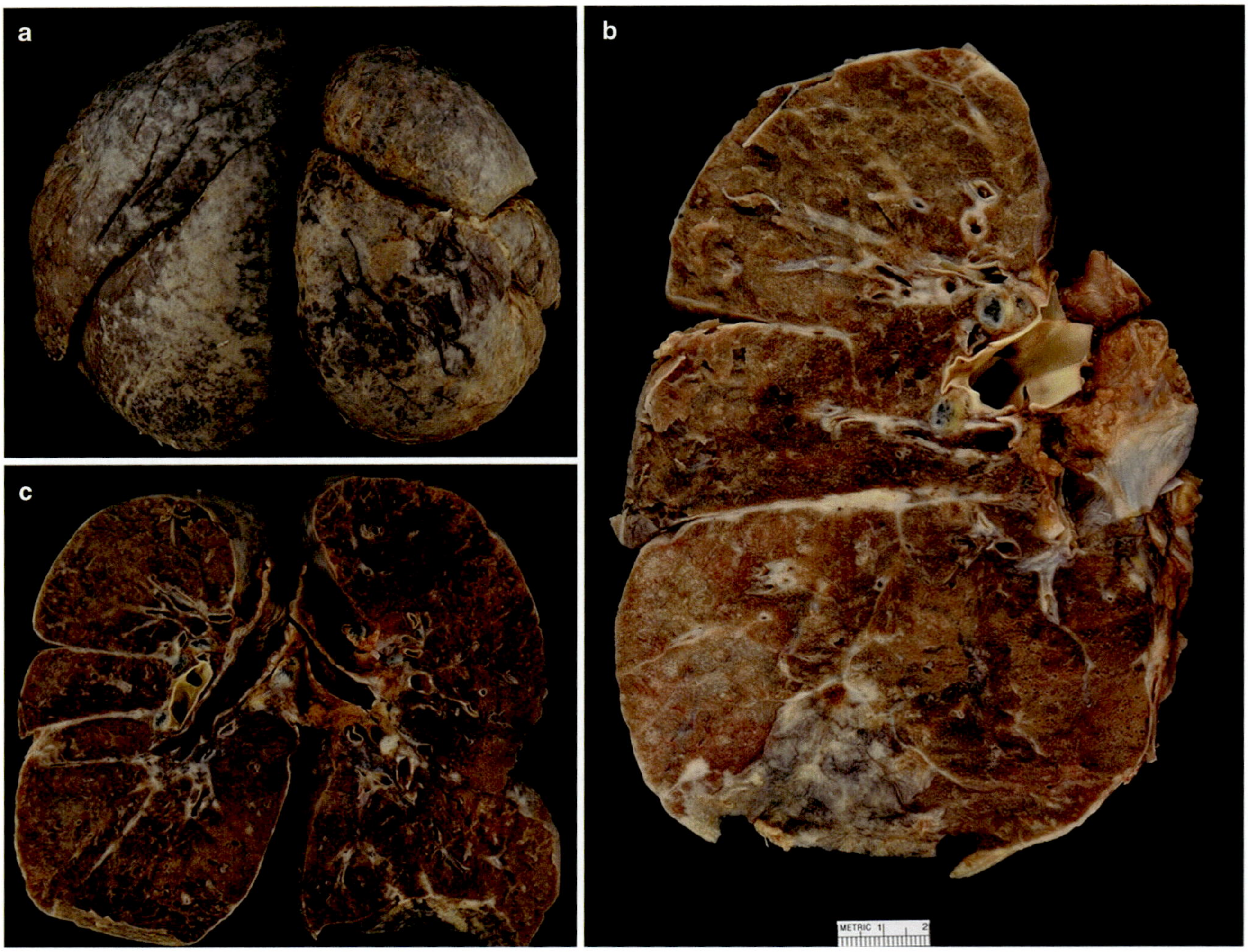

Fig. 21.3 (**a**) Gross evaluation from an autopsy specimen of a patient with pleural EHE shown here caking the pleural surface (posterior and superior view). (**b**) Cut surface shows multiple small nodules throughout both lungs. (**c**) The pleura is diffusely thickened including the fissures as well as multiple intrapulmonary tumor nodules

What Is the Prognosis of Epithelioid Hemangioendothelioma?

The prognosis of soft tissue EHE is generally indolent; however, 20–30% experience metastases, and approximately 15% of patients die of their disease [1–3]. The prognosis of thoracic EHE is worse with a 5-year survival of 60% [9–11]. Negative prognostic indicators include extensive intrapulmonary and pleural spread, weight loss, anemia, and hemorrhagic pleural effusions. Most patients eventually die of respiratory failure due to replacement of pulmonary parenchyma by tumor. EHE arising from the pleura is invariably aggressive; most patients survive less than 1 year and often succumb to uncontrolled local spread followed by systemic disease [9, 10].

What Are the Most Common Differential Diagnoses of Pulmonary Epithelioid Hemangioendothelioma?

The most common differential diagnosis is metastatic or primary carcinoma [1]. Primary lung carcinoma typically presents in older patients with a smoking history. Both tumors

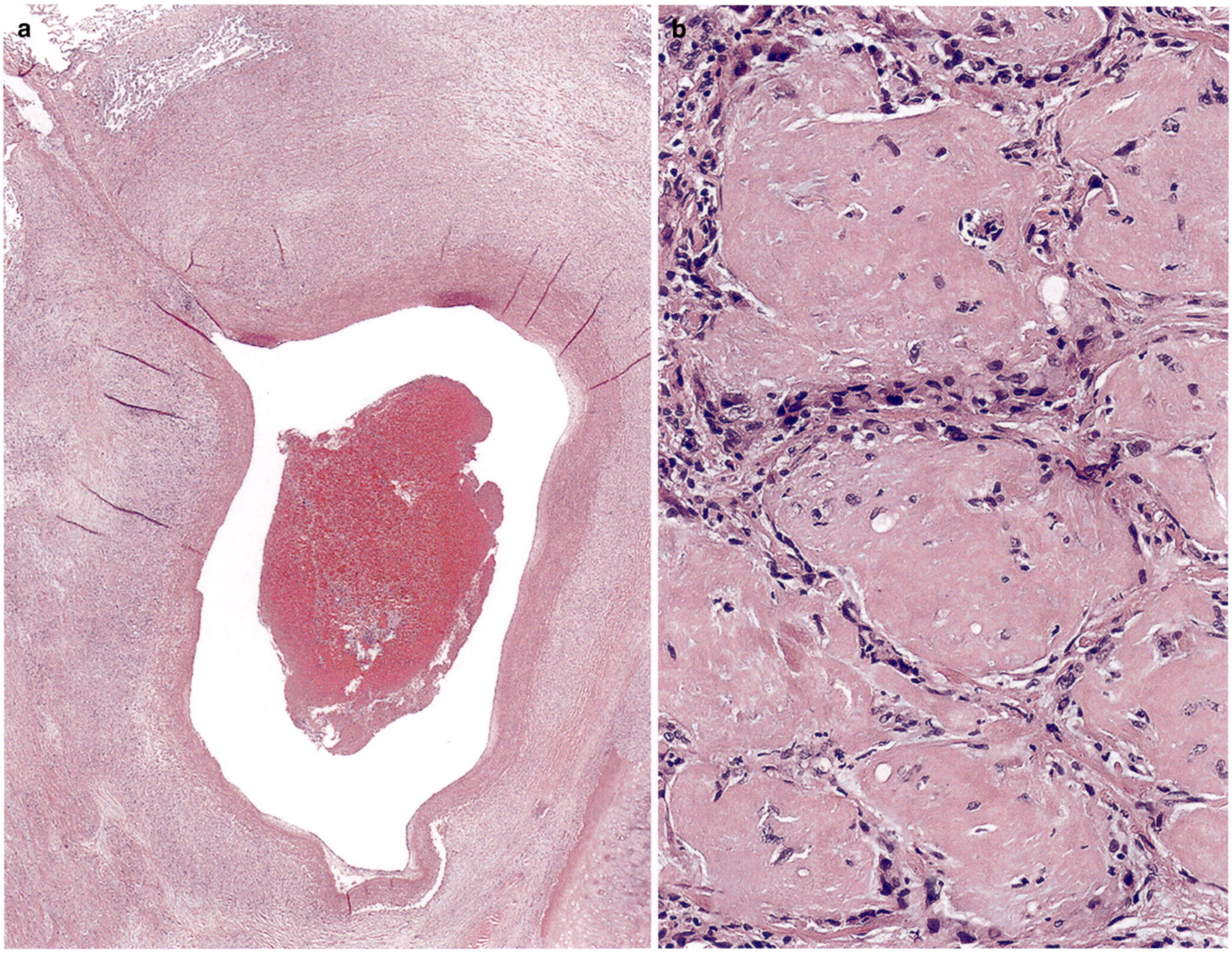

Fig. 21.4 (**a**) PEHE is often associated with large blood vessels. (**b**) Epithelioid tumor cells in a sclerotic, eosinophilic background matrix filling the alveoli

may show cytokeratin positivity; however, diffuse expression for keratins as well as TTF-1 or p40/p63, in concert with the lack of expression of endothelial antigens, is helpful to exclude PEHE. In addition, carcinomas do not harbor the t(1;3)(p36;q23–25) *WWTR1-CAMTA1* or *YAP1-TFE3* translocations seen in epithelioid hemangioendothelioma [4–8].

In addition to carcinoma, the differential diagnosis includes other epithelioid vascular neoplasms. Epithelioid hemangioma typically has a lobular architecture composed of well-formed plump epithelioid-to-histiocytoid endothelial cells lining the vascular channels with an admixed chronic inflammatory infiltrate often rich with eosinophils. In addition, many cases of epithelioid hemangioma harbor *FOS* gene rearrangements and show FOS/FOSB expression by immunohistochemistry [14]. Epithelioid hemangiomas are negative for CAMTA1 and TFE3 [8, 13, 14].

Epithelioid angiosarcoma (EAS) is another epithelioid vascular neoplasm that deserves consideration [8, 15]. Histologically, epithelioid angiosarcoma typically contains sheets or nodules of large epithelioid cells with overt nuclear pleomorphism lining irregular vascular spaces. Furthermore, abundant mitotic activity and tumor necrosis is often present. The immunophenotype of EAS may overlap with epithelioid hemangioendothelioma; however, EAS is negative for CAMTA1 and TFE3 [8, 13, 15].

Epithelioid sarcoma and EHE have an overlapping immunophenotype and occasionally show similar morphologic features. Epithelioid sarcoma most commonly presents in the

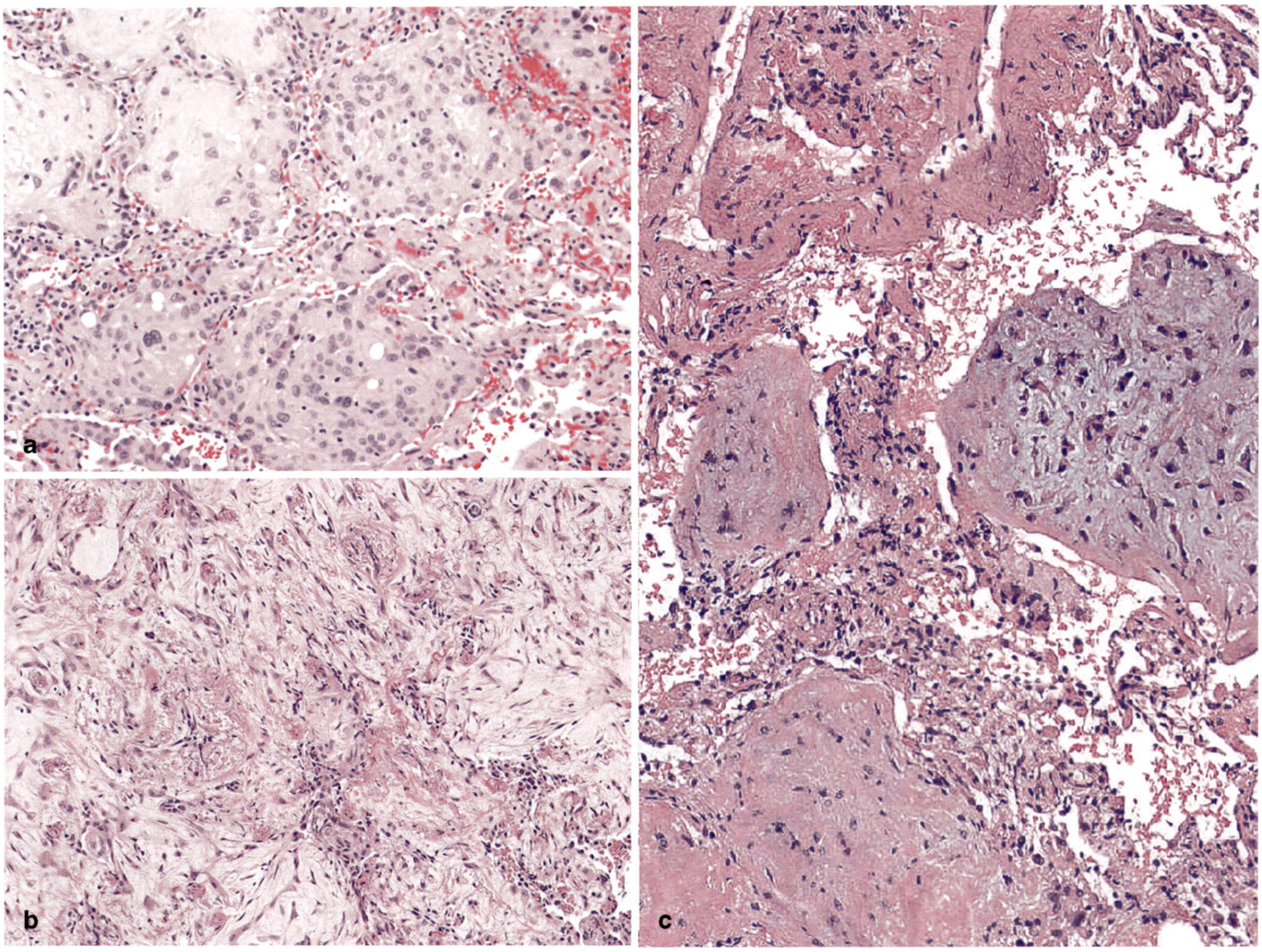

Fig. 21.5 (**a**) PEHE growing in an alveolar filling pattern with epithelioid or (**b**) spindled cells within (**c**) a distinctive myxohyaline stroma

distal extremities of younger patients (classic or distal-type) or in the proximal trunk of middle-aged adults (proximal-type) [16]. Epithelioid sarcoma often shows a prominent granuloma-like pattern with central necrosis (distal-type) or large, plump rhabdoid cells with ample cytoplasm (proximal-type). Epithelioid sarcoma is rare in the lungs. Epithelioid sarcoma often shows expression of keratins as well as CD34 positivity in about 50% of cases. Epithelioid sarcoma, however, is negative for CAMTA1 and also shows loss of nuclear expression of INI1 (SMARCB1) by immunohistochemistry [13, 16].

Finally, when PEHE presents with diffuse pleural plaques and/or surface nodules, mesothelioma is an important diagnostic consideration. Furthermore, the presence of bland epithelioid to spindle cells may cause further diagnostic challenges especially in limited sampling. Immunohistochemistry is valuable as mesothelioma will typically express WT1 (nuclear) and calretinin, whereas it will not express endothelial markers [12, 17].

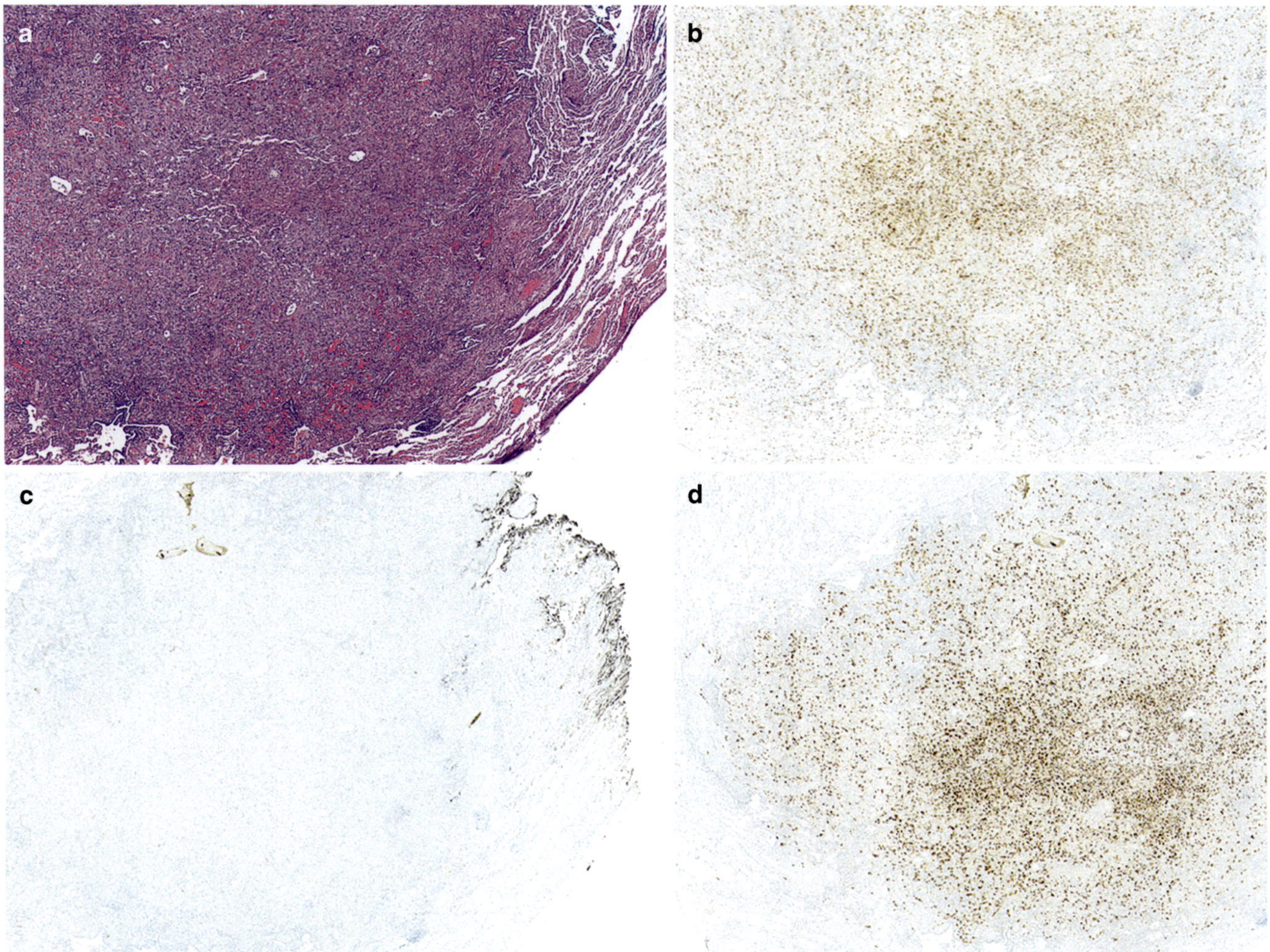

Fig. 21.6 (**a**) A subset of EHE will harbor *YAP1-TFE3* gene fusions instead of *WWTR1-CAMTA1* like this PEHE shown here. (**b**) Immunohistochemistry is positive for ERG. (**c**) CAMTA1 is negative; however, (**d**) TFE3 is diffusely positive

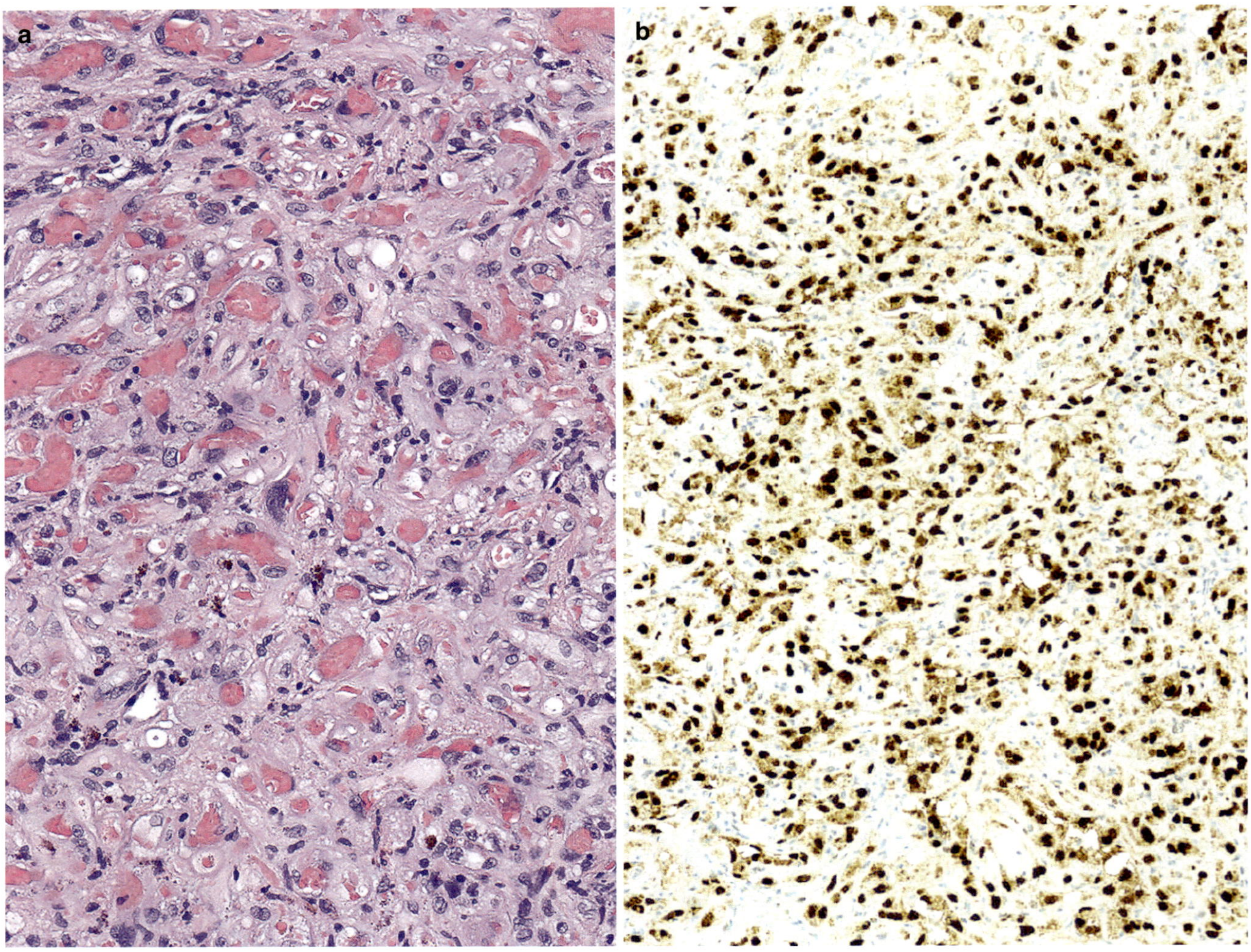

Fig. 21.7 (**a**) PEHE with *YAP1-TFE3* gene rearrangement often shows more prominent vasoformation. (**b**) TFE3 immunohistochemistry shows strong nuclear staining

References

1. Weiss SW, Enzinger FM. Epithelioid hemangioendothelioma: a vascular tumor often mistaken for a carcinoma. Cancer. 1982;50(5):970–81.
2. Mentzel T, Beham A, Calonje E, Katenkamp D, Fletcher CD. Epithelioid hemangioendothelioma of skin and soft tissues: clinicopathologic and immunohistochemical study of 30 cases. Am J Surg Pathol. 1997;21(4):363–74.
3. Deyrup AT, Tighiouart M, Montag AG, Weiss SW. Epithelioid hemangioendothelioma of soft tissue: a proposal for risk stratification based on 49 cases. Am J Surg Pathol. 2008;32(6):924–7.
4. Mendlick MR, Nelson M, Pickering D, Johansson SL, Seemayer TA, Neff JR, et al. Translocation t(1;3)(p36.3;q25) is a nonrandom aberration in epithelioid hemangioendothelioma. Am J Surg Pathol. 2001;25(5):684–7.
5. Tanas MR, Sboner A, Oliveira AM, Erickson-Johnson MR, Hespelt J, Hanwright PJ, et al. Identification of a disease-defining gene fusion in epithelioid hemangioendothelioma. Sci Transl Med. 2011;3(98):98ra82.
6. Errani C, Zhang L, Sung YS, Hajdu M, Singer S, Maki RG, et al. A novel WWTR1-CAMTA1 gene fusion is a consistent abnormality in epithelioid hemangioendothelioma of different anatomic sites. Genes Chromosomes Cancer. 2011;50(8):644–53.
7. Patel NR, Salim AA, Sayeed H, Sarabia SF, Hollingsworth F, Warren M, et al. Molecular characterization of epithelioid haemangioendotheliomas identifies novel WWTR1-CAMTA1 fusion variants. Histopathology. 2015;67(5):699–708.
8. Antonescu CR, Le Loarer F, Mosquera J-M, Sboner A, Zhang L, Chen C-L, et al. Novel YAP1-TFE3 fusion defines a distinct subset of epithelioid hemangioendothelioma. Genes Chromosomes Cancer. 2013;52(8):775–84.
9. Anderson T, Zhang L, Hameed M, Rusch V, Travis WD, Antonescu CR. Thoracic epithelioid malignant vascular tumors: a clinicopathologic study of 52 cases with emphasis on pathologic grading and molecular studies of WWTR1-CAMTA1 fusions. Am J Surg Pathol. 2015;39(1):132–9.
10. Bagan P, Hassan M, Le Pimpec BF, Peyrard S, Souilamas R, Danel C, et al. Prognostic factors and surgical indications of pulmonary epithelioid hemangioendothelioma: a review of the literature. Ann Thorac Surg. 2006;82(6):2010–3.
11. Mesquita RD, Sousa M, Trinidad C, Pinto E, Badiola IA. New insights about pulmonary epithelioid hemangioendothelioma: review of the literature and two case reports. Case Rep Radiol. 2017;2017:5972940.

12. Bahrami A, Allen TC, Cagle PT. Pulmonary epithelioid hemangioendothelioma mimicking mesothelioma. Pathol Int. 2008;58(11):730–4.
13. Doyle LA, Fletcher CDM, Hornick JL. Nuclear expression of CAMTA1 distinguishes epithelioid hemangioendothelioma from histologic mimics. Am J Surg Pathol. 2016;40(1):94–102.
14. Huang SC, Zhang L, Sung YS, Chen CL, Krausz T, Dickson BC, et al. Frequent FOS gene rearrangements in epithelioid hemangioma: a molecular study of 58 cases with morphologic reappraisal. Am J Surg Pathol. 2015;39(10):1313–21.
15. Cao Y, Zou SM, Zhang KT, Lu N, Liu Y, Feng L, et al. Genetic alterations in pulmonary epithelioid hemangioendothelioma and epithelioid angiosarcoma. Histol Histopathol. 2011;26(4):491–6.
16. Hornick JL, Dal Cin P, Fletcher CD. Loss of INI1 expression is characteristic of both conventional and proximal-type epithelioid sarcoma. Am J Surg Pathol. 2009;33(4):542–50.
17. McGregor SM, Dunning R, Hyjek E, Vigneswaran W, Husain AN, Krausz T. BAP1 facilitates diagnostic objectivity, classification, and prognostication in malignant pleural mesothelioma. Human Pathol. 2015;46(11):1670–8.

Epithelioid Malignant Mesothelioma Versus Adenocarcinoma

22

Anshu Bandhlish and Haodong Xu

Case Presentation

The patient is an 80-year-old male with a history of being a shipyard worker for 25 years and with a sporadic presence in shipyard facilities subsequently. He is a former smoker with a history of one pack per day for 6–8 years, who quitted 25 years ago. He developed rapidly progressive dyspnea on excretion, and the workup revealed a large pleural effusion. Chest computed tomography (CT) demonstrated a large pleural effusion with thickening (Fig. 22.1a). A positron-emission tomography (PET)-CT confirmed mild abnormal fluorodeoxyglucose (FDG) uptake within the pleura and circumferential nodules (Fig. 22.1b). No lung nodules were identified. He underwent thoracentesis.

Pleural fluid was submitted for cytopathologic evaluation, and immunocytochemical stains were performed on the cell block. The atypical epithelioid cells (Fig. 22.2a, b) are positive for multiple mesothelial markers (CK5, D2-40, and WT-1) (Fig. 22.2c–e) with weak variable positivity for calretinin (Fig. 22.2f); they are also positive for epithelial marker MOC-31 (Fig. 22.2g) with loss of BAP-1 nuclear staining (Fig. 22.2h). A diagnosis of epithelioid malignant mesothelioma was rendered. Subsequently, the patient underwent a video-assisted thoracoscopic surgical pleural biopsy. Histological sections show a malignant epithelioid cell proliferation in solid sheets, nests and singly, infiltrating into the fibrous tissue. The malignant cells have high nuclear-to-cytoplasmic ratios with abundant eosinophilic cytoplasm with conspicuous nucleoli. They are positive for AE1/AE3, CK5, D2-40, calretinin, WT-1, and MOC-31 and negative for m-CEA, TTF-1, and p40 (Fig. 22.3a–j).

A. Bandhlish (✉) · H. Xu
Department of Laboratory Medicine and Pathology, University of Washington Medical Center, Seattle, WA, USA
e-mail: anshuba@uw.edu

H. Xu et al. (eds.), *Practical Lung Pathology*, Practical Anatomic Pathology, https://doi.org/10.1007/978-3-031-14402-8_22

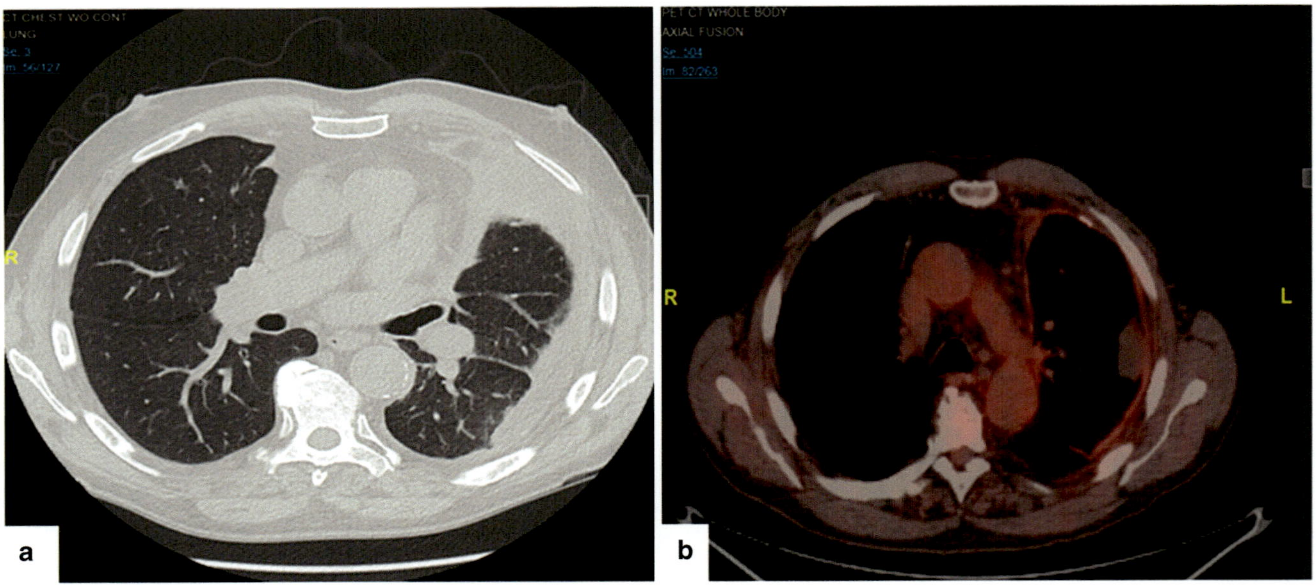

Fig. 22.1 (**a**) Chest CT without contrast shows left pleural effusion and thickening. (**b**) PET-CT demonstrates mild abnormal FDG uptake within the pleura

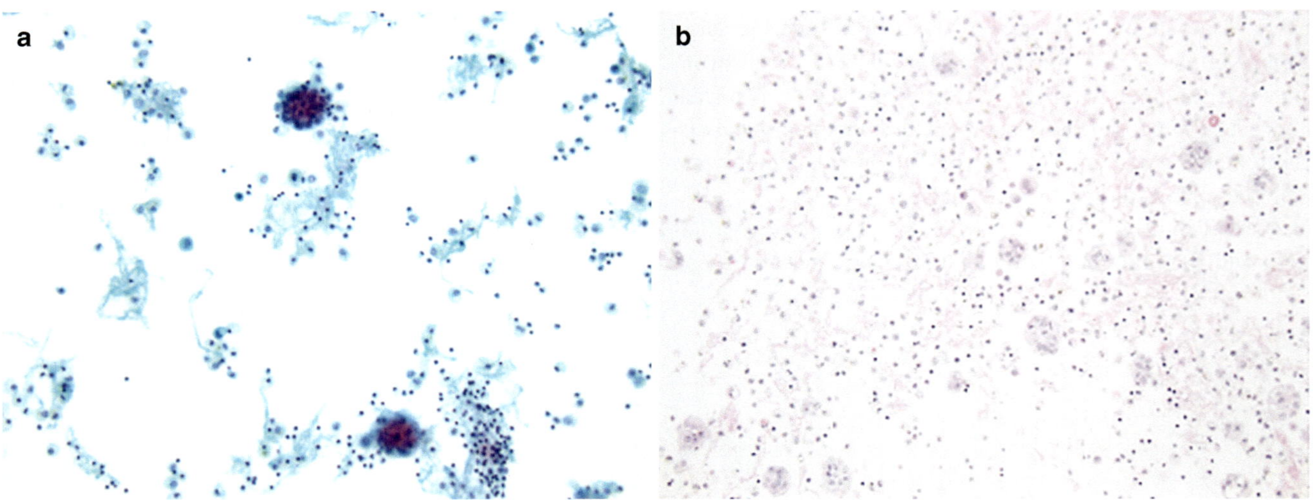

Fig. 22.2 Cytopathology and immunocytochemistry of epithelioid malignant mesothelioma. (**a**, **b**) Pleural fluid cytology with Pap smear and a section from the cell block demonstrate cohesive clusters of atypical epithelioid cells with a moderate amount of cytoplasm and round-to-ovoid nuclei with prominent nucleoli (100×). (**c**–**f**) Immunostaining results show that atypical epithelioid cells and background scattered single cells are positive for CK5 (**c**), D2–40 (**d**), WT-1 (**e**), calretinin (variably) (**f**), and MOC-31 (**g**) with loss of nuclear staining for BAP-1 (**h**). IHC: 200×

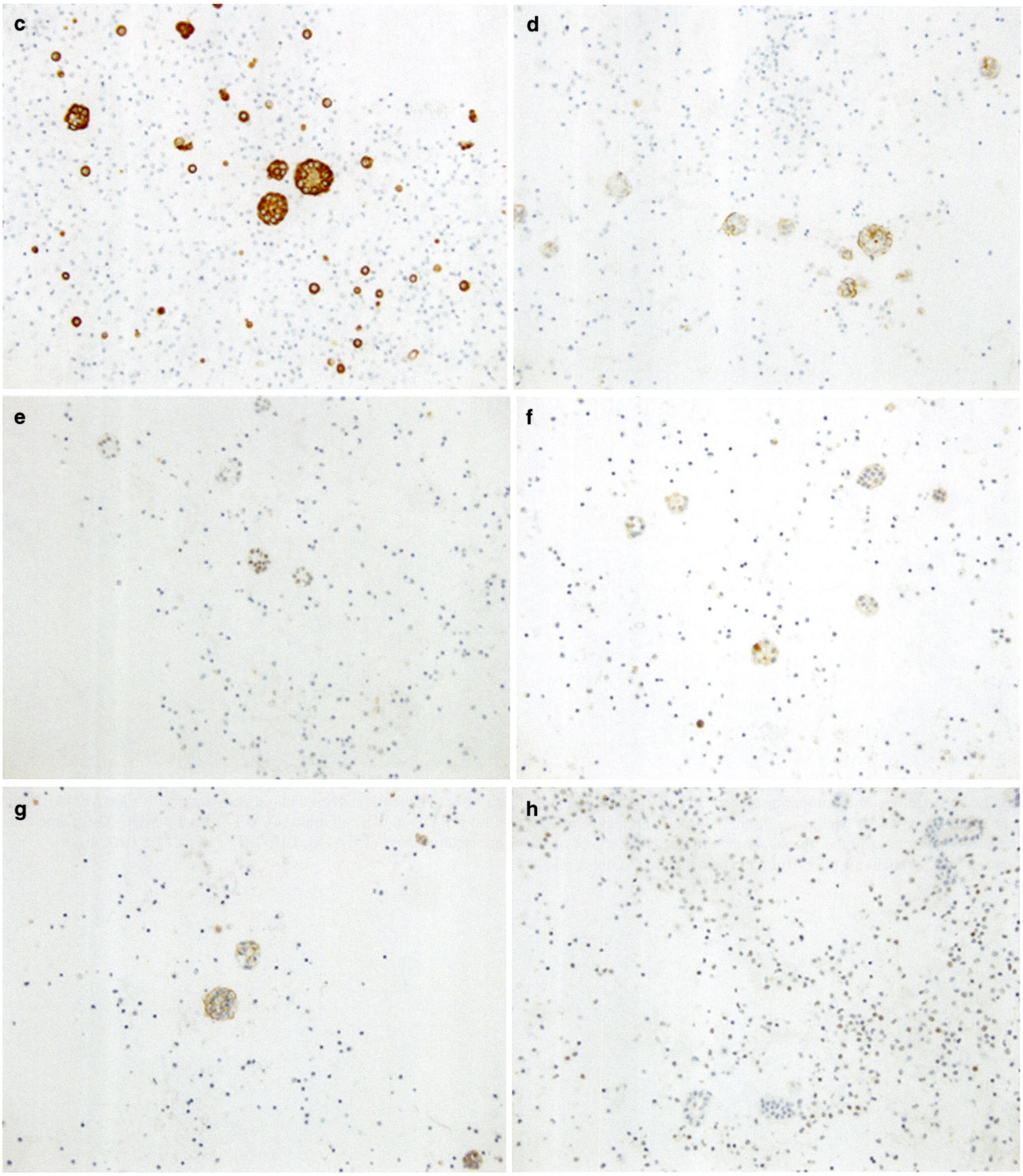

Fig. 22.2 (continued)

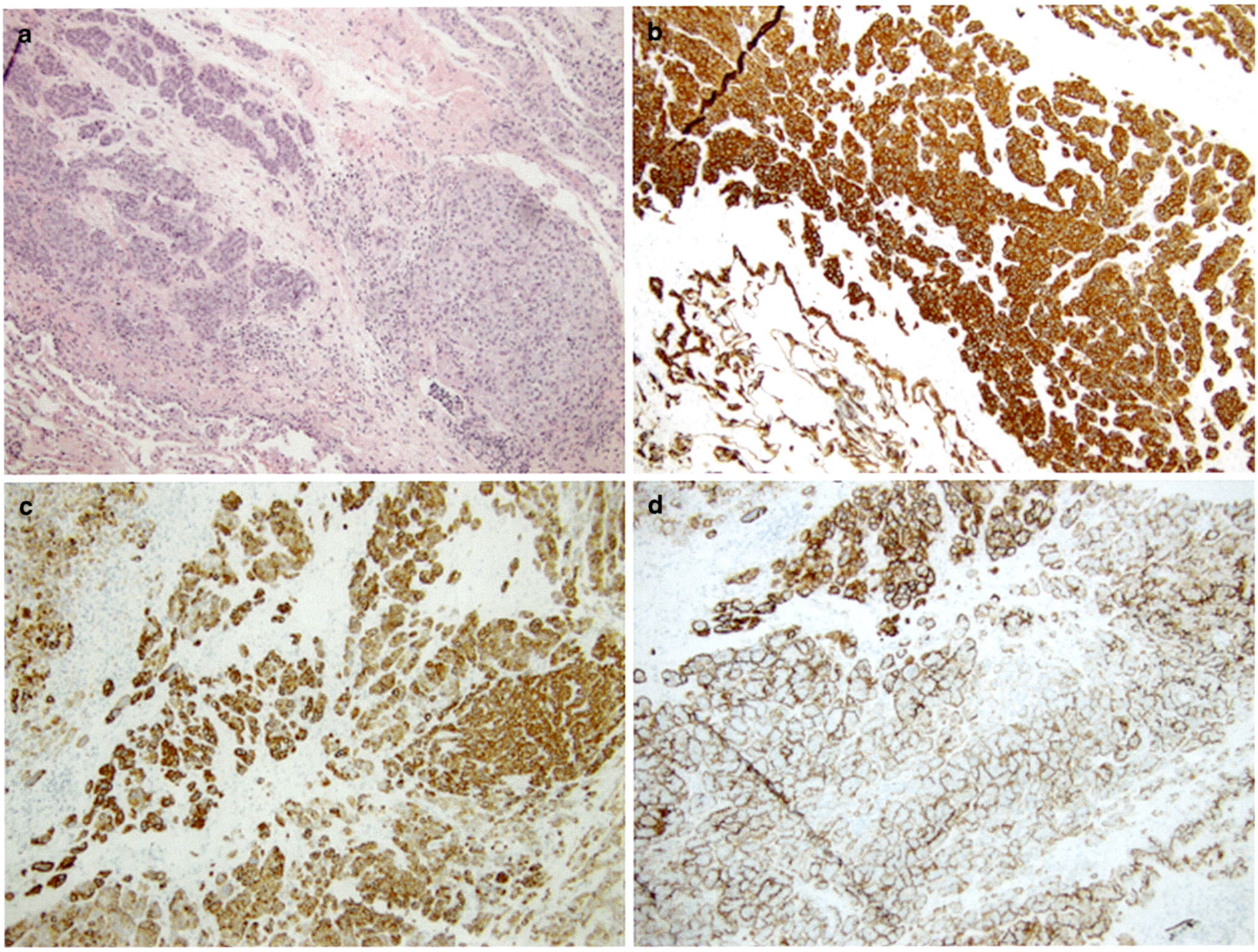

Fig. 22.3 Histology and immunohistochemistry of epithelioid malignant mesothelioma. (**a**) Malignant epithelioid cells arranged in nests and sheets infiltrating in the fibrous tissue without involvement of the adjacent lung parenchyma (40×). Immunohistochemical staining results show that the malignant epithelioid cells are positive for AE1/AE3 (**b**), CK5 (**c**), D2-40 (**d**), calretinin (**e**), WT-1 (**f**), and MOC-31 (**g**), and they are negative for m-CEA (**h**), TTF-1 (**i**), and p40 (**j**). IHC: 100×

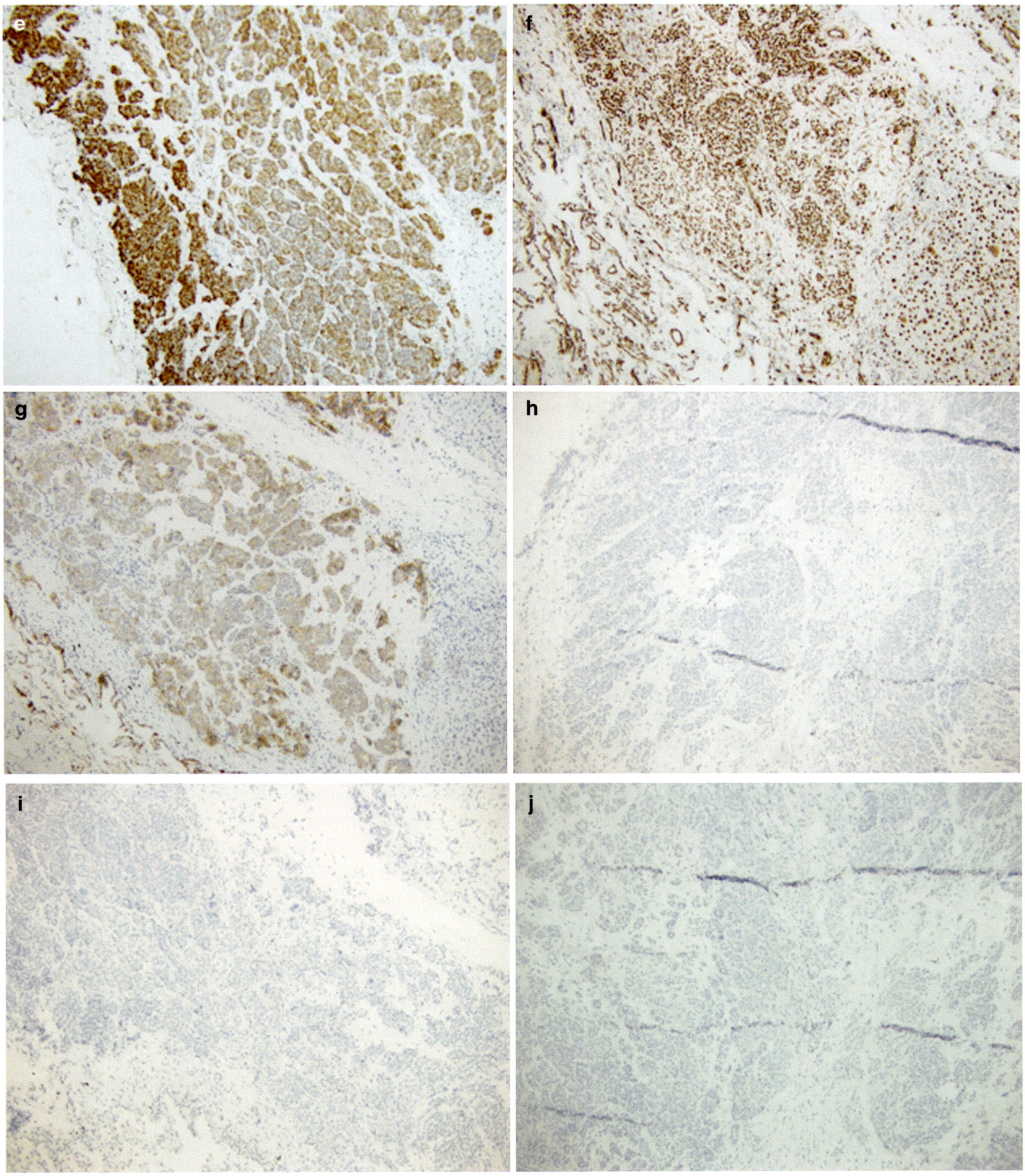

Fig. 22.3 (continued)

Pathologic Diagnosis: Epithelioid Malignant Mesothelioma

What Are the Panels of Mesothelial and Epithelial Markers to Separate Epithelioid Malignant Mesothelioma from Adenocarcinoma?

Immunohistochemical studies for the diagnosis of malignant mesothelioma and non-mesothelial tumors have evolved. A panel of immunohistochemical stains for evaluation of mesothelial and epithelial lineage is one of the most important steps for an accurate diagnosis.

Per guidelines of the International Mesothelioma Interest Group, the distinction between epithelioid mesothelioma and adenocarcinoma should include both positive and negative markers (at least two mesothelial markers and two epithelial markers with a broad-spectrum cytokeratin), which can be tailored depending on the differential diagnosis [1, 2]. Mesothelial markers (calretinin, cytokeratin 5 or 5/6, WT-1, and D2-40) and epithelial markers (claudin-4, MOC-31, BerEP4, and monoclonal CEA) along with TTF-1 and napsin-A for lung adenocarcinoma are considered good markers in distinguishing epithelioid malignant mesotheliomas from adenocarcinoma [2]. The significance of positivity by a single marker should be interpreted with caution due to extensive overlap of staining patterns [1].

Immunohistochemical stains utilized should have greater than 80% sensitivity or specificity for the lesion being tested. Interpretation of a positive stain depends not only on the pattern of immunostaining (nuclear versus cytoplasmic) but also on the percentage of cells staining (greater than 10% for cytoplasmic and membranous markers) [1].

What Are the Pitfalls of the Various Mesothelial and Epithelial Markers Utilized to Distinguish Epithelioid Malignant Mesothelioma from Adenocarcinoma?

Markers of mesothelial lineage such as calretinin with approximately 80–100% sensitivity in epithelioid mesotheliomas can also be expressed in a subset of carcinoma of lung, breast, ovarian, and squamous cell carcinomas among others [2–4]. CK5/6 is another mesothelial marker with sensitivity ranging from 51 to 100% and can also be expressed in lung adenocarcinoma (less than 5% of cases) and poorly differentiated squamous cell carcinoma [5, 6]. Podoplanin (D2-40) with its characteristic membranous staining pattern identified in 80–100% of epithelioid mesotheliomas is also positive in squamous cell carcinoma, seminoma, epithelioid angiosarcoma, and serous ovarian carcinoma [2, 5, 7]. Entrapped lymphatics with membranous staining for D2-40 can be mistakenly interpreted as mesothelial cells if accurate correlation with the morphology is not made [1]. Lung adenocarcinoma usually lacks true strong membranous staining with D2-40.

WT-1 with its strong nuclear staining pattern has a reported sensitivity of approximately 70–100% in epithelioid mesotheliomas. Ovarian serous carcinomas, along with a small percentage of breast carcinomas, lung squamous cell carcinomas, and renal cell carcinomas, can also be positive for WT-1, while lung adenocarcinomas can be usually negative [1, 2].

GATA-3 is often positive in breast carcinoma, but strong and diffuse GATA-3 nuclear positivity has been demonstrated in up to one third to one half of epithelioid mesotheliomas [4, 8].

P63 and p40, usually positive in lung squamous cell carcinoma, can also be expressed in a small percentage of cases of epithelioid mesothelioma. However, the staining pattern is usually focal (approximately 1–10% of positive cells) [7, 9]. The sensitivity and specificity of p40 are higher than that of p63 for distinguishing between epithelioid mesothelioma and squamous cell carcinoma [10]. TTF-1 and napsin-A have a high specificity for lung adenocarcinoma [9].

Claudin-4 is emerging as one of the more reliable epithelial markers currently in use. In an immunohistochemical study (on tissue microarrays) of 68 epithelioid mesotheliomas, 31 sarcomatoid mesotheliomas, and 147 non-small-cell lung carcinomas, claudin-4 stained 0 of 68 (0%), MOC-31 stained 22 of 68 (32%), and Ber-EP4 stained 24 of 68 (35%) epithelioid mesotheliomas, highlighting a high specificity (100%) for claudin-4 in the diagnosis of epithelioid malignant mesothelioma. In this study, the sensitivities of claudin-4, MOC-31, and Ber-EP4 for non-small-cell lung carcinomas were comparable [11].

What Biomarkers Are Useful in Differentiating Malignant Mesothelioma from Reactive Mesothelial Cells?

Sensitivity of cytology for the diagnosis of mesothelioma ranges from 30% to 75% due to various aspects such as morphologic and immunocytochemical overlap between benign reactive and malignant mesothelioma cells and, most importantly, the lack of ability to assess invasion of the surrounding tissue, one of the most important diagnostic findings in malignant mesotheliomas [12]. Utilization of immunohistochemistry and molecular markers in cytologic specimens and small biopsies has increased the accuracy of diagnosis of malignant mesothelioma [1].

Utilization of BAP1 (BRCA-associated protein 1) immunomarker and *CDKN2A* encoding p16 fluorescence in situ hybridization (FISH) have been reported as reliable markers of malignancy in small biopsies and effusion cytology specimens. BAP1 is considered the most commonly acquired germline mutation in malignant mesothelioma [13, 14]. The sensitivity of BAP1 loss by immunohistochemistry to differentiate between malignant mesothelioma and reactive mesothelial proliferations is between 61% and 67% with a specificity of 100% [15, 16]. BAP1 loss can also be observed in a melanoma as well as carcinomas of the breast, lung, and kidney; therefore, confirmation of a mesothelial lineage is important before interpreting BAP1 immunohistochemistry [17, 18].

The homozygous deletion of the 9p21 locus involves a cluster of genes such as *CDKN2A*, *CDKN2B*, and *MTAP* (methylthioadenosine phosphorylase). Loss of p16 is seen commonly due to homozygous deletion of the *CDKN2A* locus (9p21) and is considered diagnostic of malignancy once the mesothelial origin has been established [13, 19].

Deletion of *CDKN2A* has been reported in up to 80% of malignant mesotheliomas, including 90–100% of cases with sarcomatoid morphology and approximately 70% of those with biphasic and epithelioid morphology [1]. In contrast, BAP1 loss is more frequently observed with epithelioid morphology, and some biphasic mesotheliomas, while being mostly retained in sarcomatoid and desmoplastic subtypes [20].

The *MTAP* gene exists near the *CDKN2A* locus at 9p21. Both genes have been reported to be co-deleted, with a high degree of concordance between MTAP loss by IHC and *CDKN2A*p16 deletion (9p21) by FISH [2].

A combination of MTAP and BAP1 IHC has a reported sensitivity of approximately 77.8%, higher than BAP1 IHC alone or p16 FISH alone (62.2%), in distinguishing malignant mesothelioma from reactive mesothelial proliferations [21].

Can We Reliably Distinguish Malignant Mesothelioma from Metastatic Adenocarcinoma on Imaging?

Imaging studies play an important role in the evaluation of patients suspected with malignant mesothelioma, especially in patients unfit for invasive biopsy procedures. Few of the commonly identified findings on CT in malignant mesotheliomas include circumferential lung encasement by multiple nodules, pleural thickening with irregular pleuro-pulmonary margins, and pleural thickening with superimposed nodules [22].

Sensitivity and specificity of these findings are variable, as detection can be highly operator-dependent; additionally, CT cannot reliably differentiate malignant mesothelioma from metastatic neoplasms, although circumferential/rind-like pleural thickening and mediastinal pleural involvement are more frequently observed in malignant mesothelioma [22, 23]. As much as imaging is important in the diagnosis and staging of pleural malignancies, it has its own limitations, especially in cases with minimal or absent pleural thickening. Various benign pleural diseases such as empyema and tuberculous pleurisy as well as various asbestos-related advanced pleural abnormalities can demonstrate significant radiologic overlap with malignant mesothelioma [24].

PET-CT comprises high-resolution CT scanning with injection of radioactive metabolic tracer, e.g., 18-fluoro-deoxy-glucose (FDG), reported as standardized uptake values (SUV). The maximum SUV is higher in malignant mesothelioma than in benign disease, and a threshold of 2 is quite reliable in differentiating between malignant and benign disease [25]. False-positive results can be observed in inflammatory disorders such as rheumatoid pleuritis, tuberculous pleurisy, and prior pleurodesis [24].

How Can Electron Microscopy Help in the Diagnosis of Malignant Mesothelioma?

Electron microscopic features of malignant mesotheliomas are well described. The role of electron microscopy for the diagnosis of malignant mesothelioma is limited as immunohistochemistry is more accessible, faster, and cheaper [26]. With the advent of biomarkers such as BAP1 and MTAP IHC and *CDKN2A* FISH, the role of electron microscopy is even more restricted. Electron microscopy is useful in cases where the immunohistochemical results are equivocal or additional finding to support the diagnosis of a malignant mesothelioma is needed. Electron microscopy is extremely useful in diagnosing epithelioid mesotheliomas which have characteristically long microvilli, not covered by glycocalyx. They are not associated with rootlets and frequently demonstrate large desmosomes and prominent junctional complexes. A single finding is usually not diagnostic of mesothelioma; rather, a combination of several features is more useful [26]. A caveat to these findings is that sarcomatoid mesothelioma does not demonstrate the specific ultrastructural feature as seen in epithelial mesotheliomas [1].

References

1. Husain AN, Colby TV, Ordóñez NG, et al. Guidelines for pathologic diagnosis of malignant mesothelioma 2017 update of the consensus statement from the international mesothelioma interest group. Arch Pathol Lab Med. 2018;142(1):89–108.
2. Chapel DB, Schulte JJ, Husain AN, Krausz T. Application of immunohistochemistry in diagnosis and management of malignant mesothelioma. Transl Lung Cancer Res. 2020;9(Suppl 1):S3–S27.
3. Ordóñez NG. Role of immunohistochemistry in distinguishing epithelial peritoneal mesotheliomas from peritoneal and ovarian serous carcinomas. Am J Surg Pathol. 1998;22(10):1203–14.

4. Ordóñez NG, Sahin AA. Diagnostic utility of immunohistochemistry in distinguishing between epithelioid pleural mesotheliomas and breast carcinomas: a comparative study. Hum Pathol. 2014;45(7):1529–40.
5. Comin CE, Novelli L, Cavazza A, et al. Expression of thrombomodulin, calretinin, cytokeratin 5/6, D2-40 and WT-1 in a series of primary carcinomas of the lung: an immunohistochemical study in comparison with epithelioid pleural mesothelioma. Tumori. 2014;100(5):559–67.
6. King JE, Thatcher N, Pickkering CAC, Hasleton PS. Sensitivity and specificity of immunohistochemical markers used in the diagnosis of epithelioid mesothelioma: a detailed systematic analysis using published data. Histopathology. 2006;48(3):223–32.
7. Kushitani K, Amatya VJ, Okada Y, et al. Utility and pitfalls of immunohistochemistry in the differential diagnosis between epithelioid mesothelioma and poorly differentiated lung squamous cell carcinoma. Histopathology. 2017;70(3):375–84.
8. Miettinen M, McCue PA, Sarlomo-Rikkala M, et al. GATA3: a multispecific but potentially useful marker in surgical pathology: a systematic analysis of 2500 epithelial and nonepithelial tumors. Am J Surg Pathol. 2014;38(1):13–22.
9. Mawas AS, Amatya VJ, Kushitani K, et al. MUC4 immunohistochemistry is useful in distinguishing epithelioid mesothelioma from adenocarcinoma and squamous cell carcinoma of the lung. Sci Rep. 2018;8(1):134.
10. Bishop JA, Teruya-Feldstein J, Westra WH, et al. p40 (ΔNp63) is superior to p63 for the diagnosis of pulmonary squamous cell carcinoma. Mod Pathol. 2012;25(3):405–15.
11. Naso JR, Churg A. Claudin-4 shows superior specificity for mesothelioma vs non-small-cell lung carcinoma compared with MOC-31 and Ber-EP4. Hum Pathol. 2020;100:10–4.
12. Henderson DW, Reid G, Kao SC, van Zandwijk N, Klebe S. Challenges and controversies in the diagnosis of mesothelioma: part 1. Cytology-only diagnosis, biopsies, immunohistochemistry, discrimination between mesothelioma and reactive mesothelial hyperplasia, and biomarkers. J Clin Pathol. 2013;66(10):847–53.
13. Rozitis E, Johnson B, Cheng YY, Lee K. The use of immunohistochemistry, fluorescence in situ hybridization, and emerging epigenetic markers in the diagnosis of malignant pleural mesothelioma (MPM): a review. Front Oncol. 2020;10:1742.
14. Nasu M, Emi M, Pastorino S, et al. High incidence of somatic BAP1 alterations in sporadic malignant mesothelioma. J Thorac Oncol. 2015;10(4):565–76.
15. Hida T, Hamasaki M, Matsumoto S, et al. BAP1 immunohistochemistry and p16 FISH results in combination provide higher confidence in malignant pleural mesothelioma diagnosis: ROC analysis of the two tests. Pathol Int. 2016;66(10):563–70.
16. Berg KB, Dacic S, Miller C, Cheung S, Churg A. Utility of methylthioadenosine phosphorylase compared with BAP1 immunohistochemistry, and CDKN2A and NF2 fluorescence in situ hybridization in separating reactive mesothelial proliferations from epithelioid malignant mesotheliomas. Arch Pathol Lab Med. 2018;142(12):1549–53.
17. Bott M, Brevet M, Taylor BS, et al. The nuclear deubiquitinase BAP1 is commonly inactivated by somatic mutations and 3p21.1 losses in malignant pleural mesothelioma. Nat Genet. 2011;43(7):668–72.
18. Carbone M, Ferris LK, Baumann F, et al. BAP1 cancer syndrome: malignant mesothelioma, uveal and cutaneous melanoma, and MBAITs. J Transl Med. 2012;10:179.
19. Chiosea S, Krasinskas A, Cagle PT, et al. Diagnostic importance of 9p21 homozygous deletion in malignant mesotheliomas. Mod Pathol. 2008;21(6):742–7.
20. Hwang HC, Pyott S, Rodriguez S, et al. BAP1 immunohistochemistry and p16 FISH in the diagnosis of sarcomatous and desmoplastic mesotheliomas. Am J Surg Pathol. 2016;40(5):714–8.
21. Kinoshita Y, Hida T, Hamasaki M, et al. A combination of MTAP and BAP1 immunohistochemistry in pleural effusion cytology for the diagnosis of mesothelioma. Cancer Cytopathol. 2018;126(1):54–63.
22. Metintas M, Ucgun I, Elbek O, et al. Computed tomography features in malignant pleural mesothelioma and other commonly seen pleural diseases. Eur J Radiol. 2002;41(1):1–9.
23. Bibby AC, Tsim S, Kanellakis N, et al. Malignant pleural mesothelioma: an update on investigation, diagnosis and treatment. Eur Respir Rev. 2016;25(142):472–86.
24. Treglia G, Sadeghi R, Annunziata S, et al. Diagnostic accuracy of 18F-FDG-PET and PET/CT in the differential diagnosis between malignant and benign pleural lesions: a systematic review and meta-analysis. Acad Radiol. 2014;21(1):11–20.
25. Yildirim H, Metintas M, Entok E, et al. Clinical value of fluorodeoxyglucose-positron emission tomography/computed tomography in differentiation of malignant mesothelioma from asbestos-related benign pleural disease: an observational pilot study. J Thorac Oncol. 2009;4(12):1480–4.
26. Hammar SP. Macroscopic, histologic, histochemical, immunohistochemical, and ultrastructural features of mesothelioma. Ultrastruct Pathol. 2006;30(1):3–17.

Pleomorphic Carcinoma Versus Sarcomatoid Malignant Mesothelioma

23

Marina K Baine, Guoping Cai, and Xuchen Zhang

Case Presentation

A 78-year-old man, former smoker, presented with a history of worsening cough and dyspnea for 8 months. Initial computed tomography (CT) imaging of the chest revealed a large (6.5 × 6.1 cm) mass in the left upper lobe of the lung with pleural involvement (Fig. 23.1). Core-needle biopsy of the mass showed a neoplasm composed of a dual population of malignant spindle and pleomorphic giant cells (Fig. 23.2a, b). Both cell populations were positive for pan-cytokeratin and TTF-1 immunohistochemical stains (Fig. 23.2c, d) but negative for p40. Based on these findings, the diagnosis of non-small-cell carcinoma with spindle and giant cells was rendered.

A subsequent left upper lobectomy and mediastinal lymph node dissection were performed. The resection specimen was a left upper lung lobe with an area of puckered pleura. Sectioning of the specimen revealed a 6.5 × 6.1 × 4.3 cm friable, tan-yellow, fleshy mass with foci of hemorrhage and necrosis (Fig. 23.3a). Microscopically, the tumor showed a mixture of spindle and giant tumor cells (Fig. 23.3b, c). A small focus of adenocarcinoma (5%) was present (Fig. 23.3d). Similar to the prior biopsy, both the spindle and giant tumor cells were positive for pan-cytokeratin and TTF-1. Visceral pleural invasion was present and confirmed by Elastica-van Gieson (EVG) stain. One of the hilar lymph nodes showed tumor metastasis.

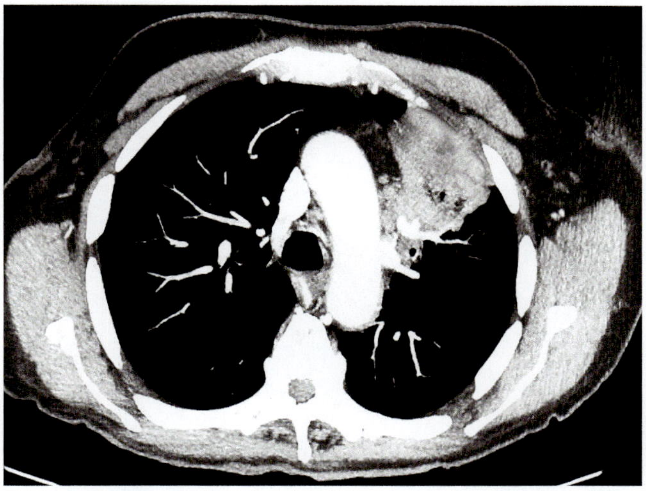

Fig. 23.1 CT image of a large mass in the left upper lobe of the lung with pleural involvement

M. K Baine
Department of Pathology and Laboratory Medicine, Memorial Sloan Kettering Cancer Center, New York, NY, USA

G. Cai · X. Zhang (✉)
Department of Pathology, Yale University School of Medicine, New Haven, CT, USA
e-mail: xuchen.zhang@yale.edu

H. Xu et al. (eds.), *Practical Lung Pathology*, Practical Anatomic Pathology, https://doi.org/10.1007/978-3-031-14402-8_23

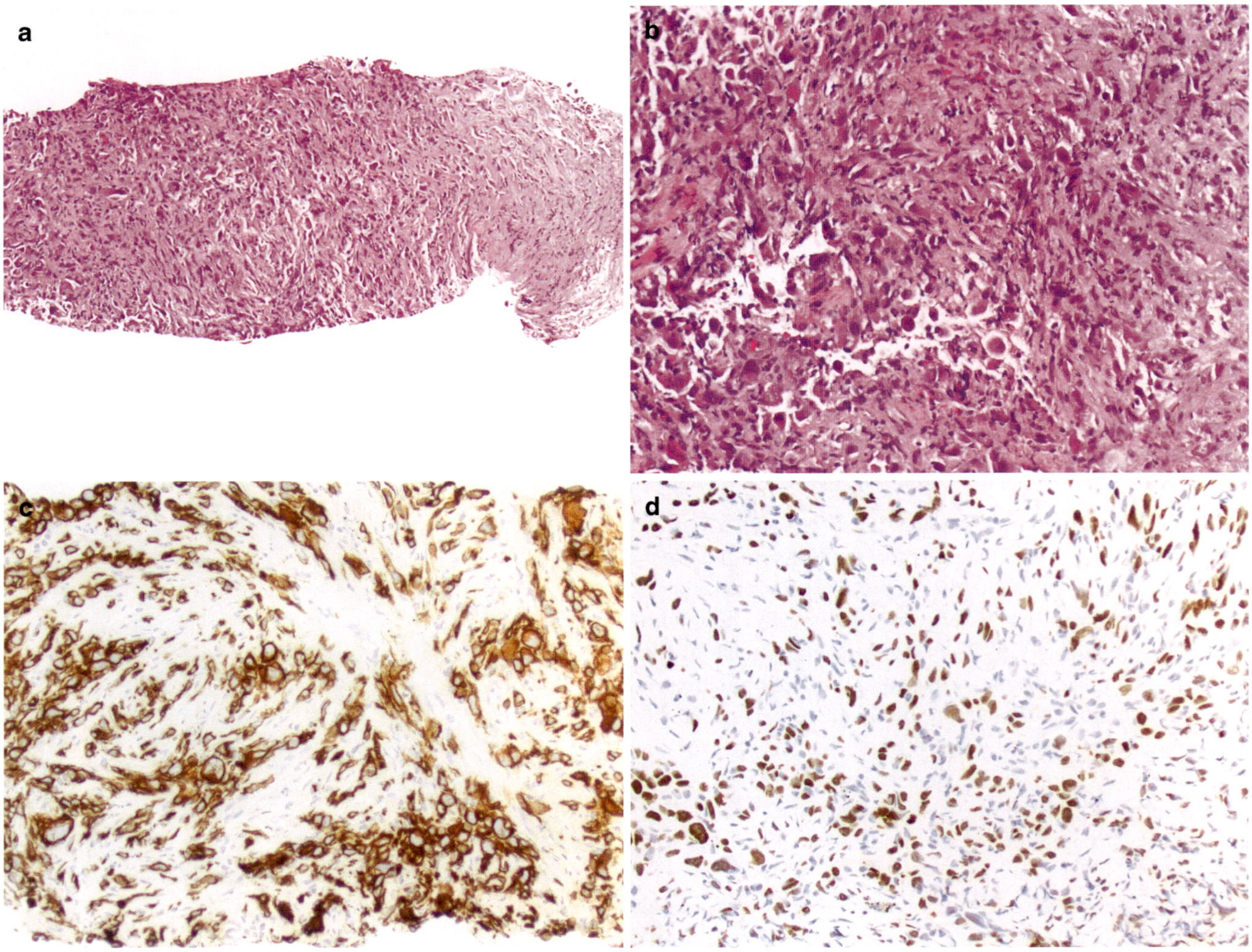

Fig. 23.2 Histology and immunohistochemistry of pleomorphic carcinoma. (**a** and **b**) Histologic sections of the left upper lobe mass biopsy show that the tumor consists of mainly spindle cells admixed with large pleomorphic/giant cells (hematoxylin and eosin, H & E; **a**, 100×; **b**, 200×). (**c**) Both spindle and giant cells are positive for pan-cytokeratin (IHC, 200×). (**d**) Both spindle and giant cells are positive for TTF-1 (IHC, 200×)

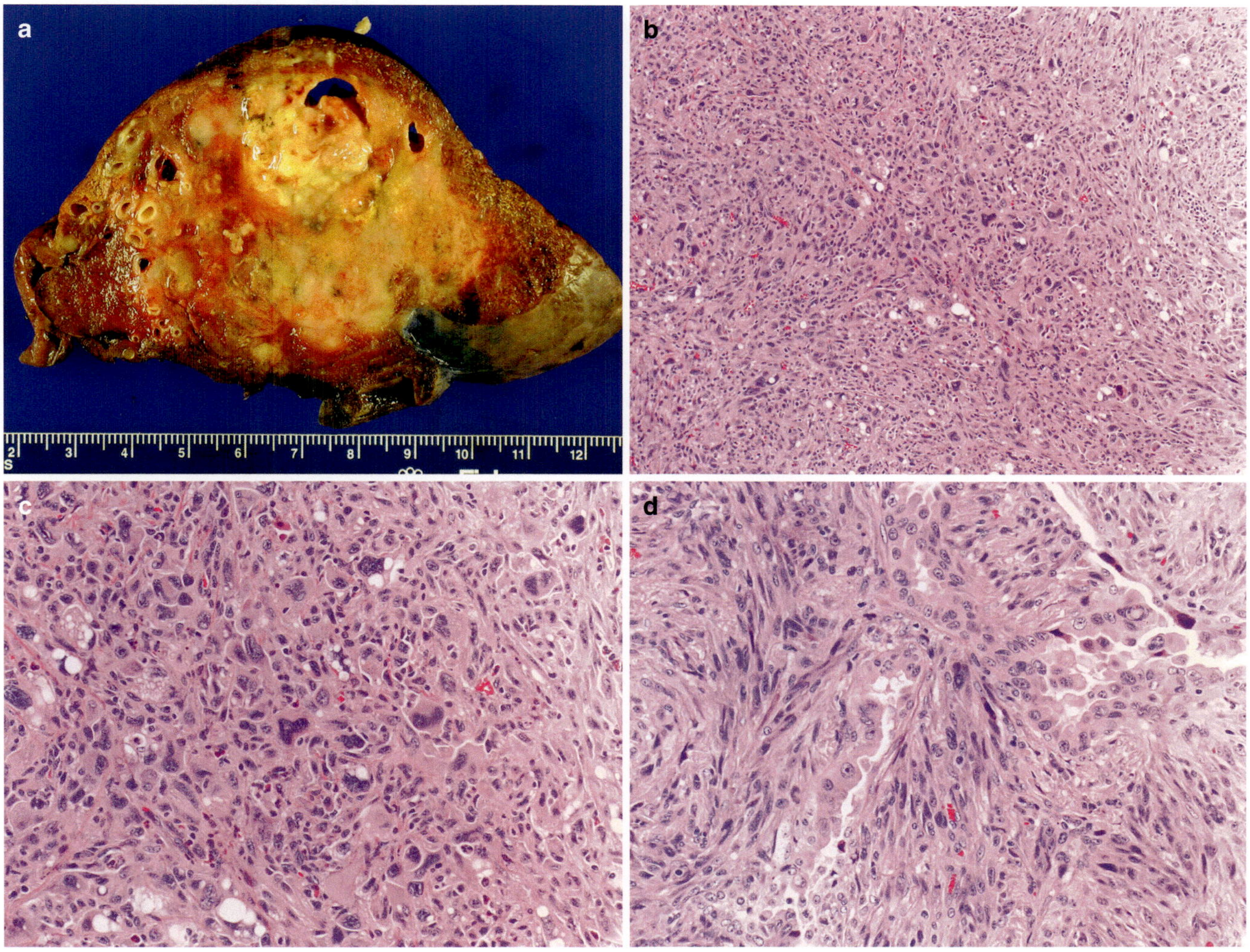

Fig. 23.3 Gross and histologic examination of the lung mass. (**a**) Gross image shows a 6.5 cm friable, tan-yellow, fleshy mass with foci of hemorrhage and necrosis. (**b**) Histologic sections show that the tumor consists of spindle cells admixed with giant cells. Scattered lymphoplasmacytic infiltration is present (**b**, hematoxylin and eosin, H & E; 100×). (**c**) Higher magnification histologic section highlights marked pleomorphism of the giant tumor cells, with cytomegaly and large irregular multilobated and hyperchromatic nuclei (H & E, 200×). (**d**) Histologic section showing a focus of adenocarcinoma admixed with malignant spindle cells (**d**, H & E, 200×)

Final Pathologic Diagnosis: Pleomorphic (Spindle and Giant Cell) Carcinoma with Adenocarcinoma Component (pT3 N1)

What Is the Definition of Pleomorphic Carcinoma of the Lung?

Pleomorphic carcinoma of the lung is a general term used to refer to a spectrum of histologically heterogeneous group of tumors with loss of morphologic features of epithelial differentiation. These may be classified as pure spindle cell carcinoma, pure giant cell carcinoma, or pleomorphic carcinoma with both spindle and giant cell carcinoma and/or conventional non-small cell lung carcinoma (NSCLC) components, in which spindle and/or giant cells constitute at least 10% of total resected tumor [1]. Although "sarcomatoid carcinoma" is an acceptable alternative term for pleomorphic carcinoma, the 2021 WHO classification of Thoracic Tumours [2] more clearly defines sarcomatoid carcinoma as a term encompassing a broader range of tumors, which includes pleomorphic carcinoma, pulmonary blastoma and carcinosarcoma.

What Are the Clinical, Radiographic, and Prognostic Features of Pleomorphic Carcinoma of the Lung?

Pleomorphic carcinoma of the lung is a rare histologic subtype of NSCLC accounting for 0.5–0.8% of all lung cancers. Most patients are tobacco smokers with a median age of 68.5 years (range 33–88 years) and predominantly male (~4:1 male-to-female ratio) [1, 3–5]. Presenting symptoms are similar to those of other NSCLCs and include chest pain, cough, and hemoptysis. The typical imaging finding at the time of presentation is a large peripheral mass (2.0–17.0 cm), usually in one of the upper lobes, with areas of cavitation or low central attenuation on CT (Fig. 23.1). These tumors often invade into the overlying pleura. Otherwise, the imaging study findings are similar to those of other NSCLCs. Overall, patients with pleomorphic carcinoma of the lung present with more advanced stage and have a high risk for relapse and worse survival outcomes than patients with other forms of NSCLCs [1, 4, 6].

What Are the Pathologic Features of Pleomorphic Carcinoma of the Lung?

Gross Examination

Pleomorphic carcinomas of the lung are usually well circumscribed, often large (median size 5 cm), and most frequently located at the periphery of the upper lobes. They often have involvement of the pleura and even the chest wall or mediastinum. Tumor necrosis and hemorrhage with or without cavitation are common. The cut surface may be somewhat heterogeneous with both firm and soft areas, some of which may be grayish gelatinous or "fish-flesh" in appearance (Fig. 23.3a).

Histology

While giant cell and spindle cell carcinomas consist almost entirely of tumor giant cells or spindle cells, respectively, the term pleomorphic carcinoma is used to refer to tumors with mixed morphology. Specifically, pleomorphic carcinoma is a poorly differentiated NSCLC, most commonly adenocarcinoma (Fig. 23.4a), followed by squamous cell carcinoma (Fig. 23.4b) or undifferentiated carcinoma containing a spindle cell and/or giant cell component. The spindle/giant cell component should comprise at least 10% of the tumor cells. In addition, tumors composed of a mixture of malignant spindle and giant cells in the absence of recognizable adenocarcinoma or squamous cell carcinoma components are also classified as pleomorphic carcinomas. The presence of epithelial components, either squamous cell carcinoma or adenocarcinoma, should be reported in the final pathologic diagnosis. Although rare, if a component of small-cell carcinoma is present, the tumor is classified as a combined small cell carcinoma, with mention of the specific NSCLC components present. Since pleomorphic carcinoma often has a larger size, at least 1 section/cm of the tumor mass should be submitted for histologic examination. If there is suspicion for the presence of a differentiated epithelial component in a sarcomatoid tumor, more thorough sampling to identify areas of adenocarcinoma or squamous cell carcinoma may help in making the diagnosis. In small biopsy specimens, the possibility of pleomorphic carcinoma may be suggested if spindle cell and/or giant cell components are present, but a diagnosis of pleomorphic carcinoma cannot be made due to the requirement of at least 10% neoplastic spindle and/or giant cells in a resection specimen. Accordingly, a biopsy diagnosis of NSCLC (mention if adenocarcinoma or squamous cell carcinoma is present) with spindle cell and/or giant cell features has been suggested [2, 7].

As alluded to above, spindle cell carcinoma is defined as carcinoma consisting of an almost pure population of malignant spindle cells arranged in a fascicular or storiform pattern (Fig. 23.5a, b) without differentiated carcinomatous components or heterologous elements with recognizable cartilaginous, osteogenic, myogenic, or vascular differentiation.

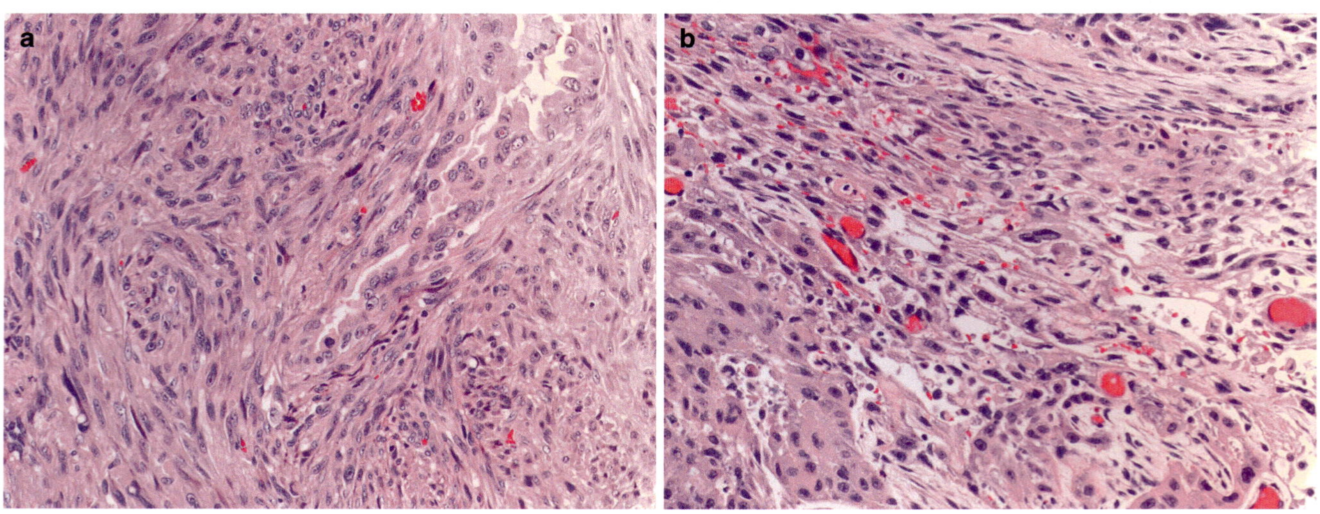

Fig. 23.4 (**a**) Histology of pleomorphic carcinoma of the lung. (**a**) Histologic sections demonstrate a pleomorphic carcinoma with malignant spindle cells admixed with adenocarcinoma (**a**, H & E, 200×). (**b**) Histologic sections show a pleomorphic carcinoma with malignant spindle cells admixed with squamous cell carcinoma (**b**, H & E, 200×)

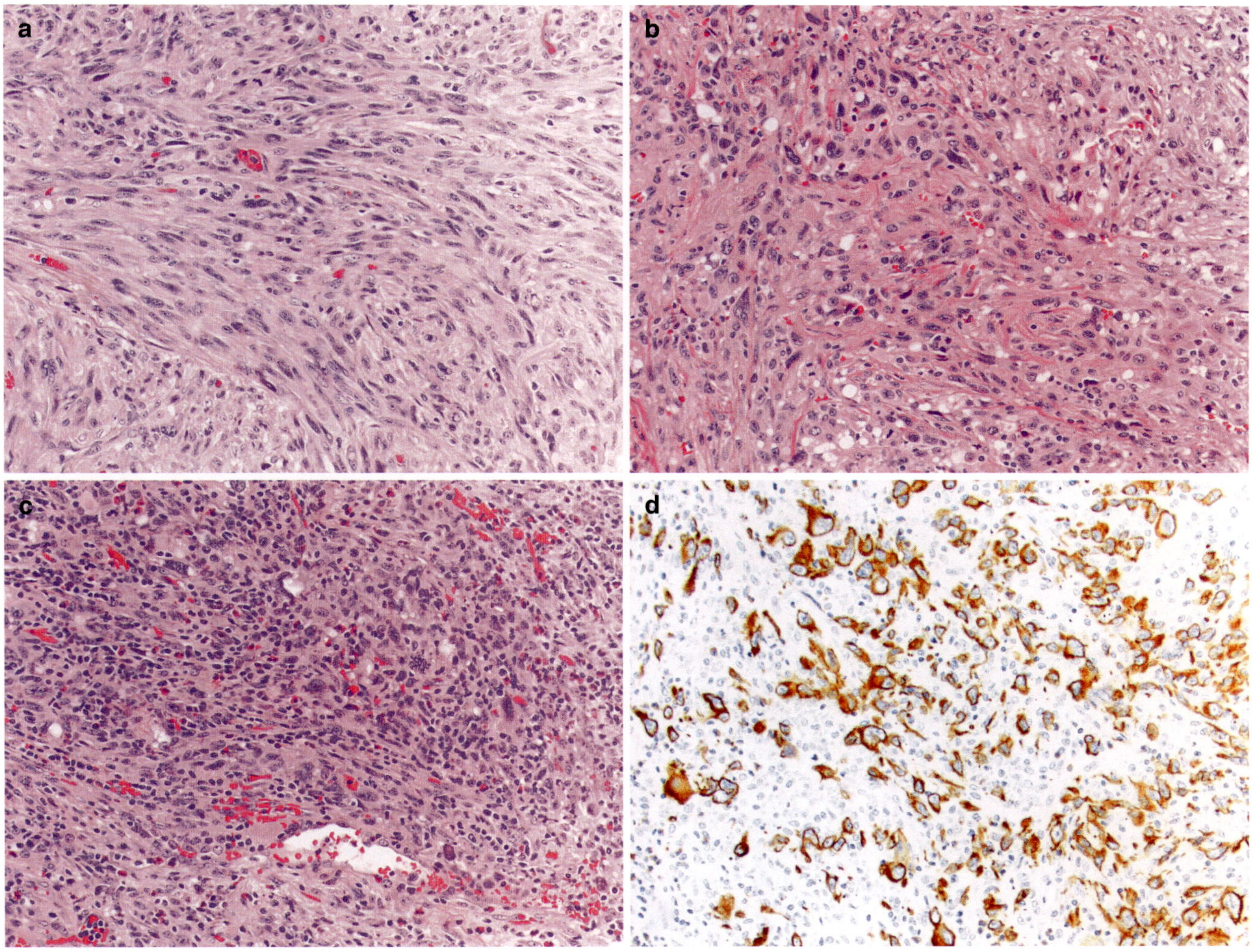

Fig. 23.5 Histology and immunohistochemistry of spindle cell carcinoma of the lung. Histology of spindle cell carcinoma shows malignant spindle cells in a fascicular pattern with hyperchromatic nuclei and prominent nucleoli in a hyalinized stroma (**a**, H & E, 200×), malignant spindle cells in a storiform pattern with hyperchromatic nuclei and prominent nucleoli (**b**, H & E, 200×), and a prominent inflammatory stroma (**c**, H & E, 200×); immunohistochemistry shows malignant spindle cells staining with cytokeratin in the background of inflammatory cells (**d**, IHC, 200×)

Small biopsies with foci of spindle cells are generally insufficient for the diagnosis. Rare cases may show prominent inflammatory stroma (Fig. 23.5c), often leading to confusion with other inflammatory lesions, such as necrotizing granulomas or inflammatory myofibroblastic tumors. Immunohistochemical stain for cytokeratin is very helpful in distinguishing tumor-associated desmoplasia and inflammatory lesions from spindle cell carcinoma (Fig. 23.5d).

Giant cell carcinoma consists almost entirely of pleomorphic tumor giant cells (including multinucleated cells) without differentiated carcinomatous components. The giant cells are large and discohesive with eosinophilic cytoplasm and bizarre shapes, as well as large irregular single or multiple nuclei with prominent nucleoli and coarse or vesicular chromatin (Fig. 23.6a). Positive diffuse cytokeratin expression by immunohistochemistry can help differentiate giant cell carcinoma from most types of sarcoma (Fig. 23.6b). Intratumoral neutrophilic infiltration and emperipolesis may be seen in some cases.

Immunohistochemistry

The diagnosis of pleomorphic carcinoma of the lung is mainly based on morphology; however, the use of immunohistochemistry (IHC) can help recognize different tumor components and to differentiate it from other mimics if needed. Of note, positive cytokeratin expression is not required in the spindle/giant cell component if non-pleomorphic carcinomatous components are unequivocally recognized. Cytokeratins and lineage-specific markers such as TTF-1, napsin A, p63, p40, and CK5/6 can be variably expressed in pleomorphic components. The tumoral giant cells may morphologically resemble syncytiotrophoblast and

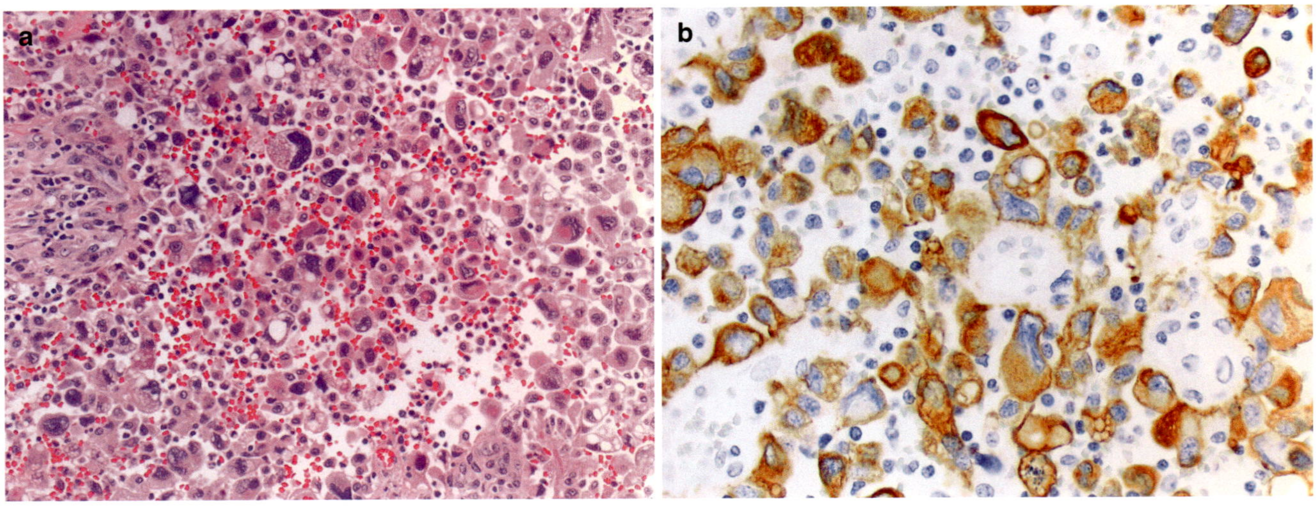

Fig. 23.6 Histology and immunohistochemistry of giant cell carcinoma. (**a**) Histology of giant cell carcinoma shows malignant giant cells with eosinophilic cytoplasm and bizarre shapes, as well as large, irregular, single, and multiple nuclei (**a**, H & E, 200×). (**b**) Immunohistochemistry of giant cell carcinoma shows that the malignant giant cells are positive for pan-cytokeratin (**b**, IHC, 400×)

show immunoreactivity for human chorionic gonadotropin (HCG). However, this finding should not be interpreted as primary lung choriocarcinoma [8, 9], as up to 84% lung cancers can ectopically produce any of the placental glycoproteins [10]. Morphologically, the absence of two distinct trophoblast cell forms and the presence of overall greater cytologic pleomorphism are features that favor the diagnosis of giant cell carcinoma. Although cases of primary lung choriocarcinoma have been reported [9, 11], most cases actually represent giant cell carcinomas with ectopic production of HCG [7].

What Are the Genetic and/or Molecular Features of Pleomorphic Carcinoma of the Lung?

Compared to other NSCLCs, only a few studies have explored the genetic and molecular profiles of pleomorphic carcinomas of the lung. One recent study demonstrated genomic alterations of p53 in 74%, *KRAS* in 34%, *MET* in 13.6%, *EGFR* in 8.8%, *BRAF* in 7.2%, *HER2* in 1.6%, and *RET* in 0.8% of pleomorphic carcinomas of the lung [3]. Several studies have demonstrated an overrepresentation of *MET* exon 14 skipping mutations in pleomorphic carcinomas when compared to pulmonary adenocarcinoma [12, 13]. Anaplastic lymphoma kinase (*ALK*) rearrangements have also been reported, with one case of successful treatment with ALK tyrosine kinase inhibitor, crizotinib [6]. In addition, pleomorphic carcinomas of the lung show slightly higher tumor mutational burdens compared to other NSCLCs (>20 mutations vs. 14 mutations/Mb) [3].

What Are the Differential Diagnoses for Pleomorphic Carcinoma of the Lung?

The differential diagnosis includes poorly differentiated squamous cell carcinoma or adenocarcinoma, carcinoma with reactive desmoplastic stroma, inflammatory myofibroblastic tumor, carcinosarcoma, lung primary or metastatic sarcoma, metastatic malignant melanoma, and sarcomatoid malignant mesothelioma (SMM). IHC staining with cytokeratins, TTF-1/napsin A, and p63/p40 can aid in the distinction of pleomorphic carcinoma from sarcoma or reactive stromal cells. Clinical history and IHC with melanocytic markers such as SOX10, Melan A, or HMB45 can help make the diagnosis of metastatic malignant melanoma. Of note, synovial sarcoma may closely resemble spindle cell carcinoma, even by electron microscopy and IHC. The marked propensity of synovial sarcoma to affect children, adolescents, and young adults, its typical SS18-SSX gene fusion/X;18 translocation, which can now be detected by fusion-specific IHC, nuclear staining with TLE1, and lack of TTF-1 expression are important features for distinguishing it from spindle cell carcinoma of the lung.

Carcinosarcoma is a malignant tumor that consists of a mixture of NSCLC (typically squamous cell carcinoma or adenocarcinoma) and sarcoma, with the latter component often containing malignant heterologous elements of skeletal muscle, cartilage, or bone origin [2]. Among the heterologous components, rhabdomyosarcoma is the most common, followed by chondrosarcoma and osteosarcoma. Combination of these heterologous components is also common. As previously mentioned, pleomorphic carcinoma differs from carcinosarcoma in that it lacks the mesenchymal heterologous component. Extensive sampling (at least 1 section/cm) of a resected tumor mass should be submitted for histologic examination to rule out the possibility of heterologous components in a pleomorphic carcinoma.

Due to its frequent peripheral location and pleural involvement, pulmonary pleomorphic carcinoma can be mistaken for a malignant tumor of pleural origin with lung parenchymal involvement, particularly sarcomatoid malignant mesothelioma (SMM).

What Are the Clinicopathologic Features of Sarcomatoid Malignant Mesothelioma?

Malignant mesothelioma (MM) can be either localized or diffuse depending on its extent of pleural involvement (gross appearance), and it can be categorized into epithelioid, biphasic, or sarcomatoid subtypes; both of these features are important for prognosis and treatment decisions. Epithelioid MM is the most common histologic subtype, composed mainly of tubulopapillary, solid, and trabecular architectural patterns and less frequently micropapillary and adenomatoid (microcystic) patterns [2]. Epitheliod MM can also show a spectrum of cytologic features, including deciduoid, small cell, clear cell, and signet ring, which bear no prognostic implications, lymphohistiocytoid, which is considered prognostically favorable, and rhabdoid and pleomorphic, which are associated with adverse clinical outcomes. In fact, MMs composed entirely of diffuse/solid sheets of anaplastic or prominent giant cells have been designated as "pleomorphic mesotheliomas," a variant of epithelioid MM that behaves more like sarcomatoid and biphasic variant MMs [2, 5].

Sarcomatoid MM (SMM) comprises approximately 10% of MMs. Similar to pleomorphic carcinoma of the lung, patients diagnosed with SMM are more commonly male (83% male versus 17% female). However, SMM is slightly more prevalent in older patients (median 74 years, range 40–90 years) [5]. SMM is defined by the 2021 WHO classification as a proliferation of spindle cells arranged in fascicles or in a haphazard pattern with a wide range of morphologic features from plump to thin long cells. Nuclear atypia and mitotic activity can vary from minimal to marked. SMM often involves the adipose tissue of the parietal pleura and the adjacent lung parenchyma [2]. Desmoplastic mesothelioma, a variant of SMM, is characterized by hyalinized bundles of collagen arranged in a storiform pattern ("patternless pattern") and separated by plump hyperchromatic spindle cell nuclei, with this pattern involving $\geq$ 50% of the tumor. In addition to spindle-shaped neoplastic cells, SMMs can have heterologous osteosarcomatous, chondrosarcomatous, and/or rhabdomyosarcomatous components. Biphasic MMs are composed of both epithelioid and sarcomatoid/desmoplastic components, with at least 10% of each pattern required for diagnosis [2].

How Does One Differentiate Pleomorphic Carcinoma of the Lung from Sarcomatoid Malignant Mesothelioma?

The differential diagnosis between epithelioid MM, including pleomorphic mesothelioma, and pleomorphic carcinoma of the lung can often be resolved with the use of IHC for mesothelial markers (such as calretinin, WT1, and/or D2-40) and markers of carcinoma (such as claudin-4, Ber-EP4, MOC31, monoclonal CEA, Leu M1 (CD15), B72.3). However, the distinction of sarcomatoid and desmoplastic MMs from pleomorphic carcinomas of the lung may be difficult, since both types of tumors can be morphologically indistinguishable and are frequently only positive for pancytokeratin. A frequently useful initial IHC panel includes one or more cytokeratins such as AE1/AE3, OSCAR, CK18, or CAM 5.2, which can be used to exclude the possibility of sarcoma. Mesothelial markers (such as WT1 and CK5/6) tend to be negative in SMMs, while epithelial markers (such as claudin 4, MOC31, BER-EP4, and monoclonal CEA) are often not helpful in distinguishing different sarcomatoid tumors. Therefore, IHC for these markers may be unfruitful, and should be avoided when there is limited tissue. Podoplanin (D2-40) (74%, range 47.7–89.9%) and calretinin (53.9%, range 41.8–65.6%) are commonly positive in SMMs, but the positivity may be extremely focal, and can also be seen in 20.1% (14.2–27.7%) and 37.1% (14.1–68.0%) of pleomorphic carcinomas of the lung, respectively [5, 14]. GATA3, a marker that is frequently positive in breast and urothelial carcinomas, has been reported in one study as strong and diffuse in sarcomatoid/desmoplastic MMs and negative in sarcomatoid carcinomas with only rare cases showing weak and patchy staining [15].

Although IHC is broadly used to distinguish SMMs from pleomorphic carcinomas of the lung, there are still no clear guidelines on how to interpret cases that show overlapping or equivocal IHC findings. Recently, a systematic meta-analysis was performed by the International Mesothelioma Panel and the MESOPATH National Reference Center, and best evidence diagnostic guidelines were proposed [5]. In this proposed guidelines, three panels of antibodies are recommended to use to differentiate SMM and sarcomatoid carcinomas: keratins (> 1 antibody), mesothelial markers (WT1, D2-40, calretinin), and carcinoma markers (claudin 4, Ber-EP4, TTF-1, and others). For example, if both keratin and mesothelial markers are positive, but carcinoma markers are negative, the recommended diagnosis is SMM; if keratin markers are positive, but mesothelial and carcinoma markers are negative, the recommended diagnosis is probable SMM, and other keratin-expressing tumors such as vascular tumors, synovial sarcoma, and others should be excluded; if mesothelial markers are positive, but keratin and carcinoma markers are negative, the recommended diagnosis is possible

SMM, and a careful review of the clinical history and imaging studies is suggested to exclude the possibility of tumors other than SMM. If both keratin and carcinoma markers are positive, but mesothelial markers are negative, the recommended diagnosis is pleomorphic carcinoma of the lung; if carcinoma markers are positive, but keratins and mesothelial markers are negative, the recommended diagnosis is probable pleomorphic carcinoma of the lung. If keratins are positive, but mesothelial and carcinoma markers are negative, the recommended diagnosis is possible pleomorphic carcinoma of the lung or SMM, but this immunoprofile is unusual, and IHC should probably be repeated to exclude laboratory errors. If all the three panels of markers are negative, the recommended diagnosis is undifferentiated sarcomatoid neoplasm, and the possibility of sarcoma should be excluded [5].

Are There Any Molecular Markers that Can Help Differentiate Sarcomatoid Malignant Mesothelioma from Pleomorphic Carcinoma of the Lung?

The most common molecular alterations in MM are acquired or germline mutations of BRCA1-associated protein 1 (BAP1) and homozygous deletion of 9p21 locus within a cluster of genes including *CDKN2A* (*p16INK4A*), *CDKN2B*, and *methylthioadenosine phosphorylase* (*MTAP*). Homozygous deletion of *p16INK4A* detected by fluorescence in situ hybridization (FISH) and/or loss of BAP1 expression detected by IHC are the features that help distinguish pleural MMs from reactive mesothelial proliferations. BAP1 loss is absent or rarely seen in pleomorphic carcinoma of the lung, but is found more commonly in epithelioid MMs (40–60%) than in SMMs (<20%) [16–18]. In contrast, homozygous deletion of *p16INK4A* is more commonly seen in SMMs (90–100%) than in epithelioid MMs (up to 70%) [14]. *MTAP* gene, which is also located on the 9p21 locus, is frequently co-deleted with *p16INK4A* in some MMs, allowing MTAP loss by IHC to serve as a surrogate marker of p16INK4A deletion. Recently, a combination of MTAP and BAP1 loss detected by IHC was shown to detect MM with a higher sensitivity than BAP1 IHC alone or 9p21/*p16INK4A* FISH alone [19]. Although these markers are excellent in differentiating pleural MMs from reactive mesothelial proliferations, they, especially *p16INK4A FISH and MTAP* IHC, are not particularly useful in distinguishing MMs from carcinomas of the lung, since genetic alteration of 9p21 is one of the most frequent events in other tumors, including NSCLC, melanoma, and sarcomas [14, 20].

References

1. Rahouma M, Kamel M, Narula N, Nasar A, Harrison S, Lee B, et al. Pulmonary sarcomatoid carcinoma: an analysis of a rare cancer from the surveillance, epidemiology, and end results database. Eur J Cardiothorac Surg. 2018;53(4):828–34.
2. WHO Classification of Tumours Editorial Board. Thoracic tumours. Lyon (France): International Agency for Research on Cancer; 2021. (WHO classification of tumours series, 5th ed.; vol. 5). https://publications.iarc.fr/595.
3. Schrock AB, Li SD, Frampton GM, Suh J, Braun E, Mehra R, et al. Pulmonary sarcomatoid carcinomas commonly harbor either potentially targetable genomic alterations or high tumor mutational burden as observed by comprehensive genomic profiling. J Thorac Oncol. 2017;12(6):932–42.
4. Steuer CE, Behera M, Liu Y, Fu C, Gillespie TW, Saba NF, et al. Pulmonary sarcomatoid carcinoma: an analysis of the National Cancer Data Base. Clin Lung Cancer. 2017;18(3):286–92.
5. Marchevsky AM, LeStang N, Hiroshima K, Pelosi G, Attanoos R, Churg A, et al. The differential diagnosis between pleural sarcomatoid mesothelioma and spindle cell/pleomorphic (sarcomatoid) carcinomas of the lung: evidence-based guidelines from the international mesothelioma panel and the MESOPATH National Reference Center. Hum Pathol. 2017;67:160–8.
6. Chen X, Zhang Y, Lu J, Xu C, Liang J, Wang F, et al. Pulmonary sarcomatoid carcinoma with ALK rearrangement: frequency, clinical-pathologic characteristics, and response to ALK inhibitor. Transl Oncol. 2017;10(2):115–20.
7. Travis WD. Sarcomatoid neoplasms of the lung and pleura. Arch Pathol Lab Med. 2010;134(11):1645–58.
8. Boucher LD, Yoneda K. The expression of trophoblastic cell markers by lung carcinomas. Hum Pathol. 1995;26(11):1201–6.
9. Attanoos RL, Papagiannis A, Suttinont P, Goddard H, Papotti M, Gibbs AR. Pulmonary giant cell carcinoma: pathological entity or morphological phenotype? Histopathology. 1998;32(3):225–31.
10. Wilson TS, McDowell EM, McIntire KR, Trump BF. Elaboration of human chorionic gonadotropin by lung tumors: an immunocytochemical study. Arch Pathol Lab Med. 1981;105(4):169–73.
11. Ikura Y, Inoue T, Tsukuda H, Yamamoto T, Ueda M, Kobayashi Y. Primary choriocarcinoma and human chorionic gonadotrophin-producing giant cell carcinoma of the lung: are they independent entities? Histopathology. 2000;36(1):17–25.
12. Liu X, Jia Y, Stoopler MB, Shen Y, Cheng H, Chen J, Mansukhani M, Koul S, Halmos B, Borczuk AC. Next-generation sequencing of pulmonary sarcomatoid carcinoma reveals high frequency of actionable MET gene mutations. J Clin Oncol. 2016;10;34(8):794–802. https://doi.org/10.1200/JCO.2015.62.0674. Epub 2015 Jul 27. PMID: 26215952.
13. Awad MM, Oxnard GR, Jackman DM, Savukoski DO, Hall D, Shivdasani P, Heng JC, Dahlberg SE, Jänne PA, Verma S, Christensen J, Hammerman PS, Sholl LM. MET exon 14 mutations in non-small-cell lung cancer are associated with advanced age and stage-dependent MET genomic amplification and c-Met overexpression. J Clin Oncol. 2016;1;34(7):721–30. https://doi.org/10.1200/JCO.2015.63.4600. Epub 2016 Jan 4. PMID: 26729443.
14. Husain AN, Colby TV, Ordonez NG, Allen TC, Attanoos RL, Beasley MB, et al. Guidelines for pathologic diagnosis of malignant mesothelioma 2017 update of the consensus statement from the international mesothelioma interest group. Arch Pathol Lab Med. 2018;142(1):89–108.

15. Berg KB, Churg A. GATA3 immunohistochemistry for distinguishing sarcomatoid and desmoplastic mesothelioma from Sarcomatoid carcinoma of the lung. Am J Surg Pathol. 2017;41(9):1221–5.
16. Hwang HC, Pyott S, Rodriguez S, Cindric A, Carr A, Michelsen C, et al. BAP1 immunohistochemistry and p16 FISH in the diagnosis of sarcomatous and desmoplastic mesotheliomas. Am J Surg Pathol. 2016;40(5):714–8.
17. Owen D, Sheffield BS, Ionescu D, Churg A. Loss of BRCA1-associated protein 1 (BAP1) expression is rare in non-small cell lung cancer. Human Pathol. 2017;60:82–5.
18. Yoshimura M, Kinoshita Y, Hamasaki M, Matsumoto S, Hida T, Oda Y, et al. Diagnostic application of BAP1 immunohistochemistry to differentiate pleural mesothelioma from metastatic pleural tumours. Histopathology. 2017;71(6):1011–4.
19. Hida T, Hamasaki M, Matsumoto S, Sato A, Tsujimura T, Kawahara K, et al. Immunohistochemical detection of MTAP and BAP1 protein loss for mesothelioma diagnosis: comparison with 9p21 FISH and BAP1 immunohistochemistry. Lung Cancer. 2017;104:98–105.
20. Su CY, Chang YC, Chan YC, Lin TC, Huang MS, Yang CJ, et al. MTAP is an independent prognosis marker and the concordant loss of MTAP and p16 expression predicts short survival in non-small cell lung cancer patients. Eur J Surg Oncol. 2014;40(9):1143–50. https://doi.org/10.1016/j.ejso.2014.04.017.

Primary Sarcoma (Unclassified) Versus Sarcomatoid Mesothelioma/Carcinoma

24

Amir Qorbani, Gregory A. Fishbein, and Scott D. Nelson

Case Presentation

A 66-year-old man presented in clinic with 15-pound weight loss, night sweats, and right-sided chest wall pain. Initial workup revealed normocytic anemia and a right pulmonary mass on chest X-ray (Fig. 24.1). Computed tomography (CT) scan demonstrated a large heterogeneous mass within the right lung base that measured 15 × 13.6 × 6.2 cm. Positron-emission tomography (PET)/CT scan showed an enhancing mass with intense fluorodeoxyglucose (FDG) uptake (standardized update value, SUV max 22.3), abutting the right hemidiaphragm and extending into the rib interspaces, most prominently at the right seventh/eighth rib interspace (Fig. 24.2). He subsequently underwent CT-guided biopsy that revealed a poorly differentiated malignant neoplasm (Fig. 24.3). The tumor did not show any line of differentiation by histology or immunohistochemistry studies (negative staining for pan-cytokeratin, calretinin, TTF1, S100 protein, SOX10, MART1, desmin, CD34, EMA, CAM5.2, and caldesmon). He underwent surgical resection of the right chest wall and the right lower and middle lobes. Gross examination showed a well-circumscribed mass with light tan and firm cut surfaces, measuring 17.5 cm × 6.5 cm × 1.5 cm and abutting the rib without gross evidence of invasion (Fig. 24.4). Microscopic examination showed spindle-to-epithelioid neoplastic cells arranged in storiform and fascicular patterns, with large, pleomorphic nuclei with prominent nucleoli and moderate amounts of cytoplasm, as well as brisk mitotic activity and areas of necrosis and hemorrhage (Fig. 24.5a–d). The neoplastic cells did not show any immunoreactivity to epithelial, mesothelial, or glandular markers, evidenced by negative staining for pan-cytokeratin, CAM5.2, keratin 5/6, p63, calretinin, WT1, D2-40, TTF1, S100, SOX10, MART1, HMB45, desmin, caldesmon, EMA, CD34, STAT6, C-Kit, DOG1, myogenin, MyoD1, CD21, CD23, CD35, chromogranin, TLE1, BCL2, and CD99 (Fig. 24.6). All surgical margins were free of malignancy, and no lymph node metastases were identified. The patient was scheduled for adjuvant chemotherapy using an alkylating agent and radiation therapy.

A. Qorbani (✉)
UCSF Medical Center at Mission Bay, Pathology Department, University of California, San Francisco (UCSF), San Francisco, CA, USA
e-mail: amir.qorbani@ucsf.edu

G. A. Fishbein
Department of Pathology and Laboratory Medicine, David Geffen School of Medicine at UCLA, Los Angeles, CA, USA
e-mail: GFishbein@mednet.ucla.edu

S. D. Nelson
UCLA Santa Monica and Orthopedic Hospital, University of California, Los Angeles (UCLA), Santa Monica, CA, USA
e-mail: SDNelson@mednet.ucla.edu

H. Xu et al. (eds.), *Practical Lung Pathology*, Practical Anatomic Pathology, https://doi.org/10.1007/978-3-031-14402-8_24

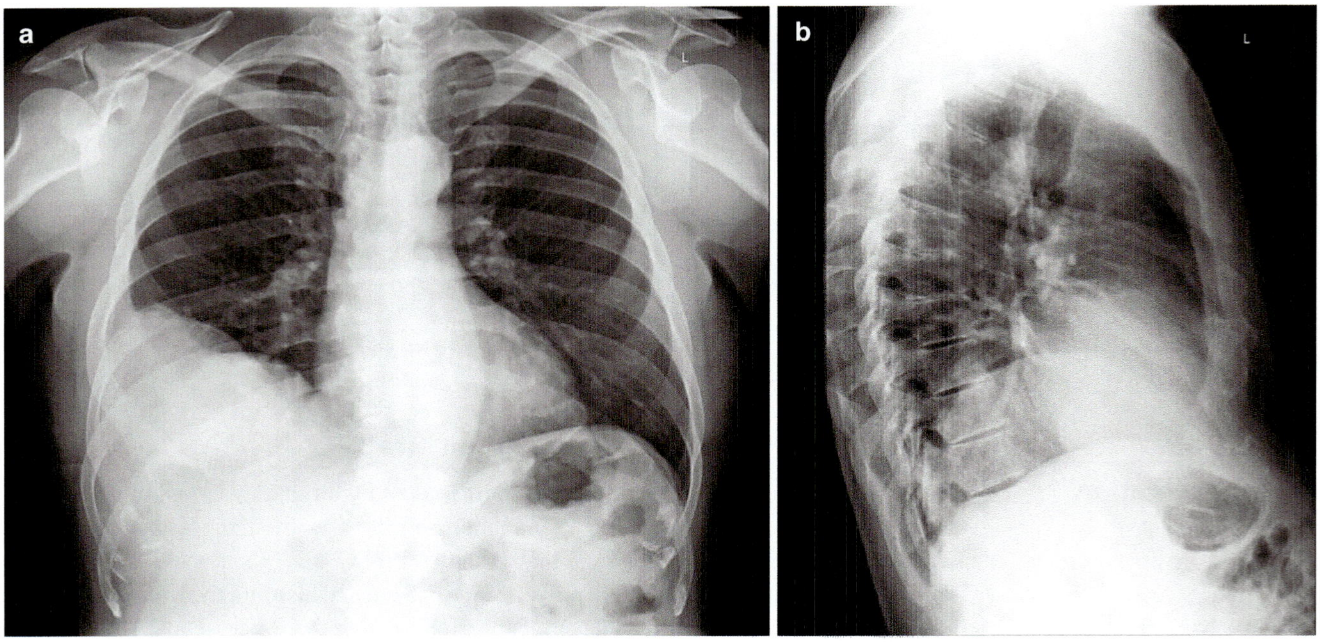

Fig. 24.1 Chest X-ray (**a**) anteroposterior view; (**b**) lateral view showing a large right lower lung mass. Reprinted from Qorbani A, Nelson SD. Primary pulmonary undifferentiated pleomorphic sarcoma (PPUPS). Autops Case Rep. 2019 Aug 22;9(3):e2019110. doi: 10.4322/acr.2019.110. PMID: 31528627; PMCID: PMC6709651 [1]

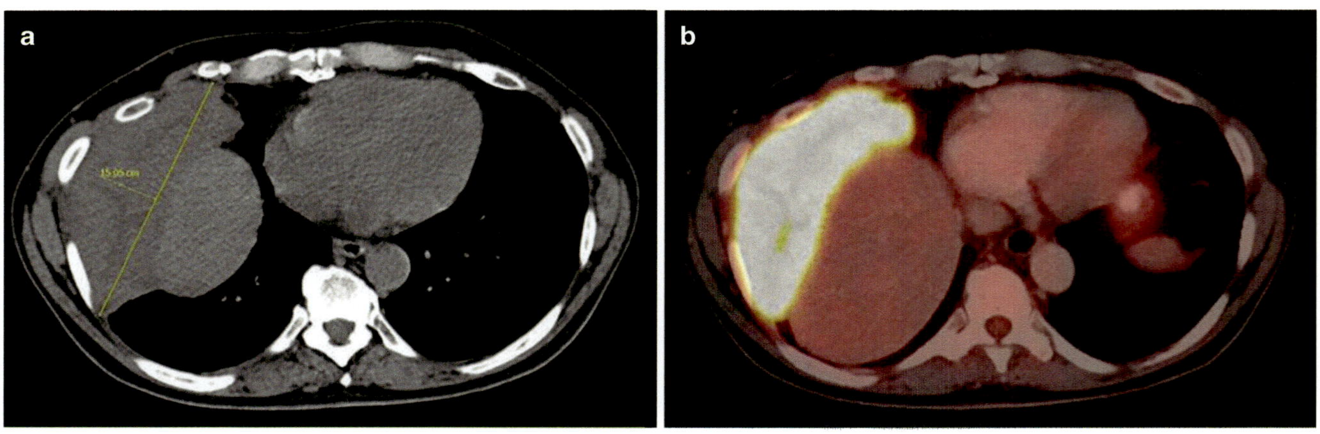

Fig. 24.2 Imaging study of the thorax. CT scan (**a**, axial plane; **c**, coronal plane) shows a 15 × 6 cm poorly circumscribed right lower lung mass protruding into the eighth and ninth intercostal spaces. (**b**, axial plane; **d**, coronal plane) PET scan shows a 15 cm right inferior lung mass and a 6 cm right superior paramediastinal mass with a high FDG uptake. Reprinted from Qorbani A, Nelson SD. Primary pulmonary undifferentiated pleomorphic sarcoma (PPUPS). Auops Case Rep. 2019 Aug 22;9(3):e2019110. doi: 10.4322/acr.2019.110. PMID: 31528627; PMCID: PMC6709651 [1]

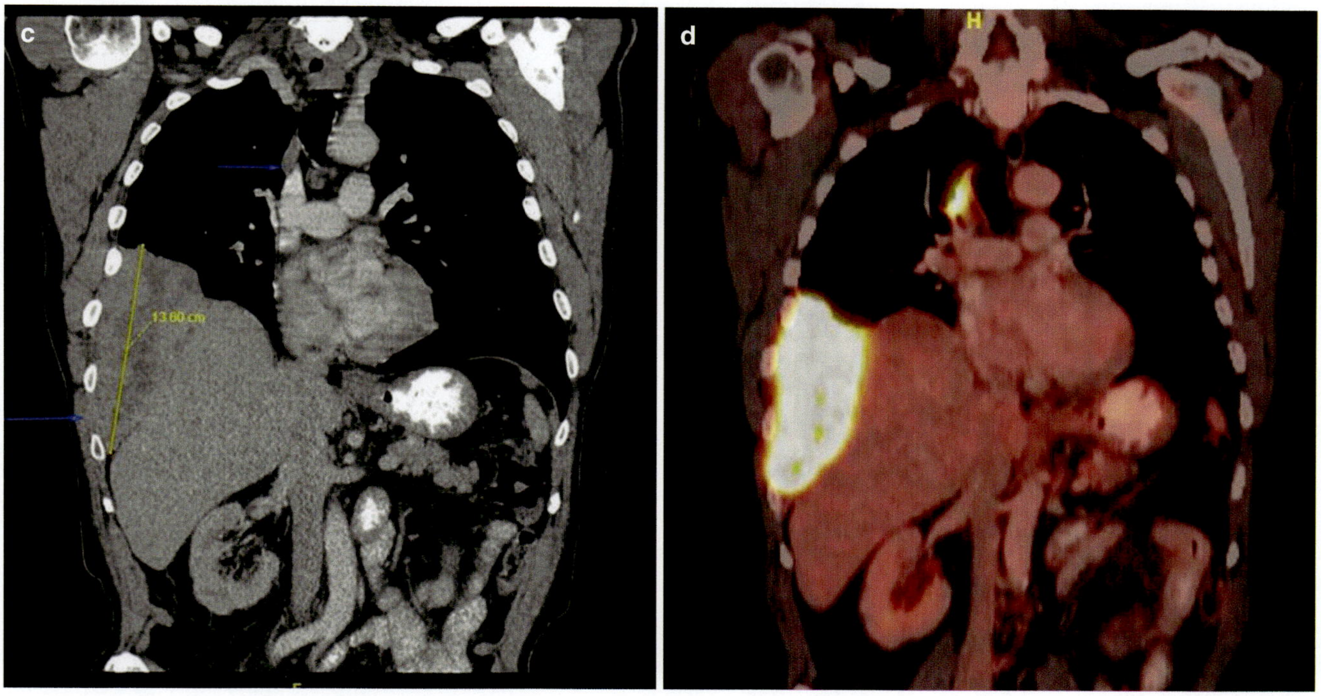

Fig. 24.2 (continued)

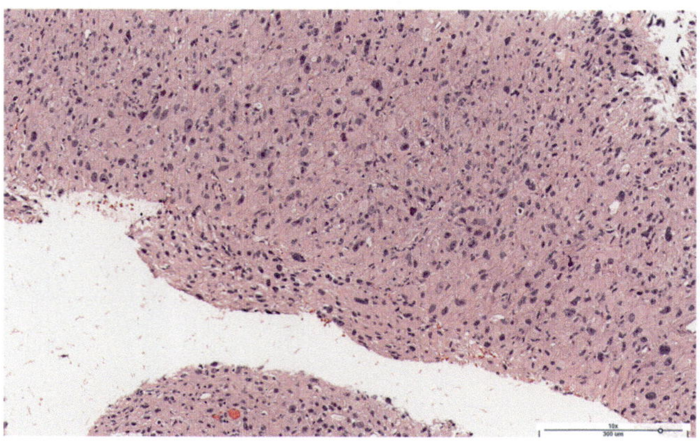

Fig. 24.3 CT-guided biopsy showed a poorly differentiated malignant epithelioid neoplasm (magnification 100×)

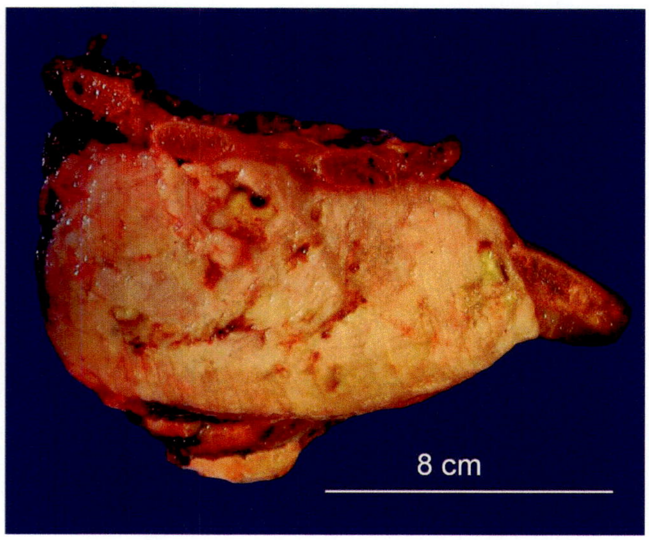

Fig. 24.4 Gross examination of the lung mass resection. 17.5 cm × 6.5 cm × 1.5 cm mass abutting the rib without direct invasion. Reprinted from Qorbani A, Nelson SD. Primary pulmonary undifferentiated pleomorphic sarcoma (PPUPS). Autops Case Rep. 2019 Aug 22;9(3):e2019110. doi: 10.4322/acr.2019.110. PMID: 31528627; PMCID: PMC6709651 [1]

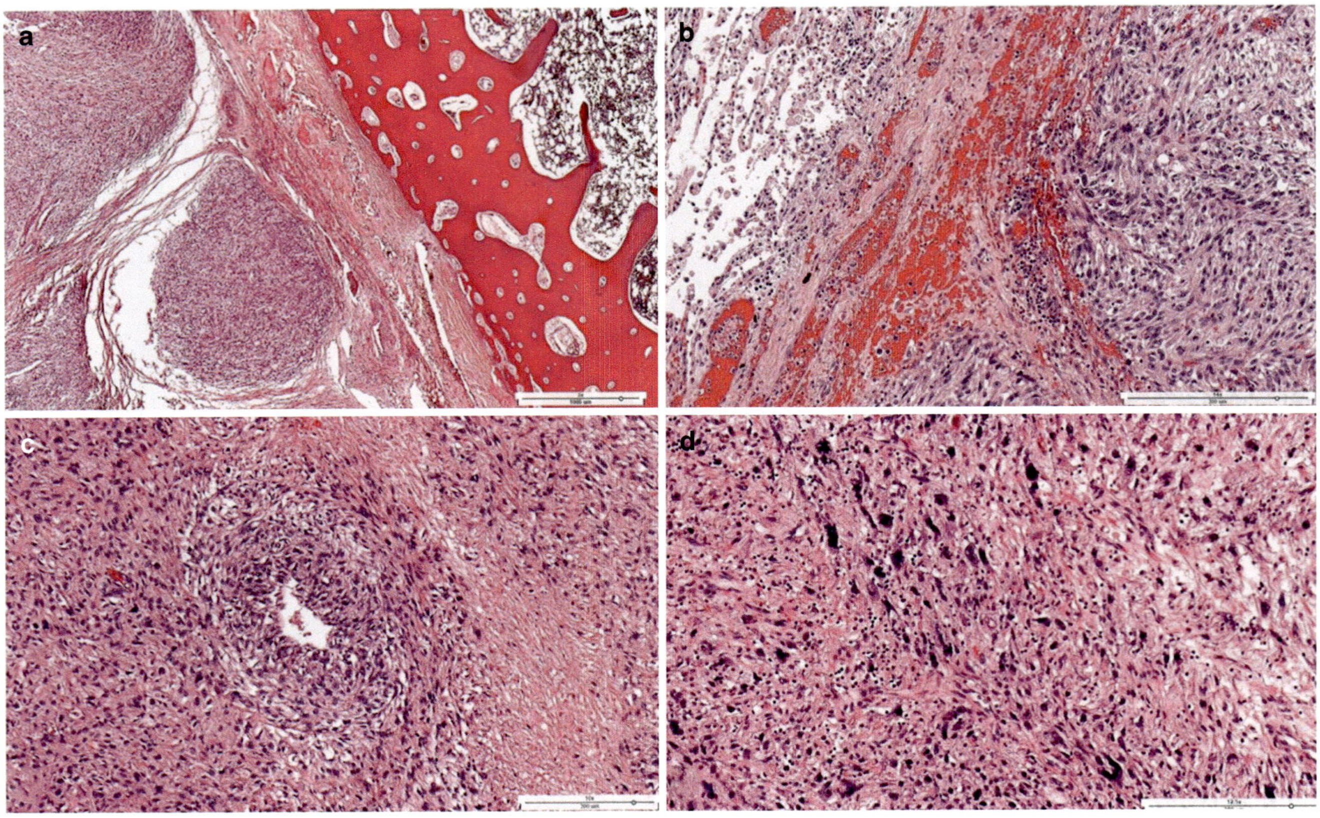

Fig. 24.5 Photomicrographs of the tumor showing in: (**a**) vaguely nodular high-grade spindle-to-epithelioid neoplasm with adjacent rib bone (H&E, 30×); (**b**) neoplastic cells with adjacent normal lung parenchyma (H&E, 140×); (**c**) undifferentiated pleomorphic sarcoma with areas of necrosis (H&E, 100×); (**d**) pleomorphic cells with a high mitotic activity, atypical mitoses, chronic inflammatory cell infiltrate, and focal necrosis (H&E, 125×). Reprinted from Qorbani A, Nelson SD. Primary pulmonary undifferentiated pleomorphic sarcoma (PPUPS). Autops Case Rep. 2019 Aug 22;9(3):e2019110. doi: 10.4322/acr.2019.110. PMID: 31528627; PMCID: PMC6709651 [1]

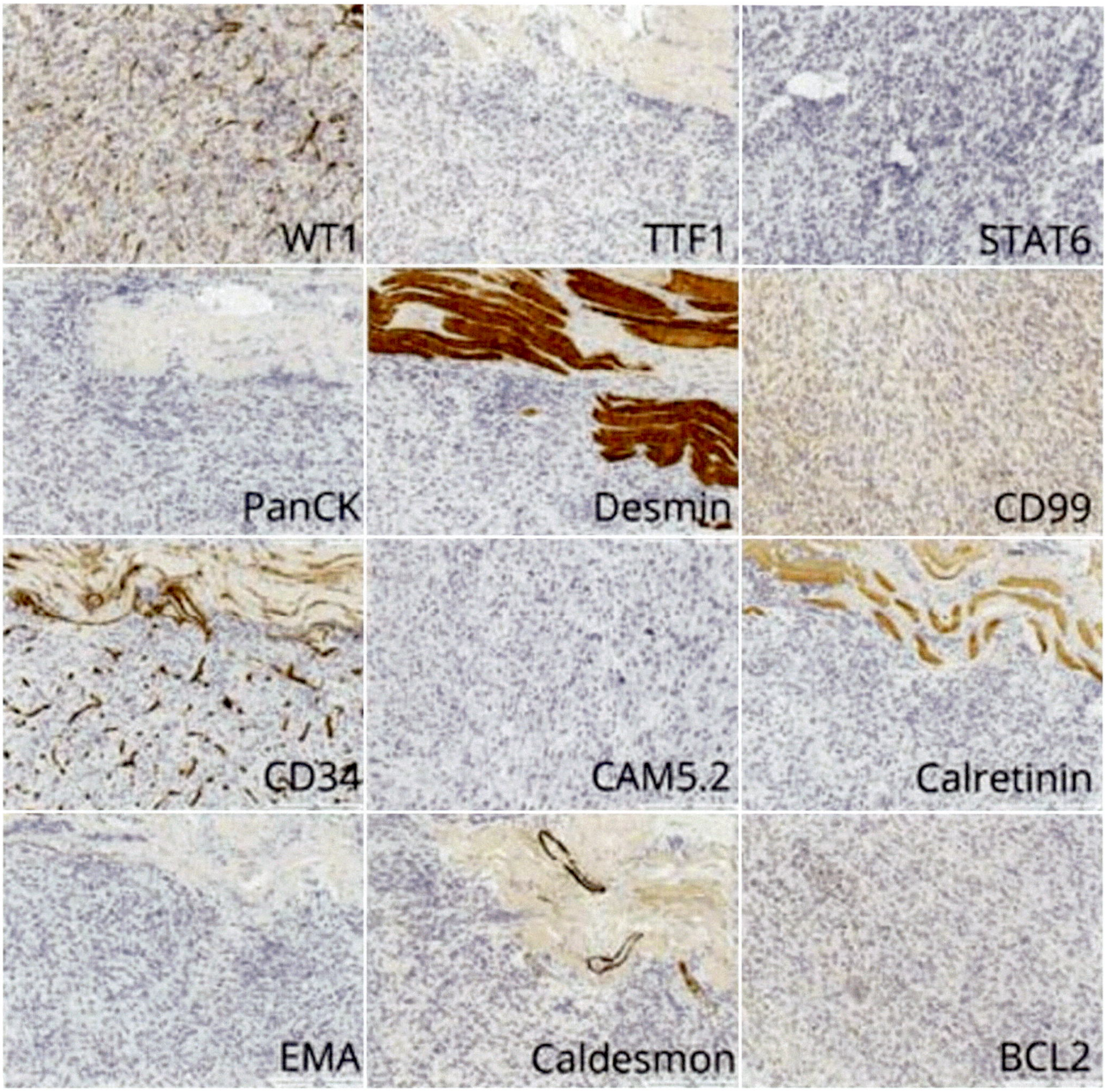

Fig. 24.6 Photomicrographs of the tumor. Immunohistochemistry studies show no line of differentiation (magnification 100×). Reprinted from Qorbani A, Nelson SD. Primary pulmonary undifferentiated pleomorphic sarcoma (PPUPS). Autops Case Rep. 2019 Aug 22;9(3):e2019110. doi: 10.4322/acr.2019.110. PMID: 31528627; PMCID: PMC6709651 [1]

Final Pathologic Diagnosis: Primary Pulmonary Undifferentiated Pleomorphic Sarcoma (PPUPS)

What Are the Clinical Features of PPUPS, and How Do They Differ from Sarcomatoid Mesothelioma/Carcinoma?

In general, primary lung sarcomas affect middle-aged to elderly patients with a slight male predominance. They account for less than 0.5% of all lung neoplasms. Primary pulmonary undifferentiated pleomorphic sarcoma (PPUPS) (formerly primary pulmonary malignant fibrous histiocytoma (MFH)) is exceptionally rare, with less than 75 reported cases in the English literature. Originally, it was thought that these tumors are derived from fibrohistiocytic origin, but gradually due to advanced immunohistochemical techniques, and electron microscopy, it became clear that there was no real scientific evidence for a "fibrohistiocytic" line of differentiation. Therefore, in 2012, the World Health Organization (WHO) declassified MFH as a diagnostic entity, replacing it with "undifferentiated pleomorphic sarcoma" [2]. UPSs usually occur in middle-aged to elderly adults (median age of 54 years) with no consistent gender predilection. In 1978, Weiss and Enzinger first described MFH in 200 cases [3]. One year later, Bedrossian et al. reported the first case of primary pulmonary MFH in a 51-year-old man [4]. Nascimento AG et al. reported four examples of primary pulmonary MFH in the Mayo Clinic archives among 10,134 cases of tumors arising in the lung [5]. Qorbani et al. reported the only case of PPUPS that has been diagnosed at UCLA from 2002 to 2018 [1]. Yousem and Hochholzer reported the most extensive series of primary malignant fibrous histiocytomas in the lung in 1987, describing 22 patients ranging from 18 to 80 years old [6]. Previous irradiation is a known pathogenic risk factor for UPS tumors arising in soft tissue, and few reports in the literature are available regarding patients who develop PPUPS years after radiation therapy for another tumor [6, 7]. Such tumors may alternatively be considered radiation-associated sarcomas.

Primary pulmonary sarcomas often present as a large peripheral or hilar well-circumscribed mass. However, they also can present as endobronchial tumors in 10% of cases [6], usually with symptoms of bronchial obstruction (chest pain, cough, hemoptysis, etc.). Radiologic findings can show post-obstructive effects (recurrent pneumonia, bronchiectasis, lobar or segmental atelectasis) and in some cases with extraluminal growth and/or local invasion into adjacent structures. Endobronchial masses have a more favorable prognosis compared to other sites [8]. The clinical course of these tumors is generally rapidly progressive, and metastasis is common [6]. The majority of patients die within a period of 1–72 months.

Sarcomatoid mesothelioma typically occurs in older adults (mean age of 70 years). These lesions usually present as progressive shortness of breath, unilateral chest pain, weight loss, and unilateral pleural effusion. Diffuse pleural thickening or, less commonly, a single pleural mass may be observed [9].

Clinical presentations are more dependent on the tumor location than the histological type. Therefore, clinical and radiographic features of PPUPS, sarcomatoid mesothelioma/carcinoma, or even more common epithelial tumors of the lung can be identical.

What Are the Pathologic Features of PPUPS and Sarcomatoid Mesothelioma/Carcinoma?

Gross

PPUPSs are usually well circumscribed but not encapsulated with light tan and firm cut surfaces. Areas of necrosis and hemorrhage are frequently seen in these tumors. The size of these tumors may range from 1 cm to more than 10 cm in greatest dimension [6]. Mesotheliomas usually present as solitary, circumscribed mass attached to the pleura or other serosal surfaces.

Histology

UPS is characterized by spindle-to-epithelioid neoplastic cells arranged in a storiform, fascicular, or medullary pattern, with a cartwheel-like pattern around the vessels. The presence of large, bizarre pleomorphic cells with moderate amounts of cytoplasm, round-to-oval nuclei, and prominent nucleoli is the hallmark of these tumors. These larger cells also may be multinucleated, mimicking Reed-Sternberg cells and/or osteoclast-like giant cells. Mitotic figures are readily identified, and areas of necrosis or hemorrhage can be seen. In some cases, myxoid and hemangiopericytic-like areas are present. An inflammatory infiltrate composed of plasma cells and lymphocytes may be observed. Vascular invasion has been reported in approximately 50% of cases of pulmonary UPS. By definition, undifferentiated sarcomas should have no discernible microscopic evidence of any specific form of differentiation (e.g., lipoblasts, bone formation, epithelial structures). So, careful examination of tissue and generous sampling of the specimen are essential for the correct diagnosis.

Sarcomatoid mesothelioma contains malignant oval-to-spindle-shaped cell proliferations, and they cytologically mimic other tumors of mesenchymal origin, such as UPS. Therefore, immunohistochemical studies play an important role in diagnosis, as described below.

How Can Ancillary Tests Be Used to Distinguish UPS Versus Sarcomatoid Mesothelioma/Carcinoma?

Immunohistochemistry

UPS characteristically shows positive staining for histiocytic markers, including CD68 and α1-antichymotrypsin, as well as vimentin. However, these findings are nonspecific and do not help in establishing this diagnosis. Staining for TTF1, S100 protein, desmin, actin, myoglobin, caldesmon, D2-40, and calretinin is negative. In some cases, keratin staining may be positive, which makes it difficult to differentiate from sarcomatoid carcinomas (SCs). However, SCs usually display stronger cytokeratin staining and, to a variable extent, more differentiated carcinomatous elements, as well as immunoreactivity to other epithelial markers. A wider-than-usual panel of immunohistochemical studies is necessary to rule out other neoplasms that can resemble UPS, including other types of sarcomas, sarcomatoid carcinoma, melanoma, or mesothelioma (see Table 24.1) [1].

Table 24.1 Helpful ancillary tests to differentiate tumors with sarcomatoid features

Tumor	IHC	Molecular
Sarcomatoid carcinoma (SC)	P63, P40, pankeratin, TTF1, epithelial markers (MOC31, BerEP4, BG8, B72.3, monoclonal CEA)	Gains at chromosomes 8q, 7, 1q, 3q, and 19. KRAS mutation, EGFR mutation
Sarcomatoid mesothelioma	WT1, CK5/6, D2-40, calretinin	Inactivation of CDKN2A at 9p21 on PCR
Angiomatoid fibrous histiocytoma (AFH)	Desmin+/–, CD68+/–, EMA+/–	EWSR1-CREB1, EWSR1-ATF1, or FUS-ATF1 fusion
Synovial sarcoma (SS)	TLE1, keratin, EMA, S100+/–, CD56, CD99, calretinin+/–	t(X;18) involving SS18 (SYT) gene
Epithelioid sarcoma (ES)	Loss INI, EMA+, keratin+/–, CD34+/–	SMARCB1 (INI1) gene alterations on (22q11)
Dedifferentiated liposarcoma (DDLPS)	MDM2, CDK4, SMA+/–, desmin+/–	Ring and giant marker chromosomes derived from amplification of 12q13–15 (variable amplification of MDM2, SAS, CDK4, HMGA2)
Anaplastic large-cell lymphoma (ALCL)	CD45+, CD30+, ALK+/–	TCR gene rearrangement, rearrangement of 2p23 (ALK)
Inflammatory myofibroblastic tumor (IMT)	ALK+/–, SMA+/–, desmin+/–	Rearrangement of 2p23 (ALK)
Ewing sarcoma	FLI1+, CD99+	t(11;22) and other translocations involving EWSR1 gene
Melanoma	S100+, SOX10, Melan A/MART1, MITF, tyrosinase	BRAF, ARID2, BAP1, GNAQ, HRAS, KIT, NF1, NRAS, and PTEN mutations
Malignant peripheral nerve sheath tumors (MPNST)	S100+/–, GFAP+/–. CD34+/–	Complex
Solitary fibrous tumor (SFT)	STAT6, CD34, BCL2, CD99	NAB2-STAT6 fusion
Leiomyosarcoma (LMS)	SMA, desmin, caldesmon	Complex
Rhabdomyosarcoma (RMS)	Desmin, myogenin, MyoD1	Complex
Angiosarcoma	Vascular markers (CD31, CD34, FLI1, ERG), keratin + in epithelioid angiosarcoma	MYC (8q24) or FLT4 (VEGFR3) (5q35) amplification, upregulation of vascular-specific receptor tyrosine kinases (TIE1, KDR, TEK, FLT1)
Kaposi sarcoma	HHV8 (LANA), vascular markers, lymphatic markers (D2-40, LYVE1, Prox1)	KSHV/HHV8 with PCR
Epithelioid hemangioendothelioma (EHE)	Vascular markers, TFE3+/–, keratin +/–	WWTr1-CAMTA1 fusion, YAP1-TFE1 fusion
Alveolar soft part sarcoma (ASPS)	TFE3, desmin+/–	der(17)t(X;17)(p11.2;q25) translocation (ASPSCR1-TFE3 fusion)
Perivascular epithelioid cell tumor (PEComa)	SMA+, desmin+, HMB45+, MITF+, MART1+	TSC2 mutations, TFE3 gene fusions

Reprinted from "Qorbani A, Nelson SD. Primary pulmonary undifferentiated pleomorphic sarcoma (PPUPS). Autops Case Rep. 2019 Aug 22;9(3):e2019110. https://doi.org/10.4322/acr.2019.110. PMID: 31528627; PMCID: PMC6709651." [1]

Molecular Testing

The genetic profile of primary pulmonary mesenchymal tumors is identical to that of their soft tissue counterparts, showing complex and nonspecific cytogenetic aberrations. However, molecular studies can be helpful to rule out other tumors with similar histological findings (Table 24.1) [1]. Molecular mechanisms responsible for primary pulmonary UPS formation and progression are unknown [10].

What Is the Most Specific Test for Diagnosing PPUPS?

There is no specific test for the diagnosis of UPS. It is a diagnosis of exclusion, and generous tissue sampling and adequate contextually interpreted immunohistochemistry are required to rule out other tumors with sarcomatoid features. In a retrospective study, Fletcher CD re-evaluated 159 tumors and showed that only 26% of cases previously diagnosed as MFH were "true" UPS, while more than half of these cases had an identifiable line of differentiation [11]. Some authors believe that the category of UPS serves primarily as a "wastebasket" for a heterogeneous group of unclassifiable neoplasms with pleomorphic morphology [12].

What Are the Helpful Immunohistochemical Stains Used in Diagnosing Sarcomatoid Mesothelioma?

Given that the expression of immunohistochemical markers of mesothelial differentiation is often lost in sarcomatoid mesothelioma, a broad panel of stains must be employed to make this diagnosis. Although no markers are 100% specific, immunoreactivity for calretinin, CK5/6, D2-40, and WT1 is useful to make this diagnosis. Recognition of the appropriate pattern of staining is crucial. Calretinin immunoreactivity must be nuclear and cytoplasmic; D2-40 must be membranous; and WT1 must be nuclear to be considered positive. Loss of BAP-1 correlates with a worse prognosis in malignant mesothelioma. Some authors suggested that it also may be useful for the early diagnosis of malignant mesothelioma; however, loss of BAP-1 is more observed in epithelioid mesothelioma than in the sarcomatoid subtype [13].

Homozygous deletion of p16 gene can be seen in malignant mesothelioma and is useful in differentiating it from reactive mesothelial cells or reactive mesenchymal spindle cells [14].

What Are the Helpful Immunohistochemical Stains Used in Diagnosing Sarcomatoid Carcinoma?

Immunoreactivity to pulmonary adenocarcinoma markers (e.g., TTF1, napsin-A, surfactant protein A), squamous markers (e.g., p63, p40), and/or epithelial markers (e.g., MOC31, BerEP4, BG8, B72.3, monoclonal CEA, CD15, and claudin 4) supports a diagnosis of sarcomatoid carcinoma.

What Is the Next Step if You Find a True UPS in the Lung?

Search for an extrapulmonary origin of metastatic disease. Since most UPSs in the lung are metastatic from a soft tissue origin [1], it is essential to exclude extrapulmonary lesions before diagnosing the tumor as primary pulmonary UPS.

References

1. Qorbani A, Nelson SD. Primary pulmonary undifferentiated pleomorphic sarcoma (PPUPS). Autops Case Rep. 2019;9(3):e2019110. https://doi.org/10.4322/acr.2019.110.
2. Fletcher CDM, Bridge JA, Hogendoorn PCW, et al. WHO classification of tumours of soft tissue and bone. Lyon: IARC Press; 2013.
3. Weiss SW, Enzinger FM. Malignant fibrous histiocytoma: an analysis of 200 cases. Cancer. 1978;41:2250–66.
4. Bedrossian CW, Verani R, Unger KM, Salman J. Pulmonary malignant fibrous histiocytoma. Light and electron microscopic studies of one case. Chest. 1979;75(2):186–9. https://doi.org/10.1378/chest.75.2.186.
5. Nascimento AG, Unni KK, Bernatz PE. Sarcomas of the lung. Mayo Clin Proc. 1982;57(6):355–9.
6. Yousem SA, Hochholzer L. Malignant fibrous histiocytoma of the lung. Cancer. 1987;60(10):2532–41. https://doi.org/10.1002/1097-0142(19871115)60:10<2532::aid-cncr2820601031>3.0.co;2-5. PMID: 2822221
7. Nonaka M, Kadokura M, Ohkubo F, Kushihashi T, Kunimura T, Kataoka D, Yamamoto S, Takaba T. Post radiation inflammatory malignant fibrous histiocytoma arising from the chest wall. Ann Thorac Cardiovasc Surg. 2001;7(6):371–4.
8. Kim JH, Cho SH, Kim EK, Lee JH, Jeong HC. Endobronchial malignant fibrous histiocytoma: case report of an unusual presentation and palliative flexible bronchoscopic resection. Respir Care. 2013;58(8):e92–4. https://doi.org/10.4187/respcare.01996.
9. Klebe S, Brownlee NA, Mahar A, Burchette JL, Sporn TA, Vollmer RT, Roggli VL. Sarcomatoid mesothelioma: a clinical-pathologic correlation of 326 cases. Mod Pathol. 2010;23(3):470–9. https://doi.org/10.1038/modpathol.2009.180. Epub 2010 Jan 15. PMID: 20081811
10. Goldblum JR, Folpe AL, Weiss SW. Enzinger and Weiss's soft tissue tumors. 6th ed. Philadelphia: Elsevier; 2014.

11. Fletcher CD. Pleomorphic malignant fibrous histiocytoma: fact or fiction? A critical reappraisal based on 159 tumors diagnosed as pleomorphic sarcoma. Am J Surg Pathol. 1992;16(3):213–28.
12. Hornick JL. Practical soft tissue pathology: a diagnostic approach. 2nd ed. Philadelphia: Elsevier; 2019.
13. Pulford E, Huilgol K, Moffat D, Henderson DW, Klebe S. Malignant mesothelioma, BAP1 immunohistochemistry, and VEGFA: does BAP1 have potential for early diagnosis and assessment of prognosis? Dis Markers. 2017;2017:1310478. https://doi.org/10.1155/2017/1310478.
14. Chapel DB, Schulte JJ, Husain AN, Krausz T. Application of immunohistochemistry in diagnosis and management of malignant mesothelioma. Transl Lung Cancer Res. 2020;9(Suppl 1):S3–S27. https://doi.org/10.21037/tlcr.2019.11.29.

Synovial Sarcoma Versus Solitary Fibrous Tumor

25

Hui Zhu

Case Presentation

A 25-year-old female initially presented with multiple episodes of spontaneous pneumothorax more than 10 years ago. She underwent a left lobe wedge resection, with a pathologic diagnosis of unremarkable lung tissue, and was subsequently treated with repeated mechanical pleurodesis. Currently the patient presented with non-productive cough and chest pain. Computed tomography (CT) scan showed a large cystic and solid mass in the left upper lobe (Fig. 25.1). Fine-needle aspiration was attempted but was nondiagnostic due to scant material. Given the the large size of the mass, left upper lobectomy was performed along with a portion of the parietal pleura.

Pathologic examination showed a 7.1 cm well-circumscribed cystic and hemorrhagic mass involving both the lung parenchyma and parietal pleura. Microscopic examination showed a large blood-filled cyst between the parietal and visceral pleura. While the majority of the cystic wall appeared fibrous, compact hypercellular areas were present. The tumor cells had monotonous spindled-to-oval nuclei with coarse chromatin and scant cytoplasm. Scattered mitotic figures were seen. Focal necrosis was present (see Fig. 25.2).

The differential diagnosis of this pleural-based mass is broad and includes both benign and malignant processes. Such considerations include SFT, endometriosis (given the patient's age, long history of pneumothorax, and the hemorrhagic appearance of the cyst), endometrial stromal sarcoma, and other benign and malignant spindle cell neoplasms.

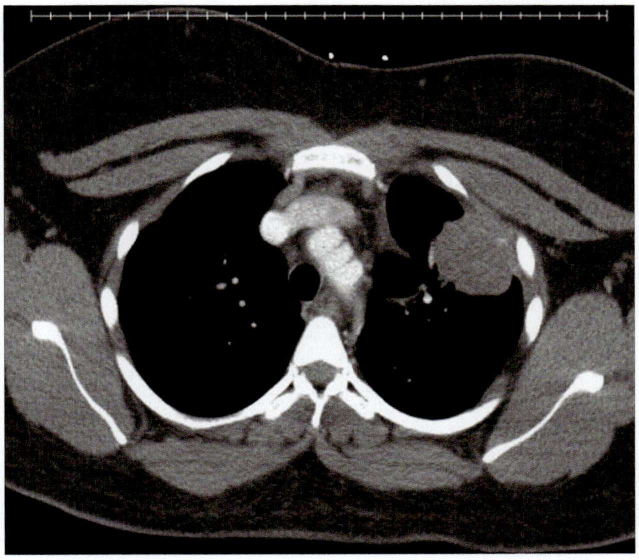

Fig. 25.1 CT scan showed a large pleural-based mass in the left upper lobe

Immunohistochemical staining showed that the tumor cells were focally positive for AE1/AE3, EMA, and CK7 (Fig. 25.2). CD99, BCL2, S100, CD10, ER, PR, inhibin, CD34, and ERG were negative. A diagnosis of synovial sarcoma was favored. Fluorescent in situ hybridization showed break-apart in the *SYT* gene, confirming the diagnosis of synovial sarcoma.

H. Zhu (✉)
Pathology and Laboratory Services, Forward Pathology Solutions, HCA North Cypress Medical Center, Cypress, TX, USA
e-mail: huizhu@hcaheathcare.com

H. Xu et al. (eds.), *Practical Lung Pathology*, Practical Anatomic Pathology, https://doi.org/10.1007/978-3-031-14402-8_25

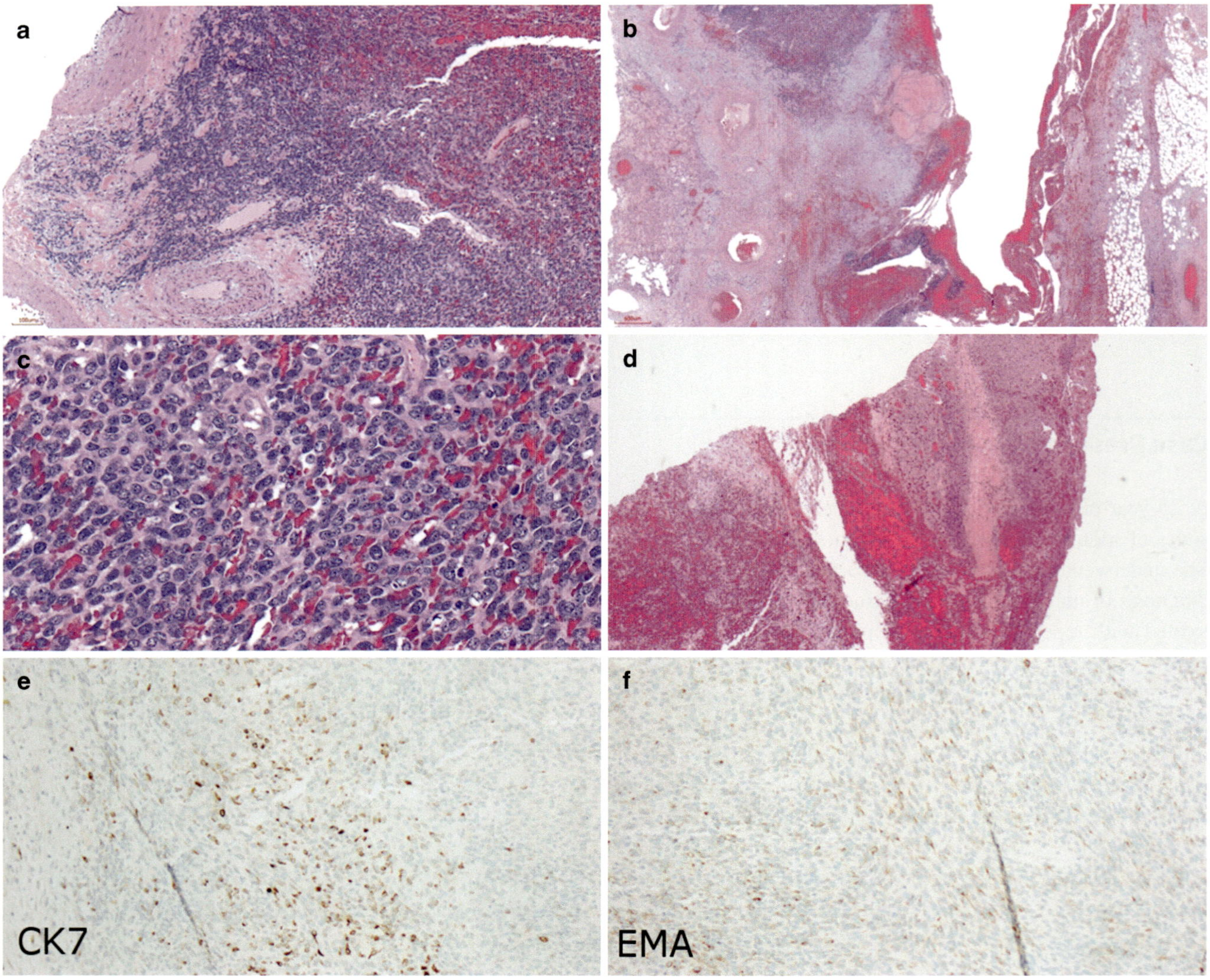

Fig. 25.2 (**a**) A densely cellular area of the mass with associated hemorrhage (100×). (**b**) Large hemorrhagic cyst-like area between the parietal and visceral pleura. Lung alveoli were visible at the left side of the image (20×). (**c**) Higher-power view of a hypercellular area of monotonous spindle cells with high N/C ratio and mitotic figures (400×). (**d**) Focal necrosis was present (40×). Immunohistochemical staining for (**e**) CK7 and (**f**) EMA was focally positive in the tumor cells (100×)

Final Diagnosis: Synovial Sarcoma

What Are the Clinical and Prognostic Features of SS, and How Do They Differ from SFT?

SS can be seen at any age but is most common in adolescents and young adults. SS most often occurs in the extremities and head and neck region but less commonly can present as a visceral primary. Primary pulmonary SS usually presents as a pleural-based solid tumor [1]. Calcification and/or ossification, seen in less than 20% of cases, as evidenced by multiple small, spotty radiopacities on radiologic studies, may be helpful to suggest a preoperative diagnosis of SS [2]. A significant subset of pulmonary SS is cystic and presents as recurrent pneumothorax. These cases can be difficult to diagnose clinically and pathologically [3–6]. SS generally behaves in an aggressive manner. The prognosis of pulmonary SS is especially poor with frequent local recurrences and distal metastasis. Five-year survival is about 30%, and the median survival time is only 14.5 months [1, 7].

SFT is predominantly seen in middle-aged adult patients and is rare in children and adolescents. Pleural SFT is usually asymptomatic and discovered incidentally on imaging studies. Occasionally, SFT can cause hypoglycemia due to tumor production of insulin-like growth factor. This is most commonly seen in tumors located in the pelvis and retroperitoneum but is rare in pulmonary cases [8]. On imaging studies, a majority of SFT are pleural-based solid masses with smooth borders [8]. Rare tumors can show cystic degeneration or necrosis. Overall, pleural SFT has an indolent clinical behavior with 10% recurrence rate and metastasis in 5–10% of cases [9].

What Are the Pathologic Features of SS? How Do They Differ from SFT?

SS can be biphasic or monophasic. The biphasic type is generally readily recognizable by the presence of both epithelial and spindle cell components. The epithelial cells can form solid nests or glandular structures. The spindle cell component of biphasic SS is identical to the spindle cells in monophasic SS. These tumor cells have oval, hyperchromatic nuclei and scant cytoplasm. Mitotic figures are variable (from 2 to >20 per 10 HPFs), and necrosis is present in most cases [1]. The tumor cells are characteristically monotonous and arranged in dense cellular sheets or vague fascicles with a herringbone pattern. Areas with myxoid change and hyalinization can be seen (Fig. 25.3).

Usually, these changes are focal and unlikely to cause diagnostic difficulty. When diffuse, it can mimic less aggressive or even benign neoplasms such as SFT, leiomyoma, or schwannoma. Many cases of SS have prominent staghorn-like vasculature resembling that of SFT. As previously mentioned, the histologic presence of calcification and/or ossification can be a diagnostic clue for SS.

Rare cases of pulmonary SS are cystic and present as recurrent spontaneous pneumothorax. In a few cases, a very large SS was found after multiple episodes of pneumothorax, bullectomy, pleural abrasion, and mechanical pleurodesis, raising the possibility that SS was not recognized in the original bullectomy specimen [5] (Fig. 25.1). Morphologically, the cyst wall can be predominantly fibrotic and benign looking. Areas of compact hypercellular spindle cell proliferation are invariably present and reveal the true nature of this lesion (Fig. 25.2). A majority of these cystic SS cases are monophasic, but rare biphasic form can also be seen [3]. Careful histopathologic examination of resected bullectomy specimens is crucial for the correct diagnosis.

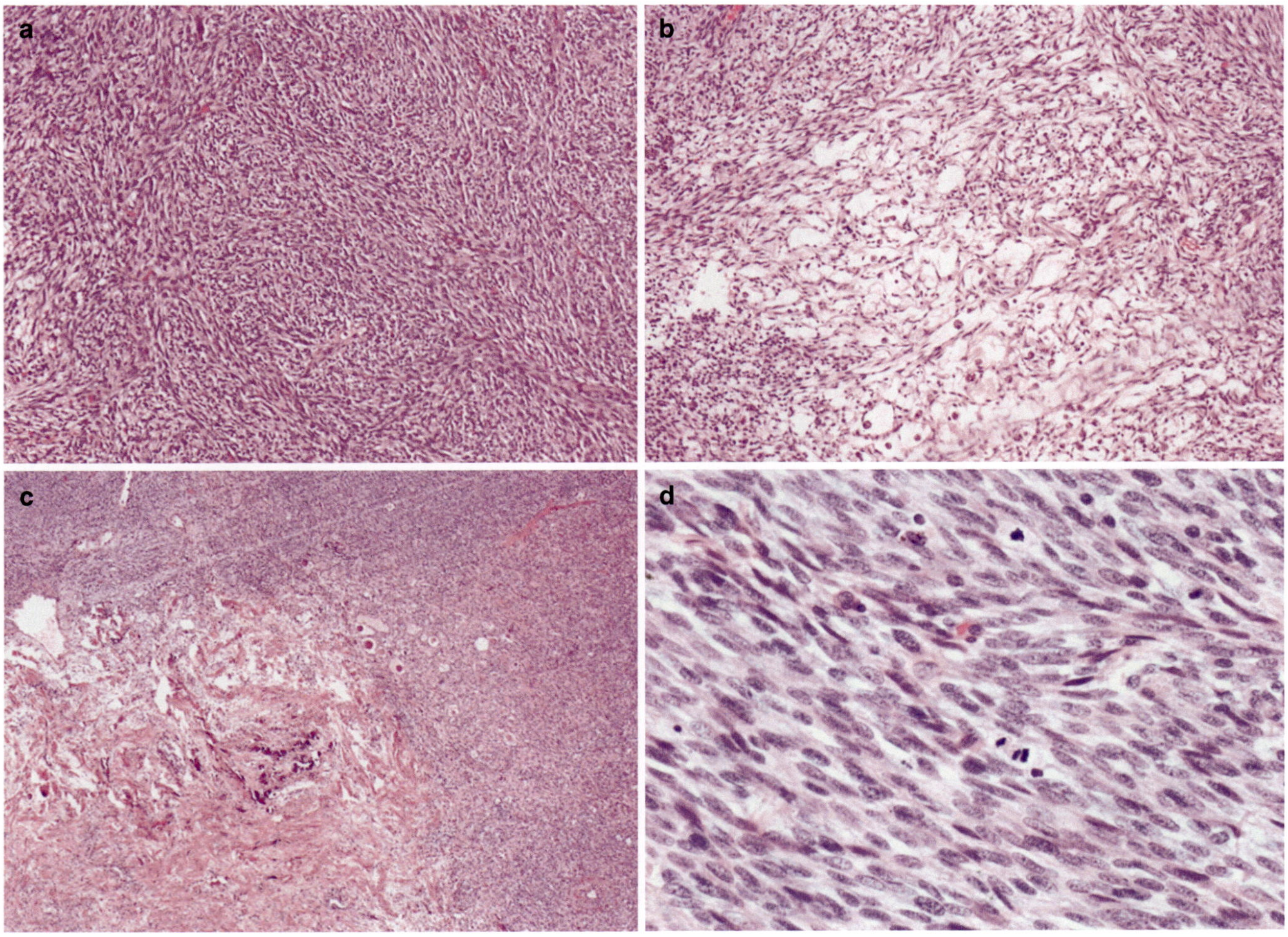

Fig. 25.3 (**a**) Typical morphology of monophasic SS: monotonous spindle cells with focal herringbone pattern (100×). (**b**) Focal myxoid change in SS. When diffuse, it can mimic SFT and other benign spindle cell tumors (100×). (**c**) Calcification and ossification are important morphologic clues for SS (40×). (**d**) Mitotic figures are typically easy to identify (400×)

SFT can have a broad range of histopathologic features with variable proportions of cells and fibrous stroma. Some tumors are hypocellular with extensive hyalinized collagen stroma, while others are hypercellular with scant collagen (Fig. 25.4). A majority of cases have alternating cellular and fibrous areas. The typical morphology of SFT consists of bland spindle cells arranged in a "patternless" pattern, surrounded by ropey collagen bundles. Thin-walled branching "staghorn" vasculature is a helpful, yet nonspecific, finding. The tumor cells have vesicular chromatin, pale eosinophilic cytoplasm, and indistinct cell borders. Mitoses are generally absent or sparse. Unusual histologic features include myxoid change, microcyst formation, ossification, and even adipose tissue components, which can cause diagnostic confusion. Recognizing areas of more typical SFT morphology and immunohistochemical stains can be key to diagnosis in such cases.

Less than 10% of pleural SFT are malignant. Predictors of aggressive behavior include older age, large tumor size, necrosis, and increased mitotic activity (>4/10 high-power fields) [10] (Fig. 25.4). Malignant SFT can morphologically mimic synovial sarcoma, round cell, and pleomorphic sarcomas [8, 9].

How Can Immunohistochemistry and Molecular Testing Be Used to Distinguish SS from SFT?

Immunohistochemically, the epithelial component of biphasic SS shows strong immunoreactivity with EMA and cytokeratins, while the spindle cell component is typically only focally positive for these epithelial markers. Staining for S100 is seen in about 30% of cases. CD99 and BCL2, while nonspecific, are positive in the majority of SS [2]. TLE1 has emerged as a somewhat useful marker for SS, with diffuse strong nuclear staining seen in a majority of SS cases. However, recent studies have found that strong diffuse staining for TLE1 can be seen in SFT, malignant peripheral nerve sheath tumor, rhabdomyosarcoma, and others [11]. In

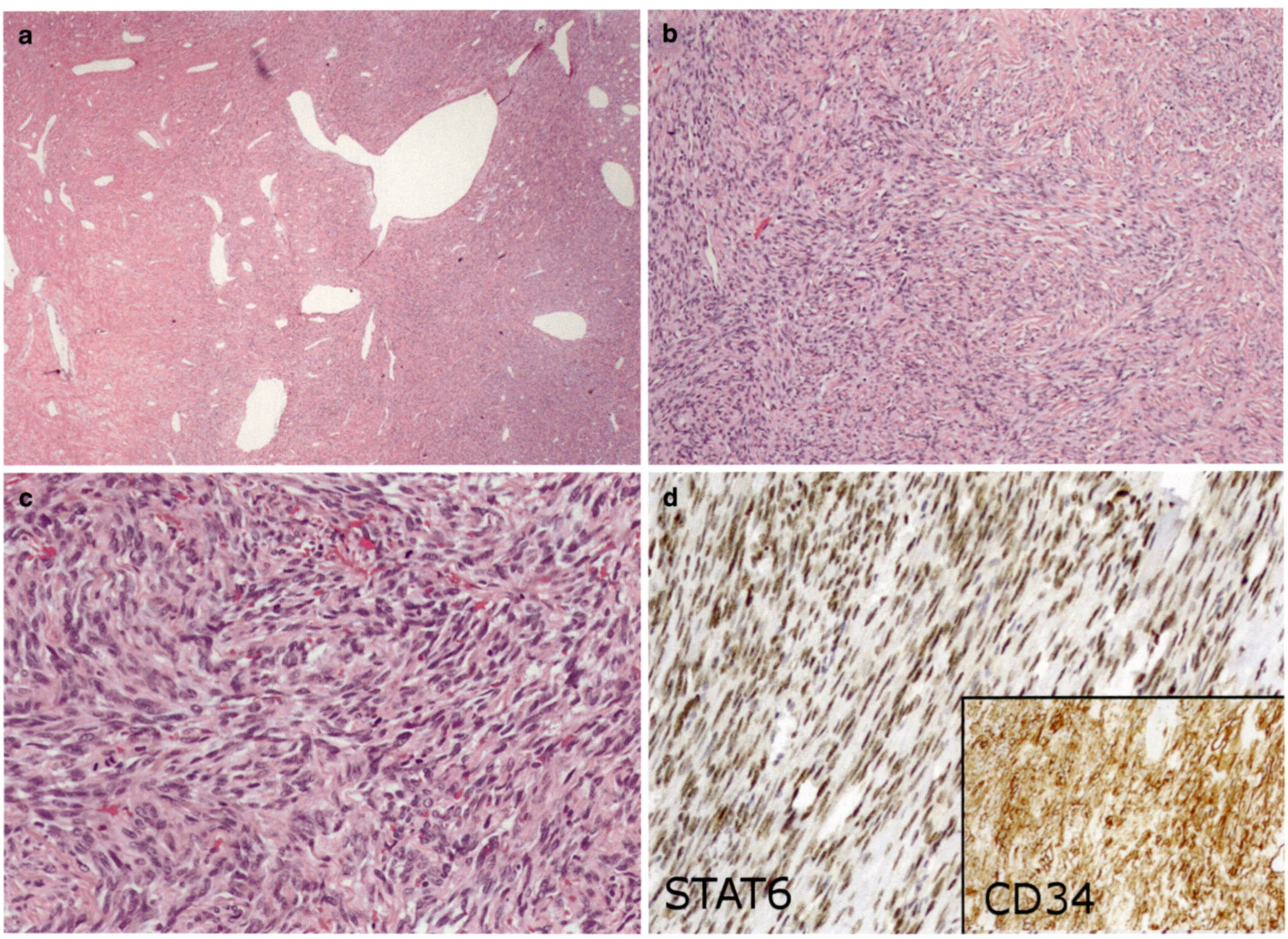

Fig. 25.4 (**a**) Morphologic features of solitary fibrous tumor, including prominent "staghorn" vessels (20×) and (**b**) "patternless" architecture with variable collagen deposition (100×). (**c**) Features of aggressive behavior include mitotic activity >4 /10 HPFs (200×). (**d**) Tumor cells are diffusely positive for STAT6 (nuclear expression) and CD34 (inset) (200×)

contrast to SFT and many other mesenchymal neoplasms, CD34 immunoreactivity is very rare in SS.

SS is characterized by the consistent and specific t(X;18)(p11; q11) translocation, which leads to a gene fusion involving *SYT* and one of the *SSX* genes (*SSX1*, *SSX2*, or *SSX4*) [2]. This fusion can be detected by multiple methods, such as FISH or RT-PCR. Detection of this rearrangement is generally considered the gold standard for the diagnosis of SS.

Immunohistochemically, SFT is diffusely positive for CD34 in up to 95% of cases. CD99, BCL2, SMA, and EMA can all be variably positive, while S100 and cytokeratins are typically negative in SFT. Nuclear expression of STAT6 by immunohistochemistry, which results from a *NAB2-STAT6* fusion gene, is highly sensitive and specific for SFT [12, 13]. However, immunoreactivity for STAT6 can be seen a subset of dedifferentiated liposarcomas, which may also show SFT-like morphologic features [14]. Detection of *MDM2* amplification, a hallmark of dedifferentiated liposarcoma, is useful for appropriately classifying such tumors. Expression of STAT6 in this subset is likely due to amplification of the *STAT6* gene, which is located in proximity to *MDM2* and *CDK4* [15].

References

1. Fletcher CDM, Dacic S, Ladanyi M. Synovial sarcoma. In: Travis WD, Brambilla E, Burke AP, Marx A, Cicholson AG, editors. WHO classification of tumours of the lung, pleura, thymus, and heart. 4th ed. Lyon: IARC Press; 2015.
2. Goldblum JR, Folpe AL, Weiss SW. Other malignant soft tissue tumors, including those of uncertain type. In: Enzinger & Weiss's soft tissue tumors. 7th ed. Amsterdam: Elsevier; 2019: 175-1270.
3. Cummings NM, Desai S, Thway K, Stewart S, Hill DA, Priest JR, et al. Cystic primary pulmonary synovial sarcoma presenting as recurrent pneumothorax: report of 4 cases. Am J Surg Pathol. 2010;34(8):1176–9.
4. Johnson ED, Downs-Kelly E, Bull DA, Gulbahce HE. Primary cystic pleuropulmonary synovial sarcoma presenting as recurrent pneumothorax. Case Rep Oncol. 2017;10(2):660–5.
5. Guo C, Liu C, Pu Q, Lin F, Liu L. Occult primary pulmonary synovial sarcoma presenting as recurrent spontaneous pneumothorax and explosive progression. Thorac Cancer. 2017;8(2):121–3.
6. Petrosyan A, Bergeron P. Extensive surgical treatment of primary pulmonary synovial sarcoma after recurrent pneumothorax. Ann Thorac Surg. 2015;100(5):1893–5.
7. Lan T, Chen H, Xiong B, Zhou T, Peng R, Chen M, et al. Primary pleuropulmonary and mediastinal synovial sarcoma: a clinicopathologic and molecular study of 26 genetically confirmed cases in the largest institution of Southwest China. Diagn Pathol. 2016;11(1):62.
8. Goldblum JR, Folpe AL, Weiss SW. Soft tissue tumors of intermediate malignancy of uncertain type. In: Enzinger & Weiss's soft tissue tumors. 7th ed. Amsterdam: Elsevier; 2019: 107-1174.
9. Fletcher CDM, Gibbs A. Solitary fibrous tumor. In: Travis WD, Brambilla E, Burke AP, Marx A, Cicholson AG, editors. WHO classification of tumours of the lung, pleura, thymus, and heart. 4th ed. Lyon: IARC Press; 2015.
10. Demicco EG, Wagner MJ, Maki RG, Gupta V, Iofin I, Lazar AJ, Wang WL. Risk assessment in solitary fibrous tumors: validation and refinement of a risk stratification model. Mod Pathol. 2017;30(10):1433–42.
11. Kosemehmetoglu K, Vrana JA, Folpe AL. TLE1 expression is not specific for synovial sarcoma: a whole section study of 163 soft tissue and bone neoplasms. Mod Pathol. 2009;22(7):872–8.
12. Demicco EG, Harms PW, Patel RM, Smith SC, Ingram D, Torres K, et al. Extensive survey of STAT6 expression in a large series of mesenchymal tumors. Am J Clin Pathol. 2015;143(5):672–82.
13. Robinson DR, Wu YM, Kalyana-Sundaram S, Cao X, Lonigro RJ, Sung YS, et al. Identification of recurrent NAB2-STAT6 gene fusions in solitary fibrous tumor by integrative sequencing. Nat Genet. 2013;45(2):180–5.
14. Creytens D, Libbrecht L, Ferdinande L. Nuclear expression of STAT6 in dedifferentiated liposarcomas with a solitary fibrous tumor-like morphology: a diagnostic pitfall. Appl Immunohistochem Mol Morphol. 2015;23(6):462–3.
15. Doyle LA, Tao D, Mariño-Enríquez A. STAT6 is amplified in a subset of dedifferentiated liposarcoma. Mod Pathol. 2014;27(9):1231–7.

Inflammatory Myofibroblastic Tumor Versus Organizing Pneumonia

26

Omer Abdelaziz Mohammed Saeed and Chen Zhang

Case Presentation

A 22-year-old male presents with shortness of breath and cough for 2 months. He denies hemoptysis, fever, wheezing, or weight loss. Physical examination shows a well-nourished male with no palpable masses, lymphadenopathy, or organomegaly. Chest X-ray and computed tomography (CT) scan show right upper lung lobe collapse with a questionable underlying mass (Fig. 26.1). Bronchoscopy shows an obstructing friable endobronchial mass in the right main bronchus. Endobronchial biopsy is performed.

The endobronchial biopsy shows a tumor composed of spindle cells with mixed chronic inflammatory infiltrate (Fig. 26.2). The spindle cells are arranged in a fascicular pattern without significant cytologic atypia or mitotic activity. The spindle cells are positive for anaplastic lymphoma kinase (ALK, clone D5F3) and negative for pancytokeratin AE1/AE3, smooth muscle actin (SMA), and desmin. A right upper lobectomy was performed, containing a lesion with similar histologic features, which measures approximately 1.2 cm in maximum dimension and involves the bronchial cartilaginous structures (Fig. 26.3). Surgical margins are negative. The patient is currently doing well.

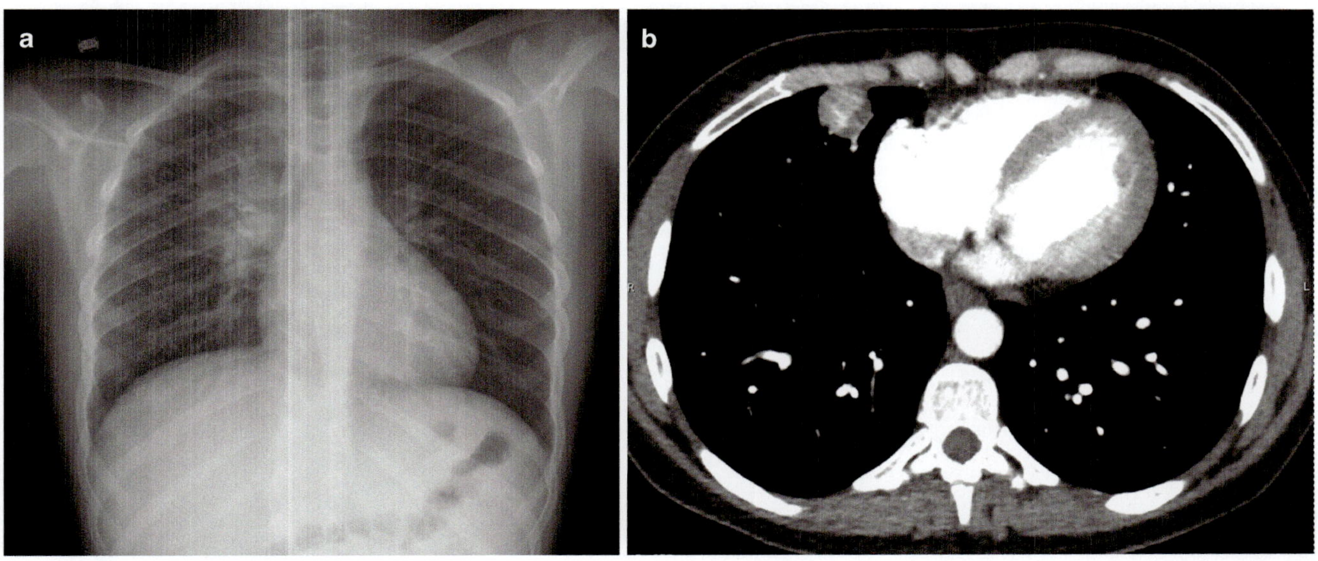

Fig. 26.1 Imaging features of IMT. (**a**) Chest X-ray showing right upper lung collapse with a questionable underlying mass. (**b**) Chest CT scan from a different patient with a parenchyma IMT showing a solitary well-demarcated right upper lobe mass with somewhat irregular borders

O. A. M. Saeed
Department of Pathology and Laboratory Medicine, Indiana University School of Medicine, Indianapolis, IN, USA

C. Zhang (✉)
Weill Cornell Medicine, Department of Pathology and Laboratory Medicine, New York, NY, USA
e-mail: fjr9007@med.cornell.edu

H. Xu et al. (eds.), *Practical Lung Pathology*, Practical Anatomic Pathology, https://doi.org/10.1007/978-3-031-14402-8_26

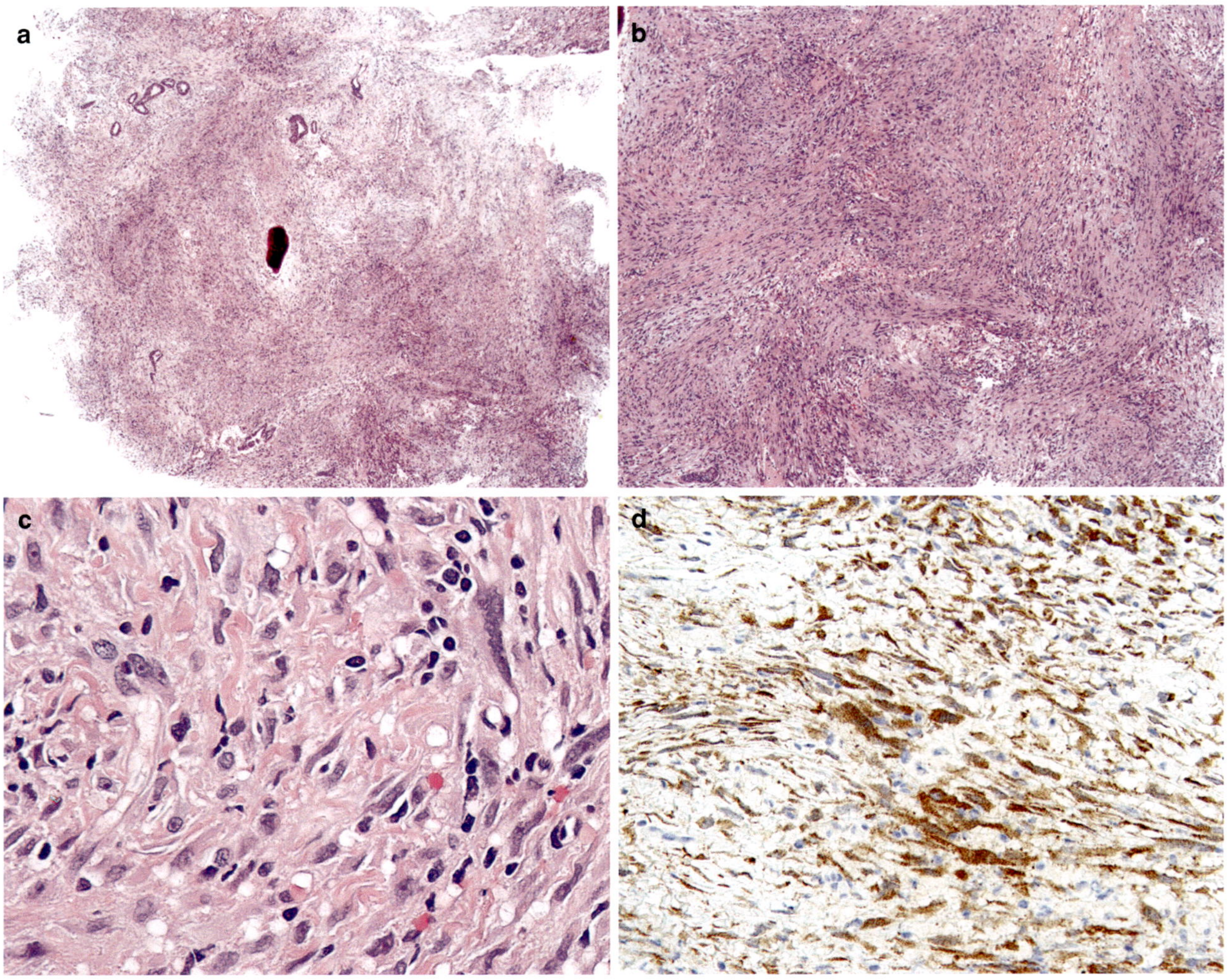

Fig. 26.2 Histological features of IMT on the transbronchial biopsy. (**a**) Low-magnification photomicrograph showing a spindle cell lesion with a collagenous and focally myxoid background. Residual/entrapped bronchial submucosal glands and ducts are seen. H&E, 20×. (**b**) Intermediate magnification of the lesion showing the fascicular growth of spindly tumor cells in a collagenous to myxoid stroma (fasciitis-like pattern). H&E, 100×. (**c**) High-magnification photomicrograph showing spindle cells with plump eosinophilic cytoplasm and vesicular nuclei, admixed with lymphoplasmacytic infiltrate. The spindle cells show mild cytological atypia, and no mitosis or necrosis is seen. H&E, 400×. (**d**) A majority of the spindle cells stain positive with ALK immunohistochemical stain. 200×

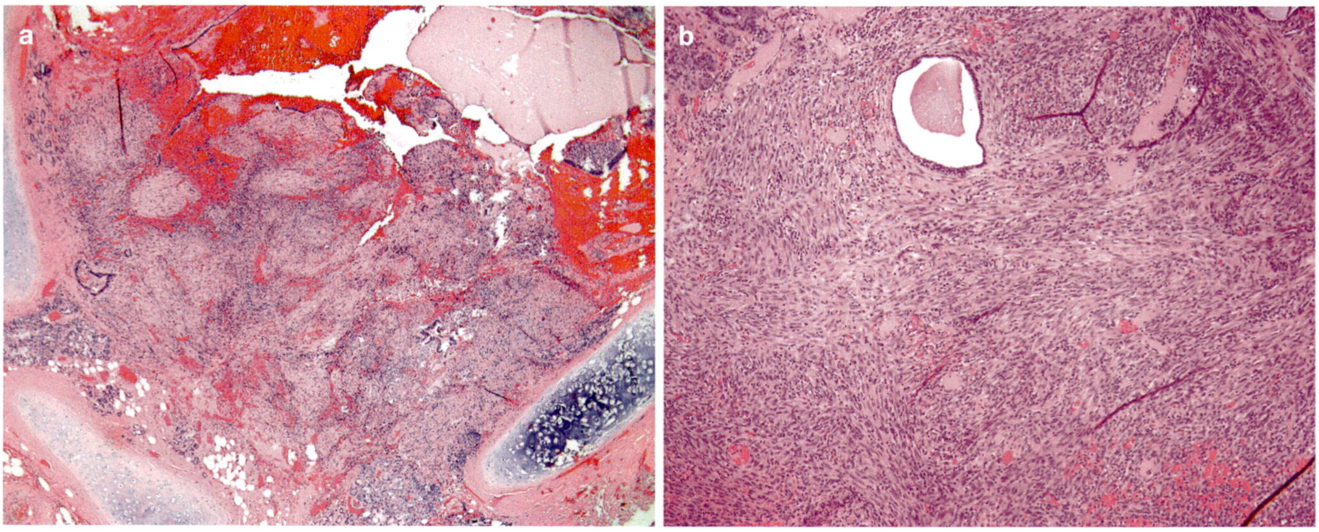

Fig. 26.3 Histological features of IMT on the resection specimen. (**a**) Low magnification showing the tumor involving a cartilaginous airway (bronchus). H&E, 20×. (**b**) Higher magnification showing that the tumor consists of fascicular spindle cell proliferation in a collagenous-to-myxoid stroma, admixed with inflammatory cell infiltrate. H&E, 100×

Diagnosis: Inflammatory Myofibroblastic Tumor

What Is the Definition, Epidemiology, and Clinical Presentation of Inflammatory Myofibroblastic Tumor (IMT), and How Does It Differ from Organizing Pneumonia (OP)?

IMT, formerly designated "inflammatory pseudotumor," is a neoplasm composed of myofibroblastic spindle cells admixed with inflammatory infiltrate [1–3]. IMT was first described in the lung by Brunn et al. in 1939 [4] and then was described in extrapulmonary sites [2, 5]. Our knowledge has evolved over time, from considering IMTs as a reparative/reactive inflammatory process to benign tumors, and currently they are thought of as neoplasms of intermediate biological behavior [1, 2].

Most cases of IMT occur in patients younger than 40 years. However, cases have been described up to the eighth decade of life. IMTs has no gender predilection [6]. IMT is the most common pulmonary neoplasm in children [7], and clinically, more than half of the patients are asymptomatic [6]. The most common symptoms in patients with lung and/or endobronchial IMTs are cough and dyspnea [6, 8]. In one study by Thistlethwaite et al., 45% of the patients with endobronchial presented with lung collapse/pneumonia [8].

OP, on the other hand, is a nonspecific histologic pattern used to describe a proliferation of loose connective tissue/granulation tissue within alveolar structures with or without bronchiolar component [9, 10]. OP can be idiopathic (cryptogenic organizing pneumonia) or secondary to a variety of etiologies, including drug reaction, viral infection, radiation, and others. OP pattern can also be seen adjacent to other lesions, such as tumors [10].

Do IMT and OP Look Differently on Radiographic Imaging?

IMTs usually present on imaging as a solitary nodule or mass lesion [11]. These lesions usually have a well-demarcated border but can sometimes have irregular peripheral edges. IMTs can be avid on 18F-fludeoxyglucose-positron emission tomography (18F-FDG-PET) scan [12] raising concern for malignancy. When IMTs have an endobronchial location, they can still appear as a distinct mass; however, lung collapse may be the only finding in some cases, obscuring the underlying mass [8].

The radiographic appearance of OP varies according to the underlying etiology. In the idiopathic form, the most common radiographic appearance of COP is patchy consolidation resembling pneumonia; this can be unilateral or bilateral, and usually in a peripheral location [9, 10].

What Are the Pathological Features of IMT and OP? What Are the Similarities and Differences? Can Immunohistochemical Studies Help in Differentiating These Two?

Grossly, IMT of the lung, like their counterparts in other locations, are white, firm or fleshy, and well-circumscribed lesions that range from 1 to 10 cm in maximum dimension [11, 13]. OP, on the other hand, looks like patchy areas of consolidation [10].

The term "inflammatory pseudotumors of the lung" was used in the old literature as a synonymous term with IMT. The term is now discouraged by the World Health Organization (WHO) classification since it represents a heterogeneous family of lesions rather than a single entity. This family includes reparative/reactive changes, IgG4-related lesions, IMT, and secondary organizing pneumonia [2]. IMTs of the lung have historically been classified into three histologic patterns: organizing pneumonia, fibrohistiocytic, and lymphoplasmacytic [14]. As our understanding that IMT is a specific entity evolves, more accurate histologic classifications emerged. Coffin et al., in his paper describing extrapulmonary IMTs, detailed three microscopic appearances [15]. The first is fasciitis-like pattern. In this pattern, the tumor consists of loose spindle cell proliferation in a myxoid background with prominent vascularity and inflammatory cell infiltrate in the form of neutrophils and eosinophils. The second pattern is compact cellular pattern, in which the myofibroblasts have a fascicular arrangement in a background of collagenous tissue and lymphoplasmacytic infiltrate. The third is hypocellular pattern which resembles fibromatosis [13, 15]. The cells in IMTs are uniformly spindled with plump eosinophilic cytoplasm and vesicular nuclei. The cells can show mild atypia, and mitosis is usually low [2].

OP is a patchy process consisting of loose, polypoid connective tissue filling up the bronchiolar and/or alveolar spaces, with spindle cell proliferation in a mucopolysaccharide-rich loose background with occasional lymphoplasmacytic infiltrate [9]. Differentiating OP from IMT is easy on surgical resection specimens but might be challenging on small biopsy in the absence of clinical and radiographic data. Distinguishing IMTs from the other "inflammatory pseudotumor" depends on observing the microscopic features that favor reactive processes. For instance, noticing the presence of granulomas or neutrophilic abscesses at the edge of the lesion argues against a diagnosis of IMT [2].

Immunohistochemical stains can be helpful in differentiating IMTs from a reactive/reparative process. Vimentin is usually diffusely positive in both reactive processes and IMT, and smooth muscle actin highlights the myofibroblastic element in both. Keratin positivity is reported in up to one third of IMTs [2]. Positivity for ALK, when present, is specific for IMTs but is only detected in about 50–60% of the cases [2, 5, 13].

What Are the Genetic/Molecular Findings of IMT?

Approximately half of IMTs show a characteristic rearrangement of the *ALK* gene, located in chromosome 2p23 [16, 17]. The most common fusion partners are *TPM3*, *TPM4*, and *CTLC* [18]. A recent study by Lovly et al. reports the presence of kinase gene fusions in approximately 85% of IMT, including rearrangements in *ROS1* and *PDGFRB* [19].

What Are the Treatment Modalities for Pulmonary IMTs, and What Is the Prognosis?

Surgical resection, such as wedge resection or lobectomy, is the treatment of choice of pulmonary IMT [6, 8, 20], with a recurrence rate ranging from 6 to 13% [8, 21]. Other treatment modalities such as steroids, chemotherapy, radiation, and tyrosine kinase inhibitors have a limited role in the management of IMT [19, 22].

IMTs are classified as tumors of uncertain malignant potential [1], with a risk of local recurrence, and rarely metastatic disease [8, 20].

References

1. Travis W, Brambilla E, Burke A, Marx A, Nicholson A. WHO classification of tumors of the lung, pleura, thymus and heart. 4th ed. Lyon: International Agency for Research on Cancer (IARC); 2015. p. 121–2.
2. Gleason BC, Hornick JL. Inflammatory myofibroblastic tumours: where are we now? J Clin Pathol. 2008;61(4):428–37.
3. Panagiotopoulos N, Patrini D, Gvinianidze L, Woo WL, Borg E, Lawrence D. Inflammatory myofibroblastic tumour of the lung: a reactive lesion or a true neoplasm? J Thorac Dis. 2015;7(5):908–11.
4. Brunn H. Two interesting benign lung tumors of contradictory histopathology; remarks on necessity for maintaining chest tumor registry. J Thorac Surg. 1939;9:199.
5. Saeed O, Saxena R. Primary mesenchymal liver tumors of childhood. Semin Diagn Pathol. 2017;34(2):201–7.
6. Melloni G, Carretta A, Ciriaco P, Arrigoni G, Fieschi S, Rizzo N, et al. Inflammatory pseudotumor of the lung in adults. Ann Thorac Surg. 2005;79(2):426–32.
7. Bahadori M, Liebow AA. Plasma cell granulomas of the lung. Cancer. 1973;31(1):191–208.
8. Thistlethwaite PA, Renner J, Duhamel D, Makani S, Lin GY, Jamieson SW, et al. Surgical management of endobronchial inflammatory myofibroblastic tumors. Ann Thorac Surg. 2011;91(2):367–72.
9. European RS, Society AT. American Thoracic Society/European Respiratory Society international multidisciplinary consensus classification of the idiopathic interstitial pneumonias. This joint statement of the American Thoracic Society (ATS), and the European Respiratory Society (ERS) was adopted by the ATS board of directors, June 2001 and by the ERS executive committee, June 2001. Am J Respir Crit Care Med. 2002;165(2):277–304.
10. Travis WD. Non-neoplastic disorders of the lower respiratory tract. Washington, DC: American Registry of Pathology: Armed Forces Institute of Pathology; 2002.
11. Agrons G, Rosado-de-Christenson M, Kirejczyk W, Conran R, Stocker J. Pulmonary inflammatory pseudotumor: radiologic features. Radiology. 1998;206(2):511–8.
12. Takeda S-i, Onishi Y, Kawamura T, Maeda H. Clinical spectrum of pulmonary inflammatory myofibroblastic tumor. Interact Cardiovasc Thorac Surg. 2008;7(4):629–33.
13. Coffin CM, Hornick JL, Fletcher CD. Inflammatory myofibroblastic tumor: comparison of clinicopathologic, histologic, and immunohistochemical features including ALK expression in atypical and aggressive cases. Am J Surg Pathol. 2007;31(4):509–20.
14. Matsubara O, Tan-Liu NS, Kenney RM, Mark EJ. Inflammatory pseudotumors of the lung: progression from organizing pneumonia to fibrous histiocytoma or to plasma cell granuloma in 32 cases. Hum Pathol. 1988;19(7):807–14.
15. Coffin CM, Watterson J, Priest JR, Dehner LP. Extrapulmonary inflammatory myofibroblastic tumor (inflammatory pseudotumor). A clinicopathologic and immunohistochemical study of 84 cases. Am J Surg Pathol. 1995;19(8):859–72.
16. Coffin CM, Patel A, Perkins S, Elenitoba-Johnson KS, Perlman E, Griffin CA. ALK1 and p80 expression and chromosomal rearrangements involving 2p23 in inflammatory myofibroblastic tumor. Mod Pathol. 2001;14(6):569–76.
17. Griffin CA, Hawkins AL, Dvorak C, Henkle C, Ellingham T, Perlman EJ. Recurrent involvement of 2p23 in inflammatory myofibroblastic tumors. Cancer Res. 1999;59(12):2776–80.
18. Tavora F, Shilo K, Ozbudak IH, Przybocki JM, Wang G, Travis WD, et al. Absence of human herpesvirus-8 in pulmonary inflammatory myofibroblastic tumor: immunohistochemical and molecular analysis of 20 cases. Mod Pathol. 2007;20(9):995–9.
19. Lovly CM, Gupta A, Lipson D, Otto G, Brennan T, Chung CT, et al. Inflammatory myofibroblastic tumors harbor multiple potentially actionable kinase fusions. Cancer Discov. 2014;4(8):889–95.
20. Cerfolio RJ, Allen MS, Nascimento AG, Deschamps C, Trastek VF, Miller DL, et al. Inflammatory pseudotumors of the lung. Ann Thorac Surg. 1999;67(4):933–6.
21. Lee HJ, Kim JS, Choi YS, Kim K, Shim YM, Han J, et al. Treatment of inflammatory myofibroblastic tumor of the chest: the extent of resection. Ann Thorac Surg. 2007;84(1):221–4.
22. Kubo N, Harada T, Anai S, Otsubo K, Yoneshima Y, Ijichi K, et al. Carboplatin plus paclitaxel in the successful treatment of advanced inflammatory myofibroblastic tumor. Intern Med. 2012;51(17):2399–401.

27 Metastatic Malignant Epithelioid Melanoma Versus Poorly Differentiated Carcinoma

Hui Zhu

Case Presentation

A 60-year-old male presented with seizure and altered mental status. Computed tomography (CT) scan found a solitary large lung mass and multiple brain masses, concerning for metastatic malignancy (Fig. 27.1). Due to the patient's mental status, his past medical history was unknown.

Core-needle biopsy of the lung mass demonstrated a neoplasm composed of epithelioid cells with nested and sheet-like growth pattern. The tumor cells had a moderate amount of eosinophilic cytoplasm, pleomorphic nuclei with fine chromatin, and inconspicuous nucleoli. Brisk mitotic activity was present. Immunohistochemical stains showed that the tumor cells were diffusely positive for AE1/3, CAM5.2, and S100 (Fig. 27.2) and negative for synaptophysin and chromogranin. Additional immunohistochemical stains showed that the tumor cells were positive for Melan-A, HMB45, and SOX10 (Fig. 27.2). Upon further investigation, the patient had a remote history of "melanocytic tumor" removed from his thigh.

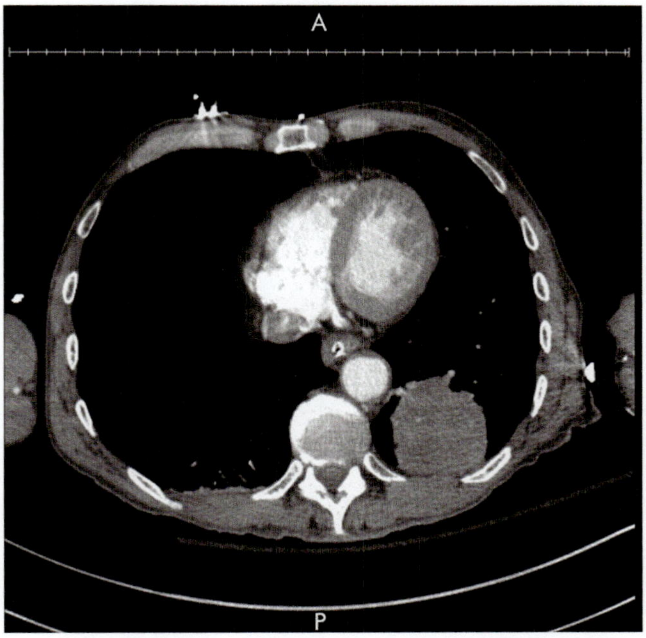

Fig. 27.1 Metastatic melanoma presented as a solitary large pulmonary mass. CT scan showed a single large (5.7 cm) mass in the lower lobe of the left lung. The patient had a remote history of a "melanocytic tumor" removed from the thigh

H. Zhu (✉)
Pathology and Laboratory Services, Forward Pathology Solutions,
HCA North Cypress Medical Center, Cypress, TX, USA
e-mail: huizhu@hcaheathcare.com

H. Xu et al. (eds.), *Practical Lung Pathology*, Practical Anatomic Pathology, https://doi.org/10.1007/978-3-031-14402-8_27

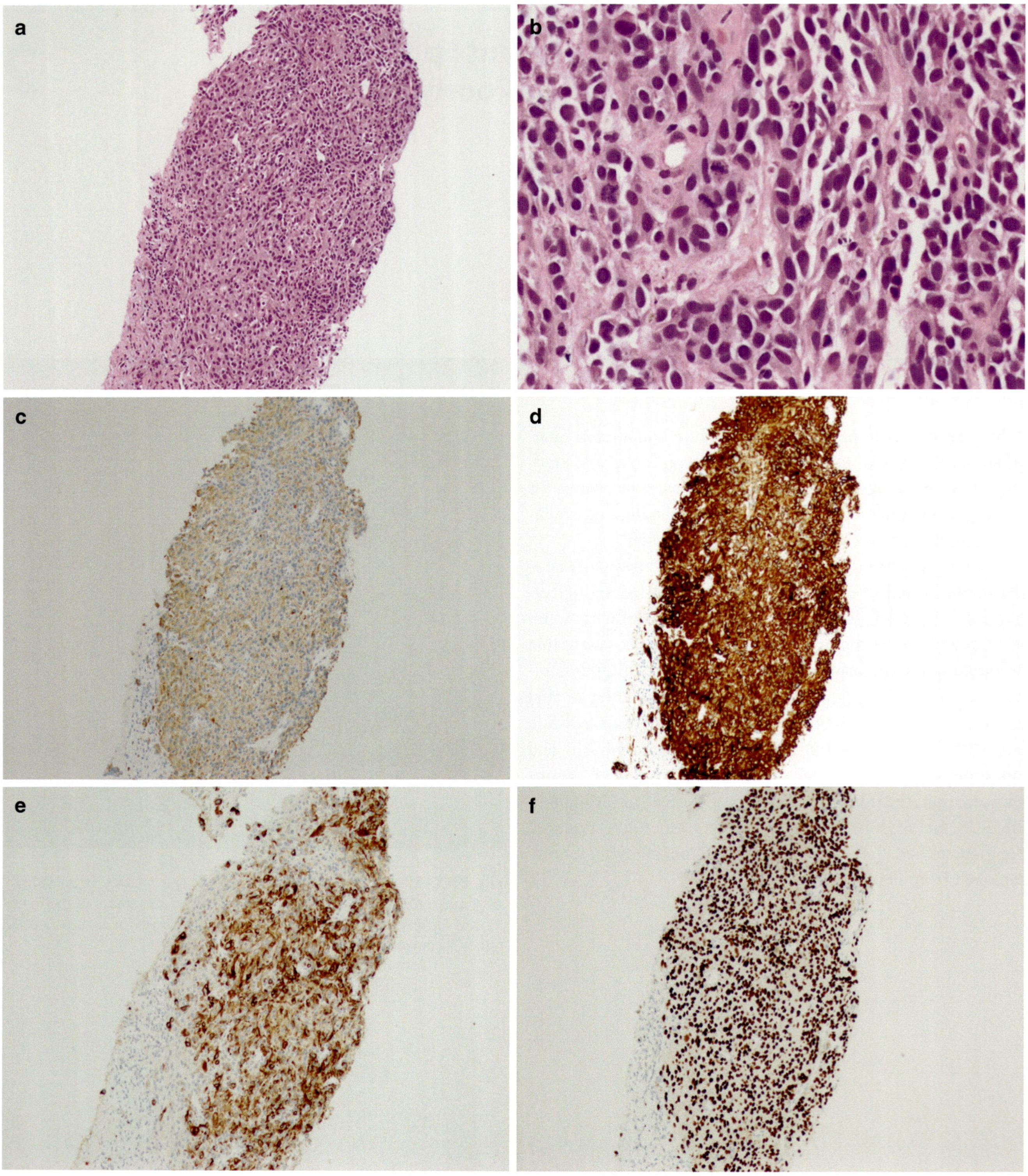

Fig. 27.2 (**a**) Biopsy of the mass showed epithelioid tumor cells with a moderate amount of eosinophilic cytoplasm with nested growth pattern (H&E, original magnification 100×). (**b**) Brisk mitotic activity was present. Focal melanin pigment was also seen (H&E, original magnification 400×). Immunohistochemically, melanoma cells showed diffuse weak AE1/AE3 staining (**c**) and strong CAM5.2 staining (**d**). Melanocytic markers were diffusely and strongly positive in tumor cells, including Melan-A (**e**), SOX-10 (**f**), HMB-45, and S100 (not shown) (immunohistochemistry, original magnification 100×)

Final Diagnosis: Metastatic Melanoma

What Are the Clinical Presentations of Pulmonary Metastatic Melanoma, and How Do They Differ from Primary Carcinoma?

Metastatic neoplasms are more common than primary neoplasms in the lung [1]. Virtually any malignancy can spread to the lungs. The most common presentation for metastatic lung tumors is the presence of bilateral small (<2 cm) lung nodules in patients with known extrapulmonary malignancies. Solitary metastasis occurs in less than 10% of all metastases to the lungs [2, 3]. Large solitary metastasis (more than 5 cm) is less common and is often confused with primary neoplasms, especially when the primary site is not identified. Very rarely, metastatic tumors can form endobronchial masses, which are particularly challenging to distinguish from primary bronchogenic tumors [4]. Melanoma is one of the tumors that can form large solitary lung and endobronchial metastases [5].

Melanoma is one of the leading causes of cancer death, and the incidence is continuously rising [6, 7]. The lung is the most commonly involved visceral organ for metastatic melanoma. A majority of patients with lung metastases have a known history of melanoma; however, a minority (~4%) of patients present with pulmonary metastases as the initial presentation of stage-IV disease [8]. Pulmonary metastasis can occur several months to more than 25 years after the initial melanoma diagnosis [9]. The typical presentation is multiple bilateral lung nodules; single metastatic melanoma mass, however, is not uncommon. In a study of 1720 patients with pulmonary metastatic melanoma, 72% of patients had multiple masses, and 28% of patients had single metastasis [10]. Metastatic melanomas are predominantly small nodules (less than 3 cm, with a medium size of 1.5 cm); however, large (>5 cm) solitary metastasis can occasionally occur (Fig. 27.1) [8]. Diagnosis of solitary large metastases, endobronchial metastases, or metastasis with no or remote history of primary melanoma can be particularly challenging. At times, there is no way to distinguish primary from secondary tumors with absolute certainty. Management for primary pulmonary melanoma does not differ much from single metastatic lesion, with surgical excision being the treatment of choice, and prognosis for both primary and metastatic lung melanoma is equally poor. On the other hand, management and prognosis for patients with melanoma are very different from those with poorly differentiated carcinoma [10]. Thus, distinguishing melanoma from poorly differentiated carcinoma is crucial for patient care.

What Are the Pathologic Features of Metastatic Melanoma and Poorly Differentiated Carcinoma? How Can Immunohistochemistry and Molecular Testing Be Used to Distinguish These Two Entities?

Similar to cutaneous melanoma, metastatic melanoma in the lung can have a great variety of microscopic appearances. The cells can be epithelioid, spindled, or anaplastic. Their size can vary from small lymphocyte-like (small blue cell tumor) to multinucleated giant cells. The cytoplasm can be eosinophilic, foamy, vacuolated, or clear. Cytologic atypia can vary from mild with bland cells and low mitotic rate to anaplastic cells with brisk mitotic activity. A great variety of growth patterns including pseudoglandular, pseudopapillary, trabecular, nested, solid sheet, and discohesive single cells can be seen. The stroma can be fibrotic, myxoid, or rich in lymphocytes [9]. Thus, histomorphological findings are less of a link to the correct diagnosis (Fig. 27.2).

The presence of melanin pigment is perhaps the most helpful morphologic clue for the diagnosis. However, in many cases melanin can be scant and difficult to identify or even absent (amelanotic melanoma). Known as the great mimicker, melanoma is often included in the differential diagnosis for poorly differentiated carcinoma, sarcoma, and lymphoma. Given the different clinical management for melanoma from carcinoma and sarcoma, it is important to rule out melanoma before considering the diagnosis of high-grade carcinoma or sarcoma, NOS.

Immunohistochemistry is a valuable diagnostic tool. S100, HMB-45, Melan-A, SOX-10, and microphthalmia transcription factor (MITF) are commonly used as melanocytic markers that are expressed in a majority of melanoma cases. Of these, S100 and SOX-10 are the most sensitive markers for melanocytic differentiation and are positive in more than 97% of melanomas. S100 is an acidic dimeric calcium-binding protein with both cytoplasmic and nuclear location. Thus, an apparently positive stain showing only cytoplasmic or nuclear pattern should be questioned (Fig. 27.2). SOX-10 is a transcription factor implicated in melanocyte tumorigenesis with a nuclear staining pattern. S100 and SOX-10 are expressed in all melanoma subtypes. However, S-100 is nonspecific and is expressed in a wide variety of tumors including dendritic cell tumor, cartilage tumor, nerve sheath tumors, myoepithelial tumors, etc. SOX-10 is a relatively recently recognized marker that is more specific than S100, but it is also positive in clear cell sarcoma, nerve sheath tumors, and some breast and salivary gland carcinomas. Melan-A and HMB-45 are specific markers for melanocytic tumors with cytoplasmic staining pattern. However, the sensitivity for both markers is lower than S100 and SOX-10, especially for metastatic melanoma. Sensitivity for metastatic melanoma is 70–90% and 57–92% for HMB-45 and Melan-A, respectively. In addition, HMB-45 and Melan-A are not entirely specific for melanoma. HMB-45 is also expressed in PEComa, melanocytic schwannoma, some ovarian stromal tumors, and some renal cell carcinoma. Melan-A is also expressed in PEComa, adrenocortical tumor, ovarian sex-cord stromal tumor, and clear cell sarcoma. MITF is another marker with nuclear staining pattern. MITF is expressed in most melanomas (up to 80%). Its utility is limited by low specificity. MITF is present in a wide variety of neoplasms, including mesenchymal tumors and lymphoid neoplasms, as well as some carcinomas [11].

In contrast to the dogma that positivity for keratin immunohistochemical staining defines epithelial differentiation and rules out the possibility of melanoma, metastatic melanoma can express epithelial markers including keratins and EMA [12]. One study has shown that focal cytokeratin 8 and cytokeratin 18 staining is present in most metastatic melanoma cases [13]. Low-molecular-weight keratins are more frequently positive and often show stronger positivity than high-molecular-weight keratins (Fig. 27.2). The staining pattern is typically focal and weak, but diffuse strong positivity can also be seen (Fig. 27.2). Diagnostic difficulties are often encountered when patient's history of melanoma is unknown and/or with imaging study showing a solitary large mass and clinical suspicion of a primary lung neoplasm. With the assumption that what is dealt with is a primary lung neoplasm, S100 and other melanocytic markers are usually not included in the initial antibody panel. Positivity for cytokeratin stain can lead to misdiagnosis of poorly differentiated primary lung carcinoma.

Metastatic melanoma can lose the expression of one or more melanocytic markers, and occasional cases may display loss of all of the melanocytic markers. In these cases, molecular testing with *BRAF/NRAS/KIT* genotyping can be helpful in establishing the correct diagnosis [14].

As mentioned above, due to the great phenotypic diversity, morphologic findings are less of a clue to correct diagnosis of melanoma. Epithelioid melanoma can be a perfect mimicker of poorly differentiated carcinoma (Fig. 27.3).

Poorly differentiated primary pulmonary carcinoma is often positive only for pancytokeratin and lacks expression of adenocarcinoma markers such as TTF-1, napsin-A, and CK7 or squamous markers such as p40, p63, and CK5/6 [15]. Similarly, metastatic melanoma can be positive for cytokeratin and is negative for other adenocarcinoma or squamous cell carcinoma markers. Before making the diagnosis of poorly differentiated primary pulmonary carcinoma, clinical and radiologic correlation and melanocytic markers are essential to exclude the possibility of metastatic melanoma, especially for patients with known history of melanoma.

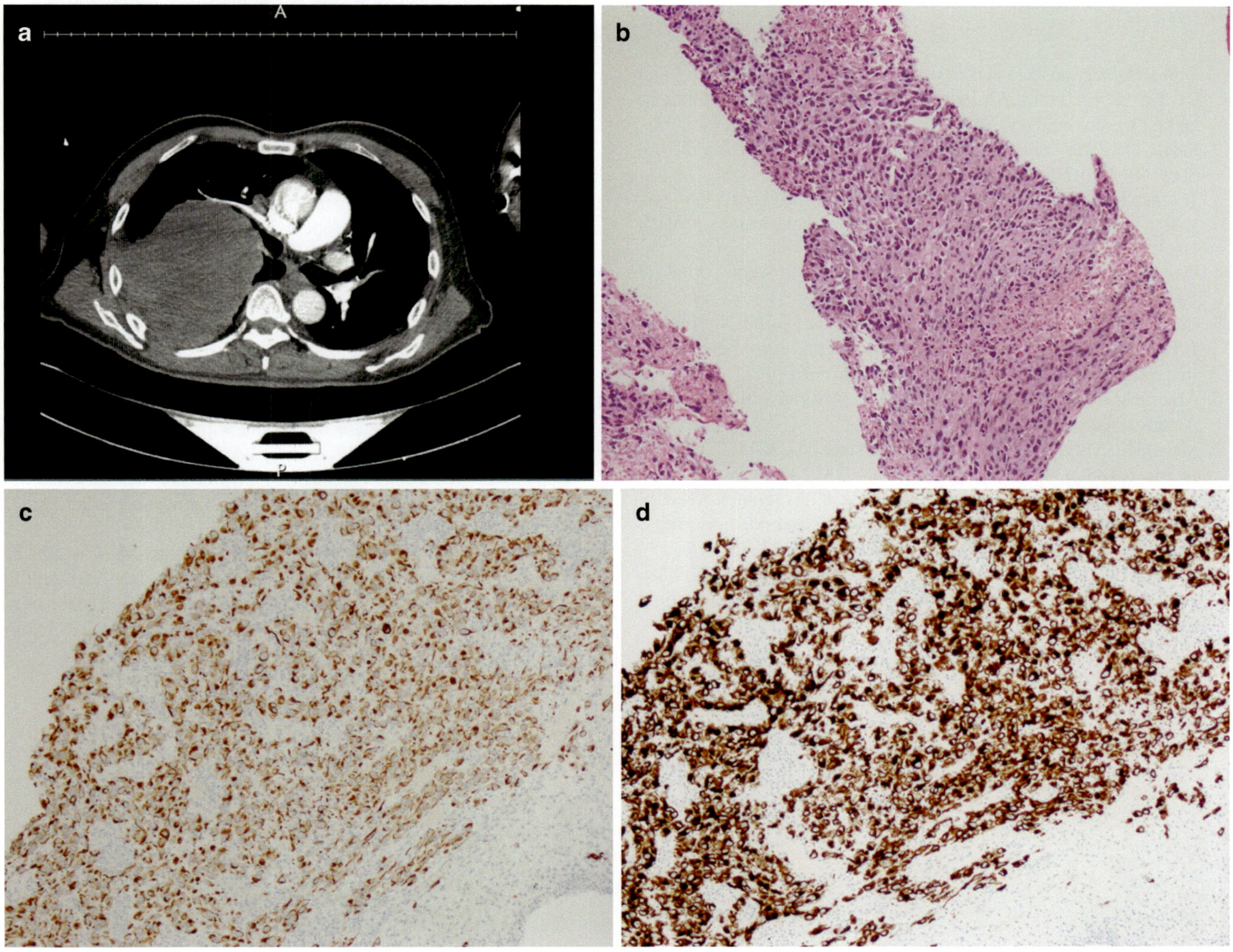

Fig. 27.3 Poorly differentiated primary lung carcinoma. (**a**) CT scan showed a single large mass occupying the upper lobe of the right lung. (**b**). Tumor cells have abundant eosinophilic cytoplasm and prominent red nucleoli (H&E, original magnification 100×). Clinical and morphological features are similar to the metastatic melanoma case shown in Figs. 27.1 and 27.2. The tumor cells are diffusely strongly positive for CAM5.2 (**c**) and AE1/3 (**d**). Melanocytic markers, as well as TTF-1 and p40, are negative. Immunohistochemistry, original magnification 100×

Key Points for Differentiating Epithelioid Metastatic Melanoma from Poorly Differentiated Primary Carcinoma

A history of melanoma is perhaps the most important clue to the correct diagnosis. For any high-grade neoplasm presented in a patient with known history of melanoma, the possibility of metastatic melanoma needs to be excluded. A misdiagnosis can be avoided in the challenging cases if S100 and other melanocytic markers are included in the antibody panel.

Although often scant or even absent, the presence of melanin pigment is the most helpful morphologic feature for melanoma diagnosis. Melanoma is one of the few tumors that produce melanin pigment. The presence of melanin pigment in a high-grade malignant neoplasm is highly suggestive, if not diagnostic, of melanoma.

Immunohistochemically, S100 and SOX-10 are the two most sensitive markers for melanocytic differentiation. It is also important to keep in mind that a significant number of metastatic melanomas can show positivity for keratin staining, especially low-molecular-weight keratins. Rare cases can show diffuse strong keratin positivity. Positivity for keratin does not exclude the diagnosis of melanoma.

Molecular testing for BRAF/NRAS/KIT genotyping can be of great value for rare dedifferentiated/undifferentiated melanoma cases with loss of all melanocytic markers.

References

1. Dail DH. Metastasis to and from the lung. In: Tomashefski J, Cagle PT, Farver CF, Fraire AE, editors. Dail and Hammar's pulmonary pathology. 3rd ed. New York: Springer; 2008.
2. Steele JD. The solitary pulmonary nodule. J Thorac Cardiovasc Surg. 1963;46:21–39.
3. Toomes H, Delphendahl A, Manke HG, Vogt-Moykopf I. The coin lesion of the lung: a review of 955 resected coin lesions. Cancer. 1983;51:534–7.
4. Fitzgerald RH. Endobronchial metastases. South Med J. 1977;79:440–3.
5. Chaussende A, Hermant C, Tazi-Mezalek R, Favrolt N, Hureaux J, Fournier C, et al. Endobronchial metastases from melanoma: a survival analysis. Clin Respir J. 2017;11(6):1006–11.
6. American Cancer Society. Cancer facts & figures 2018. Atlanta: American Cancer Society; 2018.
7. Siegel RL, Miller KD, Jemal A. Cancer statistics, 2018. CA Cancer J Clin. 2018;68(1):7–30. https://doi.org/10.3322/caac.21442.
8. Neuman HB, Patel A, Hanlon C, Wolchok JD, Houghton AN, Coit DG. Stage-IV melanoma and pulmonary metastases: factors predictive of survival. Ann Surg Oncol. 2007;14(10):2847–53.
9. Bastian BC, Lazar A. Melanoma. In: Calonje JE, Brenn T, Lazar AJ, Billings SD, editors. McKee's pathology of the skin. 4th ed. Philadelphia: Saunders; 2011.
10. Petersen RP, Hanish SI, Haney JC, Miller CC 3rd, Burfeind WR Jr, Tyler DS, et al. Improved survival with pulmonary metastasectomy: an analysis of 1720 patients with pulmonary metastatic melanoma. J Thorac Cardiovasc Surg. 2007;133(1):104–10.
11. Ordóñez NG. Value of melanocytic-associated immunohistochemical markers in the diagnosis of malignant melanoma: a review and update. Hum Pathol. 2014;45(2):191–205. [Am J Surg Pathol. 2016; 40(2); 181–91]
12. Achilles E, Schröder S. Positive cytokeratin results in malignant melanoma. Pitfall in differential immunohistologic diagnosis of occult neoplasms. Pathologe. 1994;15(4):235–41.
13. Safadi RA, Bader DH, Abdullah NI, Sughayer MA. Immunohistochemical expression of keratins 6, 7, 8, 14, 16, 18, 19, and MNF-116 pancytokeratin in primary and metastatic melanoma of the head and neck. Oral Surg Oral Med Pathol Oral Radiol. 2016;121(5):510–9.
14. Agaimy A, Specht K, Stoehr R, Lorey T, Märkl B, Niedobitek G, et al. Metastatic malignant melanoma with complete loss of differentiation markers (undifferentiated/dedifferentiated melanoma): analysis of 14 patients emphasizing phenotypic plasticity and the value of molecular testing as surrogate diagnostic marker. Am J Surg Pathol. 2016;40(2):181–91.
15. Nicholson AG, Brambila E, Beasley MB, Caporaso NE, Carvalho L, Dalurzo ML, et al. Large cell carcinoma. In: Travis WD, Brambilla E, Burke AP, Marx A, Nicholson AG, editors. WHO classification of tumours of the lung, pleura, thymus and heart. 4th ed. Lyon: IARC Press; 2015.

28 Pulmonary Epithelioid Angiosarcoma Versus Carcinoma

John M. Gross and Robert W. Ricciotti

Case Presentation

A 68-year-old male with a past medical history of coronary artery disease status post-coronary angioplasty 5 years ago presents with symptoms of increasing dyspnea, chest pain, intermittent night sweats, and occasional hemoptysis. A chest radiograph, EKG, troponins, D-dimer, CBC, and BMP are unremarkable. A subsequent CT scan reveals an ill-defined 1.5 cm nodule in the left lung involving the pleura that was not present on prior examinations. Extensive workup reveals no other sites of disease.

A diagnostic lung wedge biopsy is obtained revealing a neoplasm composed of epithelioid cells with large nuclei and prominent nucleoli. Some areas of the neoplasm demonstrate solid, sheetlike growth, while other areas suggest vasoformation (Fig. 28.1). By immunohistochemistry, the malignant cells express CD31, CD34, FLI1, and ERG (Fig. 28.2).

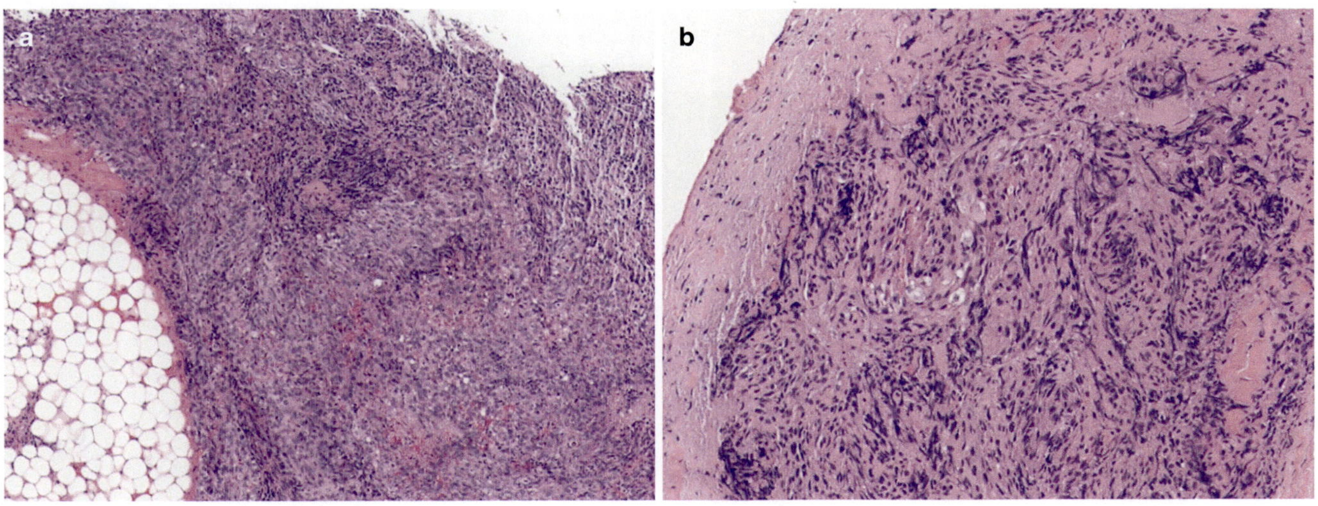

Fig. 28.1 (**a**) Malignant epithelioid neoplasm involving the pleural adipose tissue and (**b**) pleural surface (**c**) growing in solid sheets with (**d**) focal vasoformation

J. M. Gross
Division of Anatomic Pathology, The Johns Hopkins Medical Institute, Baltimore, MD, USA

R. W. Ricciotti (✉)
Department of Laboratory Medicine and Pathology, University of Washington Medical Center, Seattle, WA, USA
e-mail: ricciott@uw.edu

H. Xu et al. (eds.), *Practical Lung Pathology*, Practical Anatomic Pathology, https://doi.org/10.1007/978-3-031-14402-8_28

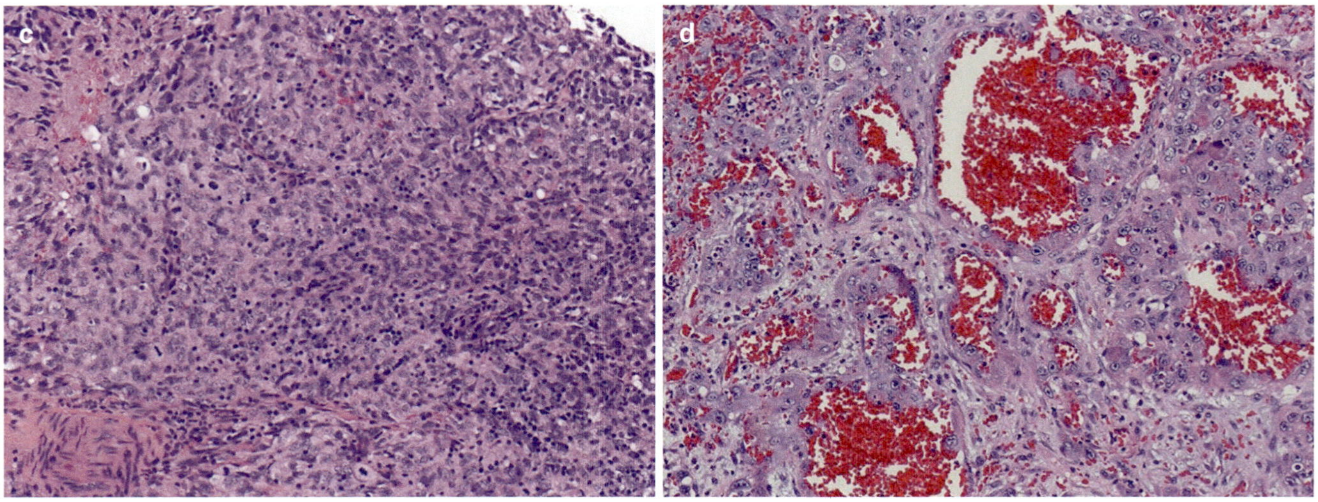

Fig. 28.1 (continued)

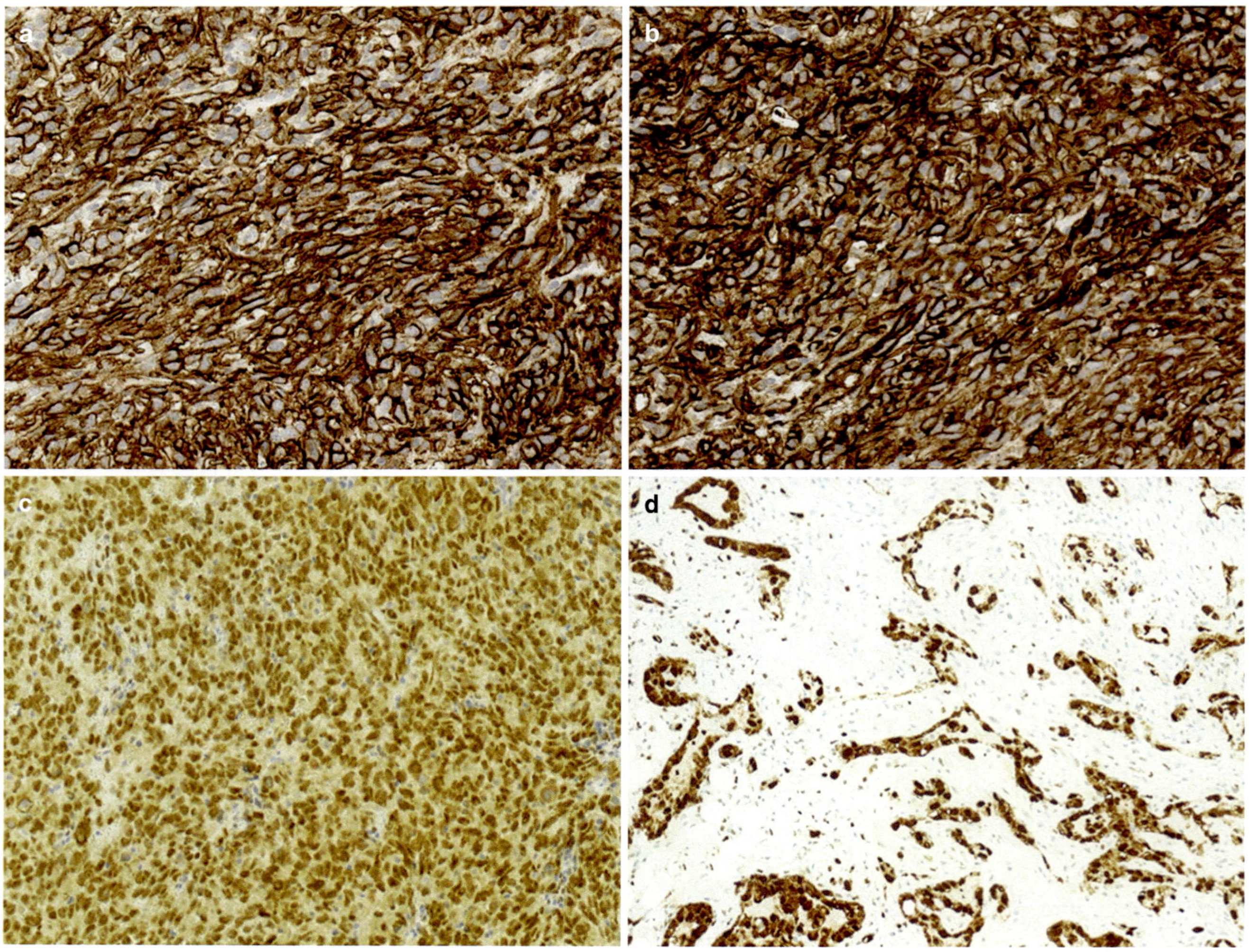

Fig. 28.2 Immunohistochemistry demonstrating strong expression of (**a**) CD31, (**b**) CD34, (**c**) and FLI1 in areas of sheetlike growth as well as (**d**) ERG in vasoformative areas, supporting endothelial differentiation

Pathologic Diagnosis: Epithelioid Angiosarcoma

What Is Epithelioid Angiosarcoma? What Are the Clinical, Demographic, Treatment, and Prognostic Features?

Epithelioid angiosarcoma (EAS) is a high-grade sarcoma of endothelial differentiation. EAS generally presents in the deep soft tissues but may rarely occur in the skin and subcutis or in visceral sites including the lung and pleura [1, 2]. Pulmonary EAS has no gender predilection and generally affects adults in the sixth to seventh decade [2–4]. The rarity of pulmonary EAS contributes to the difficulty in this clinical diagnosis as patients often present with nonspecific respiratory (cough, dyspnea, chest pain) and general symptoms (malaise, night sweats, weight loss). Approximately 40–50% of patients will experience unexplained hemoptysis and/or hemothorax; however, 20% of patients are entirely asymptomatic [2, 5].

A multidisciplinary approach to treatment is necessary with considerations of surgery, chemotherapy, and radiation. The prognosis of pulmonary angiosarcoma is poor as most patients die of disease within months of initial presentation. The presence of pleural involvement is a negative prognostic factor [2].

What Are the Radiologic Features of Primary Pulmonary Angiosarcoma?

Radiologically, primary pulmonary EAS may occur as either multifocal or solitary nodules. When the involvement is multifocal, chest radiographs show bilateral reticulonodular or alveolar infiltrates with or without pleural effusions. When a solitary nodule is present, especially if located in a centrilobular pattern with ground-glass changes, differentiation from pulmonary carcinoma is quite challenging [5].

What Are the Histologic and Immunophenotypic Features of Epithelioid Angiosarcoma?

Histologically, EAS typically consists of sheets or nodules of malignant cells with moderate amounts of eosinophilic cytoplasm and often eccentrically placed nuclei imparting an epithelioid-to-rhabdoid/plasmacytoid appearance. Some areas may show spindled cells. The nuclei often contain peripherally marginated chromatin yielding a pale vesicular appearance frequently with prominent nucleoli. The cells may grow in a syncytial pattern or appear discohesive. Vasoformation and/or blood lakes may be only focal or even absent, and some examples may show complex, irregular anastomosing channels. Mitotic activity is generally abundant, and necrosis is often identified. The various histologic features are shown in Figs. 28.3 and 28.4. By immunohistochemistry, the malignant cells show evidence of endothelial differentiation with expression of CD31, CD34, ERG, and FLI-1. Keratin and CAM5.2 expression are seen in approximately half of the cases of EAS, which is a potential diagnostic pitfall [2, 6, 7].

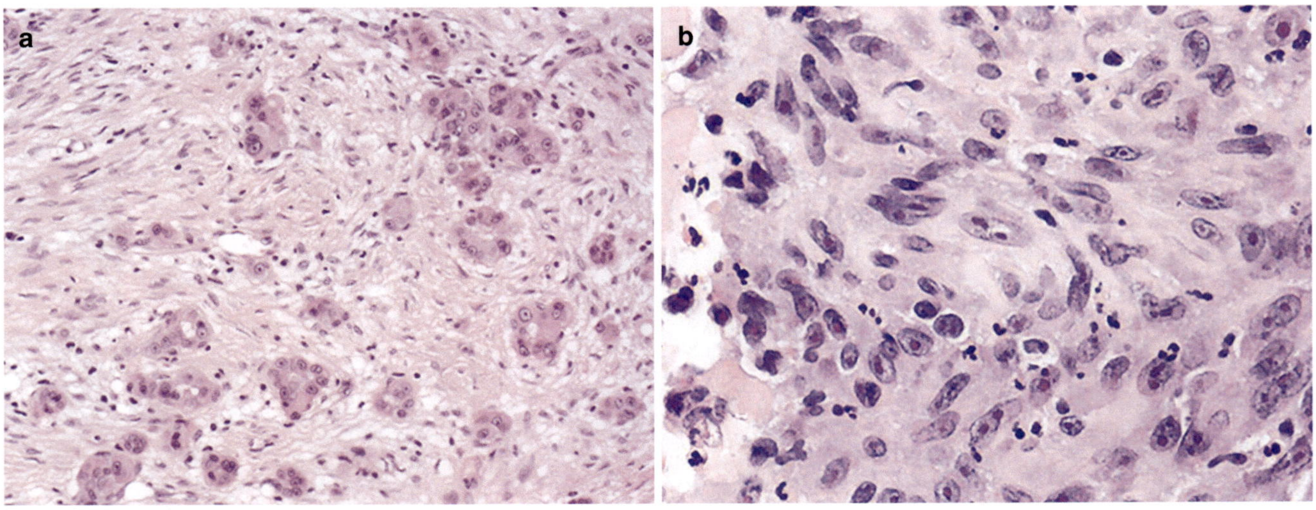

Fig. 28.3 (**a**) Epithelioid angiosarcoma often shows a variety of histologic patterns including infiltrative epithelioid cells forming vascular channels, (**b**) sheets of plump spindle cells, (**c**) discohesive epithelioid cells with prominent nuclei showing a "cracking" artifact, and (**d**) dense eosinophilic cytoplasm with eccentric nuclei assuming a rhabdoid/plasmacytoid morphology

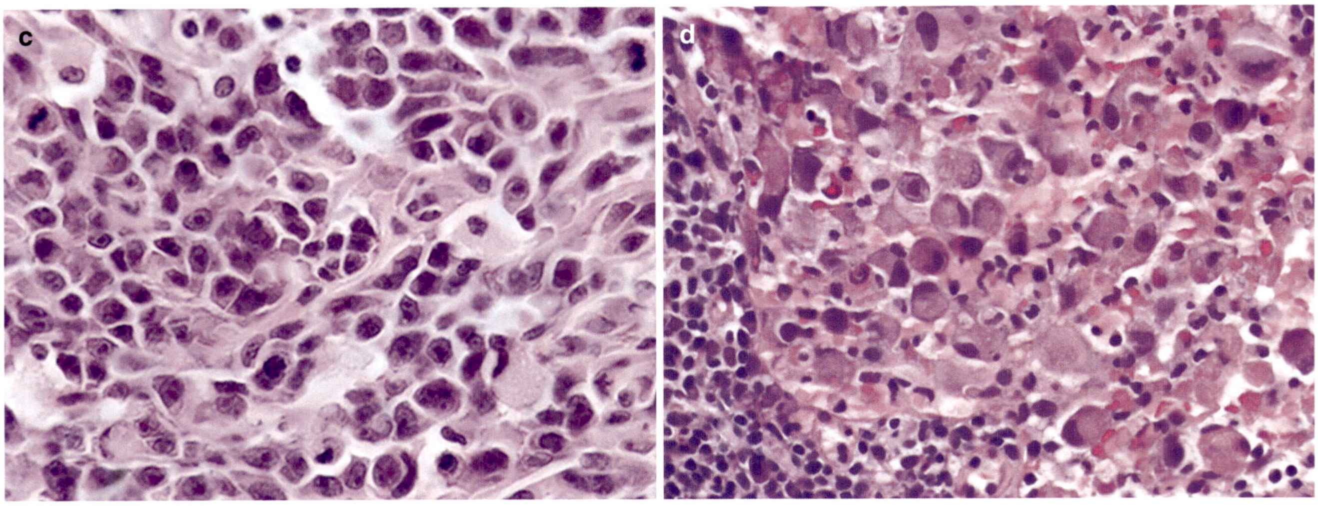

Fig. 28.3 (continued)

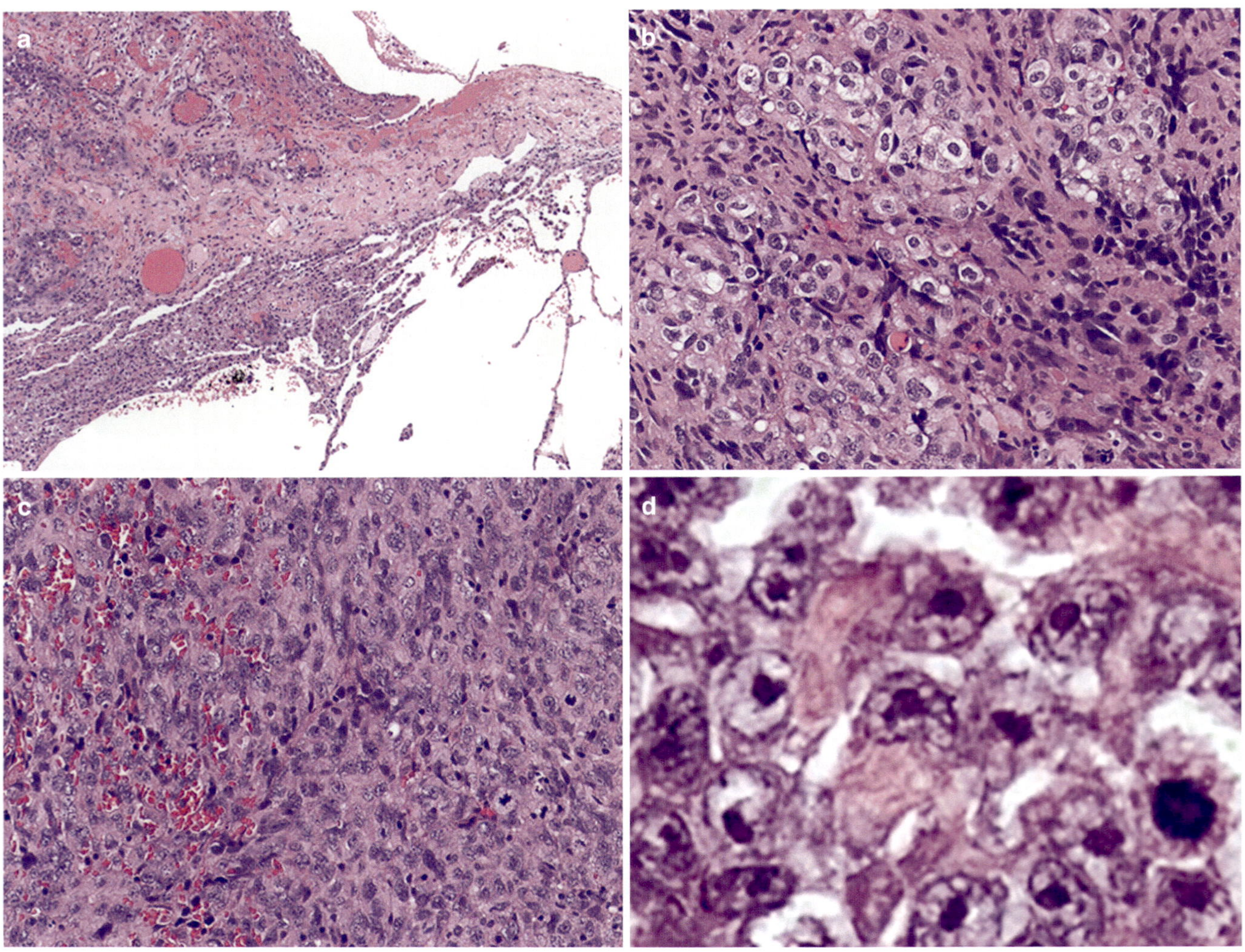

Fig. 28.4 (**a**) Pulmonary epithelioid angiosarcoma forming vascular spaces within the lung parenchyma. (**b**) Higher power showing solid growth of epithelioid cells. (**c**) An area showing poorly formed vascular spaces (left). (**d**) Prominent nucleoli and a peripherally marginated chromatin pattern are common

Does Angiosarcoma Have Any Recurrent Molecular Abnormalities?

While the majority of radiation-associated angiosarcomas (AS) show *MYC* gene amplifications with a subset showing *KDR*, *PLCG1*, and *FLT4* mutations, the genetic signature of primary AS remains poorly defined. A recent study identified *CIC* mutations and rearrangements in a subset (9%) of primary AS, some of which showed epithelioid morphology. Tumors with *CIC* abnormalities demonstrated a predilection for younger patients as well as inferior disease-free survival. In the same study, *PLCG1* and *KDR* mutations were identified in both primary and secondary AS with a predilection for breast and bone/visceral locations, regardless of *MYC* status. AS with *FLT4*-amplification showed variable epithelioid morphology but occurred predominantly in tumors related to radiotherapy for breast cancer or lymphedema. Such tumors most often showed co-amplification of *MYC*, lacked *PLCG1/KDR* mutations, and were associated with a worse prognosis [8].

What Is the Differential Diagnosis of Pulmonary Epithelioid Angiosarcoma?

In the setting of multiple lung lesions, metastatic disease is the most important diagnosis to consider. A thorough clinical history and a careful review of imaging studies are paramount.

Clinically, the differential diagnosis of pulmonary AS includes a variety of etiologies depending on the clinical presentation and site of disease. Patients may present with pulmonary hemorrhage including hemothorax and general symptoms such as night sweats and weight loss. Radiologic presentation can vary, often with nonspecific findings, as pulmonary AS may occur as a solitary mass or as multifocal lesions with nodular or alveolar infiltrates. The clinicoradiologic differential diagnoses may include primary lung carcinoma, mesothelioma, metastatic disease, necrotizing vasculitis, infectious processes (tuberculosis, fungus), pneumonia, or abscesses [5].

Histologically, the sheetlike growth and epithelioid appearance, along with frequent cytokeratin expression, make distinguishing carcinoma (primary or metastatic) from EAS challenging. Morphologic features favoring EAS include intracellular lumina (which may or may not contain fragmented erythrocytes) and a cracked appearance of poorly formed vascular channels. Carcinomas will typically not express immunohistochemical markers of endothelial differentiation such as CD31, CD34, ERG, or FLI1. If aberrant endothelial marker expression in a carcinoma is suspected, confirmation with a second vascular marker may be helpful. Furthermore, AS may lose some endothelial markers, so that staining with multiple markers may be necessary to provide evidence of endothelial differentiation. Epithelioid hemangioendothelioma (EHE) has an overlapping immunophenotype with EAS (endothelial markers and keratin expression); however, EHE typically shows less severe cytologic atypia and grows in cords or singly within a dense myxohyaline matrix [2]. Table 28.1 summarizes the most relevant differential diagnoses with pulmonary EAS.

Although rare, proximal-type epithelioid sarcoma could be a diagnostic consideration as this tumor shows a distinctly high-grade epithelioid-to-rhabdoid morphology and expresses keratins and occasionally ERG; however, nuclear INI1 (SMARCB1) expression is lost in proximal-type epithelioid sarcoma, whereas it is retained in most cases of epithelioid angiosarcoma [4, 9]. Likewise, SMARCA4-deficient thoracic tumors also show malignant epithelioid-to-rhabdoid cells, and approximately half express CD34 and keratins (CK AE1/AE3, EMA); however, SMARCA4 (BRG1) will be lost, and INI1 (SMARCB1) is retained [9].

Finally, melanoma, mesothelioma, and anaplastic large-cell lymphoma can be diagnostic considerations as they may display histologic features reminiscent of epithelioid angio-

Table 28.1 Differential diagnoses of pulmonary epithelioid angiosarcoma

Diagnosis	Pulmonary EAS	Pulmonary EHE	Pulmonary carcinoma	Metastatic carcinoma
Clinical	Adults, nonspecific symptoms	Adults, nonspecific symptoms	Adults, smokers	Adults, prior cancer history
Tumor focality	Solitary or multiple	Solitary or multiple	Usually solitary	Often multiple masses
Histology	Epithelioid cells, solid or vasoformative, pleomorphism, mitotic activity, necrosis	Epithelioid cells, intraluminal RBCS, chondromyxoid stroma	Variable; adenocarcinoma or squamous	Variable epithelioid morphology
Immunohistochemistry	+ CD31, CD34, ERG, FLI1, +/− keratin expression	+ CD31, CD34, ERG, FLI1, +/− keratin, most CAMTA1+, subset TFE3+	Positive for keratins, negative for endothelial markers (CD31, CD34, ERG, FLI1)	Positive for keratins, negative for endothelial markers (CD31, CD34, ERG, FLI1)
Molecular genetics	Poorly defined; subset with *CIC* abnormalities	WWTR1-CAMTA1; subset with YAP1-TFE3	Variable; ALK, EGFR, ROS1, KRAS	Variable

sarcoma necessitating the use of immunohistochemistry to classify them [4]. Unlike EAS, melanoma will express S100, SOX10, Melan-A, and HMB45; mesothelioma will express calretinin and nuclear WT-1; and anaplastic large-cell lymphoma will express CD45, CD30, and typically at least one pan-T-cell marker [4].

References

1. Ko JS, Billings SD. Diagnostically challenging epithelioid vascular tumors. Surg Pathol Clin. 2015;8(3):331–51.
2. Anderson T, Zhang L, Hameed M, Rusch V, Travis WD, Antonescu CR. Thoracic epithelioid malignant vascular tumors: a clinicopathologic study of 52 cases with emphasis on pathologic grading and molecular studies of WWTR1-CAMTA1 fusions. Am J Surg Pathol. 2015;39(1):132–9.
3. Zhang Y, Huang X, Peng C, Wang Y, Wu Q, Wu Z, et al. Primary pulmonary epithelioid angiosarcoma: a case report and literature review. J Cancer Res Ther. 2018;14(Supplement):S533–S5.
4. Hart J, Mandavilli S. Epithelioid angiosarcoma: a brief diagnostic review and differential diagnosis. Arch Pathol Lab Med. 2011;135(2):268–72.
5. Eichner R, Schwendy S, Liebl F, Huber A, Langer R. Two cases of primary pulmonary angiosarcoma as a rare cause of lung haemorrhage. Pathology. 2011;43(4):386–9.
6. Fletcher CD, Beham A, Bekir S, Clarke AM, Marley NJ. Epithelioid angiosarcoma of deep soft tissue: a distinctive tumor readily mistaken for an epithelial neoplasm. Am J Surg Pathol. 1991;15(10):915–24.
7. Deshpande V, Rosenberg AE, O'Connell JX, Nielsen GP. Epithelioid angiosarcoma of the bone: a series of 10 cases. Am J Surg Pathol. 2003;27(6):709–16.
8. Huang S-C, Zhang L, Sung Y-S, Chen C-L, Kao Y-C, Agaram NP, et al. Recurrent CIC gene abnormalities in angiosarcomas: a molecular study of 120 cases with concurrent investigation of PLCG1, KDR, MYC, and FLT4 gene alterations. Am J Surg Pathol. 2016;40(5):645–55.
9. Perret R, Chalabreysse L, Watson S, Serre I, Garcia S, Forest F, et al. SMARCA4-deficient thoracic sarcomas: Clinicopathologic study of 30 cases with an emphasis on their nosology and differential diagnoses. Am J Surg Pathol. 2019;43(4):455–65.

29 Epithelioid Sarcoma Versus Large-Cell (Undifferentiated) Carcinoma

Amir Qorbani, Gregory A. Fishbein, and Scott D. Nelson

Case Presentation

A 24-year-old male presented with a painful mass in the right hand that was gradually increasing in size. Magnetic resonance imaging (MRI) of the right hand showed expansion and diffuse signal abnormality of the flexor pollicis brevis muscle (Fig. 29.1).

Ultrasound-guided biopsy was performed and was nondiagnostic; only a fibroblastic/myofibroblastic proliferation with histiocytes was seen. The clinical team performed an excisional biopsy and removed three separate nodules. Histologic sections showed a highly infiltrative proliferation of atypical epithelioid and plump to spindle-shaped cells arranged in nodules and infiltrative cords through the collagen and muscle fibers. These cells had round nuclei, vesicular chromatin, small nucleoli, and relatively abundant amounts of eosinophilic cytoplasm. Mitotic count was one per ten high-power fields. The infiltrative nodules had central degeneration and necrosis (Fig. 29.2).

Immunohistochemistry studies showed diffuse immunoreactivity to EMA and CAM5.2 as well as focal positive reactivity to pan-cytokeratin. The tumor cells showed loss of INI-1 immunoreactivity. Desmin, myogenin, CD163, S100, and HMB-45 were negative. He was diagnosed with epithelioid sarcoma (ES) and started on a selective multi-targeted receptor tyrosine kinase inhibitor, pazopanib. A couple of months later, he presented with chest pain. Chest X-ray (CXR) showed a left apical pneumothorax (Fig. 29.3).

The clinical team was primarily concerned that his symptoms were either a side effect of pazopanib, which has been linked with increased risk of pneumothorax, or secondary to parenchymal lung disease. Subsequent computed tomography (CT) scan showed a left pneumothorax as well as multiple bilateral pulmonary micronodules, up to 3 mm (Fig. 29.4).

The patient underwent flexible bronchoscopy, left video-assisted thoracic surgery (VATS) for left lower and upper lobe wedge resections, chemical pleurodesis with doxycycline, and mechanical pleurodesis. Histologic sections revealed lung parenchyma with multiple foci of highly atypical, large epithelioid cells in the interstitial compartment (Fig. 29.5).

Immunohistochemical stains showed that these epithelioid cells were positive for EMA (Fig. 29.6a) and CAM5.2 and they were negative for pan-cytokeratin (Fig. 29.6b), CK7, and TTF1. INI immunoreactivity is retained in lung parenchyma but is lost in epithelioid sarcoma (Fig. 29.6c). A diagnosis of primary pulmonary large-cell undifferentiated carcinoma was considered. However, due to the prior history, further workup revealed loss of INI immunoreactivity in the atypical cells, establishing a diagnosis of metastatic epithelioid sarcoma (Fig. 29.6c).

A. Qorbani (✉)
UCSF Medical Center at Mission Bay, Pathology Department, University of California, San Francisco (UCSF), San Francisco, CA, USA
e-mail: amir.qorbani@ucsf.edu

G. A. Fishbein
Department of Pathology and Laboratory Medicine, David Geffen School of Medicine at UCLA, Los Angeles, CA, USA
e-mail: GFishbein@mednet.ucla.edu

S. D. Nelson
UCLA Santa Monica and Orthopedic Hospital, University of California, Los Angeles (UCLA), Santa Monica, CA, USA
e-mail: SDNelson@mednet.ucla.edu

H. Xu et al. (eds.), *Practical Lung Pathology*, Practical Anatomic Pathology, https://doi.org/10.1007/978-3-031-14402-8_29

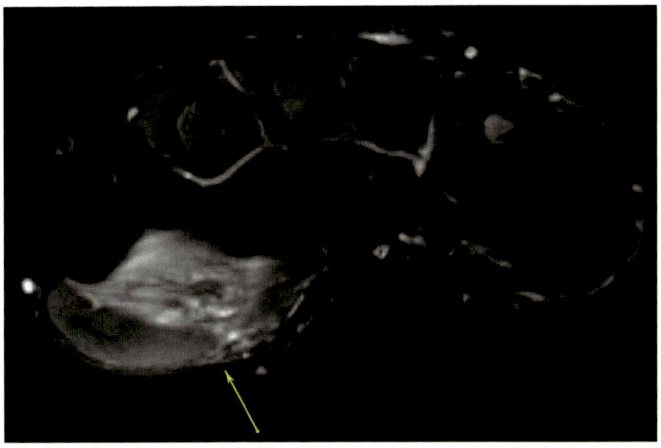

Fig. 29.1 MRI from the right hand: expansion and diffuse signal abnormality of the flexor pollicis brevis muscle

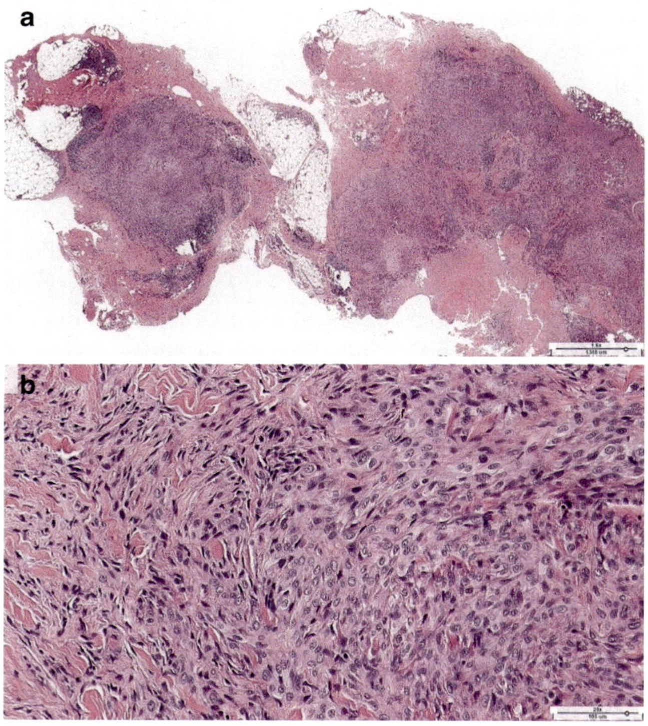

Fig. 29.2 Histologic sections of the right hand mass show a nodular infiltrating growth pattern with areas of necrosis (**a**, magnification 40×), and the tumor cells are epithelioid to spindle-shaped with round vesicular nuclei and abundant eosinophilic cytoplasm (**b**, magnification 200×)

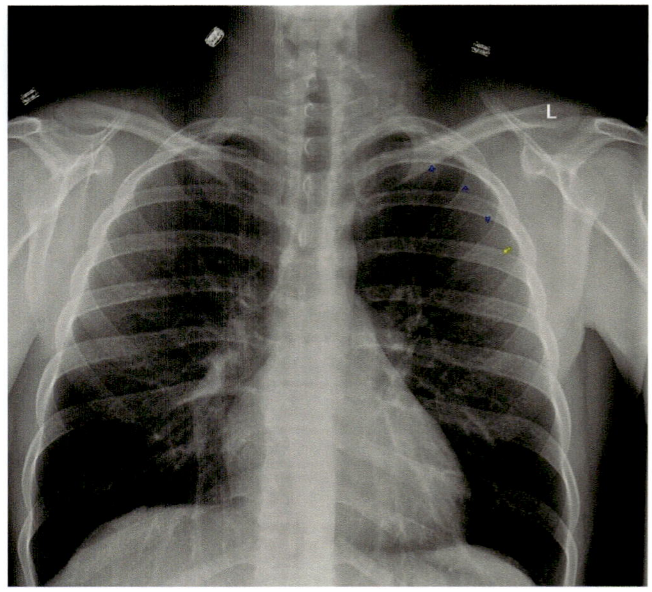

Fig. 29.3 CXR showing left apical pneumothorax. Pleural line is marked by arrows

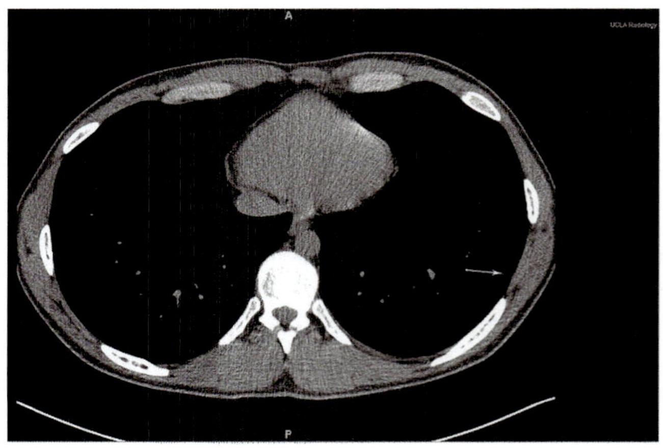

Fig. 29.4 CT scan showed a small left pneumothorax and multiple bilateral micronodules (less than 0.3 cm); one is shown at the tip of the arrow

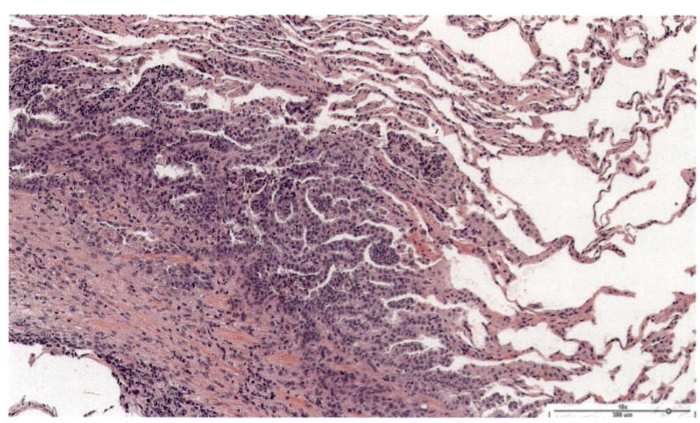

Fig. 29.5 Histologic sections of the lung mass show epithelioid to spindle cells with adjacent reactive parenchyma (magnification 100×)

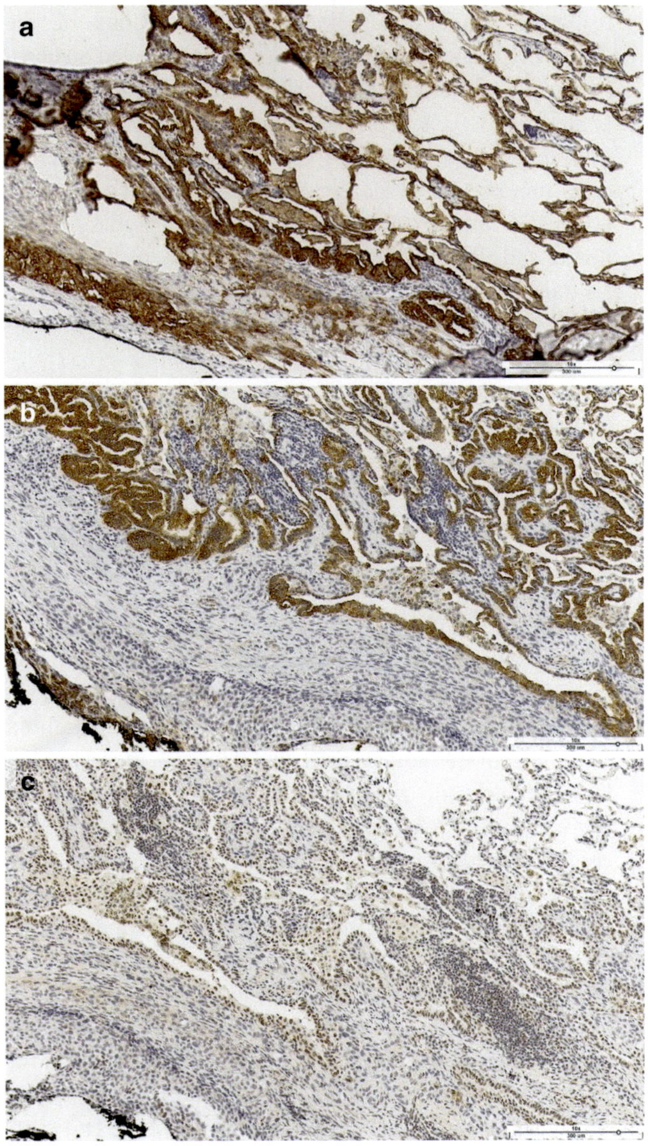

Fig. 29.6 Immunohistochemical stains were performed. EMA immunostains highlight both reactive lung parenchyma and epithelioid neoplastic cells (**a**). Pan-cytokeratin immunostains just highlight reactive lung parenchyma but not epithelioid sarcoma (**b**). INI immunoreactivity is retained in lung parenchyma but is lost in epithelioid sarcoma (**c**). (**a**)–(**c**) magnification 100×

Final Pathologic Diagnosis: Metastatic Epithelioid Sarcoma

What Are the Clinical Features of Epithelioid Sarcoma, and How Do They Differ from Large-Cell (Undifferentiated) Carcinoma?

Epithelioid sarcomas are recognized in two clinicopathological subtypes:

- Conventional (classic) type: first described in 1970 by Enzinger as a distinctive malignant neoplasm that involves the distal extremities, shows epithelioid morphology, and mimics a benign granulomatous process [1]. It typically involves the distal extremities (especially forearm, wrist, and hand) of young adults (median age, 30 years); males are affected more than females. It is the most common sarcoma of the distal extremities and typically presents as a slow-growing, often painless, intradermal or subcutaneous nodules(s) or plaque, more frequently on the flexor surfaces. It may appear to "track" up the limb or as a nonhealing ulcer and clinically may be mistaken for an inflammatory process. It is an aggressive sarcoma and can recur locally (>70%) or as metastasis in almost half of cases [2].
- Proximal type: Guillou et al. described a "proximal-type" epithelioid sarcoma in 1997, showing more tendency to occur in the proximal sites (trunk, genitalia, head and neck, or even mediastinum) of somewhat older adults (median age, 40 years), with a more aggressive behavior. Patients often present with a large infiltrative mass in the deep soft tissue that grows more rapidly than classic-type epithelioid sarcoma and can metastasize in up to 75% of cases (usually to the lymph node and lung) [3].

Lung involvement by ES is usually due to metastasis from an extrapulmonary site, presenting as multifocal lung nodules in young adults with a prior history of ES. Large-cell carcinomas are considered a primary lung cancer and usually occur as a large (more than 4 cm) peripheral mass in older adults (50–70 years old), with male gender predilection. Depending on the extent of disease, both can present with weight loss, respiratory symptoms (cough, hemoptysis, etc.), or chest pain. Clinical history (age, gender, prior cancer history, etc.) and imaging studies (CXR, CT, and MRI) can be helpful in differentiating one from another; however, the specific diagnosis requires proper tissue examination.

What Are the Pathologic Features of Epithelioid Sarcoma and Large-Cell (Undifferentiated) Carcinoma?

Gross

Primary ES, conventional type, usually presents as an indurated dermal or subcutaneous poorly defined multinodular mass with infiltrating margins, ranging in size from 0.5 to 5 cm. Deep-seated tumors can be larger (up to 15 cm) and involve tendons or fascia. The cut surfaces are gray-white with focal areas of hemorrhage and necrosis. The proximal subtype can also be single or multiple whitish deep soft tissue nodules and can be up to 20 cm in size [4].

Lung involvement by ES is usually due to metastasis, typically presenting as multifocal small nodules. Primary pulmonary large-cell carcinoma presents mostly as a unifocal, peripheral, well-defined lobulated mass with gray-white cut surfaces.

Histology

- Epithelioid sarcoma: Histological finding of the metastatic epithelioid sarcoma in the lung is similar to those of soft tissue counterparts and can be divided into two types:
  - Conventional type: The tumor nodules demonstrate central necrosis, which can mimic a granulomatous process at low magnification. The tumoral cells are medium-sized and epithelioid to spindle-shaped, with deeply eosinophilic cytoplasm, atypical nuclei, and small nucleoli, admixed with spindle cells and mixed chronic inflammation in a collagenous stroma. A pseudoglandular or pseudoangiomatous pattern, metaplastic bone formation, and/or osteoclast-like giant cells can be seen [4].
  - Proximal type: Deep-seated multinodular mass with infiltrative borders, consisting of large polygonal cells with abundant eosinophilic cytoplasm, vesicular nuclei, prominent nucleoli, and sometimes rhabdoid morphology. A high mitotic rate, necrosis, and hemorrhage are common [4].
- Large-cell undifferentiated carcinoma: By definition, it is a primary pulmonary malignant epithelial tumor with large atypical cells that does not show adenocarcinoma, squamous cell, or neuroendocrine differentiation (or any other line of differentiation). Therefore, careful examination of the entire tumor along with broad immunohistochemistry is required for the diagnosis. This diagnosis should only be rendered on resection specimens and should not be made on small biopsies [5].

How Can Ancillary Tests Be Used to Distinguish Epithelioid Sarcoma Versus Large-Cell (Undifferentiated) Carcinoma?

Immunohistochemistry

- Epithelioid sarcomas (ES) characteristically lack nuclear immunohistochemical staining of INI1 protein as the result of mutation or homozygous deletions of the *SMARCB1* gene, a tumor suppressor gene located on chromosome 22. Hornick et al. found the complete loss of INI1 expression in 91% of conventional-type and 95% of proximal-type ES [6]. Loss of INI1 expression is also seen in other tumors such as malignant rhabdoid tumor of infancy, atypical teratoid/rhabdoid tumor, renal medullary carcinoma, and SMARCB1-deficient carcinoma of the sinonasal tract, as well as 50% of epithelioid malignant peripheral nerve sheath tumors, 15% of extraskeletal myxoid chondrosarcomas, and 9% myoepithelial carcinomas [6, 7].
- Epithelioid sarcomas can show immunoreactivity to epithelial markers; almost all cases show positive EMA staining, and most show cytokeratin positivity (both low and high molecular weights), especially CK8 and CK19. However, expression of p63 and cytokeratin 5/6 is rare in ES, which can be helpful to distinguish them from squamous cell carcinomas. A subset of ES can show positivity of vascular markers; approximately half of cases have CD34 positivity (more often in proximal types), and one third can show positive staining for ERG, which poses a possible diagnostic pitfall when differentiating epithelioid sarcomas from tumors with endothelial differentiation. However, ESs do not harbor ERG-involving translocations, and other vascular markers (such as FLI1 and CD31) are not expressed in these tumors [8]. Occasional reactivity for SMA and S100 protein has also been reported [9]. Useful immunohistochemistry and molecular findings that may be helpful to differentiate tumors with epithelioid morphology are pointed out in Table 29.1.
- Large-cell undifferentiated carcinoma (LCC) can show positive immunoreactivity to cytokeratins but are negative for lineage-specific markers of glandular, squamous, or neuroendocrine differentiation. Per the 2021 WHO classification, LCC may be subclassified as (1) LCC (null immunophenotype), when showing negative TTF1 and p40 immunoreactivity; (2) LCC (unclear immunophenotype), when staining does not provide a clear answer; and (3) LCC (unclear immunophenotype), when immunohistochemistry cannot be performed due to a lack of available blocks or unstained slides [5].

Table 29.1 Helpful ancillary tests to differentiate tumors with epithelioid features

Tumors	IHC	Molecular alteration
Epithelioid sarcoma (ES)	Loss of INI, EMA+, keratin+/−, CD34+/−	Translocations or loss of heterogeneity involving SMARCB1 (INI1) on (22q11)
Large-cell (undifferentiated) carcinoma	Keratin +/−, EMA+, TTF1−, p63/p40−, INI+ (retained)	EGFR, KRAS, and TP53 mutations
Squamous cell carcinoma	P63+, P40, CK5/6+, TTF1−	TP53, CDKN2A, PTEN, PIK3CA, etc. mutations
Adenocarcinoma	TTF1+, napsin A+	EGFR, KRAS, and BRAF mutations and ALK gene rearrangement
SMARCA4-deficient undifferentiated tumor	Loss of SMARCA4, INI retained, EMA+, CK+, SOX2+	SMARCA4 mutations
Extrarenal malignant rhabdoid tumor	Loss INI1, keratin+, EMA+, SALL4+, CD34-	Deletion of SMARCB1 (INI1)

Table 29.1 (continued)

Tumors	IHC	Molecular alteration
Epithelioid malignant peripheral nerve sheath tumor (MPNST)	S100+, SOX10+, GFAP+/−. CD34+/−, loss of INI in 2/3 cases	Multiple genetic alterations
Epithelioid schwannoma	S100+, SOX10+, CD34−, EMA−	Somatic NF2 gene mutations
Melanoma	S100 protein+, SOX10+, Melan A/MART1, MITF, tyrosinase	BRAF, ARID2, BAP1, GNAQ, HRAS, KIT, NF1, NRAS, and PTEN mutations
PEComa	SMA+, desmin+, HMB45+, MITF+, MART1+	TSC2 mutations, TFE3 gene fusions
Granular cell tumor	S100+, SOX10+, TFE3+, calretinin+, CD68+, inhibin+, HMB45−	N/A
Synovial sarcoma, epithelial variant	TLE1, keratin, EMA, S100 protein+/−, CD56+, CD99+, calretinin+/−	t(X;18) involving SS18 (SYT) gene
Alveolar soft part sarcoma	TFE3+, desmin+/−	der(17)t(X;17)(p11.2;q25) translocation (ASPSCR1-TFE3 fusion)
Epithelioid angiosarcoma	Vascular markers (CD31, FLI1, ERG, etc.), keratin+ in half of cases, retained INI1	MYC (8q24) or FLT4 (VEGFR3) (5q35) amplification, upregulation of vascular-specific receptor tyrosine kinases (TIE1, KDR, TEK, FLT1)
Epithelioid hemangioendothelioma	Vascular markers, TFE3+/−, keratin +/−	WWTR1-CAMTA1 fusion, YAP1-TFE1 fusion
Pseudomyogenic hemangioendothelioma	EMA−, CD34−, CD31+, ERG+, CK+, retained INI1	t(7;19)(q22;q13) results in SERPINE1–FOSB fusion

Molecular Testing

The SMARCB1 (INI1) tumor suppressor gene, located at 22q11, is inactivated in both proximal and conventional types of epithelioid sarcomas, which correlates with the loss of immunoreactivity to the protein. It is suggested that SMARCB1 gene deletions or mutations are central in the pathogenesis of epithelioid sarcoma, as it is in malignant rhabdoid tumor of infancy (MRT) and atypical teratoid/rhabdoid tumor [4]. However, the pattern of inactivity in these tumors is different. Epithelioid sarcomas usually are a result of loss of heterozygosity or translocations involving the long arm of chromosome 22. Deletion of 22q is also seen in a small subset of epithelioid sarcomas. This contrasts with MRT, in which biallelic SMARCB1 gene deletions and point mutations are common [10]. Chromosomal gains (11q, 1q, 6p, 9q) or losses (9p, 13q) are also reported in epithelioid sarcomas [11].

What Is the Most Specific Test for Diagnosing Epithelioid Sarcomas?

In immunohistochemistry, nuclear INI1 protein expression is lost in ES but retained in pulmonary lung epithelial carcinomas including large-cell carcinoma. ES is a distinctive malignant mesenchymal neoplasm with epithelioid cytomorphology and loss of INI1 immunoreactivity. It is a rare aggressive soft tissue tumor with a high tendency to metastasize. Primary pulmonary epithelioid sarcomas are exceptionally rare; only three cases of primary pulmonary epithelioid sarcoma have been reported in the English literature [12]. So, a careful evaluation to exclude other tumors with epithelioid features and/or a possible extrapulmonary site of origin is necessary before diagnosing primary pulmonary epithelioid sarcoma. Due to positive staining for epithelial markers such as EMA and cytokeratins, and the rarity of epithelioid sarcomas, the diagnosis may be challenging. Loss of INI expression along with negative staining for TTF1, p40, and p63 is helpful to distinguish epithelial sarcoma from primary pulmonary epithelial neoplasms (see Table 29.1).

What Is the Most Specific Test for Diagnosing Large-Cell (Undifferentiated) Carcinoma?

There is no available specific test for the diagnosis of large-cell (undifferentiated) carcinoma, and it is essentially a diagnosis of exclusion. Based on the current WHO classification of the tumors, large-cell carcinoma (LCC) is an undifferentiated non-small-cell carcinoma (NSCC) that lacks the cytological, architectural, immunohistochemical, and histochemical features of other lung carcinomas, such as small-cell carcinoma, adenocarcinoma, and squamous cell carcinoma (SCC), in addition to giant cell, spindle cell, or pleomorphic carcinomas [5].

Therefore, the diagnosis is established only after excluding metastases and other non-small-cell lung cancers. Large-cell undifferentiated carcinoma lacks lineage-specific architectural and immunohistochemical features of other tumors with similar cytomorphology. Therefore, the diagnosis requires a thoroughly sampled resected tumor and cannot be rendered on a biopsy or cytology specimen.

What Is the Best Approach If You Find a Lung Tumor with Atypical Large Epithelioid Cytology?

It is important to consider primary epithelial lung neoplasms first due to their prevalence and location. Adenocarcinomas show mucin-producing cells and/or positive immunoreactivity to TTF1 or napsin A. Squamous cell carcinomas can present as TTF1-negative tumors with overt keratinization and/or positive p40, p63, and/or CK5/6 immunostaining. If these studies fail to pinpoint the diagnosis, then one should consider other neoplasms with epithelioid morphology before diagnosing large-cell (undifferentiated) carcinoma. The differential diagnosis includes, but is not limited to, melanoma, epithelioid MPNST, epithelioid angiosarcoma, epithelioid sarcoma, alveolar soft part sarcoma (ASPS), and thoracic SMARCA4-deficient undifferentiated tumor (see Table 29.1). If the tumor has non-small-cell morphology and cytokeratin positivity, and if all available studies fail to further classify the tumor, then large-cell (undifferentiated) carcinoma is the proper diagnosis, as long as metastatic disease of extrapulmonary origin is excluded clinically.

References

1. Enzinger FM. Epitheloid sarcoma. A sarcoma simulating a granuloma or a carcinoma. Cancer. 1970;26(5):1029–41. https://doi.org/10.1002/1097-0142(197011)26:5<1029::aid-cncr2820260510>3.0.co;2-r. PMID: 5476785
2. Chase DR, Enzinger FM. Epithelioid sarcoma. Diagnosis, prognostic indicators, and treatment. Am J Surg Pathol. 1985;9(4):241–63.
3. Guillou L, Wadden C, Coindre JM, Krausz T, Fletcher CD. "Proximal-type" epithelioid sarcoma, a distinctive aggressive neoplasm showing rhabdoid features. Clinicopathologic, immunohistochemical, and ultrastructural study of a series. Am J Surg Pathol. 1997;21(2):130–46. https://doi.org/10.1097/00000478-199702000-00002. PMID: 9042279
4. Goldblum JR, Folpe AL, Weiss SW. Enzinger and Weiss's soft tissue tumors. 6th ed. Philadelphia: Elsevier; 2014.
5. Rossi G, Nicholson AG, Leighl NB, Lu S, Smit EF, et al. Large cell carcinoma. WHO classification of tumours editorial board. Thoracic tumours. 5th ed. Lyon: IARC Press; 2021.
6. Hornick JL, Dal Cin P, Fletcher CD. Loss of INI1 expression is characteristic of both conventional and proximal-type epithelioid sarcoma. Am J Surg Pathol. 2009;33(4):542–50. https://doi.org/10.1097/PAS.0b013e3181882c54.
7. Kohashi K, Oda Y, Yamamoto H, Tamiya S, Oshiro Y, Izumi T, Taguchi T, Tsuneyoshi M. SMARCB1/INI1 protein expression in round cell soft tissue sarcomas associated with chromosomal translocations involving EWS: a special reference to SMARCB1/INI1 negative variant extraskeletal myxoid chondrosarcoma. Am J Surg Pathol. 2008;32(8):1168–74. https://doi.org/10.1097/PAS.0b013e318161781a. PMID: 18580682
8. Miettinen M, Wang Z, Sarlomo-Rikala M, Abdullaev Z, Pack SD, Fetsch JF. ERG expression in epithelioid sarcoma: a diagnostic pitfall. Am J Surg Pathol. 2013;37(10):1580–5. https://doi.org/10.1097/PAS.0b013e31828de23a. PMID: 23774169; PMCID: PMC3772974
9. Miettinen M, Fanburg-Smith JC, Virolainen M, Shmookler BM, Fetsch JF. Epithelioid sarcoma: an immunohistochemical analysis of 112 classical and variant cases and a discussion of the differential diagnosis. Hum Pathol. 1999;30(8):934–42. https://doi.org/10.1016/s0046-8177(99)90247-2.
10. Kohashi K, Izumi T, Oda Y, Yamamoto H, Tamiya S, Taguchi T, Iwamoto Y, Hasegawa T, Tsuneyoshi M. Infrequent SMARCB1/INI1 gene alteration in epithelioid sarcoma: a useful tool in distinguishing epithelioid sarcoma from malignant rhabdoid tumor. Hum Pathol. 2009;40(3):349–55. https://doi.org/10.1016/j.humpath.2008.08.007. Epub 2008 Oct 29. PMID: 18973917
11. Lushnikova T, Knuutila S, Miettinen M. DNA copy number changes in epithelioid sarcoma and its variants: a comparative genomic hybridization study. Mod Pathol. 2000;13(10):1092–6. https://doi.org/10.1038/modpathol.3880203. PMID: 11048803
12. Saha D, Basu A, Maiti A, Rodriguez E. Primary proximal epithelioid sarcoma of the lung successfully treated with pneumonectomy and adjuvant chemotherapy. BMJ Case Rep. 2016;2016:bcr2015213966. https://doi.org/10.1136/bcr-2015-213966. PMID: 27045049; PMCID: PMC4840621

30 Intimal Sarcoma Versus Other Spindle Cell Neoplasms

John M. Gross and Robert W. Ricciotti

Case Presentation

A 49-year-old female without a significant past medical history had multiple recent hospital admissions for acute-onset chest tightness, intermittent hemoptysis, and dyspnea in the setting of progressive fatigue over a 6-month period. A chest CT scan demonstrated a mass within the right ventricular outflow tract (Fig. 30.1a). Despite no known risk factors, the patient was diagnosed with pulmonary thromboembolism and was treated with anticoagulation. A subsequent bilateral lower-extremity venous duplex scan and thrombophilia workup were both negative. Furthermore, the thrombus was refractory to therapeutic anticoagulation. A subsequent cardiac MRI with contrast revealed a heterogeneously enhancing mass which was later shown to be PET avid (Fig. 30.1b) within the left main pulmonary artery. A left pneumonectomy was performed, at which time the mass within the main pulmonary artery showed proximal extension into the main pulmonary trunk with adherence to the pulmonary valvular cusp. Gross pathologic examination revealed an occlusive, gelatinous mass measuring 6.0 × 2.2 × 1.5 cm originating from within, and expanding, the left main pulmonary artery with extension into the segmental pulmonary artery branches (Fig. 30.1c). Histologic evaluation revealed a high-grade spindle cell neoplasm arising from the tunica intima of the pulmonary artery with ony focal extension into the pulmonary parenchyma. A myxofibrosarcoma-like pattern was seen consisting of high-grade spindle cells floating in a myxoid stroma containing prominent, arcuate vasculature (Fig. 30.2). By immunohistochemistry, the neoplastic cells were negative for desmin, AE1/AE3, and S100. FISH studies showed *MDM2* gene amplification (Fig. 30.2). Further SNP microarray analysis revealed gene amplification of *PDGFRA*, *EGFR*, *DDIT3*, *CDK4*, *MDM2*, and *CCNE1* as well as numerous other copy number alterations. The patient's postoperative course was uneventful, and she was discharged home in stable condition.

J. M. Gross
Division of Anatomic Pathology, The Johns Hopkins Medical Institute, Baltimore, MD, USA

R. W. Ricciotti (✉)
Department of Laboratory Medicine and Pathology, University of Washington Medical Center, Seattle, WA, USA
e-mail: ricciott@uw.edu

H. Xu et al. (eds.), *Practical Lung Pathology*, Practical Anatomic Pathology, https://doi.org/10.1007/978-3-031-14402-8_30

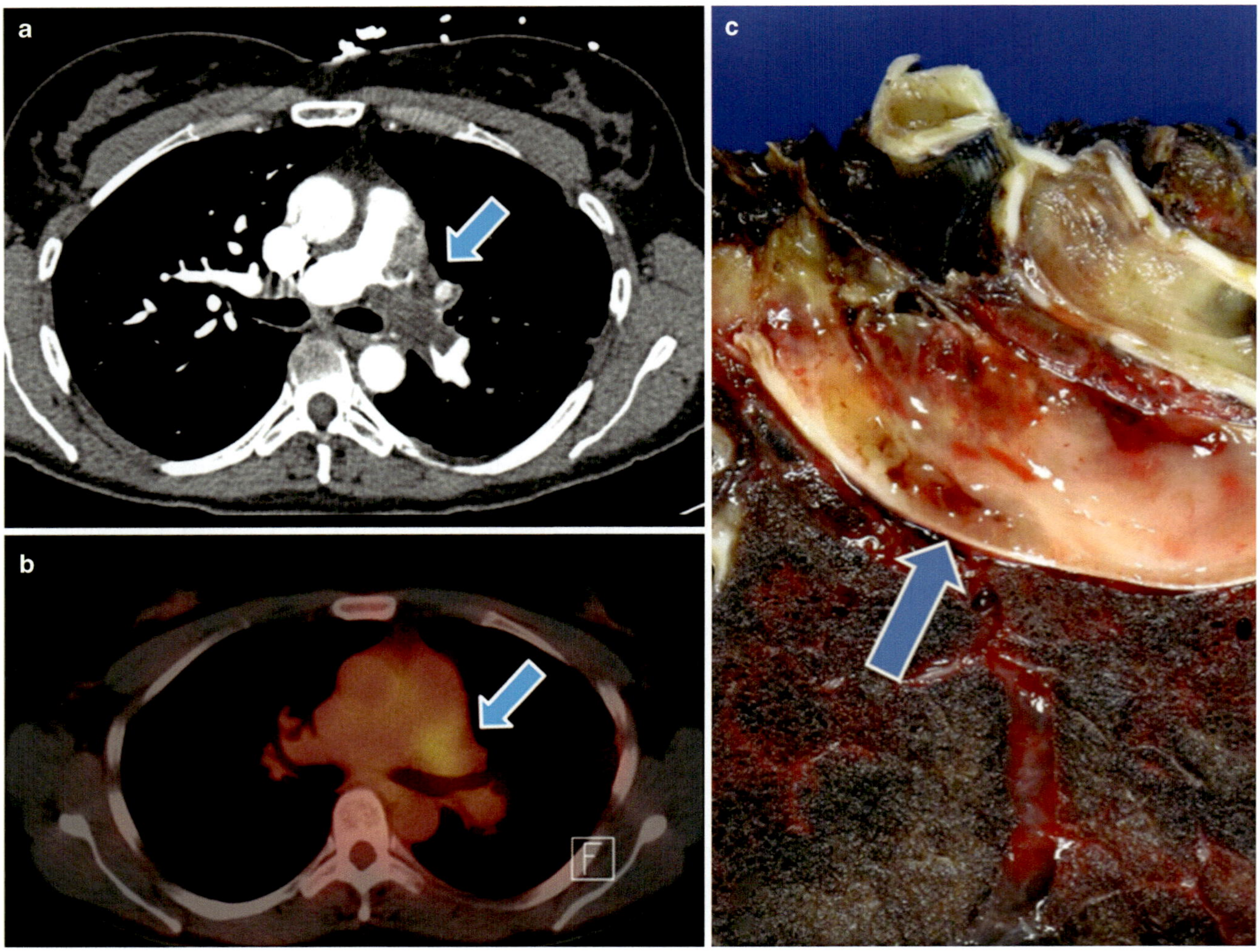

Fig. 30.1 (**a**) CT scan demonstrates a mass filling the left main pulmonary artery. (**b**) PET CT shows mild hypermetabolic activity. (**c**) Gross examination of the pneumonectomy specimen reveals a gelatinous mass occupying and expanding the pulmonary artery

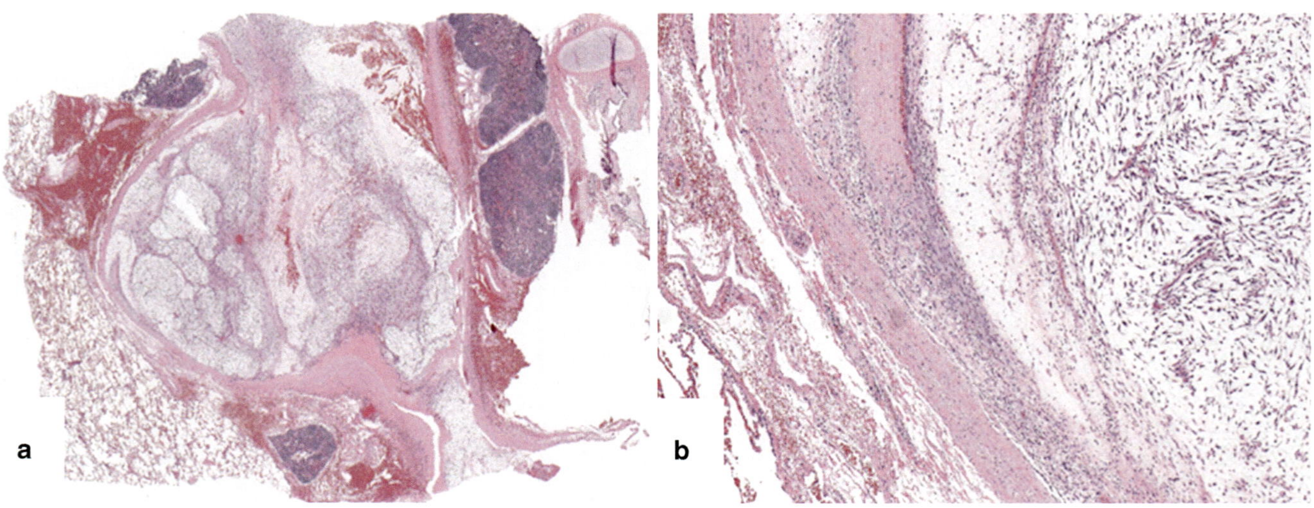

Fig. 30.2 (**a**) Myxoid neoplasm filling and expanding the pulmonary artery lumen. (**b**) Tumor arising from vascular intima with myxofibrosarcoma-like morphology. (**c**) Pleomorphic spindle cells floating in myxoid stroma with perivascular condensation. (**d**) *MDM2* gene amplification is confirmed by fluorescence in situ hybridization (FISH)

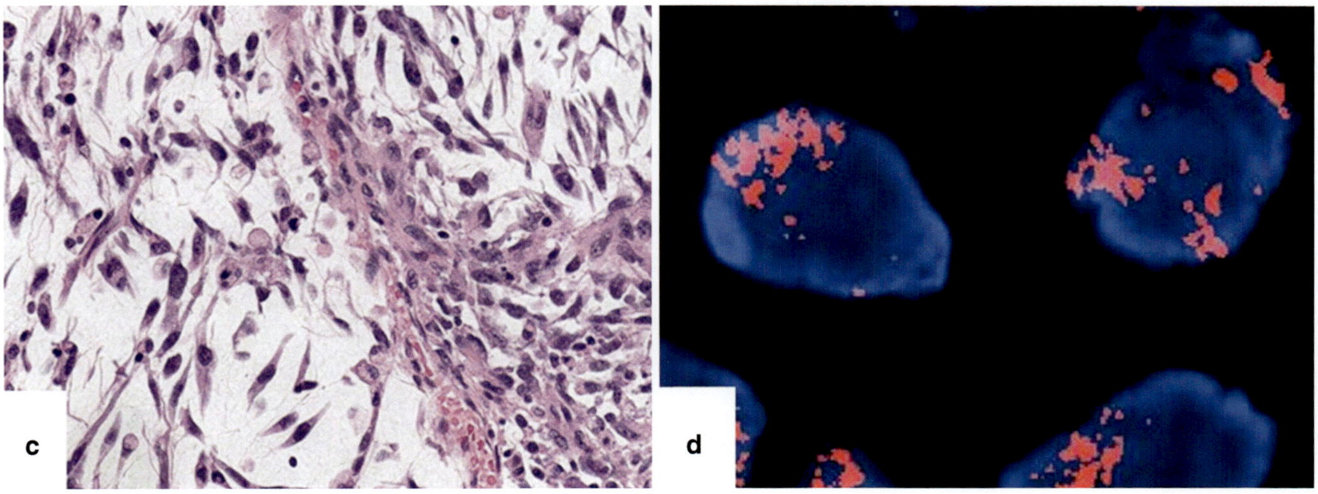

Fig. 30.2 (continued)

Pathologic Diagnosis: Intimal Sarcoma

What Is the Definition of Intimal Sarcoma?

The term "intimal sarcoma" is reserved for sarcomas arising within the large blood vessels such as the pulmonary artery and aorta as well as the heart. As these malignant tumors show a sine qua non feature of intraluminal growth, they commonly present with embolic phenomenon and eventually luminal obstruction [1, 2].

What Are the Epidemiologic Factors?

Intimal sarcomas are very rare and account for fewer than 1% of all sarcomas [3]. Intimal sarcomas most commonly arise in the pulmonary artery but may also occur in the aorta. Additionally, in a series of 100 cardiac sarcomas, intimal sarcoma was the most frequent primary cardiac sarcoma (42%) [3]. In that study, there was no clear gender preference, and tumors most commonly occured in middle-aged adults during their fifth to seventh decade [3].

What Are the Clinical Considerations of Intimal Sarcoma?

The clinical presentation of intimal sarcoma is often nonspecific and most commonly related to tumor emboli [1]. The diagnosis of intimal sarcoma of the pulmonary artery is often delayed or made postmortem as these patients are usually thought to have pulmonary thromboemboli and began on anticoagulation therapy [1, 3, 4]. On the other hand, some patients present with symptoms of acute or chronic pulmonary hypertension. Intimal sarcoma of the aorta often presents with signs and symptoms of emboli such as claudication, absent pulses, back pain, abdominal angina, malignant hypertension, or rupture of aneurysm [1, 3, 4]. In addition, other presenting complaints include dyspnea, cough, hemoptysis, and unexpected weight loss [1, 3, 4].

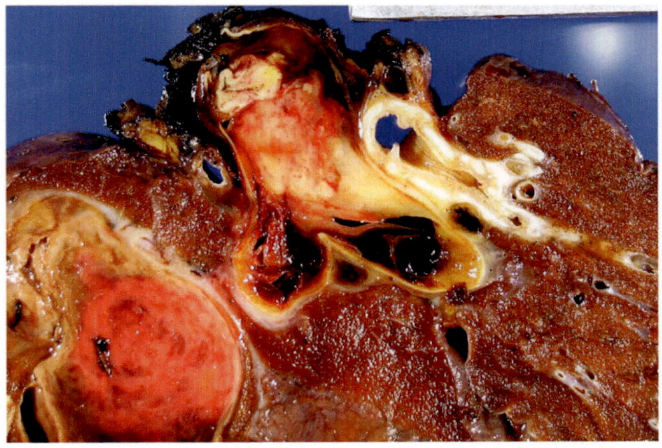

Fig. 30.3 Cut section of a lung and pulmonary vessels reveals an intraluminal mass occluding and expanding the pulmonary artery with a gelatinous to fleshy appearance

Conventional imaging techniques are often nonspecific; however, PET, MRI, and CT scans can sometimes help define the neoplastic nature of the occlusive tissue [4].

What Are the Gross Macroscopic Features of Intimal Sarcoma?

Intimal sarcomas are mostly intravascular masses attached to the vessel wall, grossly resembling thrombi and extending proximally and distally along the branches of the involved vessels. The gross consistency is often gelatinous to fleshy (Fig. 30.3); however, occasionally heterologous osteosarco-

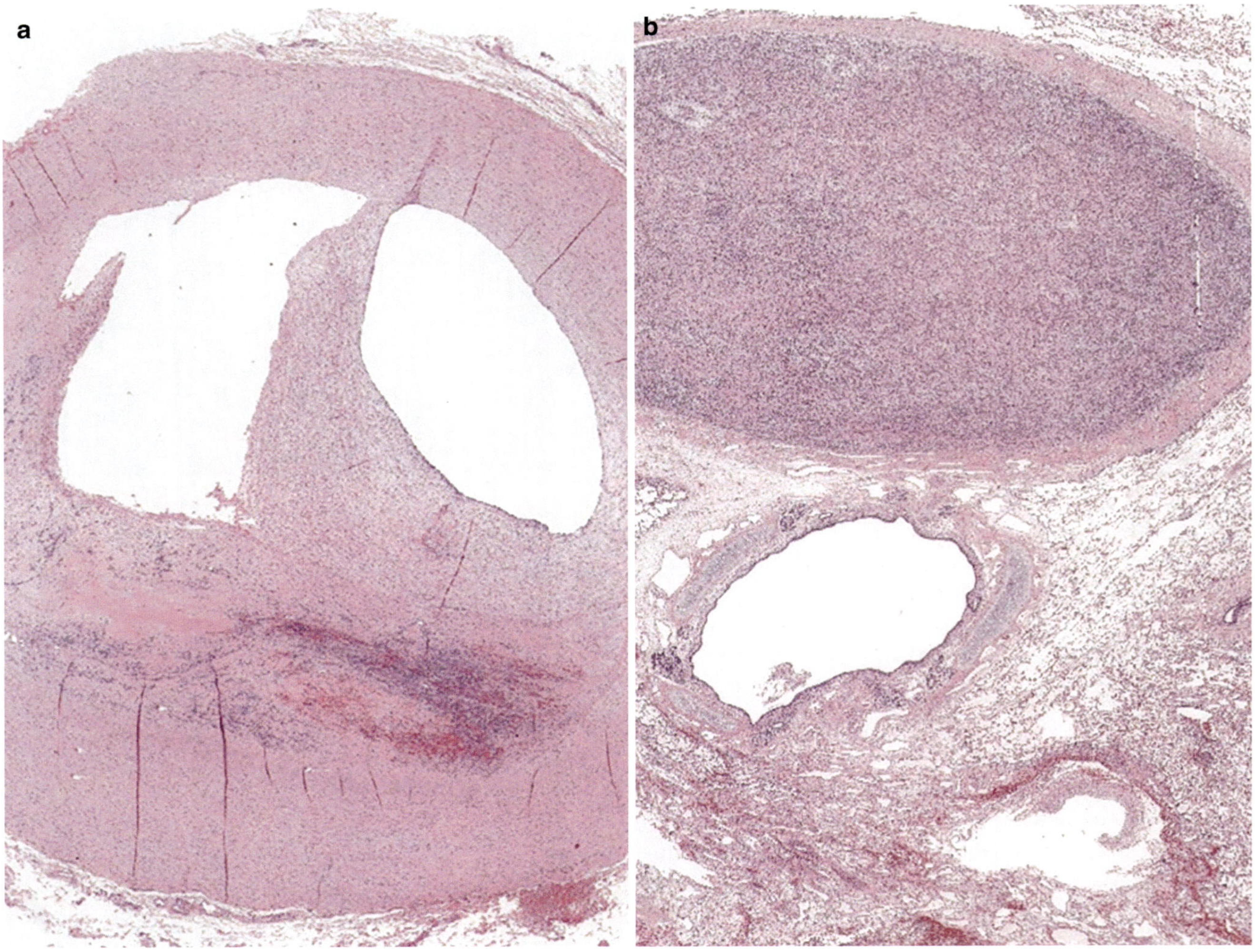

Fig. 30.4 (**a**) Low-power cross section of pulmonary artery shows an intimal sarcoma arising from subendothelium, (**b**) pulmonary artery intimal sarcoma filling and occluding the vessel

matous and chondrosarcomatous elements may be present, grossly resembling bone and cartilage, respectively. In addition, some tumors may form an adherent plaque grossly mimicking atherosclerosis [1, 3, 5].

What Are the Histologic and Immunophenotypic Features of Intimal Sarcoma?

The histologic spectrum of intimal sarcoma is widely variable; however, most intimal sarcomas show features of a high-grade spindle cell sarcoma with varying degrees of mitotic activity, necrosis, and nuclear pleomorphism. Some tumors demonstrate myxoid areas reminiscent of myxofibrosarcoma. Others may contain epithelioid and low-grade spindle cell morphology. Prominent spindling and fascicular growth may be present. Approximately 15% of cases will demonstrate heterologous elements such as rhabdomyosarcomatous, osteosarcomatous, chondrosarcomatous, and angiosarcomatous differentiation [1, 3, 5] (see Figs. 30.4, 30.5, and 30.6).

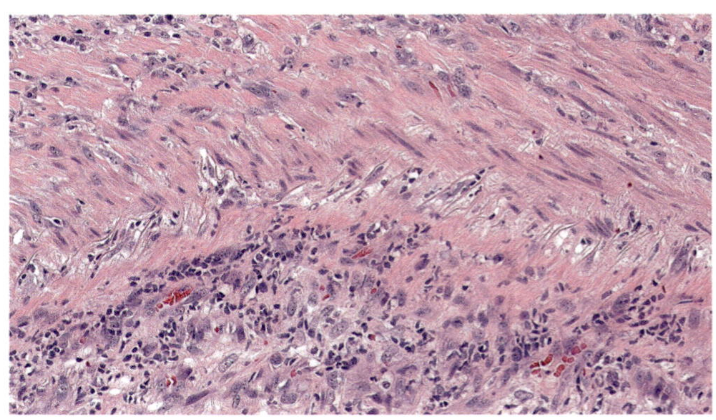

Fig. 30.5 Neoplastic cells originating from the subendothelial layer

The immunophenotype of intimal sarcoma is nonspecific with variable SMA and rare desmin expression reported. Most cases are negative for cytokeratins as well as endothelial and melanocytic markers [1, 3, 5]. MDM2 and CDK4 demonstrate nuclear staining in most cases. FISH testing to demonstrate *MDM2* gene amplification is a highly sensitive and specific test [2, 3, 6, 7].

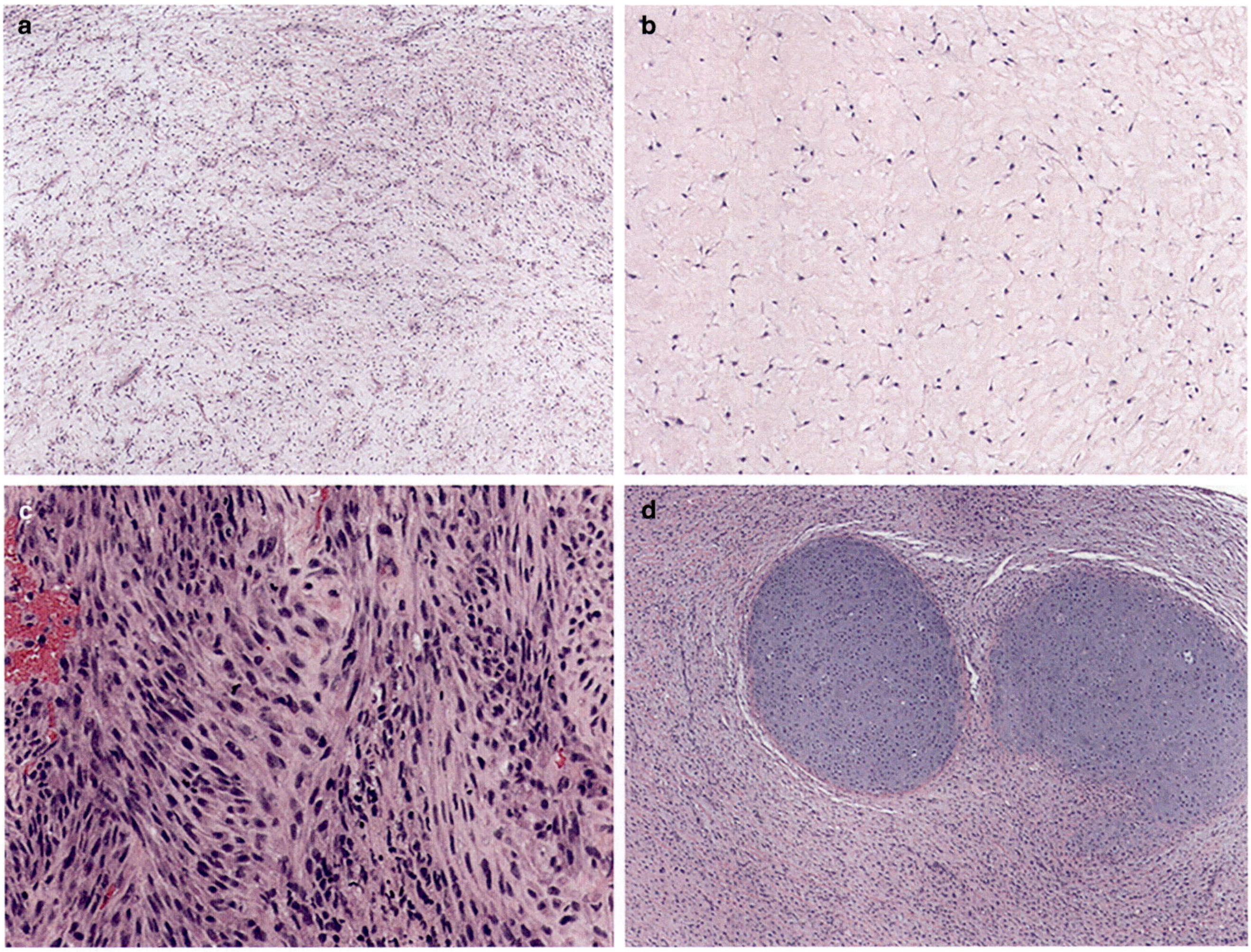

Fig. 30.6 (**a**) Myxofibrosarcoma-like pattern with myxoid stroma and prominent curvilinear vasculature, (**b**) bland spindle cells floating in myxoid background, (**c**) high-grade pleomorphic spindle cells in a herringbone pattern, and (**d**) heterologous chondrosarcomatous differentiation

What Are the Genetics of Intimal Sarcoma?

Most cases of intimal sarcoma will demonstrate regional amplification of the 12q12-15 locus including *CDK4*, *MDM2*, and other (*TSPAN31*, *GLI1*) genes. In addition, several studies report amplification or copy number gains of *PDGFR* and *EGFR* as well as numerous other structural gains and losses [2, 3, 6–9].

How Are Most Cases of Intimal Sarcoma Treated?

When possible, surgical resection is the treatment of choice. Most patients will undergo some form of adjuvant chemotherapy and/or radiation in the postoperative setting. Chemotherapy alone is reserved for inoperable tumors or patients with disseminated disease. Recent advances in the understanding of the genetics of intimal sarcoma have led to the investigation with clinical trials using *MDM2*, *CDK4*, *EGFR*, and *PDGFR* inhibitors [4, 8].

What Is the Prognosis of Intimal Sarcoma?

In general, the prognosis of intimal sarcoma is poor with a median survival of less than 2 years. Patients who undergo surgical resection of their primary tumors may have a longer survival; however, this may be explained by more advanced disease in inoperable patients. Surgery still offers the best chance of long-term survival and can provide symptomatic relief [1, 3, 4].

What Are the Most Common Differential Diagnoses of Intimal Sarcoma?

Dedifferentiated liposarcoma (DDLS) can be difficult to distinguish from intimal sarcoma as both sarcomas can have nearly identical histologic features and both characteristically have *MDM2* gene amplification. While intimal sarcoma arises from the subendothelium within large vessels, DDLS would not typically arise within the great vessels and/or heart, but instead most commonly occurs in the retroperitoneum, paratesticular region, and deep soft tissues of extremities and even the trunk. They can, however, arise within the soft tissues of the mediastinum, potentially leading to difficulty in distinction from intimal sarcoma. DDLS will frequently have an adjacent component of well-differentiated liposarcoma, which could be helpful as a distinguishing feature if present. Clinical and radiologic correlation is also frequently helpful [3].

Cardiac (atrial) myxoma may enter the differential diagnosis of intimal sarcomas; however, these benign neoplasms most commonly present as pedunculated masses in the left atrium or arise from the interatrial septum rather than within large vessels. Histologically, they often consist of bland spindle cells within a myxo-edematous background stroma. Mitotic activity is limited or absent, and FISH for *MDM2* gene amplification is negative [3].

Leiomyosarcoma most commonly arises from the tunica media of large veins as opposed to the tunica intima (subendothelium). Histologically, leiomyosarcomas grow as fascicles of elongated spindle cells with "cigar-shaped" nuclei and dense eosinophilic cytoplasm. Most cases of leiomyosarcoma are positive by immunohistochemistry for at least two myogenic markers such as smooth muscle actin (SMA), desmin, and/or h-caldesmon. *MDM2* gene amplification is not a feature of leiomyosarcoma [3].

Epithelioid hemangioendothelioma (EHE) is a malignant neoplasm often presenting as an angiocentric mass filling and occluding the vascular lumen; however, the aorta and large pulmonary arteries are uncommon sites for EHE. Histologically, EHE consists of cords of epithelioid cells with intracytoplasmic vacuoles containing erythrocytes ("blister cells") within a myxoid background matrix. EHE expresses endothelial immunohistochemical markers (CD31, CD34, ERG) and variably expresses cytokeratins. Furthermore, immunohistochemistry for CAMTA1 often shows positive staining, representing the surrogate marker for the most common fusion gene specific for EHE, t(1;3) *WWTR1-CAMTA1* [10, 11]. A subset of EHEs has *YAP1-TFE3* rearrangements and will show nuclear positivity for TFE3 by immunohistochemistry [12]. *MDM2* gene amplification is not present in EHE.

Angiosarcoma may enter the differential diagnosis of intimal sarcoma. Most angiosarcomas will show vasoformation and express endothelial markers by immunohistochemistry (CD31, CD34, ERG, FLI1). *MDM2* gene amplification is not a feature of angiosarcoma [3].

Histomorphologically, metastatic sarcomatoid carcinoma or melanoma may be diagnostic considerations; however, most cases will express markers of epithelial (keratins, EMA, p40, p63, TTF1) or melanocytic (SOX10, S100, MART1, Melan-A, HMB45) differentiation. A careful review of the patient's medical history is always prudent, and clinical correlation may be needed to exclude metastasis from a distant site.

Finally, the recently described *SMARCA4*-deficient thoracic sarcomas may enter the differential diagnosis of intimal sarcoma. These rare sarcomas are primarily thoracic rather than intravascular. Histologically, *SMARCA4*-deficient thoracic sarcomas typically have epithelioid and/or rhabdoid morphology and demonstrate loss of SMARCA4 by immunohistochemistry. *MDM2* gene amplification would not be expected in this entity [13].

References

1. Burke AP, Virmani R. Sarcomas of the great vessels. A clinicopathologic study. Cancer. 1993;71(5):1761–73.
2. Bode-Lesniewska B, Zhao J, Speel EJ, Biraima AM, Turina M, Komminoth P, et al. Gains of 12q13-14 and overexpression of mdm2 are frequent findings in intimal sarcomas of the pulmonary artery. Virchows Arch. 2001;438(1):57–65.
3. Neuville A, Collin F, Bruneval P, Parrens M, Thivolet F, Gomez-Brouchet A, et al. Intimal sarcoma is the most frequent primary cardiac sarcoma: clinicopathologic and molecular retrospective analysis of 100 primary cardiac sarcomas. Am J Surg Pathol. 2014;38(4):461–9.
4. Wong HH, Gounaris I, McCormack A, Berman M, Davidson D, Horan G, et al. Presentation and management of pulmonary artery sarcoma. Clin Sarcoma Res. 2015;5(1):3.
5. Sebenik M, Ricci A Jr, DiPasquale B, Mody K, Pytel P, Jee KJ, et al. Undifferentiated intimal sarcoma of large systemic blood vessels: report of 14 cases with immunohistochemical profile and review of the literature. Am J Surg Pathol. 2005;29(9):1184–93.
6. Zhang H, Macdonald WD, Erickson-Johnson M, Wang X, Jenkins RB, Oliveira AM. Cytogenetic and molecular cytogenetic findings of intimal sarcoma. Cancer Genet Cytogenet. 2007;179(2):146–9.
7. Zhao J, Roth J, Bode-Lesniewska B, Pfaltz M, Heitz PU, Komminoth P. Combined comparative genomic hybridization and genomic microarray for detection of gene amplifications in pulmonary artery intimal sarcomas and adrenocortical tumors. Genes Chromosomes Cancer. 2002;34(1):48–57.
8. Dewaele B, Floris G, Finalet-Ferreiro J, Fletcher CD, Coindre J-M, Guillou L, et al. Coactivated platelet-derived growth factor receptor {alpha} and epidermal growth factor receptor are potential therapeutic targets in intimal sarcoma. Cancer Res. 2010;70(18):7304–14.
9. Tamborini E, Casieri P, Miselli F, Orsenigo M, Negri T, Piacenza C, et al. Analysis of potential receptor tyrosine kinase targets in intimal and mural sarcomas. J Pathol. 2007;212(2):227–35.
10. Tanas MR, Sboner A, Oliveira AM, Erickson-Johnson MR, Hespelt J, Hanwright PJ, et al. Identification of a disease-defining gene

fusion in epithelioid hemangioendothelioma. Sci Transl Med. 2011;3(98):98ra82.

11. Doyle LA, Fletcher CDM, Hornick JL. Nuclear expression of CAMTA1 distinguishes epithelioid hemangioendothelioma from histologic mimics. Am J Surg Pathol. 2016;40(1):94–102.
12. Antonescu CR, Le Loarer F, Mosquera JM, Sboner A, Zhang L, Chen CL, et al. Novel YAP1-TFE3 fusion defines a distinct subset of epithelioid hemangioendothelioma. Genes Chromosomes Cancer. 2013;52(8):775–84.
13. Sauter JL, Graham RP, Larsen BT, Jenkins SM, Roden AC, Boland JM. SMARCA4-deficient thoracic sarcoma: a distinctive clinicopathological entity with undifferentiated rhabdoid morphology and aggressive behavior. Mod Pathol. 2017;30(10):1422–32.

Sclerosing Pneumocytoma Versus Lung Adenocarcinoma

31

Cherise Meyerson and Gregory A. Fishbein

Case Presentation

A 27-year-old female nonsmoker from China was found to have a mass in the right middle lobe on chest X-ray while undergoing a routine employment physical. She had no significant past medical history and no symptoms. Follow-up chest computed tomography (CT) showed a 2.0 × 2.0 cm well-circumscribed soft tissue mass within the right middle lobe, adjacent to the bronchovascular bundle (Fig. 31.1).

Based on the imaging findings, the differential included a low-grade neuroendocrine tumor, pulmonary hamartoma, sarcoma, granuloma, or lung adenocarcinoma. She underwent a right middle lobectomy and hilar lymph node dissection.

On gross examination, sections of the right middle lobe showed a 2.2 cm, circumscribed, homogeneous yellow-tan mass abutting the right middle lobe lateral segmental bronchus (Fig. 31.2).

No endobronchial component was present. Histologic sections showed a partially encapsulated mass compressing the surrounding lung parenchyma. The mass was composed of a proliferation of two cell populations arranged predominantly in a papillary architecture with scattered areas of sclerosis and xanthomatous histiocytes (Fig. 31.3).

One cell population appeared to line the papillae and appeared cuboidal, resembling type II pneumocytes. The second population composed the stroma of the papillae and appeared polygonal with indistinct cell borders, oval nuclei, fine chromatin, and inconspicuous nucleoli. Both cell populations were positive for thyroid transcription factor 1 (TTF-1) and epithelial membrane antigen (EMA) immunohistochemistry, while only the surface cells were positive for pancytokeratin (AE1/AE3) and napsin-A (Fig. 31.4).

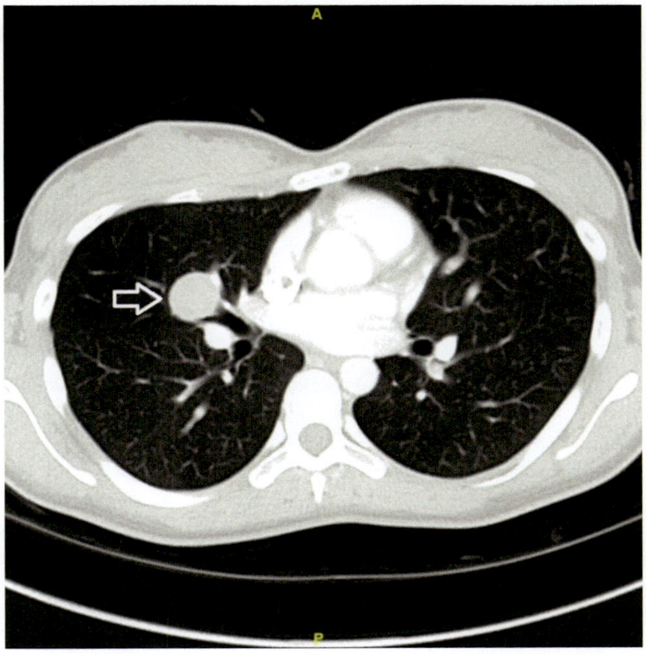

Fig. 31.1 Axial chest computed tomography shows a 2.0 cm, well-circumscribed mass in the right middle lobe (arrow)

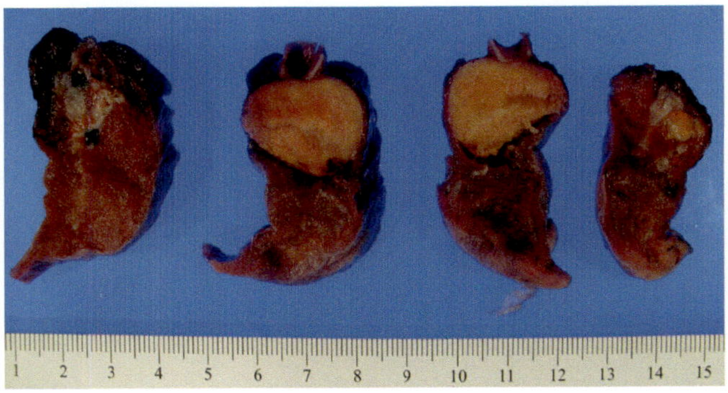

Fig. 31.2 The gross specimen shows a well-circumscribed, homogeneous tan-yellow parenchymal mass. It abuts the bronchus but does not have an endobronchial component

C. Meyerson · G. A. Fishbein (✉)
Department of Pathology and Laboratory Medicine, David Geffen School of Medicine at UCLA, University of California, Los Angeles, CA, USA
e-mail: gfishbein@mednet.ucla.edu

H. Xu et al. (eds.), *Practical Lung Pathology*, Practical Anatomic Pathology, https://doi.org/10.1007/978-3-031-14402-8_31

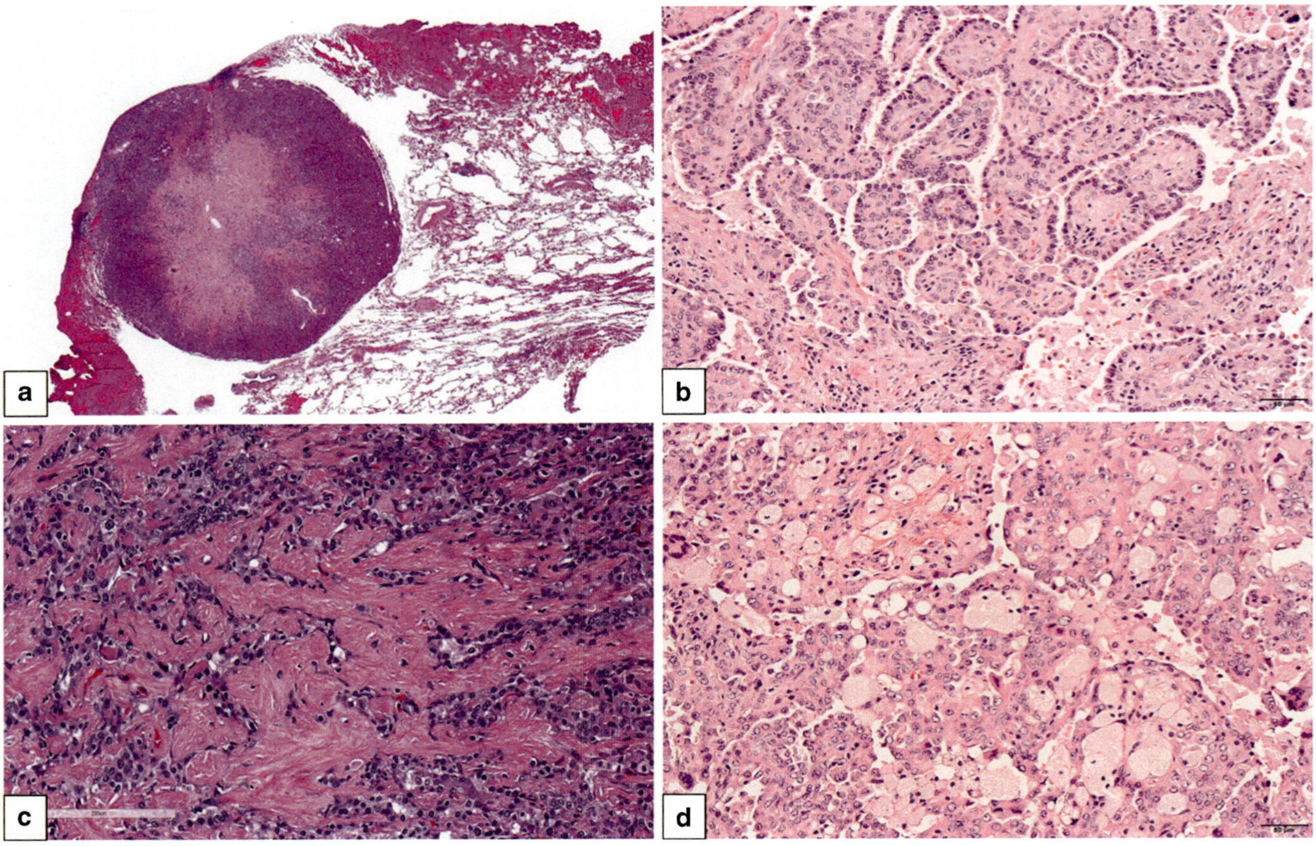

Fig. 31.3 Sclerosing pneumocytoma appears well-circumscribed at low power (**a**). Architectural patterns include papillary (**b**) and sclerotic (**c**). Xanthomatous histiocytes are also commonly seen (**d**). [Original magnifications 100× (**a**) and 200× (**b**, **c**, and **d**)]

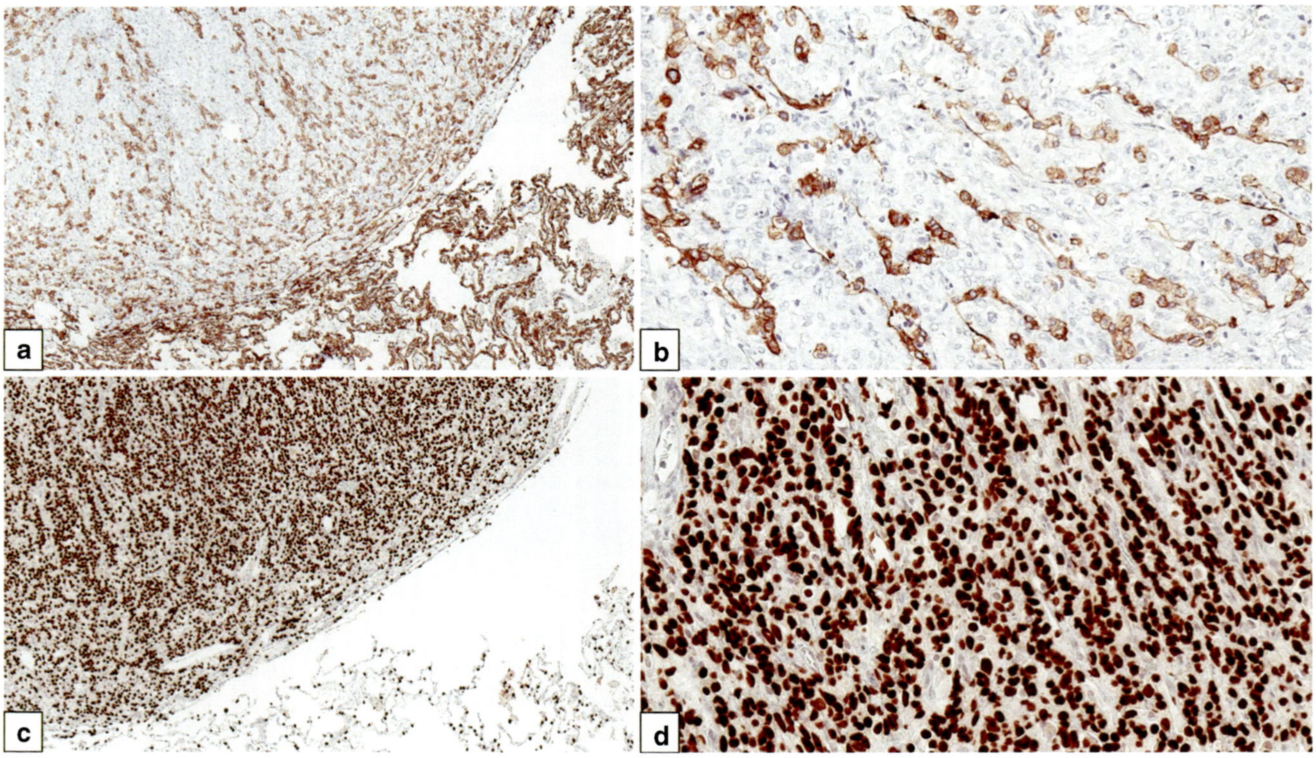

Fig. 31.4 In sclerosing pneumocytomas, pancytokeratin, AE1/AE3 (**a** and **b**), and napsin A (not shown) highlight surface cells but not stromal round cells. TTF-1 (**c** and **d**) is positive in both surface and round cells. [Original magnifications 200× (**a**, **c**) and 100× (**b**, **d**)]

Final Pathologic Diagnosis: Sclerosing Pneumocytoma

What Is the Histogenesis and Epidemiology of Sclerosing Pneumocytomas?

Sclerosing pneumocytoma, previously called "sclerosing hemangioma," was first described in 1956 by Liebow and Hubell, who hypothesized a vascular origin of this neoplasm [1]. Many subsequent theories were proposed for the histogenesis of this tumor, including mesothelial, epithelial, and neuroendocrine [2–4]. Some authors proposed that the tumor was hamartomatous [5]; however, later molecular studies demonstrated its clonal nature [6]. In the largest series to date, positive staining for TTF-1 in the both surface and round cells confirmed respiratory epithelial origin. In addition, the round cells lacked expression of surfactant protein A and B, as well as Clara cell antigen, suggesting that sclerosing pneumocytoma is derived from primitive, undifferentiated respiratory epithelium [7]. Sclerosing pneumocytoma was thus moved from the "miscellaneous tumors" group in the 1999 and 2004 World Health Organization (WHO) Classifications to the "adenomas" group in the 2015 WHO Classification [8].

Sclerosing pneumocytomas are more commonly seen in females (5:1 female to male ratio) [7], with a higher incidence in East Asia. It occurs more frequently in middle-aged women, and most patients are asymptomatic. They are considered benign lesions in which surgical resection is curative. Rare cases with lymph node metastases have been reported with no effect on prognosis [9–11].

What Are the Differential Diagnoses for Sclerosing Pneumocytoma?

The differential diagnosis includes both benign and malignant lung tumors. Benign lung tumors include clear cell "sugar" tumor and pulmonary hamartoma. Clear cell "sugar" tumor of the lung is considered part of the perivascular epithelioid cell tumor (PEComa) family and will stain with both smooth muscle and melanocytic immunohistochemical markers [e.g., smooth muscle actin (SMA), MART-1, and HMB-45]. Pulmonary hamartomas are composed of a combination of mature hyaline cartilage, fat, or smooth muscle and may contain entrapped respiratory epithelium. Malignant tumors in the differential diagnosis include lung adenocarcinoma and carcinoid tumor. The two distinct epithelial cell populations in sclerosing pneumocytoma are useful to differentiate these lesions from adenocarcinoma. The typical organoid and trabecular architecture of carcinoid tumors is not seen in sclerosing pneumocytoma, and immunohistochemical stains typically demonstrate diffuse reactivity for neuroendocrine markers in carcinoid tumor while negative in sclerosing pneumocytoma. Sometimes, however, entrapped pneumocytes within a carcinoid tumor can give the appearance of two epithelial cell populations, as seen in sclerosing pneumocytomas (Fig. 31.5).

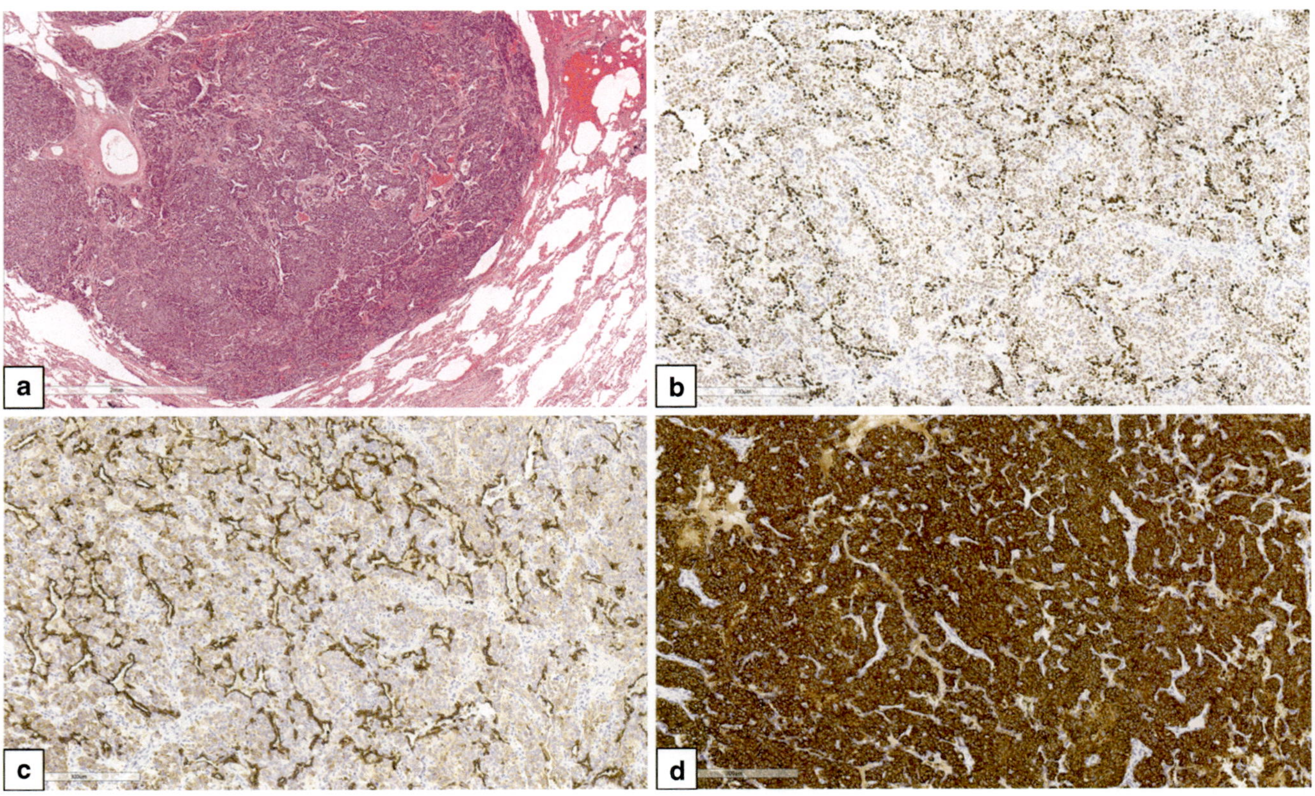

Fig. 31.5 Carcinoid tumors are also well-circumscribed lesions (**a**). Like sclerosing pneumocytomas, TTF-1 can appear to highlight two different cell populations (**b**), but pancytokeratin is also positive in both cell populations (**c**). The more darkly staining cells are therefore entrapped pneumocytes. Synaptophysin (**d**) and chromogranin (not shown) are diffusely positive, confirming neuroendocrine origin. [Original magnifications 200× (**a**) and 100× (**b**, **c**, and **d**)]

In such cases, immunohistochemistry for cytokeratins and neuroendocrine markers may be required to differentiate between these two.

How Do Sclerosing Pneumocytoma and Lung Adenocarcinoma Differ on Imaging?

Sclerosing pneumocytoma typically appears as a solitary, solid, and well-defined mass with no predilection for a particular lobe. One study of 76 patients showed that most patients had a single lesion (92.1%) with a smooth boundary (65.8%), oval shape (65.8%), and mean diameter of 2.27 cm [12]. Seventeen patients who underwent fluorodeoxyglucose positron emission tomography (FDG-PET) had hypometabolic lesions (<2.5 maximum standardized uptake value (SUVmax)). In contrast, invasive lung adenocarcinomas are usually peripheral, spiculated, poorly defined solid lesions that may be surrounded by ground-glass opacities that correspond to a lepidic-predominant pattern [13, 14]. However, one-third of the 76 sclerosing pneumocytomas had irregular boundaries and one-fifth of cases had outer ground-glass opacities, similar to those seen in lung adenocarcinomas [12]. Some studies have reported hypermetabolic sclerosing pneumocytomas on FDG-PET scans with SUVmax >2.5, which can be falsely interpreted as malignancy [15–18]. Therefore, sclerosing pneumocytomas should be considered in the differential diagnosis of FDG-PET avid solitary pulmonary nodules, and, ultimately, biopsy or surgical resection is required for definitive diagnosis.

How Do Sclerosing Pneumocytoma and Lung Adenocarcinoma Differ Grossly?

Sclerosing pneumocytomas are well-circumscribed and usually solitary lesions. They are most commonly found peripherally but can occur adjacent to a bronchus. The cut surface is usually tan to yellow and solid, though it may contain cystic [19] or hemorrhagic areas.

Lung adenocarcinomas are typically seen in the periphery of the lung parenchyma, often associated with pleural retraction [20]. Cut surfaces show irregular tan-gray lesions that may contain anthracotic pigment.

How Do Sclerosing Pneumocytoma and Lung Adenocarcinoma Differ Histologically and Immunohistochemically?

Sclerosing pneumocytoma is composed of two epithelial cell populations: the surface cells, which are cuboidal and resemble type II pneumocytes, and the round cells, which are small and polygonal. The most common architectural patterns are papillary, solid, hemorrhagic, and sclerotic. The papillary pattern is composed of surface cells covering the round cells within the papillary stalk. The solid pattern shows nests of round cells surrounded by surface cells. Sclerotic areas show hyalinized collagen within papillae or in solid areas. The hemorrhagic pattern is notable for cystic spaces filled with blood, called "blood lakes," with round cells around the periphery. Other common findings include xanthomatous histiocytes, chronic inflammation, mast cells, hemosiderin, cholesterol clefts, and calcifications [7]. TTF-1 and EMA immunohistochemistry is positive in both surface and round cells [7, 21]. The surface cells are also positive for pancytokeratin (AE1/AE3), cytokeratin 7 (CK7), Cam 5.2, surfactant proteins A and B, and napsin-A [7, 22, 23]. The round cells lack positivity for surfactant proteins and napsin-A. Cytokeratins are typically negative in the round cells, but focal expression of CK7 and Cam 5.2 may be seen.

Lung adenocarcinomas are infiltrative, gland-forming malignant epithelial neoplasms that can have different architectural patterns, including acinar, papillary, micropapillary, solid, and lepidic patterns (Fig. 31.6) [8]. They may also have mucinous or enteric differentiation.

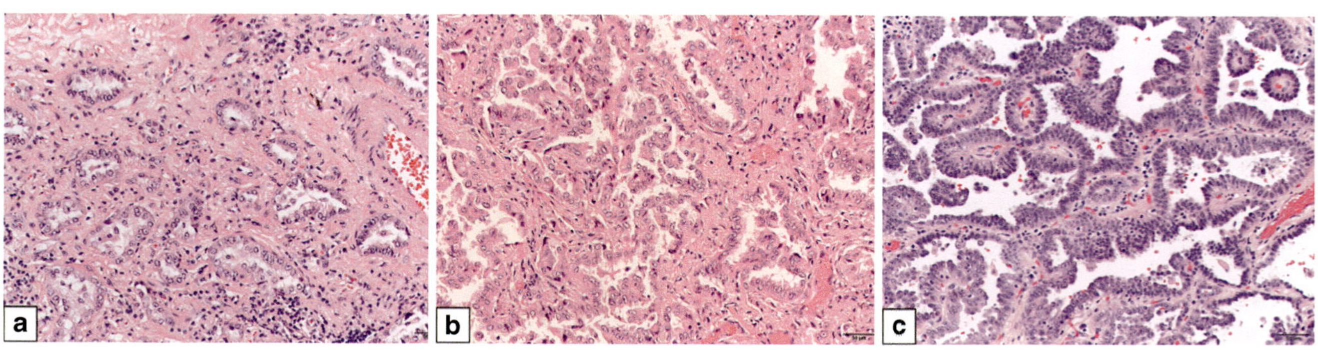

Fig. 31.6 Lung adenocarcinomas can show many different architectural patterns, including acinar (**a**), micropapillary (**b**), and papillary (**c**). The papillary pattern of adenocarcinoma superficially resembles the papillary component of sclerosing pneumocytomas (see Fig. 31.3b), but note the cytologic atypia, including prominent nucleoli, and lack of an inner round cell population within the papillary stalks. [Original magnification 200× (**a, b**, and **c**)]

Cytologically, they usually appear more atypical than sclerosing pneumocytomas with large, irregular nuclei, variably prominent nucleoli, and conspicuous mitotic figures. In contrast to sclerosing pneumocytomas, a dual-cell population is not seen, and all neoplastic cells usually stain with pancytokeratin. Pneumocyte markers, including TTF-1 and napsin-A, are positive in the majority of lung adenocarcinomas.

How Does One Differentiate Between Sclerosing Pneumocytoma and Lung Adenocarcinoma on Cytologic Specimens or Intraoperative Frozen Sections?

The cytologic diagnosis of sclerosing pneumocytoma can be challenging and usually requires recognition of a dual cell population [24]. Sheets of round cells and papillary groups may be present in a hemorrhagic background with foamy histiocytes. Definitive diagnosis by fine-needle aspiration with cell blocks and immunohistochemistry is possible [25, 26]. However, fine-needle aspiration is often inconclusive, and the most important diagnostic pitfall is well-differentiated papillary adenocarcinoma. Features that are more suggestive of adenocarcinoma include necrosis, prominent nucleoli, nuclear irregularities, high nuclear-to-cytoplasmic (NC) ratios, and three or more nuclei within tumor cells [27].

Intraoperative frozen section can be challenging as well. In one retrospective study of 59 sclerosing pneumocytomas in which frozen sections were performed, the rate of accurate diagnosis was 44.1%, the deferral rate was 15.3%, and ten cases (16.9%) were misdiagnosed as malignancy, prompting lobectomies and lymph node dissections [28]. A solid-predominant pattern was misdiagnosed more frequently than other growth patterns, and other diagnostic pitfalls included hypercellularity, glandular spaces, desmoplasia-like sclerosis, cellular atypia, and coagulative necrosis. Intraoperative cytology can provide better morphologic detail and circumvent frozen section artifact [29]. One study also found that a diagnosis of sclerosing pneumocytoma can be made intraoperatively based on tumor circumscription and variegated histological patterns [21].

How Do Sclerosing Pneumocytoma and Lung Adenocarcinoma Differ at the Molecular Level?

A loss of heterozygosity (LOH) study by Dacic et al. comparing sclerosing pneumocytoma and lepidic-predominant adenocarcinoma (formerly known as bronchioloalveolar carcinoma or BAC) analyzed microsatellite markers adjacent to tumor suppressor genes. Similar patterns of allelic loss were found for both sclerosing pneumocytoma and BAC, suggesting a common origin. Interestingly, frequent LOH of 5q (66.7% of cases) and 10q (62.5% of cases) was found in sclerosing pneumocytoma, suggesting that the *APC* and *PTEN* genes may play a role in its pathogenesis. In adenocarcinoma, 52.6% of cases showed LOH on 17p, the chromosomal arm containing *p53*, which is less frequently altered in sclerosing pneumocytomas; however, this difference is not statistically significant [30]. Similarly, mutations in *p53* gene were uncommonly reported in sclerosing pneumocytomas, in a sequencing study by Wang et al. [31].

Another study of microsatellite instability in sclerosing pneumocytoma reported allelic losses in *p16* and *Rb* loci in four and two out of nine cases, respectively. However, fluorescence in situ hybridization (FISH) and mutational analysis of *EGFR*, *HER2*, and *KRAS* did not reveal any alterations [32]. Whole exome sequencing of sclerosing pneumocytomas revealed recurrent *AKT1* and β-catenin mutations, which are not commonly found in lung adenocarcinomas [33].

References

1. Liebow AA, Hubbell DS. Sclerosing hemangioma (histiocytoma, xanthoma) of the lung. Cancer. 1956;9(1):53–75.
2. Xu HM, Li WH, Hou N, Zhang SG, Li HF, Wang SQ, et al. Neuroendocrine differentiation in 32 cases of so-called sclerosing hemangioma of the lung: identified by immunohistochemical and ultrastructural study. Am J Surg Pathol. 1997;21:1013–22.
3. Huszar M, Suster S, Herczeg E, Geiger B. Sclerosing hemangioma of the lung: immunohistochemical demonstration of mesenchymal origin using antibodies to tissue-specific intermediate filaments. Cancer. 1986;58:2422–7.
4. Katzenstein AL, Weise DL, Fulling K, Battifora H. So-called sclerosing hemangioma of the lung: evidence for mesothelial origin. Am J Surg Pathol. 1983;7:3–14.
5. Spencer H, Nambu S. Sclerosing haemangiomas of the lung. Histopathology. 1986;10:477–87.
6. Niho S, Suzuki K, Yokose T, Kodama T, Nishiwaki Y, Esumi H. Monoclonality of both pale cells and cuboidal cells of sclerosing hemangioma of the lung. Am J Pathol. 1998;152:1065–9.
7. Devouassoux-Shisheboran M, Hayashi T, Linnoila RI, Koss MN, Travis WD. A clinicopathologic study of 100 cases of pulmonary sclerosing hemangioma with immunohistochemical studies: TTF-1 is expressed in both round and surface cells, suggesting an origin from primitive respiratory epithelium. Am J Surg Pathol. 2000;24:906–16.
8. Travis WD, Brambilla E, Nicholson AG, Yatabe Y, Austin JHM, Beasley MB, et al. The 2015 World Health Organization classification of lung tumors: impact of genetic, clinical and radiologic advances since the 2004 classification. J Thorac Oncol. 2015;10:1243–60.
9. Kim K-H, Sul H-J, Kang D-Y. Sclerosing hemangioma with lymph node metastasis. Yonsei Med J. 2003;44:150–4.
10. Katakura H, Sato M, Tanaka F, Sakai H, Bando T, Hasegawa S, et al. Pulmonary sclerosing hemangioma with metastasis to the mediastinal lymph node. Ann Thorac Surg. 2005;80:2351–3.
11. Miyagawa-Hayashino A, Tazelaar HD, Langel DJ, Colby TV. Pulmonary sclerosing hemangioma with lymph node metastases: report of 4 cases. Arch Pathol Lab Med. 2003;127:321–5.

12. Shin SY, Kim MY, Oh SY, Lee HJ, Hong SA, Jang SJ, et al. Pulmonary sclerosing pneumocytoma of the lung: CT characteristics in a large series of a tertiary referral center. Medicine (Baltimore). 2015;94:1–10.
13. Austin JHM, Garg K, Aberle D, Yankelevitz D, Kuriyama K, Lee H-J, et al. Radiologic implications of the 2011 classification of adenocarcinoma of the lung. Radiology. 2013;266:62–71.
14. Gardiner N, Jogai S, Wallis A. The revised lung adenocarcinoma classification—an imaging guide. J Thorac Dis. 2014;6:S537–46.
15. Patrini D, Shukla R, Lawrence D, Borg E, Hayward M, Panagiotopoulos N. Sclerosing hemangioma of the lung showing strong FDG avidity on PET scan: case report and review of the current literature. Respir Med Case Rep. 2016;17:20–3.
16. De Luca G, Martucci N, Setola S, Rocco G. Sclerosing hemangioma of the lung mimicking pulmonary metastasis. Lung. 2015;193:447–8.
17. Lee E, Park CM, Kang KW, Goo JM, Kim MA, Paeng JC, et al. 18F-FDG PET/CT features of pulmonary sclerosing hemangioma. Acta Radiol. 2013;54:24–9.
18. Lin K-H, Chang C-P, Liu R-S, Wang S-J. F-18 FDG PET/CT in evaluation of pulmonary sclerosing hemangioma. Clin Nucl Med. 2011;36:341–3.
19. Khoury JD, Shephard MN, Moran CA. Cystic sclerosing haemangioma of the lung. Histopathology. 2003;43:239–43.
20. Moran CA. Pulmonary adenocarcinoma: the expanding spectrum of histologic variants. Arch Pathol Lab Med. 2006;130:958–62.
21. Chan ACL, Chan JKC. Pulmonary sclerosing hemangioma consistently expresses thyroid transcription factor-1 (TTF-1): a new clue to its histogenesis. Am J Surg Pathol. 2000;24:1531–6.
22. Rossi G, Cadioli A, Mengoli MC, Piccioli S, Cavazza A. Napsin a expression in pulmonary sclerosing haemangioma. Histopathology. 2012;60:361–3.
23. Schmidt LA, Myers JL, Mchugh JB. Napsin a is differentially expressed in sclerosing hemangiomas of the lung. Arch Pathol Lab Med. 2012;136:1580–4.
24. Gal AA, Nassar VH, Miller JI. Cytopathologic diagnosis of pulmonary sclerosing hemangioma. Diagn Cytopathol. 2002;26:163–6.
25. Dettrick A, Meikle A, Fong KM. Fine-needle aspiration diagnosis of sclerosing hemangioma (pneumocytoma): report of a case and review of the literature. Diagn Cytopathol. 2014;42:242–6.
26. Onorati M, Nicola M, Bianchi CL, Bini F, Bellaviti N, Di Nuovo F. Pitfalls and key features of a case of sclerosing pneumocytoma: a cytological challenge? Acta Cytol. 2016;60:85–8.
27. Iyoda A, Baba M, Saitoh H, Hoshino H, Shibuya K, Nomoto Y, et al. Imprint cytologic features of pulmonary sclerosing hemangioma. Cancer. 2002;96:146–9.
28. Yang CH, Lee LY. Pulmonary sclerosing pneumocytoma remains a diagnostic challenge using frozen sections: a clinicopathological analysis of 59 cases. Histopathology. 2018;72:500–8.
29. Wu CY, Wang J, Chang NY. A comparative study of intraoperative cytology and frozen sections of sclerosing pneumocytoma. Int J Surg Pathol. 2016;24:600–6.
30. Dacic S, Sasatomi E, Swalsky PA, Kim DW, Finkelstein SD, Yousem SA. Loss of heterozygosity patterns of sclerosing hemangioma of the lung and bronchioloalveolar carcinoma indicate a molecular pathogenesis. Arch Pathol Lab Med. 2004;128:880–4.
31. Wang Y, Dai SD, Qi FJ, Xu HT, Wang EH. P53 protein expression and genetic mutation in two primary cell types in pulmonary sclerosing haemangioma. J Clin Pathol. 2008;61:192–6.
32. Sartori G, Bettelli S, Schirosi L, Bigiani N, Maiorana A, Cavazza A, et al. Microsatellite and EGFR, HER2 and K-RAS analyses in sclerosing hemangioma of the lung. Am J Surg Pathol. 2007;31:1512–20.
33. Jung S-H, Kim MS, Lee S-H, Park H-C, Choi HJ, Maeng L, et al. Whole-exome sequencing identifies recurrent *AKT1* mutations in sclerosing hemangioma of lung. Proc Natl Acad Sci. 2016;113:10672–7.

Erdheim-Chester Disease Versus Reactive Inflammatory Infiltrates

32

Rouba Hadi and Haodong Xu

Case Presentation

A 59-year-old man with past medical history significant of knee pain resulting in knee replacement surgery, diabetes insipidus, hypogonadism, and obstructive sleep apnea presented at the Center for Interstitial Lung Disease with exacerbation of dyspnea on exertion. He reported acute worsening of dyspnea, even though it had been an ongoing symptom for a few years. He was a cigarette smoker in the past but at the time of presentation had not been smoking for over 10 years. He endorsed smoking marijuana, however, at least every other day for the past 10 years.

Pulmonary function tests at the time of presentation showed a combined obstructive and restrictive disease process, with the following reported results: FVC of 4.50 (75% predicted), FEV1 1.97(43% predicted), and a FEV1/FVC ratio of 0.44, decreased. Earlier computed tomography (CT) scans of the chest showed only subtle interstitial lung disease in the lower lobes with no obvious honeycombing. High-resolution CT performed 2 months later revealed inter- and intralobular septal thickening as well as diffuse ground-glass changes superimposed on a background of moderate centrilobular and paraseptal emphysema (Fig. 32.1).

Wedge biopsies of the lower and upper lung lobes demonstrated significant emphysematous changes in addition to marked pleural and septal thickening containing diffuse histiocytic infiltrate (Fig. 32.2a). The histiocytes had abundant, pale to foamy cytoplasm and round to oval nuclei (Fig. 32.2b). Immunohistochemical stains showed that the histiocytes were positive for CD163, CD68, Factor XIIIa (Fig. 32.2c), and variable S100 while negative for CD1a (Fig. 32.2d). While BRAF ^{V600E} by immunohistochemistry showed indeterminate, weak reactivity, molecular testing detected the presence of BRAF ^{V600E} mutation.

The pathological diagnosis is Erdheim-Chester disease (ECD). After the diagnosis, the patient was placed on steroids and immunomodulating agents, with plans for more extensive workup, including bone images, whole body positron emission tomography (PET)-CT scans, and a bone marrow biopsy to exclude a secondary hematologic malignancy.

R. Hadi · H. Xu (✉)
Department of Laboratory Medicine and Pathology, University of Washington Medical Center, Seattle, WA, USA
e-mail: xuh8@uw.edu

H. Xu et al. (eds.), *Practical Lung Pathology*, Practical Anatomic Pathology, https://doi.org/10.1007/978-3-031-14402-8_32

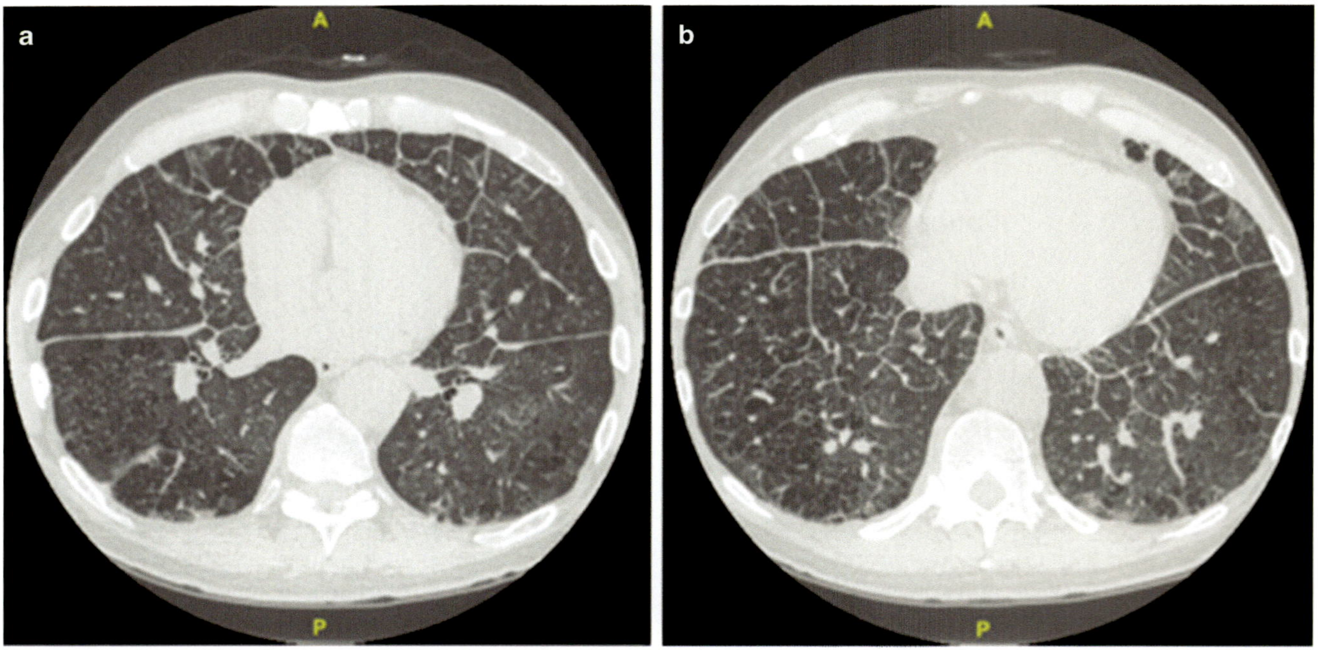

Fig. 32.1 Characteristics of chest HRCT. (**a**), (**b**) HRCT show inter- and intralobular septal thickening throughout the lungs and diffuse ground-glass opacities superimposed in a background of paraseptal and centrilobular emphysema

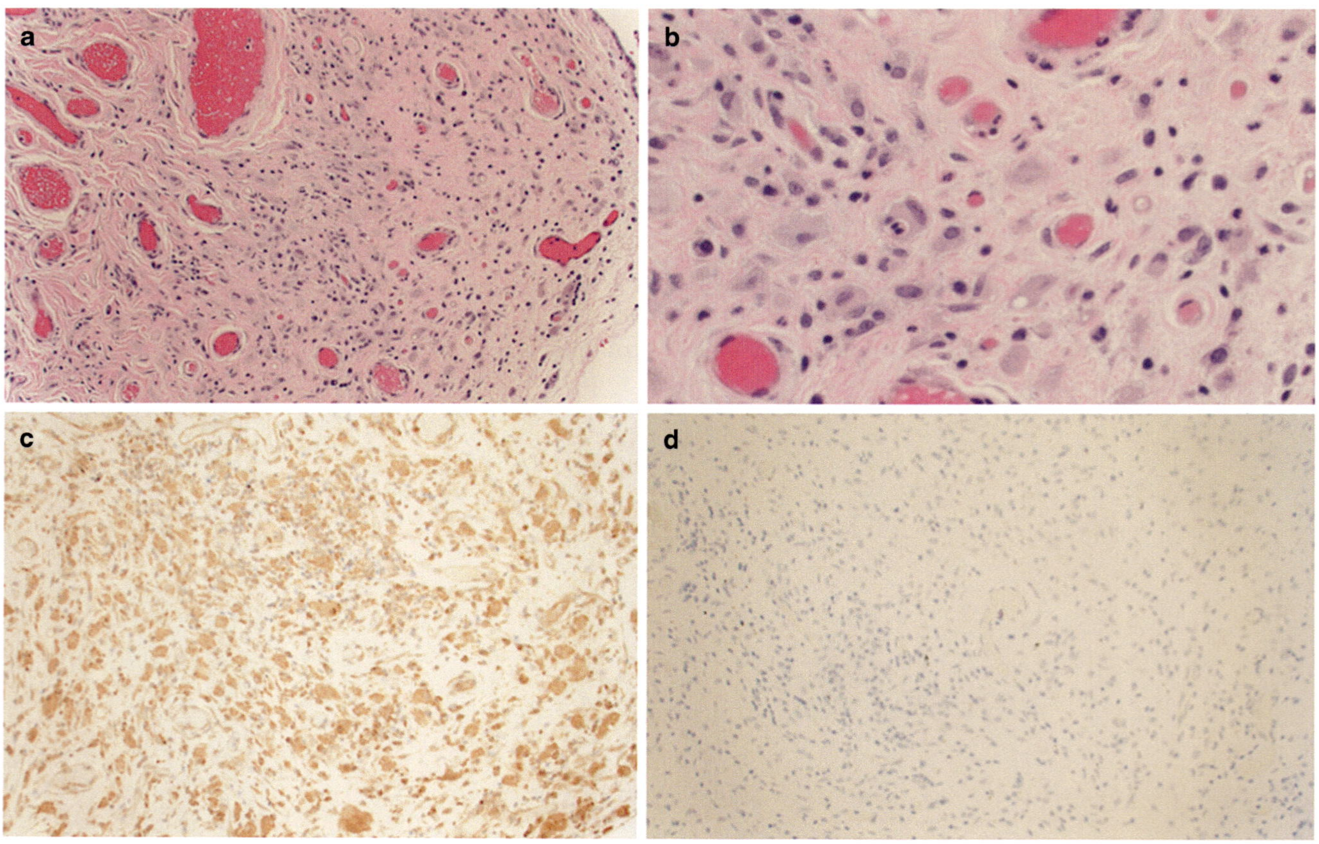

Fig. 32.2 Histologic features and immunohistological staining results. Histologic section shows a dense histiocytic infiltrate with associated septal thickening (**a**) and large histiocytes with round to oval nuclei, and abundant pale and variably foamy cytoplasm (**b**). Immunohistochemical stains show that histiocytic cells are positive for Factor XIIIa (**c**) and they are negative for CD1a (**d**). (**a**) (H&E: 200× magnification); (**b**) (H&E: 600× magnification); (**c**) (IHC: 200× magnification); (**d**) (IHC: 200× magnification)

Pathologic Diagnosis: Erdheim-Chester Disease

What Are Classic Clinical Features of Erdheim-Chester Disease?

ECD is predominantly seen in adults, usually around the fifth to seventh decades of life, with occasional cases also reported in the pediatric population [1, 2]. Its clinical presentation varies from case to case. While some reports of ECD describe a localized, more benign condition, others show systemic, multi-organ involvement that is considerably more aggressive and even fatal. Despite the variation in clinical features of ECD, bone pain is considered the most common symptom and has in some cases even been reported as an isolated one [1, 3]. Other frequently reported symptoms include diabetes insipidus, xanthelasma, exophthalmos, renal and testicular impairment, as well as generalized symptoms such as weight loss, fever, and fatigue [3, 4]. Involvement of the lungs, cardiovascular and central nervous system is also not uncommon [4]. One multicenter prospective cohort study reported up to 43% of cases to have pulmonary involvement [5]. The most common presenting symptoms in patients with pulmonary ECD are progressive dyspnea (which can be over a period of months to years) with or without dry cough [1, 6]. Pulmonary function testing may show either normal or reduced carbon monoxide diffusion capacity, usually with a mild restrictive ventilation pattern [1].

What Are the Radiographic Findings of Erdheim-Chester Disease? Can Imaging Help Distinguish Pulmonary Involvement by Erdheim-Chester from Other Interstitial Lung Disease Processes?

Imaging studies are essential in establishing a diagnosis of ECD. As bone pain is the most commonly reported clinical manifestation, it is of no surprise that a pathognomonic feature of ECD is thus specific radiological findings in long bones: bilateral cortical sclerosis/osteosclerosing lesions on plain radiographs and abnormally high tracer uptake levels of the periarticular regions/distal ends on ^{99m}Tc bone scintigraphs [1, 7]. In cases suspicious for pulmonary involvement, radiographic studies alone are not diagnostic. High-resolution CT scans of the chest may be contributory, but the overall findings are not entirely specific to the disease. Regardless, imaging findings will frequently include interlobular septal thickening (distributed mostly in the apical, anterior and peripheral lung segments), as well as possible patchy centrilobular micronodular opacities, ground-glass opacities, patchy consolidations, and/or microcysts [6, 8]. Pleural involvement is not uncommon, typically with pleural thickening and, occasionally, pleural effusion [8].

What Are the Major Histopathologic Features of Erdheim-Chester Disease and How Do They Differ from a Reactive Inflammatory Process?

While a definitive diagnosis of ECD requires correlation with radiographic and clinical findings, some histologic features of ECD (in combination with immunohistochemistry) are arguably highly specific to the disease, thus rendering histopathology essential when ECD is suspect. Histologic evaluation of wedge biopsies will show an infiltrative population of abundant xanthomatous histiocytes in a background of dense inflammation and stromal fibrosis [9]. In contrast to a reactive inflammatory infiltrate where a particular pattern of distribution may not necessarily be appreciated, histiocytic cells in ECD will tend to be seen along lymphatics. Aggregates can be present in the visceral pleura as well as surrounding bronchovascular structures and within interlobular septa [6, 9]. Furthermore, the histiocytic cells in ECD will have a particular morphology that is distinct from reactive histiocytes. Cells contain round to oval nuclei, often with a characteristic lack of nuclear grooves, and abundant foamy cytoplasm. Well-formed granulomas are uncommon, and emperipolesis, a trademark of Rosai-Dorfman disease, is typically absent. By immunohistochemistry, the histiocytic cells will usually be positive for CD68 and CD168 a lack expression of CD1a and Langerin [1, 9]. While S100 shows variable expression, a Factor XIIIa immunostain can be helpful in supporting the diagnosis of ECD as it will be strongly positive in both nuclei and the cytoplasm of the cells (as opposed to just nuclear positivity in reactive histiocytes and intra-alveolar macrophages) [6, 9]. BRAF ^{V600E} immunohistochemistry though is not as useful, as most cases show only weak and scattered positivity [9].

How Helpful Is Molecular Testing When Considering a Diagnosis of Erdheim-Chester Disease?

Studies addressing molecular testing in ECD have found a number of different genetic alterations. One common finding, however, was that most mutations affected genes encoding proteins involved in the MAPK pathway [9]. Although *BRAF* ^{V600E} is not specific for ECD, as it is also found in Langerhans cell histiocytosis, one study has reported a *BRAF* ^{V600E} mutation in over 50% of cases [10]. Over time, this has proven to be helpful in clinical management.

Targeted therapeutic agents, such the *BRAF* inhibitor vemurafenib, have shown promising results with striking improvement in patient's clinical courses who had known *BRAF* ^{V600E} mutations [1, 11].

References

1. Mazor RD, Manevich-Mazor M, Shoenfeld Y. Erdheim-Chester disease: a comprehensive review of the literature. Orphanet J Rare Dis. 2013;8:137.
2. Clerico A, Ragni G, Cappelli C, Schiavetti A, Gonfiantini M, Uccini S. Erdheim-Chester disease in a child. Med Pediatr Oncol. 2003;41(6):575–7.
3. Veyssier-Belot C, Cacoub P, Caparros-Lefebvre D, Wechsler J, Brun B, Remy M, et al. Erdheim-Chester disease. Clinical and radiologic characteristics of 59 cases. Medicine (Baltimore). 1996;75(3):157–69.
4. Haroche J, Arnaud L, Amoura Z. Erdheim-Chester disease. Curr Opin Rheumatol. 2012;24(1):53–9.
5. Arnaud L, Hervier B, Neel A, Hamidou MA, Kahn JE, Wechsler B, et al. CNS involvement and treatment with interferon-alpha are independent prognostic factors in Erdheim-Chester disease: a multicenter survival analysis of 53 patients. Blood. 2011;117(10):2778–82.
6. Rush WL, Andriko JA, Galateau-Salle F, Brambilla E, Brambilla C, Ziany-bey I, et al. Pulmonary pathology of Erdheim-Chester disease. Mod Pathol. 2000;13(7):747–54.
7. Sanchez JE, Mora C, Macia M, Navarro JF. Erdheim-Chester disease as cause of end-stage renal failure: a case report and review of the literature. Int Urol Nephrol. 2010;42(4):1107–12.
8. Arnaud L, Pierre I, Beigelman-Aubry C, Capron F, Brun AL, Rigolet A, et al. Pulmonary involvement in Erdheim-Chester disease: a single-center study of thirty-four patients and a review of the literature. Arthritis Rheum. 2010;62(11):3504–12.
9. Ozkaya N, Rosenblum MK, Durham BH, Pichardo JD, Abdel-Wahab O, Hameed MR, et al. The histopathology of Erdheim-Chester disease: a comprehensive review of a molecularly characterized cohort. Mod Pathol. 2018;31(4):581–97.
10. Haroche J, Charlotte F, Arnaud L, von Deimling A, Helias-Rodzewicz Z, Hervier B, et al. High prevalence of BRAF V600E mutations in Erdheim-Chester disease but not in other non-Langerhans cell histiocytoses. Blood. 2012;120(13):2700–3.
11. Haroche J, Cohen-Aubart F, Emile JF, Arnaud L, Maksud P, Charlotte F, et al. Dramatic efficacy of vemurafenib in both multisystemic and refractory Erdheim-Chester disease and Langerhans cell histiocytosis harboring the BRAF V600E mutation. Blood. 2013;121(9):1495–500.

Mucosal Marginal Zone Lymphoma Versus Follicular Bronchiolitis

33

Craig Dunseth and Chen Zhao

Case Presentation

A 58-year-old woman with no smoking history and nonspecific pulmonary symptoms is incidentally found to have a 23 mm nodule of the left lower lobe of the lung by high-resolution computed tomography (HRCT). Initial pulmonary function tests demonstrate a normal FEV1 and DLCO. Due to the central location of the nodule, an endobronchial biopsy is not feasible, and the patient undergoes a diagnostic wedge biopsy. An intraoperative frozen section with diff-quick smears is performed on the lung nodule, which shows a small somewhat monotonous lymphocyte population with oval/round nuclei, condensed chromatin, and moderate amounts of pale staining cytoplasm. Fresh tissue is collected for flow cytometry, which detects a CD5-negative, CD10-negative, kappa-restricted small- to intermediate-sized B-cell population.

Pathologic Diagnosis: Pulmonary Extranodal Marginal Zone Lymphoma of Mucosa-Associated Lymphoid Tissue (MALT Lymphoma)

What Is the Definition of a MALT Lymphoma? What Are Its Clinical and Prognostic Features?

Extranodal marginal zone lymphoma of mucosa-associated lymphoid tissue (MALT lymphoma) is a low-grade B-cell neoplasm composed small mature B cells, which morphologically and immunophenotypically resemble mature marginal zone cells [1].

The clinical presentation for pulmonary MALT lymphoma is nonspecific and may include dry cough and dyspnea along with weight loss, fever, and night sweats; lesions are often found incidentally by imaging studies [2, 3]. The median age of patients is >50 years old [4]. The pathogenesis is unclear; however, some lesions may be associated with chronic inflammation secondary to autoimmune or infectious diseases such as dysgammaglobulinemia, collagen vascular diseases, and AIDS [5]. A monoclonal immunoglobulin may be detected in serum by protein electrophoresis in up to 32% of patients, especially if a predominant component of neoplastic plasma cells is present [4]. Overall, these lesions show indolent growth and remain localized in the lung for long periods prior to dissemination [6]. There is no defined treatment for pulmonary marginal zone lymphoma; however, surgery, radiotherapy, and chemotherapy are available options [7]. A watch-and-wait approach may be applied if lesions are small and localized to the lung. If making the diagnosis, one should always mention the possibility of performing serum and urine protein electrophoresis especially if a predominant plasma cell population is present. Following diagnosis, patients should be fully staged to assess for extrapulmonary involvement.

What Are the Histologic and Immunophenotypic Features of MALT Lymphomas?

MALT lymphoma is composed of mature B cells that have oval or round slightly irregular nuclei, moderately dispersed chromatin, inconspicuous nucleoli, and moderate amounts of pale cytoplasm (Fig. 33.1a, b). In some MALT lymphomas, there is a marked predominance of plasma cells, resulting in resemblance to an extramedullary plasmacytoma. Dutcher bodies (nuclear pseudo-inclusions containing immunoglobu-

C. Dunseth
Department of Pathology and Laboratory Medicine, Citizens Memorial Hospital, Bolivar, MO, USA

C. Zhao (✉)
Department of Pathology and Laboratory Medicine, Case Western Reserve University/Cleveland VA Medical Center, Cleveland, OH, USA
e-mail: cxz545@case.edu

H. Xu et al. (eds.), *Practical Lung Pathology*, Practical Anatomic Pathology, https://doi.org/10.1007/978-3-031-14402-8_33

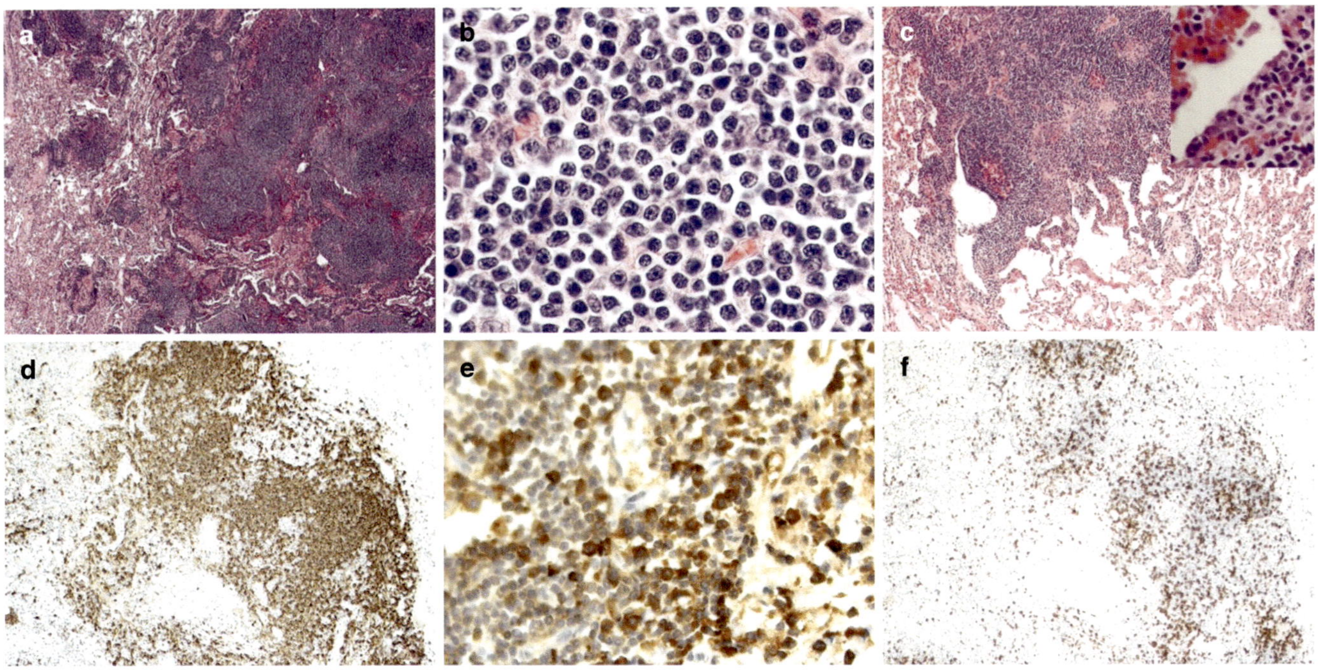

Fig. 33.1 Pulmonary MALT lymphoma. Dense nodular lymphoid infiltrates in the lung parenchyma (**a**, 40×). The lymphoid infiltrates are mainly composed of small- to medium-sized monotonous lymphocytes (**b**, 100×). The lymphocytes invaded bronchiolar epithelia [lymphoepithelial lesion (**c**, 10×; insert 600×)]. Immunostains show that these lymphocytes are predominantly CD20+ B-cells (**d**, 100×) and are kappa (**e**, 100×) but not lambda (not shown) restricted. CD3 highlights the background small T cells (**f**, 100×)

lin) may be present, indicating a neoplastic plasma cell component [8]. Amyloid deposition is seen in some cases. At low power of histological examination, MALT lymphoma may have a nodular or diffuse pattern that may extend along intact alveolar walls in a discontinuous fashion—this nodularity corresponds to residual benign germinal centers that have been colonized by neoplastic cells [9]. Destructive lymphoepithelial lesions, defined as aggregates of ≥3 marginal zone cells with distortion or destruction of the epithelium, may be present (Fig. 33.1c) and can be highlighted with a keratin immunohistochemical stain [10]. Transformed centroblast-like or immunoblast-like cells may be present in variable numbers; however, if solid or sheet-like proliferations of transformed cells are present, the lesion should be diagnosed as diffuse large B-cell lymphoma (DLBCL) and the presence of accompanying MALT lymphoma noted.

MALT lymphoma cells are positive for B-cell markers such as CD20 (Fig. 33.1d), PAX5, and CD79a. BCL2 will be positive in the majority of cases, while CD10, CD5, BCL6, cyclin D1, and CD23 will generally be negative [11]. CD43 may be helpful to reach a diagnosis of marginal zone lymphoma if positive in the neoplastic cells; however, a negative CD43 does not exclude a diagnosis of lymphoma. CD5+ or CD10+ MALT lymphomas have been reported in the literature; however, this immunophenotype is rare [12, 13]. If a plasma cell component is present, it will be positive for CD138, CD79a, or MUM1 and may have light chain restriction (Fig. 33.1e). IgD may show loss of a developed mantle cell layer [14]. CD21 or CD23 typically reveals expanded meshworks of follicular dendritic cells, corresponding to colonized follicles. CD3 is negative in tumor cells but may highlight background small benign T cells (Fig. 33.1f).

What Is the Differential Diagnosis for MALT Lymphomas?

The main differential includes reactive conditions, notably follicular bronchiolitis. Other small lymphoid lymphomas such as mantle cell lymphoma and follicular lymphoma are rare in the lung but may need to be ruled out. Abundant plasma cells are present in some MALT lymphomas, raising the differential of plasmacytoma.

What Is the Definition of Follicular Bronchiolitis (FB)? What Are Its Clinical and Prognostic Features?

The main differential in MALT lymphoma is follicular bronchiolitis (FB) which is characterized by cellular lymphoid follicles aggregated in the walls of small airways. FB is most often seen in the setting of other disease processes; however, primary (idiopathic) cases may rarely occur [15, 16]. Primary

FB is most commonly seen in middle-aged and elderly patients [17], and secondary FB is seen in a wide range of ages and is more commonly found in males than females [16]. Secondary FB can be seen in the setting of connective tissue diseases, infections, obstructive airway disease, and interstitial lung disease. Similar to MALT lymphoma, the signs and symptoms of FB are nonspecific but include worsening dyspnea, chronic cough, and recurrent pneumonias [17]. In cases of primary FB, peripheral eosinophilia may be present, suggesting an underlying hypersensitivity reaction [18]. The prognosis of follicular bronchiolitis is good, and progressive lung disease is uncommon [19]. If making the diagnosis, one should always mention the possibility of an underlying connective tissue disorders.

What Are the Histologic Features of Follicular Bronchiolitis?

FB characteristically shows multifocal well-formed lymphoid follicles within the walls of bronchioles; narrowing or complete obliteration of the bronchiolar lumen may be seen (Fig. 33.2a–d) [16, 20]. There is minimal involvement away from the bronchioles (the alveolar walls and lung spaces are uninvolved). The background lung must be assessed as FB may be seen with other processes such as obstructive pneumonia or concurrent carcinoma.

What Are the Radiographic Features of MALT Lymphomas and Follicular Bronchiolitis?

Imaging for both FB and MALT lymphoma may overlap. In FB, HRCT may show bilateral lung involvement with small centrilobular/parabronchial nodules (1–3 mm) with associated bilateral patchy ground-glass opacities and bronchial dilatation [21]. The imaging features of MALT lymphoma are diverse and may include a single consolidation, multiple nodules, bronchiectasis, or diffuse interstitial lung disease [22]. In both entities, a "tree in bud" or "cotton in bud" appearance may be seen on imaging, corresponding to lymphoid follicles becoming densely concentrated in the interstitium adjacent to bronchioles [17, 23].

How Does One Differentiate a MALT Lymphoma from Follicular Bronchiolitis?

Often, there is morphologic overlap between MALT lymphoma and follicular bronchiolitis (FB); however, large size (>1 cm) and the presence of lymphoepithelial lesions are suggestive of MALT lymphoma.

Immunohistochemistry may be needed to differentiate these two entities. Follicular bronchiolitis will show an admixture of small B cells (positive for CD20, PAX5, or

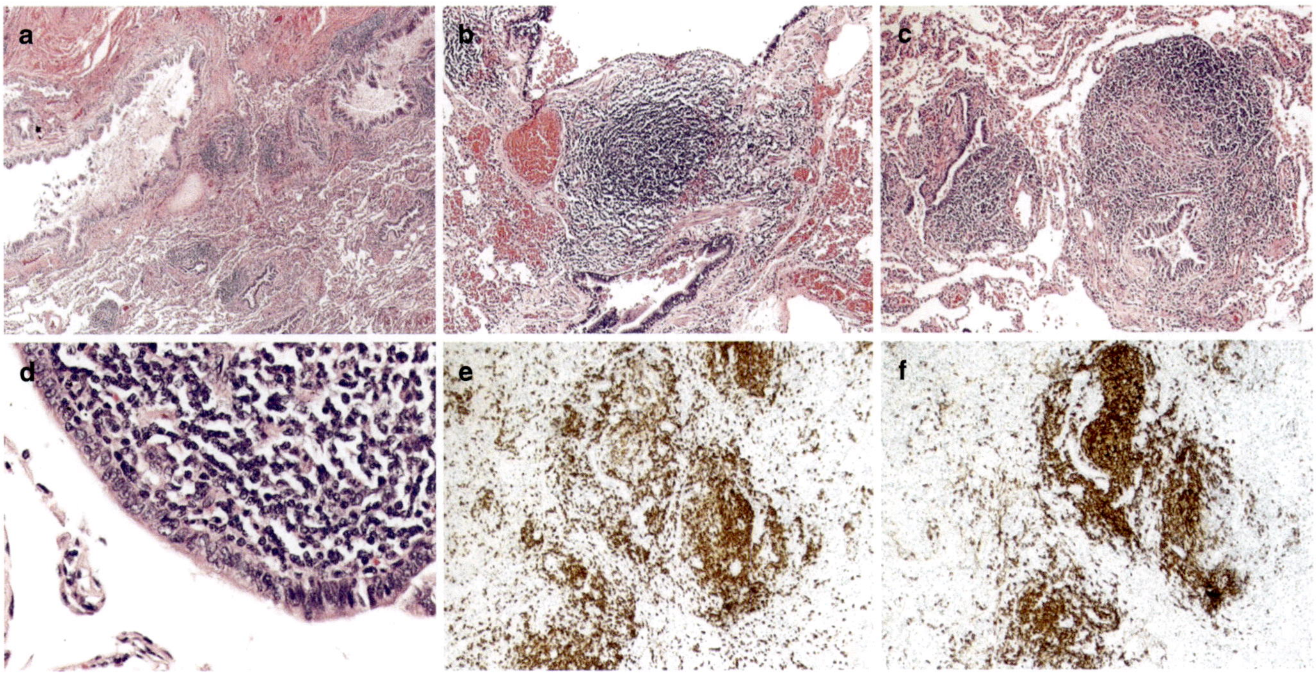

Fig. 33.2 Follicular bronchiolitis. Multifocal well-formed lymphoid aggregates are identified within or close to the bronchiolar walls (**a–c**; **a**, 40×; **b**, **c**, 100×). The bronchiolar epithelia are intact (**d**, 40×). Immunostains show that the lymphoid aggregates are composed of admixed small CD3+ T cells (**e**, 100×) and CD20+ B cells (**f**, 100×)

CD79a, predominantly in follicles) with scattered background T cells (positive for CD3) (Fig. 33.2e, f). MALT lymphoma typically shows a predominance of B cells surrounding and colonizing follicles. Immunoglobulin D highlights a well-defined mantle zone in follicular bronchiolitis as it is often lost in MALT lymphoma. In FB, CD21 and CD23 highlight the background follicular dendritic cell meshworks [10, 16], which may be expanded if follicles are colonized by MALT lymphoma.

Flow cytometry, molecular testing, and cytogenetic analysis may be performed to help differentiate reactive versus neoplastic lymphoproliferative lesions. If lesional tissue is submitted fresh, flow cytometry should be considered. MALT lymphoma characteristically shows small- to intermediate-sized B cells that are CD19+, CD20+, CD5-, CD10-, CD103-, and CD25- with light chain restriction, while FB will show polytypic B cells [24]. Clonality may also be assessed by *IGH* gene rearrangement using PCR (14). FISH studies may aid in the diagnosis as up to 40% of pulmonary MALT lymphoma cases contain a t(11;18) involving *API2/BIRC3* and MALT1 translocation [25]. Other chromosomal translocations associated with pulmonary MALT lymphomas include t(14;18)(6–10%) and t(1;14)(p22;q32)(2–7%), resulting in transcriptional deregulation of *MALT1* and *BCL10*, respectively [26].

References

1. Rubenstein JN, Beatty C, Kinkade Z, Bryan C, Hogg JP, Gibson LF, et al. Extranodal marginal zone lymphoma of the lung: evolution from an underlying reactive lymphoproliferative disorder. J Clin Exp Pathol. 2015;5(1):208.
2. O'Donnell PG, Jackson SA, Tung KT, Hassan B, Wilkins B, Mead GM. Radiological appearances of lymphomas arising from mucosa-associated lymphoid tissue (MALT) in the lung. Clin Radiol. 1998;53(4):258–63.
3. Mitchell A, Meunier C, Ouellette D, Colby T. Extranodal marginal zone lymphoma of mucosa-associated lymphoid tissue with initial presentation in the pleura. Chest. 2006;129(3):791–4.
4. Borie R, Wislez M, Thabut G, Antoine M, Rabbat A, Couderc LJ, et al. Clinical characteristics and prognostic factors of pulmonary MALT lymphoma. Eur Respir J. 2009;34(6):1408–16.
5. Lazar EB, Whitman GJ, Chew FS. Lymphoma of bronchus-associated lymphoid tissue. AJR Am J Roentgenol. 1996;167(1):116.
6. Bi L, Li J, Dan W, Lu Z. Pulmonary MALT lymphoma: a case report and review of the literature. Exp Ther Med. 2015;9(1):147–50.
7. Wang L, Xia ZJ, Zhang YJ, Huang HQ, Lin TY, Lu Y. Radical surgery may be not an optimal treatment approach for pulmonary MALT lymphoma. Tumour Biol. 2015;36(8):6409–16.
8. Molina TJ, Lin P, Swerdlow SH, Cook JR. Marginal zone lymphomas with plasmacytic differentiation and related disorders. Am J Clin Pathol. 2011;136(2):211–25.
9. Isaacson PG, Wotherspoon AC, Diss T, Pan LX. Follicular colonization in B-cell lymphoma of mucosa-associated lymphoid tissue. Am J Surg Pathol. 1991;15(9):819–28.
10. Begueret H, Vergier B, Parrens M, Lehours P, Laurent F, Vernejoux JM, et al. Primary lung small B-cell lymphoma versus lymphoid hyperplasia: evaluation of diagnostic criteria in 26 cases. Am J Surg Pathol. 2002;26(1):76–81.
11. Kurtin PJ, Myers JL, Adlakha H, Strickler JG, Lohse C, Pankratz VS, et al. Pathologic and clinical features of primary pulmonary extranodal marginal zone B-cell lymphoma of MALT type. Am J Surg Pathol. 2001;25(8):997–1008.
12. Jaso J, Chen L, Li S, Lin P, Chen W, Miranda RN, et al. CD5-positive mucosa-associated lymphoid tissue (MALT) lymphoma: a clinicopathologic study of 14 cases. Hum Pathol. 2012;43(9):1436–43.
13. Wang E, West D, Kulbacki E. An unusual nodal marginal zone lymphoma with bright CD10 expression: a potential diagnostic pitfall. Am J Hematol. 2010;85(7):546–8.
14. Bacon CM, Du MQ, Dogan A. Mucosa-associated lymphoid tissue (MALT) lymphoma: a practical guide for pathologists. J Clin Pathol. 2007;60(4):361–72.
15. Yousem SA, Colby TV, Carrington CB. Follicular bronchitis/bronchiolitis. Hum Pathol. 1985;16(7):700–6.
16. Romero S, Barroso E, Gil J, Aranda I, Alonso S, Garcia-Pachon E. Follicular bronchiolitis: clinical and pathologic findings in six patients. Lung. 2003;181(6):309–19.
17. Tashtoush B, Okafor NC, Ramirez JF, Smolley L. Follicular bronchiolitis: a literature review. J Clin Diagn Res. 2015;9(9):OE01–5.
18. Koss MN. Pulmonary lymphoid disorders. Semin Diagn Pathol. 1995;12(2):158–71.
19. Aerni MR, Vassallo R, Myers JL, Lindell RM, Ryu JH. Follicular bronchiolitis in surgical lung biopsies: clinical implications in 12 patients. Respir Med. 2008;102(2):307–12.
20. Ryu JH. Classification and approach to bronchiolar diseases. Curr Opin Pulm Med. 2006;12(2):145–51.
21. Oh YW, Effmann EL, Redding GJ, Godwin JD. Follicular hyperplasia of bronchus-associated lymphoid tissue causing severe air trapping. AJR Am J Roentgenol. 1999;172(3):745–7.
22. Hare SS, Souza CA, Bain G, Seely JM, Frcpc GMM, et al. The radiological spectrum of pulmonary lymphoproliferative disease. Br J Radiol. 2012;85(1015):848–64.
23. Lee DK, Im JG, Lee KS, Lee JS, Seo JB, Goo JM, et al. B-cell lymphoma of bronchus-associated lymphoid tissue (BALT): CT features in 10 patients. J Comput Assist Tomogr. 2000;24(1):30–4.
24. Zaer FS, Braylan RC, Zander DS, Iturraspe JA, Almasri NM. Multiparametric flow cytometry in the diagnosis and characterization of low-grade pulmonary mucosa-associated lymphoid tissue lymphomas. Mod Pathol. 1998;11(6):525–32.
25. Remstein ED, Dogan A, Einerson RR, Paternoster SF, Fink SR, Law M, et al. The incidence and anatomic site specificity of chromosomal translocations in primary extranodal marginal zone B-cell lymphoma of mucosa-associated lymphoid tissue (MALT lymphoma) in North America. Am J Surg Pathol. 2006;30(12):1546–53.
26. Swerdlow SH, Campo E, Harris NL, et al. WHO classification of tumours of haematopoietic and lymphoid tissues. Geneva: WHO Press; 2017.

Primary Pulmonary Diffuse Large B-Cell Lymphoma Versus Poorly Differentiated Carcinomas

34

Zhao Ming (David) Dong and Paul D. Simonson

Case Presentation

A 71-year-old man was incidentally found to have multiple pulmonary nodules on an X-ray performed during workup for dyspnea and congestive heart failure. He has no history of fever, night sweats, or weight loss. He had a history of coronary artery disease, status post two stents placed 1 year ago, and 50 years of smoking. A computed tomography (CT) of the chest confirmed the presence of multiple nodules of varying sizes, mainly on the right side involving the middle and lower lobes (Fig. 34.1). Positron emission tomography (PET)-CT revealed two highly PET-avid lung nodules in the right lower lobe. No uptake in mediastinum or in smaller peripheral pulmonary nodules was noted. No extrapulmonary lesion was detected. Subsequently, he underwent bronchoscopy, and an endobronchial mass located in the right lower lobe was found. Endobronchial biopsy of this mass was performed, revealing a lymphocytic proliferation consisting of clusters/sheets of large atypical lymphoid cells in a background of small lymphoid cells. Immunohistochemistry (IHC) demonstrated that these large, atypical cells were positive for CD20, BCL-6 (subset), BCL-2 (>50%), MUM-1, c-MYC (>40%), and Ki-67 (50%) and negative for CD10, CD30, CD43, CD5, and CD23 (Fig. 34.2). No CD20-positive large and atypical B cells were positive for EBV by in situ hybridization. B-cell gene rearrangement (IGH) was detected by PCR. Fluorescence in situ hybridization (FISH) studies revealed no *BCL-2*, *BCL-6*, or *c-MYC* gene rearrangement. The patient received six circles of R-CHOP. Now he is 6 years from completion of therapy and remains in complete remission.

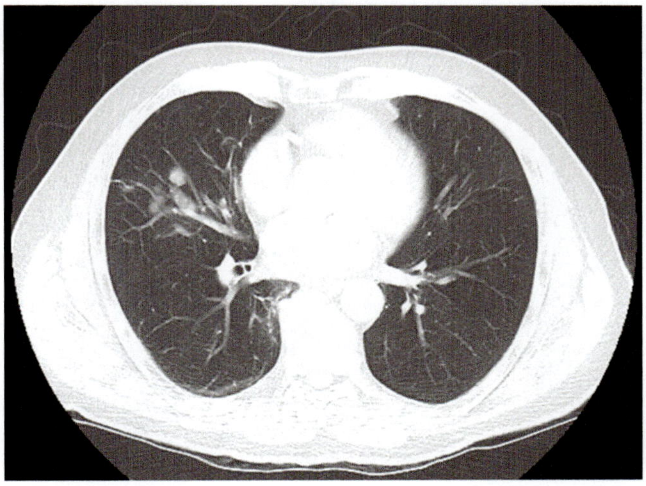

Fig. 34.1 Computed tomography (CT) of the chest image for multiple nodular lesions on the right involving middle and lower lobes

Z. Ming (David) Dong (✉)
Department of Laboratory Medicine and Pathology, Puget Sound VA Health Care System, University of Washington School of Medicine, Seattle, WA, USA
e-mail: Zhaoming.dong@va.gov

P. D. Simonson
Division of Hematopathology, Department of Pathology and Laboratory Medicine, Weill Cornell Medicine/New York-Presbyterian Hospital, New York, NY, USA

H. Xu et al. (eds.), *Practical Lung Pathology*, Practical Anatomic Pathology, https://doi.org/10.1007/978-3-031-14402-8_34

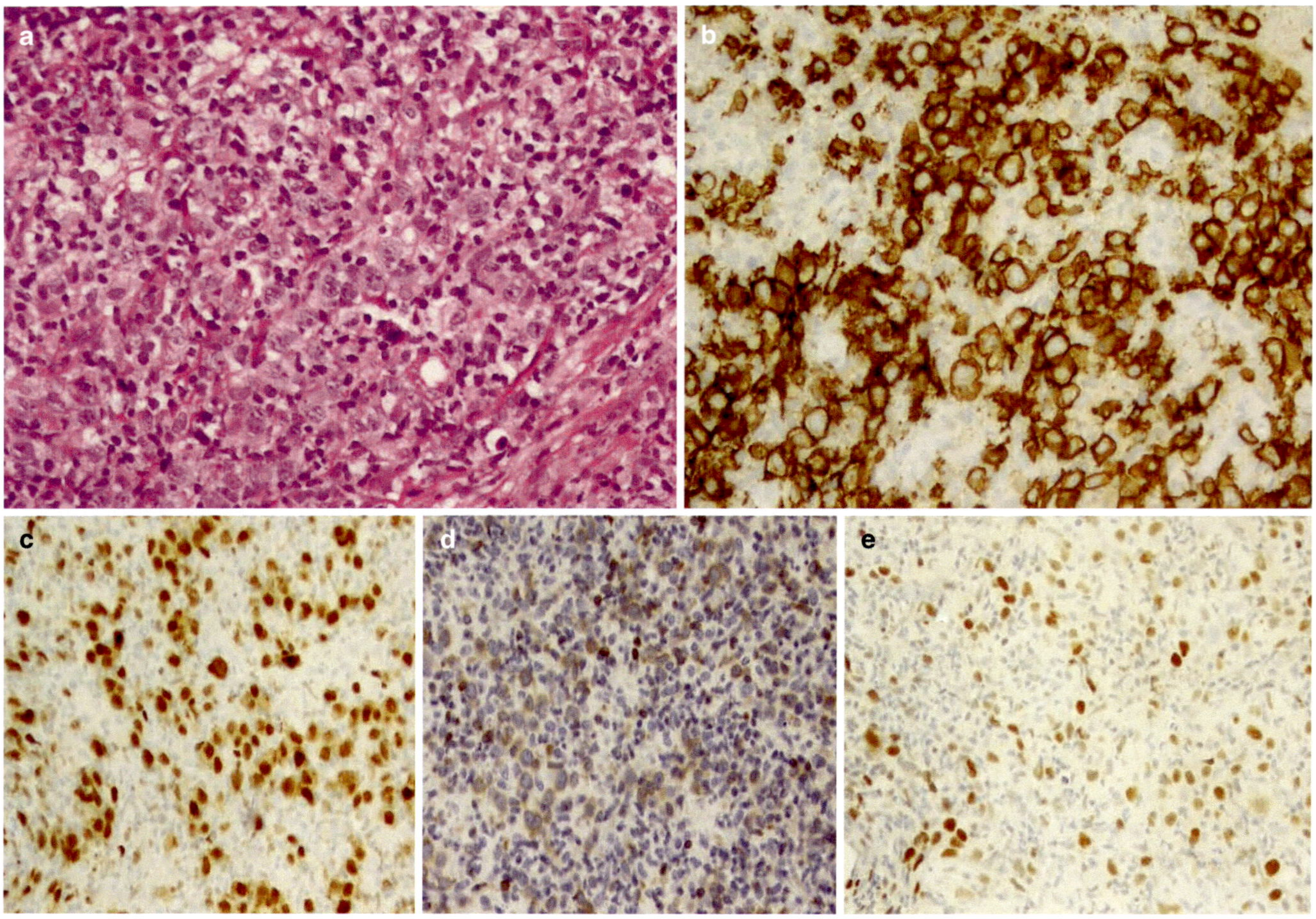

Fig. 34.2 Endobronchial biopsy of pulmonary nodule, consistent with diffuse large B-cell lymphoma, characterized by an infiltration of clusters/sheets of large atypical lymphoid cells in a background of small lymphoid cells (**a**, Hematoxylin and eosin, 200×). These atypical cells are positive for CD20 (**b**, IHC, 200×), MUM-1 (**c**, IHC, 200×), BCL-2 (**d**, IHC, 200×), and c-MYC (**e**, IHC, 200×)

Pathologic Diagnosis: Primary Pulmonary Diffuse Large B-Cell Lymphoma, Not Otherwise Specified, Non-Germinal Center (Or Activated) B-Cell Subtype, with Double-Expressor Phenotype

What Is the Definition of a Primary Pulmonary Diffuse Large B-Cell Lymphoma (PPDLBCL)?

PPDLBCL is defined as a diffuse proliferation of large B cells (i.e., B cells with a nuclear size equal to or exceeding that of a normal macrophage nucleus, or more than twice the size of a normal lymphocyte), affecting one or both lungs (parenchyma and/or bronchi) in a patient with no previous extrapulmonary involvement by DLBCL at the time of diagnosis or during the subsequent 3 months.

PPDLBCL is a rare disease, but it accounts for 5–20% of all primary pulmonary lymphomas (PPL) and is the second most common subtype after extranodal marginal zone mucosa-associated lymphoid tissue lymphoma (MALT-PPL). However, due to its rapid spread into the mediastinum and extrapulmonary locations, the true incidence of this lymphoma may be underestimated. About half of the PPDLBCL cases arise de novo, and the other half arise from transformation of preexisting or concurrent indolent PPL, such as MALT-PPL [1].

What Are the Clinical, Radiographic, and Prognostic Features and Treatment of PPDLBCL?

PPDLBCL can be seen in both immunocompromised and immunocompetent patients. It commonly affects adults in the sixth and seventh decades of life, excluding HIV-positive and chronically immunosuppressed patients who can present as a younger age. There is no sex predisposition. Patients with this disease have no overt symptoms during the initial stages; however, as the disease progresses, they are likely to present with nonspecific symptoms, including dyspnea, cough, chest pain, and other obstructive and infectious symptoms, as well as fever and weight loss [2]. Consequently, the diagnosis of PPDLBCL, in particular, in a primary care setting, is challenging and often leads to misdiagnosis and delayed treatment.

PPDLBCL can present as a single well-defined rounded solid mass or multiple masses on chest CT. These lesions tend to be located peripherally in the lower lobes. Features of MALT-PPL and PPDLBCL can overlap where solitary or multiple nodules or areas of consolidation can be seen. Cavitation and/or central necrosis on chest CT is seen in 50% of the cases and is a feature more common in PPDLBCL compared to MALT-PPL [3]. Pleural effusion and, rarely, direct chest wall invasion are also seen. Two recent cases of PPDLBCL described radiographic findings of consolidation of multiple pulmonary nodules with air bronchograms and haloes of ground-glass shadowing at lesion margins [4]. Fludeoxyglucose (FDG)-PET usually demonstrates metabolic activity. Radiologically, it is extremely difficult to differentiate PPDLBCL from more common lung malignancies, such as bronchogenic carcinoma. Cases with unilateral pulmonary involvement are considered stage IE, and cases with regional lymph node (hilar/mediastinal) involvement are IIE. Bilateral pulmonary involvement constitutes stage IV disease.

Using the current WHO classification, most of PPDLBCL should be classified as DLBCL, not otherwise specified (DLBCL-NOS), since other types of specialized DLBCL are extremely rare entities of this disease. Prognostic subtyping of DLBCL-NOS into germinal center B-cell (GCB) subtype and non-germinal center B-cell (or activated B cell, ABC) subtype is required in the 2017 WHO update, which confirms the better prognosis of GCB subtype DLBCL using current therapies. In addition, the 2017 WHO update also recognizes co-expression of BCL-2 and MYC proteins as a possible prognostic immunophenotype in DLBCL-NOS (the so-called double-expressor lymphoma) [5]. Historically, PPDLBCL was thought to have a worse prognosis with reportedly widely variable median survival ranging from 3 to 10 years. However, a large case series by Neri et al. found that PPDLBCL patients treated with conventional CHOP achieved a complete response in 77 cases (94%) with 10-year PFS of 90% [6]. HIV patients and chronically immunosuppressed patients with this lymphoma have a poor prognosis, usually due to opportunistic infections.

As compared to MALT-PPL, PPDLBCL is much more aggressive and needs aggressive treatment even in the early stages. However, due to its rarity, no randomized clinical trials have been performed to establish an optimal treatment option. Different therapeutic modalities have been used in clinical practice, including watchful waiting, surgery, chemotherapy, or chemotherapy followed by radiotherapy [7]. The choice of treatment approach should be based on the biological characteristic of the tumor, stage, and performance status. Surgery may be considered in the localized form of PPDLBCL. Radiation therapy has a limited role in PPDLBCL, probably due to its high incidence of adverse effects in the lungs. Chemotherapy consists of the same multi-agent regimens as those used in nodal DLBCL, including CHOP or CHOP plus rituximab (R-CHOP).

What Are the Pathologic Features of PPDLBCL?

On gross examination, PPDLBCL has a solid appearance and is cream colored with variable areas of necrosis [8]. Histologically, they are similar to those in other sites. They commonly form confluent sheets of tumor cells and tend to destroy the normal lung parenchyma with associated necrosis and sometimes vascular invasion. Lymphoepithelial lesions are rare. The tumor is composed of large, discohesive cells with coarse chromatin, distinct nucleoli, and abundant amphophilic cytoplasm. These are usually described as centroblastic or immunoblastic, and occasionally anaplastic. Tumor cells and fibrin may fill airspaces ("tumoral pneumonia") and often show infiltration in a lymphatic distribution. Superimposed pneumonia may mask the lymphoma. The immunophenotype of the neoplastic cells is usually positive for CD45 and B-cell markers such as CD19, CD20, and CD79a. However, the CD20 phenotype may be lost after treatment with rituximab. Flow cytometric analysis generally can detect a kappa or lambda light chain restricted monoclonal B-cell population, with or without expression of CD10. However, flow cytometry may yield a false-negative result because of necrosis and/or cell fragility.

As discussed previously, due to prognostic implication, DLBCL-NOS must be separated into GCB and ABC subtypes. These two subtypes were originally identified using gene expression profiling. However, since gene arrays are not widely available, immunohistochemical studies as a surrogate for molecular profiling must be performed on all PPDLBCL cases. The most familiar method is the Hans classifier, which uses three immunohistochemical markers—CD10, BCL6, and MUM-1-for classification. In general, GCB phenotype is CD10/BCL-6 positive and MUM-1 negative, and the ABC phenotype is MUM-1 positive and CD10 negative [5].

As mentioned, the current WHO classification discusses the "double-expressor" phenotype in DLBCL-NOS due to the possible prognostic implications, independent of genetic or FISH studies for abnormalities. This refers to expression of BCL-2 proteins in ≥50% of the cells and expression of MYC protein in ≥40% of the cells. However, routine staining for MYC and BCL2 proteins is still controversial.

Since bronchoscopic examination of PPDLBCL is usually abnormal with budding or infiltrative stenosis of bronchi, histologic diagnosis via minimally invasive procedures and bronchoscopy is feasible, even with small samples, due to the presence of sheets or clusters of large, atypical cells. Multiple case reports demonstrating success of transbronchial lung biopsy and ultrasound-guided fine needle aspiration in diagnosing PPDLBCL further support this observation [9].

What Are the Differential Diagnoses of PPDLBCL?

DLBCL is comprised of various entities, including DLBCL-NOS and other specifically named large B-cell lymphomas. As discussed previously, most PPDLBCL are DLBCL-NOS. The other specialized DLBCLs, such as T-cell/histocyte-rich large B-cell lymphoma (THRLBCL) and EBV+ DLBCL are extremely rare but can be seen in the lung [10]. Therefore, the diagnosis of DLBCL-NOS in the lung also needs to exclude these rare types of specialized DLBCL.

If large, atypical B cells do not form clusters or sheets, and in the background, there is predominantly small T cells with large, neoplastic cells comprising 10% or less of the overall cellularity, the diagnosis of THRLBCL should be considered [11].

Since PPDLBCL can occur in patients with underlying immunosuppression such as HIV infection, and nearly all cases in these patients are EBV-positive, it is prudent to test for EBV in virtually all cases of PPDLBCL by in situ staining for EBER. If the neoplastic cells contain EBV but patients are negative for HIV infection and lymphoma does not fall into one of the other named EVB-positive groups such as lymphomatoid granulomatosis, the diagnosis of EBV+ DLBCL should be considered.

PPDLBCL must be distinguished from primary mediastinal large B-cell lymphoma, which is frequently associated with extension to the lung. Immunophenotypically, unlike PPDLBCL, primary mediastinal large B-cell lymphoma characteristically lacks immunoglobulin expression with CD30 expression in >80% of cases [12]. In addition, knowledge of the clinical features in primary mediastinal large B-cell lymphoma, including young age, female sex, and the presence of a mediastinal mass, is important in establishing the correct diagnosis.

Intravascular large B-cell lymphoma may show pulmonary manifestations, but this disease is regarded as an aggressive systemic lymphoma from the outset [8].

In addition, since a high-grade B-cell lymphoma with *MYC* and *BCL2* and/or *BCL6* rearrangements (the so-called double hit or triple hit lymphomas) can display morphologic features similar to DLBCL-NOS, genetic or FISH studies to evaluate *BCL2*, *MYC*, and *BCL6* gene rearrangements are also required for all suspected PPDLBCL cases. This high-grade lymphoma is associated with more clinical aggressiveness as compared to "double-expressor" DCBCL-NOS [5]. There is also a difference in therapy.

Major differential diagnosis based on morphology alone includes primary or metastatic poorly differentiated carcinoma and metastatic melanoma.

Poorly Differentiated Squamous Cell Carcinoma and Adenocarcinoma

Poorly differentiated squamous cell carcinoma may lack characteristic features of squamous cell carcinoma such as keratinization, keratin pearl formation, and/or intercellular bridges. Similarly, poorly differentiated adenocarcinoma is commonly composed of sheets of polygonal cells lacking acini, tubules, and papillae. Therefore, they can morphologically mimic DLBCL. However, appropriate and adequate immunohistochemical stains can separate these diseases.

Large Cell Undifferentiated Carcinoma

Large cell undifferentiated carcinoma is an undifferentiated non-small cell carcinoma that lacks the cytological, architectural, and immunohistochemical features of small cell carcinoma, adenocarcinoma, or squamous cell carcinoma. Recurrent DLBCL can mistakenly be diagnosed as large cell carcinoma, especially when CD20 immunostaining is negative due to previous rituximab treatment. However, large cell undifferentiated carcinoma should be positive for cytokeratin, and recurrent DLBCL should still be positive for PAX-5.

Small Cell Carcinoma (SCLC) and Large Cell Neuroendocrine Carcinoma (LCNEC)

The distinction between SCLC and LCNEC is based on cytological criteria. When needed, immunohistochemical stains for neuroendocrine differentiation (positive for CD56, synaptophysin, or chromogranin) can be performed to confirm the diagnosis. However, distinguishing between these two tumors and DLBCL can be diagnostically challenging due to potential overlap of morphologic features and variant antigen expression. PAX-5, a valuable immunohistochemical marker for recurrent CD20-negative DLBCL following rituximab therapy, is also expressed on these neuroendocrine carcinomas (79% of small cell carcinoma expresses PAX-5) [13]. Therefore, there is a pitfall of misdiagnosing these tumors as recurrent DLBCL.

Pulmonary Lymphoepithelioma-Like Carcinoma and Metastatic Undifferentiated Carcinoma of the Nasopharynx

Both carcinomas display similar morphology. To distinguish these two diseases, examination of the nasopharynx should be performed. They are characterized by nests or diffuse sheets of syncytial tumor cells, which show round to oval vesicular nuclei with prominent nucleoli, along with an admixed heavy lymphocytic and plasma cell infiltrate [14]. The heavy lymphoplasmacytic infiltration can obscure the epithelial component, causing a misdiagnosis of lymphoma. Ancillary studies show that the presence of Epstein-Barr virus in the keratin-positive tumor cells is crucial for the diagnosis.

Metastatic Melanoma

Melanoma metastasizing to the lung is a diagnostic consideration, especially when there is the absence of melanin production and cytokeratin immunostaining is negative. In these situations, immunohistochemical stains for S100, SOX-10, HMB-45, and Melan-A are helpful for readily distinguishing between PPDLBCL and melanoma.

References

1. Sohani AR, Ferry JA. Lymphomas and lymphoproliferative disease of the lung. Diagn Histopathol. 2014;20:405–14.
2. Jiang AG, Gao XY, Lu HY. Diagnosis and management of a patient with primary pulmonary diffuse large B-cell lymphoma: a case report and review of the literature. Exp Ther Med. 2014;8:797–800.
3. Hare SS, Souza CA, Bain G, Seely JM, Gomes MM, et al. The radiological spectrum of pulmonary lymphoproliferative disease. Br J Radiol. 2012;85:848–64.
4. Saitoh Y, Ohnishi-Amemiya A, Asano M, Tanaka Y, Yoshizawa S, Fujimoto H, Itoh Y, Nakamura N, Ohyashiki K. Unique radiological features of two cases of primary pulmonary diffuse large B-cell lymphoma. Thorax. 2017;72:859–60.
5. Grimm KE, O'Malley DP. Aggressive B cell lymphomas in the 2017 revised WHO classification of tumors of hematopoietic and lymphoid tissues. Ann Diagn Pathol. 2019;38:6–10.
6. Neri N, Jesus Nambo M, Aviles A. Diffuse large B-cell lymphoma primary of lung. Hematology. 2011;16:110–2.
7. Zhu Z, Liu W, Mamlouk O, O'Donnell JE, Sen D, Avezbakiev B. Primary pulmonary diffuse large B cell non-Hodgkin's lymphoma: a case report and literature review. Am J Case Rep. 2017;18:286–90.
8. William J, Variakojis D, Yeldandi A, Raparia K. Lymphoproliferative neoplasm of the lung: a review. Arch Pathol Lab Med. 2013;137:382–91.
9. Tang VK, Vijhani P, Cherian SV, Ambelil M, Estrada-Y-Martin RM. Primary pulmonary lymphoproliferative neoplasms. Lung India. 2018;35:220–3.
10. Wei EX, Silva RF, Cotelingam JD, Shackelford RE. Pediatric pulmonary Epstein-Barr virus-positive diffuse large B-cell lymphoma: a case report and review of the literature. Case Rep Pathol. 2017;2017:8946807.
11. Kommalapati A, Tella SH, Go RS, Nowakowski GS, Goyal G. T cell/histiocyte-rich large B cell lymphoma: incidence, demographic disparities, and long-term outcomes. Br J Haematol. 2019;185:140–2.
12. Higgins JP, Warnke RA. CD30 expression is common in mediastinal large B-cell lymphoma. Am J Clin Pathol. 1999;112:241–7.
13. Mhawech-Fauceglia P, Saxena R, Zhang S, Terracciano L, Sauter G, Chadhuri A, Herrmann FR, Penetrante R. PAX-5 immunoexpression in various types of benign and malignant tumors: a high-throughput tissue microarray analysis. J Clin Pathol. 2007;60:709–14.
14. Sathirareuangchai S, Hirata K. Pulmonary lymphoepithelioma-like carcinoma. Arch Pathol Lab Med. 2019;143:1027–30.

Lymphomatoid Granulomatosis Versus Granulomatosis with Polyangiitis

35

Marina K Baine and Xuchen Zhang

Case Presentation

A 45-year-old man with a longstanding history of rheumatoid arthritis treated with methotrexate over the last 4 years, presented to the Emergency Department with intractable cough and worsening dyspnea. Physical exam and laboratory workup were unremarkable except for elevated antinuclear antibodies (ANA). Chest X-ray and CT scan demonstrated multiple small bilateral pulmonary nodules, some poorly defined and some well-defined. He subsequently underwent video-assisted thoracoscopic lung wedge biopsy. The specimen showed a 1.2 cm ill-defined white lesion with punctate foci of necrosis. Microscopic examination revealed a polymorphous lymphocytic infiltrate intermixed with plasma cells, histiocytes, and large atypical lymphoid cells infiltrating vessel walls with associated infarct-like coagulative necrosis. Immunohistochemistry (IHC) demonstrated CD20 positivity in the large, atypical cells, many of which (15 per HPF) were positive for EBV-encoded small RNA (EBER) by in situ hybridization (ISH). The background immune infiltrate was composed of predominantly CD4+ T cells and scattered polyclonal (no restriction by kappa and lambda light chain IHC) CD138+ plasma cells. B-cell gene rearrangement (IGH) was detected by PCR. Methotrexate was discontinued, and the patient was treated with multiple cycles of chemotherapy, which led to a durable remission.

M. K Baine
Department of Pathology and Laboratory Medicine, Memorial Sloan Kettering Cancer Center, New York, NY, USA

X. Zhang (✉)
Department of Pathology, Yale University School of Medicine, New Haven, CT, USA
e-mail: xuchen.zhang@yale.edu

Pathologic Diagnosis: Lymphomatoid Granulomatosis, Grade 2 of 3

What Is the Definition of a Lymphomatoid Granulomatosis?

Lymphomatoid granulomatosis (LG), a misnomer first coined by Liebow in 1972 [1], is an EBV-positive B-cell lymphoproliferative disorder characterized by angiocentricity and angiodestruction in a reactive T-cell predominant inflammatory background, which is currently classified under a larger umbrella of B-cell proliferations of uncertain malignant potential [2]. Histologic grading is on a scale from 1 to 3 depending on the number of EBV-positive atypical B cells and is prognostically significant.

What Are the Clinical, Radiographic, and Prognostic Features of Pulmonary Lymphomatoid Granulomatosis?

Although LG is generally seen in adults, children and the elderly may also be affected. It is more common in men than women, with a 2:1 male-to-female ratio [1, 3, 4]. The disease more commonly occurs in patients with congenital or acquired immunodeficiency or predisposing conditions, such as Wiskott-Aldrich syndrome, human immunodeficiency virus infection (HIV), common variable immunodeficiency, X-linked hypo- or agammaglobulinemia, rheumatoid arthritis, and chronic treatment with methotrexate or other immune suppressive medications. The lung is the most commonly affected site (>90%), followed by the skin (25–50%), central nervous system (20–30%), kidneys (~30%), and occasionally liver [2]. Unlike other B-cell lymphoproliferative disorders, LG rarely involves lymph nodes, bone marrow, and spleen [2]. Patients most frequently present with respiratory symptoms including cough, dyspnea, and chest pain.

H. Xu et al. (eds.), *Practical Lung Pathology*, Practical Anatomic Pathology, https://doi.org/10.1007/978-3-031-14402-8_35

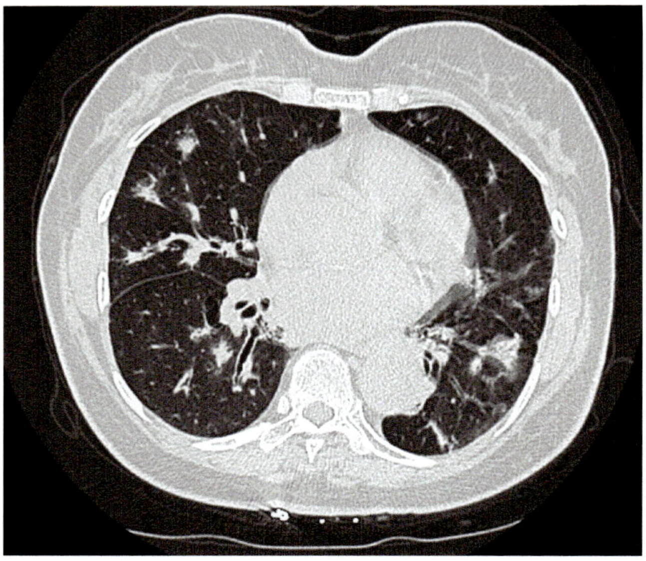

Fig. 35.1 CT scan of the chest demonstrating multiple small bilateral well-defined nodules predominantly in the low lung zones

Constitutional symptoms, such as fever, malaise, and weight loss are also common.

Pulmonary LG (PLG) appears on imaging (chest radiograph and computed tomography) as multiple bilateral poorly and/or well-defined nodules, usually <1 cm in greatest dimension but can occasionally be large and cavitating. The nodules are located along the bronchovascular structures or interlobular septa, with predilection for the mid- and lower lung fields (Fig. 35.1) [5, 6]. These findings, however, are nonspecific, and the radiographic differential diagnosis is broad and includes lymphoma, metastatic disease, lymphocytic interstitial pneumonia, sarcoidosis, cryptogenic organizing pneumonia, and granulomatosis with polyangiitis (GPA). Histopathologic evaluation of the lesions is therefore imperative for accurate diagnosis.

The prognosis of lymphomatoid granulomatosis is variable, and although most patients have progressive disease, up to 20% recover without treatment [7, 8]. The latter group is mostly composed of patients with low-grade disease and reversible immunodeficiency (e.g., medication), although spontaneous regression has also been reported in patients with high-grade disease [9]. CNS involvement and high-grade disease are associated with worse prognosis [8]. Until recently, among patients who progressed, the median survival ranged from 14 to 72 months from the time of diagnosis [7, 8]. With newly implemented chemoimmunotherapy regimens, namely, EPOCH-R (etoposide, prednisolone, oncovin/vincristine, cyclophosphamide, hydroxydaunorubicin, and rituximab/anti-CD20 monoclonal antibody) and interferon, 5-year overall survival in all-comers is now up to 70% [10, 11].

What Are the Pathologic Features of Pulmonary Lymphomatoid Granulomatosis?

Macroscopically, PLG presents as multiple bilateral, usually small (<1 cm) nodules, primarily involving the lower and mid-lung lobes. The nodules can occasionally become large and centrally necrotic. Cut surfaces have irregular and usually sharp borders, are tan-gray to yellow, and range from soft to firm depending on extent of necrosis, which may be punctate or extensive (Fig. 35.2).

Histologically, PLG is composed of a polymorphous and predominantly lymphocytic infiltrate with characteristic angiocentricity and angiodestruction (Fig. 35.3a, b). The lymphocytes infiltrate the vessel walls, compromising vascular integrity and resulting in infarct-like coagulative necrosis of the surrounding lung parenchyma. Plasma cells, immunoblasts, and histiocytes are seen in varying proportions, but neutrophils and eosinophils are absent or rare. The lesion-defining cell of this disease is an EBV-positive, usually large and atypical B cell, which may resemble an immunoblast or, rarely, a Hodgkin-like cell. The presence of central necrosis may resemble granulomatous inflammation; however, true granulomas are unusual in PLG and should raise suspicion for an infectious process or vasculitis. LG lesions in the skin, however, can elicit marked granulomatous reaction, making the identification of lesional EBV-positive B cells critical for accurate diagnosis.

Immunohistochemistry demonstrates CD45, CD20 (Fig. 35.3c), PAX5 (Fig. 35.3d), and variable CD30 (Fig. 35.3e) positivity in the large neoplastic cells, a variable number of which also express EBER by in situ hybridization (ISH) (Fig. 35.3f). The cells are negative for CD15. The background immune infiltrate is predominantly composed of CD3+ T cells, with a high CD4 to CD8 T-cell ratio.

B-cell clonality can be demonstrated in most cases of grade 2 (50%) and grade 3 (69%) disease but is not consistently identified in grade 1 lesions (up to 8%). This has been generally

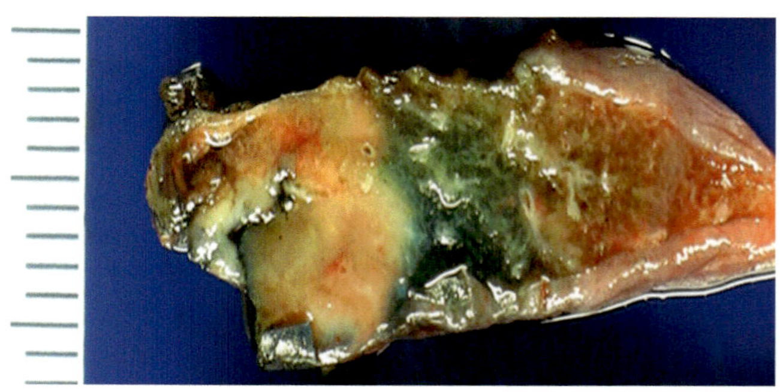

Fig. 35.2 Cut section of pulmonary lymphomatoid granulomatosis demonstrates an irregular well-demarcated pale yellow lesion, displaying central necrosis with punctate necrosis peripherally

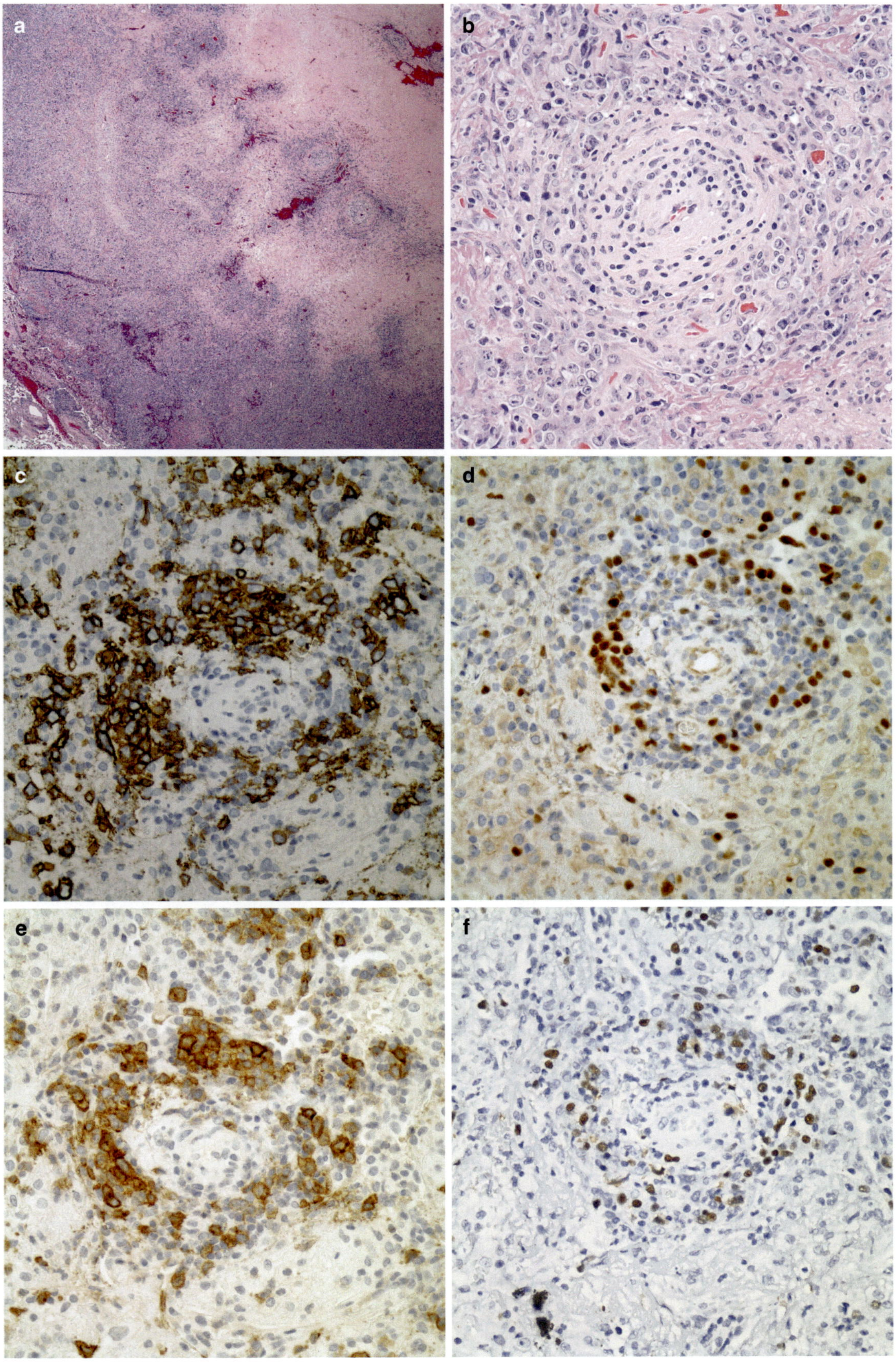

Fig. 35.3 Histologically, pulmonary lymphomatoid granulomatosis is characterized by a polymorphous lymphoid infiltrate displaying angiocentricity and angiodestruction associated with infarct-like coagulative necrosis (**a**, Hematoxylin and eosin, 40×). Admixed are large, atypical lymphocytes that penetrate through the vessel wall (**b**, Hematoxylin and eosin, 400×). These lesional cells are positive for B-cell markers CD20 (**c** DAB, 400×) and PAX5 (**d**, DAB, 400×). They can also stain with CD30 (**e**, DAB, 400×) and display variable EBV positivity (**f**, EBER ISH, 400×)

Table 35.1 Grading and histologic features of lymphomatoid granulomatosis

Grade	Polymorphous lymphocytic background	Necrosis	EBV-positive atypical B cells (average across entire lesion)[a]
1	Abundant	Absent or focal	<5 per HPF
2	Abundant	Present	5–20 per HPF[b]
3	Moderate[c]	Present, extensive	>50 per HPF[d]

Abbreviations: *HPF* high-power field, *PLG* pulmonary lymphomatoid granulomatosis, *NOS* not otherwise specified

[a] Transthoracic needle aspirates and transbronchial biopsies are too small for adequate evaluation and grading of PLG as it tends to be heterogeneous, requiring assessment of an average of EBV-positive B cells across an entire lesion. Wedge biopsy by video-assisted thoracoscopic surgery (VATS) or open thoracotomy to include at least one radiographically discrete nodule is recommended

[b] Clusters of up to 50 EBV-positive B cells may be found in grade 2 PLG

[c] In the absence of the background reactive infiltrate, the lesion should be classified as EBV-positive diffuse large B-cell lymphoma, NOS

[d] Focally, small confluent sheets of EBV-positive large B cells may be seen in grade 3 PLG. Pleomorphic and Hodgkin-like cells may also be seen in grade 3 lesions

attributed to the relative proportion of the lesional EBV-positive B cells [12]. Background T cells do not show T-cell receptor gene clonal rearrangement [12–14]. No specific oncogenic or cytogenetic abnormalities have been identified to date.

Grading of PLG is based on the number of EBV-positive B cells, determined by in situ hybridization for EBER, which is the most sensitive method (Table 35.1). Histologic features such as the amount of the background inflammatory infiltrate and degree of necrosis are helpful initial hints, but they are neither necessary nor sufficient for grading of PLG (Table 35.1). Due to lesional heterogeneity, biopsy material is insufficient for accurate grading, which should be done across the entire lesion, and therefore requires at least a wedge resection.

What Are the Main Differential Diagnoses of Pulmonary Lymphomatoid Granulomatosis?

The differential diagnosis of PLG includes other lymphomas, especially nasal-type extranodal NK/T-cell lymphoma and DLBCL. All three entities can demonstrate varying degrees of angiocentricity and angiodestruction and can involve the lung. Specifically, primary extranodal NK/T-cell lymphoma of the lung (nasal type) is very rare and highly aggressive, and it is one of the major neoplastic differential diagnoses of PLG, due to significant clinical, radiologic, and pathologic overlap. Histologically, the cells can be variable in size (small to large) with inconspicuous nucleoli and abundant pale cytoplasm. There is characteristic angioinvasion and angiodestruction with associated coagulative necrosis, and prominent inflammatory infiltrates may be present. Definitive diagnosis and differentiation from PLG require IHC with or without T-cell clonality analysis (in rare cases with T-cell rather than NK-cell origin). Although lesional cells are EBV+ and can express CD30, they lack B-cell marker expression (CD20, PAX5) and most typically display immunoreactivity with cytoplasmic CD3ε (but not surface CD3), CD56, granzyme-B, and TIA-1 [15]. Grade 3 PLG must be distinguished from EBV-positive DLBCL, the latter of which lacks background polymorphous inflammatory cells and is composed entirely of a uniform population of large atypical EBV+ B cells. Posttransplant lymphoproliferative disorder (PTLD) morphologically overlaps with PLG. Clinical history of transplantation is important to help make proper diagnosis, and PLG now is classified as PTLD in transplant recipients [2].

Nonneoplastic differential diagnoses include infection, particularly with fungal or mycobacterial organisms. Similar to PLG, angioinvasive fungal infections, including pulmonary aspergillosis and mucormycosis, affect the immunocompromised host and display angiodestruction with associated infarct-like necrosis. Definitive granulomas may be seen at the periphery but are often absent, and fungal elements may not be readily identifiable on H&E. Therefore, in nonneoplastic lung specimens with necrosis, routine examination for microorganisms is required to rule out infectious etiologies. PAS and GMS special stains can be used to highlight fungal hyphae. While *Aspergillus* has narrow (3–6 microns) uniformly septate hyphae with acute angle branching (<90°), *Mucor* has a ribbon-like appearance with broad (10–25 mm) thin-walled nonseptate hyphae with right-angle branching. However, culture confirmation of fungal species is necessary, as degenerative changes in *Aspergillus* can make it morphologically identical to *Mucor*. Identification of fruiting bodies (conidia) on histology, however, is specific for *Aspergillus*. Most importantly, invasive fungal disease has a distinct infectious clinical presentation with fever and leukocytosis evolving into sepsis. Mycobacterial infection (tuberculous and nontuberculous) can present with cavitary lesions or distinct lung nodules (uni- or multifocal) and is characterized by necrotizing granulomatous inflammation with or without multinucleated giant cells. Organisms may be detected by AFB stain, but cultures are much more sensitive and should be done on fresh tissue in cases where mycobacterial infection is suspected. In contrast to PLG, some mycobacterial lesions tend to be upper lobe predominant, due to organismal preference for higher oxygen tension and lower blood flow. AFB and/or FITE special stains can also identify *Nocardia* spp., weakly Gram-positive beaded filamentous bacteria, some of which can lead to pulmonary Nocardiosis in immunocompromised patients and can mimic PLG radiographically and histologically. However, similar to invasive fungal disease, patients with Nocardiosis have clinical signs and symptoms of infection.

Finally, one must distinguish PLG (especially grade 1 lesions that may lack clonality or EBV-positive B cells) from granulomatosis with polyangiitis (GPA) that is limited to the lung. The latter is characterized by the presence of true granulomas with palisaded histiocytes and frequently giant cells, at the periphery of areas with geographic necrosis. Serologic studies for ANCA are of additional utility in making this distinction.

How Does One Differentiate Pulmonary Lymphomatoid Granulomatosis from Granulomatosis with Polyangiitis?

Granulomatosis with polyangiitis (GPA), formerly known as Wegener granulomatosis, is a systemic vasculitis affecting small- and medium-sized vessels in multiple organs with a predilection for the upper respiratory tract and kidneys. It belongs to a group of antineutrophil cytoplasmic antibody (ANCA)-associated vasculitides, which also include microscopic polyangiitis (including renal-limited vasculitis) and eosinophilic granulomatosis with polyangiitis (aka Churg-Strauss). The disease process in GPA is mediated by ANCA, which is thought to activate neutrophils and promote their adhesion to the endothelium and degranulation, leading to direct vessel wall damage. Granulomatous tissue reaction and necrosis ensue [16, 17].

Pulmonary involvement occurs in >90% of LG cases and is the most common site of initial presentation [2], while GPA is limited to the upper respiratory tract and/or lungs in only about 25% of patients [18]. The initial clinical presentation of GPA depends on the involved organs, but patients most commonly present with rhinosinusitis and epistaxis. More than 50% of patients will also have ocular involvement with scleritis and conjunctivitis. Up to 85% of patients have kidney involvement and ultimately develop glomerulonephritis, which presents with hypertension and edema, and most progress to chronic renal failure [19–21]. Isolated pulmonary disease is extremely rare, which along with upper respiratory symptoms and positive c-ANCA serology (90% of GPA) helps to clinically distinguish GPA from PLG. Treatment with corticosteroids and cyclophosphamide is effective in most patients with severe disease (i.e., with kidney involvement), and up to 75% have complete remission [20]. However, approximately half of the patients will have disease recurrence [20].

As described above, LG patients are typically middle aged at presentation [1, 4], with a male predominance (2:1 male to female ratio). LG occurs primarily in the presence of at least some degree of immunodeficiency (congenital, acquired, or medication). Although a racial predilection has not been described, there seem to be more reported cases in Western countries compared to Asia [2].

On the other hand, patients with GPA are generally immunocompetent at presentation, older adults (although mean age at diagnosis is 55, cases in the 80s are common), and predominantly Caucasian (>90%). GPA shows no gender predilection [21].

The most common radiographic (CT) findings in GPA are bilateral, predominantly lower lobe, well-demarcated, and often spiculated nodules [22]. Cavitation of the nodules is a common feature (~50%), and the appearance of lesions can vary with time and on follow-up. GPA can also radiographically mimic a pulmonary infarct by appearing as a wedge-shaped peripheral opacity. Some cases of GPA present with pulmonary hemorrhage, which appear as diffuse infiltrates or airspace opacities. The latter two radiographic findings are not seen in PLG.

Histologically, GPA is characterized by vasculitis involving small veins and arteries, with frequent concomitant capillaritis (neutrophils within alveolar walls). The extent of vessel wall involvement varies widely even within the same lesion, with some areas demonstrating only endothelial and subendothelial injury, while others have full vessel wall involvement/obliteration. Mixed inflammatory cells including lymphocytes, plasma cells, and macrophages and/or poorly formed granulomas infiltrate the vessel walls, leading to vascular damage and necrosis. This results in geographic collagenous necrosis, another prominent feature of GPA, and one that can often be difficult to distinguish from the infarct-like coagulative necrosis of PLG. It is generally more basophilic, a characteristic imparted to GPA by the abundance of neutrophils (i.e., nucleated material). The final cardinal feature of GPA is extensive mixed inflammatory background composed of lymphocytes, plasma cells, macrophages, neutrophils (with neutrophilic microabscesses), eosinophils, and multinucleated giant cells. The latter can be found both within the involved vessels and the affected background lung parenchyma, which is another feature that can help distinguish GPA from PLG.

Immunohistochemical stains are not generally helpful for diagnosing GPA. However, CD20 IHC and EBER ISH should be done to rule out PLG in the appropriate clinical context. Elastin stain can help highlight angiocentric/angiodestructive nature of the lesion, and special stains for microorganisms (GMS, PAS, AFB) should be done to rule out fungal and mycobacterial infection.

References

1. Liebow AA, Carrington CR, Friedman PJ. Lymphomatoid granulomatosis. Hum Pathol. 1972;3(4):457–558.
2. Swerdlow SH, Campo E, Harris NL, Jaffe ES, Pileri SA, Stein H, et al. WHO classification of tumours of haematopoietic and lymphoid tissues. Lyon, France: IARC Publications; 2016.
3. Tagliavini E, Rossi G, Valli R, Zanelli M, Cadioli A, Mengoli MC, et al. Lymphomatoid granulomatosis: a practical review for

pathologists dealing with this rare pulmonary lymphoproliferative process. Pathologica. 2013;105(4):111–6.
4. Pisani RJ, DeRemee RA. Clinical implications of the histopathologic diagnosis of pulmonary lymphomatoid granulomatosis. Mayo Clin Proc. 1990;65(2):151–63.
5. Lee JS, Tuder R, Lynch DA. Lymphomatoid granulomatosis: radiologic features and pathologic correlations. AJR Am J Roentgenol. 2000;175(5):1335–9.
6. Sirajuddin A, Raparia K, Lewis VA, Franks TJ, Dhand S, Galvin JR, et al. Primary pulmonary lymphoid lesions: radiologic and pathologic findings. Radiographics. 2016;36(1):53–70.
7. Jaffe ES, Wilson WH. Lymphomatoid granulomatosis: pathogenesis, pathology and clinical implications. Cancer Surv. 1997;30:233–48.
8. Katzenstein AL, Carrington CB, Liebow AA. Lymphomatoid granulomatosis: a clinicopathologic study of 152 cases. Cancer. 1979;43(1):360–73.
9. Aiko N, Sekine A, Umeda S, Katano T, Matama G, Isomoto K, et al. The spontaneous regression of grade 3 methotrexate-related lymphomatoid granulomatosis: a case report and literature review. Intern Med. 2018;57(21):3163–7.
10. Roschewski M, Wilson WH. Lymphomatoid granulomatosis. Cancer J. 2012;18(5):469–74.
11. Wilson WH, Kingma DW, Raffeld M, Wittes RE, Jaffe ES. Association of lymphomatoid granulomatosis with Epstein-Barr viral infection of B lymphocytes and response to interferon-alpha 2b. Blood. 1996;87(11):4531–7.
12. Song JY, Pittaluga S, Dunleavy K, Grant N, White T, Jiang L, et al. Lymphomatoid granulomatosis--a single institute experience: pathologic findings and clinical correlations. Am J Surg Pathol. 2015;39(2):141–56.
13. McNiff JM, Cooper D, Howe G, Crotty PL, Tallini G, Crouch J, et al. Lymphomatoid granulomatosis of the skin and lung. An angiocentric T-cell-rich B-cell lymphoproliferative disorder. Arch Dermatol. 1996;132(12):1464–70.
14. Medeiros LJ, Peiper SC, Elwood L, Yano T, Raffeld M, Jaffe ES. Angiocentric immunoproliferative lesions: a molecular analysis of eight cases. Hum Pathol. 1991;22(11):1150–7.
15. Ding W, Wang J, Zhao S, Yang Q, Sun H, Yan J, et al. Clinicopathological study of pulmonary extranodal nature killer/T--cell lymphoma, nasal type and literature review. Pathol Res Pract. 2015;211(7):544–9.
16. Grygiel-Gorniak B, Limphaibool N, Perkowska K, Puszczewicz M. Clinical manifestations of granulomatosis with polyangiitis: key considerations and major features. Postgrad Med. 2018;130(7):581–96.
17. Nakazawa D, Masuda S, Tomaru U, Ishizu A. Pathogenesis and therapeutic interventions for ANCA-associated vasculitis. Nat Rev Rheumatol. 2019;15:91–101.
18. Stone JH, Wegener's Granulomatosis Etanercept Trial Research G. Limited versus severe Wegener's granulomatosis: baseline data on patients in the Wegener's granulomatosis etanercept trial. Arthritis Rheum. 2003;48(8):2299–309.
19. Fauci AS, Haynes BF, Katz P, Wolff SM. Wegener's granulomatosis: prospective clinical and therapeutic experience with 85 patients for 21 years. Ann Intern Med. 1983;98(1):76–85.
20. Hoffman GS, Kerr GS, Leavitt RY, Hallahan CW, Lebovics RS, Travis WD, et al. Wegener granulomatosis: an analysis of 158 patients. Ann Intern Med. 1992;116(6):488–98.
21. Seo P, Stone JH. The antineutrophil cytoplasmic antibody-associated vasculitides. Am J Med. 2004;117(1):39–50.
22. Martinez F, Chung JH, Digumarthy SR, Kanne JP, Abbott GF, Shepard JA, et al. Common and uncommon manifestations of Wegener granulomatosis at chest CT: radiologic-pathologic correlation. Radiographics. 2012;32(1):51–69.

36 Primary Pulmonary Classic Hodgkin Lymphoma Versus Other Non-Hodgkin Lymphomas

Zhao Ming (David) Dong and Paul D. Simonson

Case Presentation

A 64-year-old man presented to the emergency room with fatigue, night sweats, dry cough, lost taste for both food and cigarettes, and a 30-pound weight loss for 2 months. He had multiple risk factors for lung carcinoma including emphysema, smoking for 40 years, and likely asbestos exposure (welder for 35 years). Physical examination did not reveal clubbing, peripheral lymphadenopathy, or hepatosplenomegaly. Laboratory investigations revealed mild anemia (Hb 11.2 g/dL), thrombocytosis (platelets 527 K/μL), and leukocytosis (WBC 12.8 K/μL). There were no other hematological or biochemical abnormalities. Chest X-ray demonstrated a prominent hilum. The patient was treated with antibiotics without symptom improvement. A subsequent computed tomography (CT) of the chest showed a right upper lobe mass with extension into hilum, highly suspicious for primary lung carcinoma. Endobronchial biopsies were performed twice. At bronchoscopy, there was a large, exophytic mass in the right upper lobe apical segment and an area of irregular nodularity in the lateral wall of the bronchus intermedius. The right middle lobe and right lower lobe airways appeared normal. A biopsy was performed, which contained four fragments of bronchial tissue, one of which showed focal necrosis (Fig. 36.1a) and scattered large mononuclear Hodgkin cells and classic Reed-Sternberg cells (Fig. 36.1b) which were positive for CD30 (Fig. 36.1c), weakly positive for PAX-5 (Fig. 36.1d), and negative for CD20 (Fig. 36.1e), on a background of predominantly CD3+ T cells, plasma cells, neutrophils, histiocytes, and occasional eosinophils. The patient refused further tests for complete staging and treatment. He died 2 months after the diagnosis was made.

Z. Ming (David) Dong (✉)
Department of Laboratory Medicine and Pathology, Puget Sound VA Health Care System, University of Washington School of Medicine, Seattle, WA, USA
e-mail: Zhaoming.dong@va.gov

P. D. Simonson
Department of Pathology and Laboratory Medicine, Weill Cornell Medicine/New York-Presbyterian Hospital, New York, NY, USA

H. Xu et al. (eds.), *Practical Lung Pathology*, Practical Anatomic Pathology, https://doi.org/10.1007/978-3-031-14402-8_36

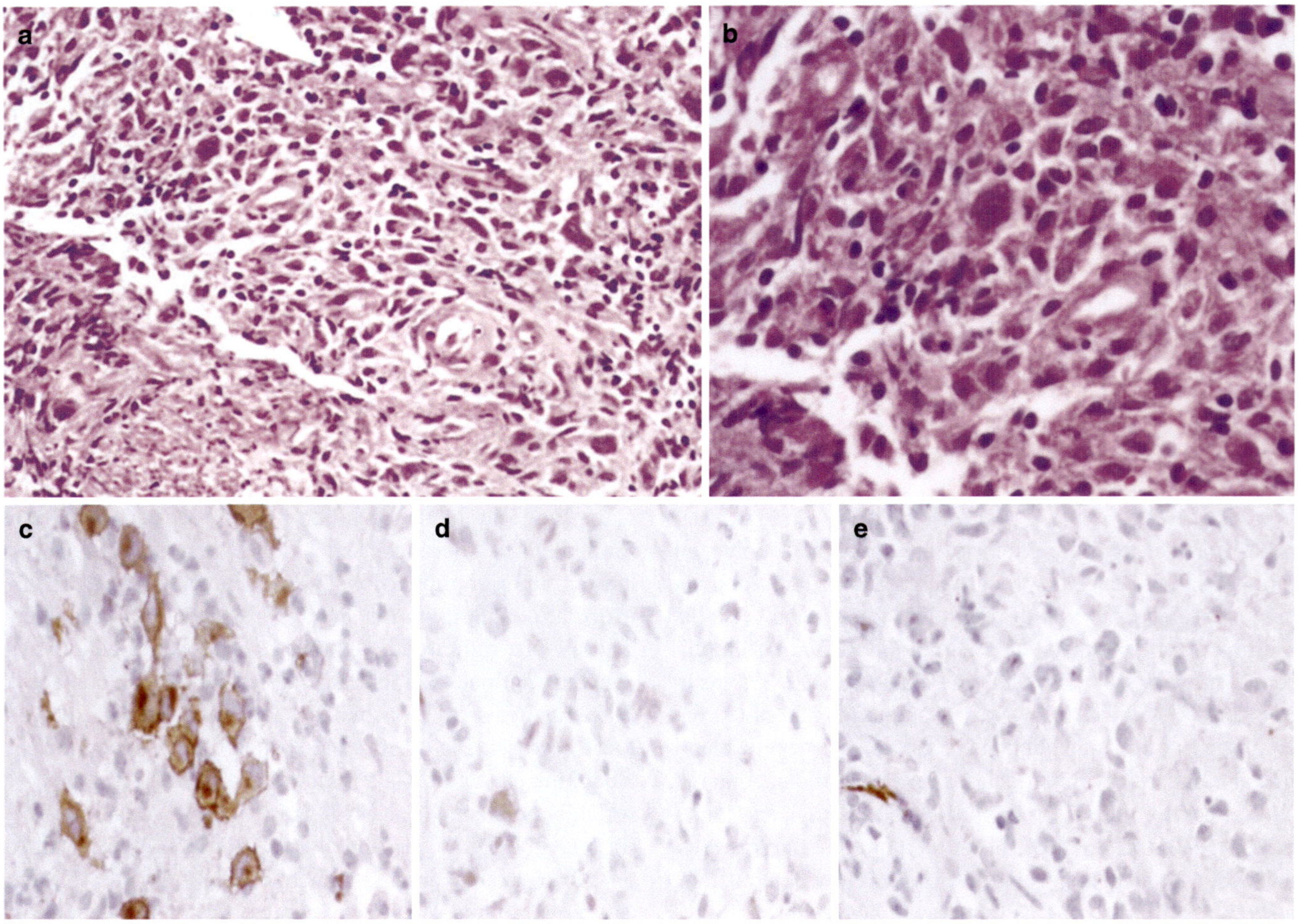

Fig. 36.1 Endobronchial biopsy of pulmonary mass, consistent with classic Hodgkin lymphoma, characterized by a polymorphous inflammatory infiltrate with focal necrosis (**a**, Hematoxylin and eosin, 200×). Admixed are large atypical mononuclear Hodgkin cells and classical Reed-Sternberg cells (**b**, Hematoxylin and eosin, 400×). These atypical cells are positive for CD30 (**c**, DAB, 400×) and PAX5 (**d**, DAB, 400×) and negative for CD20 (**e**, DAB, 400×)

Pathologic Diagnosis: Pulmonary Classic Hodgkin Lymphoma, Probably Primary

What Is the Definition of a Primary Pulmonary Classic Hodgkin Lymphoma (PPCHL)?

The criteria for the diagnosis of PPCHL include (1) histologic features of Hodgkin lymphoma; (2) restriction of the disease to the lung, with or without minimal hilar lymph node involvement; and (3) adequate clinical and/or pathological exclusion of the disease at distant sites, i.e., with no detectable extrapulmonary involvement at diagnosis or during the following 3 months. PPCHL is thought to originate from bronchial mucosa-associated lymphoid tissue or peribronchial lymph nodes and extends to the parenchyma of the lung. Our case meets two of these three criteria for diagnosis of PPCHL. However, since further tests for complete staging were not performed, secondary pulmonary involvement by nodal classic Hodgkin lymphoma (SPCHL) cannot be excluded.

SPCHL is common and occurs in 15–40% of nodal CHL cases. In contrast, PPCHL is extremely rare, with fewer than 100 cases reported worldwide. Radin AL reviewed 61 cases reported in the literature from 1927 to 1986 [1]. Most of the cases included occurred in an era when the available diagnostic imaging studies such as chest X-ray would be considered outdated by today's standard. Undoubtedly, some of the cases would not be true PPCHL if modern high-resolution computed tomography (HRCT) and positron emission tomography (PET)-CT were used to search for mediastinal and extrapulmonary disease.

What Are the Clinical, Radiographic, and Prognostic Features and Treatment of PPCHL?

Clinical presentation is nonspecific. The most common presenting symptoms are weight loss, fever, night sweats, and dry cough. Dyspnea and hemoptysis are also common. In the largest report, PPCHL showed a slight female preponderance (1.4:1 F:M), with a bimodal age distribution (<35 and >60 years; mean age 42 years).

Radiologically, PPCHL typically involves the upper lobe of the lung, whereas SPCHL shows a more random miliary distribution, without zonal predilection. Many present as a solitary mass, alveolar consolidation, multiple nodules, or cavitated lesions, and rarely as an endobronchial lesion. However, no radiological sign is pathognomonic for PPCHL [2].

Owing to the rarity of the disease and lack of survival data, prognostic factors affecting the survival of PPCHL are not well defined. However, several factors have been suggested: "B" symptoms, bilateral disease, multilobar involvement, penetration of the pleura (with or without associated pleural effusion), cavitation, age greater than 60 years, and clinical relapses [2]. Nakachi et al. found that 14 of 23 patients with PPCHL survived, and 4 relapsed or died [3].

Management plans vary in the literature. Traditionally, in cases reported prior to 1960, the modality of treatment was surgical excision. Since then a better understanding of the pathogenesis of lymphoma has led to a preference for combination chemotherapy, especially for disseminated disease throughout the lung. Some reports have suggested the use of radiation therapy for limited disease, but the risk of radiation-induced pneumonitis should be considered. Recently, immunotherapy such as monoclonal antibody brentuximab vedotin is being used to treat some cases of nodal CHL [4]. Chimeric antigen receptor (CAR) T-cell therapy is available in clinical trials. Given that most CHL is genetically programmed to overexpress PD-L1, immune checkpoint inhibitors show encouraging clinical efficacy in treatment of CHL [5]. These treatments could be applied to PPCHL.

What Are the Pathologic Features of PPCHL?

The nodal CHL can be classified into four subtypes known as nodular sclerosis, mixed cellularity, lymphocyte rich, and lymphocyte depleted. In PPCHL, the nodular sclerosis subtype is most common, followed by mixed cellularity subtype. However, if only a small biopsy is available, separating these subtypes is not practical.

PPCHL displays morphologic and immunophenotypic features similar to nodal CHL. The characteristic cell of CHL is the Reed-Sternberg cell (RS cell), a large binucleated or multinucleated cell with prominent, eosinophilic nucleoli. Mononuclear variants of RS cells (Hodgkin cells) may include pyknotic, mummified cells and lacunar variants with cytoplasmic retraction artifact. Given that both cell types are malignant, they are also referred to as HRS cells. Some cases contain these HRS cells in large clusters or sheets (called syncytial growth pattern). Background reactive cells include histiocytes, small lymphocytes, eosinophils, plasma cells, and neutrophils. Tumor nodules may show central necrosis, neutrophilic microabscesses, or granuloma-like changes. Nodular sclerosis subtype shows dense collagen bands. HRS cells are derived from clonal germinal center B (GCB) cells, having rearranged and mutated immunoglobulin variable genes; however, with the exception of PAX-5 (weakly to moderately immunopositive in almost all cases), typical B-cell surface makers (CD45, CD19, CD79a) and transcription factors (OCT-2 and BOB1) are downregulated or completely absent in HRS cells, and CD20 is expressed in only 20% of cases, with low density. In contrast, HRS cells are strongly positive for CD30 by immunohistochemical stains, with membranous and Golgi staining pattern in nearly all cases. 75–85% of cases express CD15, but in our experience, the percentage of cases expressing CD15 appears to be less than that. The variation in CD15-positivity rate most likely is due to variable CD15 expression among HRS cells, sometimes only seen in a few HRS cells. HRS cells are usually positive for MUM-1. At present, flow cytometry has not been applied to routinely immunophenotype and confirm a diagnosis of CHL. However, HRS cells can be isolated by sensitive flow cytometric gating strategies and characterized as (1) expression of CD30, CD40, and CD95; (2) increased forward and side scatter compared with normal lymphocytes; (3) lack of bright expression of CD20; (4) lack of expression of CD64; and (5) a discrete cluster in multidimensional space [6]. In our experience, flow cytometry is especially useful as an adjunct to immunohistochemical analysis in the diagnosis of CHL when only a very small biopsy is available and/or immunohistochemical stains show an equivocal phenotype.

The association between nodal CHL and Epstein-Barr virus has long been known. However, the frequency of associated EBV varies greatly. The highest rate of EBV infection is seen in mixed cellularity CHL, followed by lymphocyte-depleted CHL, lesions occurring in immunodeficient patients, and those from developing countries. There are only a few reports of PPCHL associated with EBV infection [7].

Cooksley et al. recently reviewed 20 cases of PPCHL reported in the literature from 2006 to 2014 [2]. Among these, most cases were diagnosed through wedge biopsy rather than endobronchial biopsy, since endobronchial lesions are rare. Therefore, the diagnosis of PPCHL usually requires an open thoracotomy or lung biopsy. Our presented case is a rare one, with irregular nodularity in the lateral wall of the bronchus intermedius in the right upper lobe as identified by bronchoscopic evaluation.

What Are the Differential Diagnoses for PPCHL?

Since the diagnostic process is commonly challenging, the term between initial diagnosis and final diagnosis for any primary pulmonary lymphoma reportedly is from half a month to 2 years, with a median time to the diagnosis of PPCHL of 6 months [8]. Due to its rarity and lack of specific clinical and radiological features, the initial clinical diagnoses of 20 reported cases of PPCHL from 2006 to 2014 were mainly infectious/inflammatory diseases and lung carcinomas, rather than lymphoma [2]. In some cases of PPCHL, there may be foci of central necrosis with or without cavitation, rimmed in part by histiocytes and giant cells, which can mimic other granulomatous lesions, such as tuberculosis, granulomatosis with polyangiitis, and fungal infection. The classical clinical findings of granulomatosis with polyangiitis, such as nasopharyngeal and renal involvement, and the presence of histologic and immunophenotypic features of HRS cells within granulomas in CHL should allow separation between these entities. In granulomatous infection, the caseous necrosis, lack of HRS cells, and presence of organisms help in the differential diagnosis.

Lung carcinoma and CHL usually are easily distinguished by morphology (except CHL with syncytial growth pattern). However, it has been reported that metastatic undifferentiated nasopharyngeal carcinoma (UNPC) can have striking morphologic and immunophenotypic resemblance to CHL [9]. UNPC can express CD30, while CHL can have weak expression of cytokeratin and be negative for PAX-5. In addition, CHL and UNPC can overlap clinically and etiologically. Both are associated with EBV infection and can present in adolescents and young adults as enlarged cervical lymph nodes and multiple lung nodules. Therefore, metastatic UNPC in the lung can raise diagnostic challenges for PPCHL. Clinical presentation with a nasopharyngeal lesion and/or a history of UNPC and inclusion of an extensive immunohistochemistry panel can play a critical role in distinguishing these two diseases.

When PPCHLs lack typical binucleated RS cells or show atypical immunophenotype, they can closely resemble other non-Hodgkin lymphomas (NHLs), including T-cell/histiocyte-rich large B-cell lymphoma, anaplastic large cell lymphoma, peripheral T-cell lymphoma, not otherwise specified (NOS), EBV+ diffuse large B-cell lymphoma, NOS, and lymphomatoid granulomatosis (LG). Although these NHLs are also not commonly seen in routine pathology service for lung biopsies, they have been identified as distinct entities of primary pulmonary lymphoma. Chen et al. reported 72 cases of primary pulmonary lymphoma, which consisted of 56 cases of MALT lymphoma, 8 cases of large B-cell lymphoma, 3 cases of Hodgkin lymphoma, 4 cases of T-cell lymphoma, and 1 case of intravascular large B-cell lymphoma [10]. Because of the low incidence of primary pulmonary lymphoma, a high index of suspicion is required to initiate workup and carefully select appropriate and adequate immunohistochemistry panels for distinguishing these diseases from each other. Differential features between PPCHL and these NHLs are further discussed as follows:

T-Cell/Histiocyte-Rich Large B-Cell Lymphoma (THRLBCL)

This lymphoma can be very difficult to differentiate from CHL. Like CHL, THRLBCL shows scattered, large, malignant cells resembling mononuclear Hodgkin cells in a background containing numerous small lymphocytes and/or histiocytes. The large, malignant, lymphoid cells should comprise 10% or less of the overall cellularity. However, these large, atypical cells often do not include forms with a classic binucleated RS cell appearance, and the background infiltrate lacks eosinophils and neutrophils. The phenotype differs since the tumor cells are usually positive for B-cell surface makers (CD45, CD19, CD79a, CD20) and transcription factors (OCT-2 and BOB.1) and are negative for CD15, even though they can express CD30. In our experience, there are rare cases in which definitive differentiation between the two diseases by IHC cannot be made. In this instance, flow cytometry with special gating strategies and identification of HRS cells with co-expression of CD30, CD40, and CD95 are useful, and the WHO classification of B-cell lymphoma, unclassifiable, with features intermediate between diffuse large B-cell lymphoma and classic Hodgkin lymphoma ("gray zone lymphoma") may also be considered.

Anaplastic Large Cell Lymphoma (ALCL)

This lymphoma is a CD30+ lymphoma of T or "null" cell lineage, with or without expression of ALK-1. Even though the tumor cells are typically seen in sheets and clusters, unlike the scattered tumor cells of CHL (except syncytial pattern), the morphologic spectrum of both CHL and ALCL can be similar. If one relies solely on morphology and a limited immunohistochemistry panel, ALCL may be incorrectly diagnosed. Virtually all cases of ALCL are uniformly positive for CD30 and EMA. EMA positivity can rarely be seen in CHL, and PAX5 helps distinguish between the two in most instances. In rare cases, PAX-5 expression in CHL is extremely weak; such a case can be easily misdiagnosed as ALCL with null cell phenotype. However, T-cell receptor gene rearrangement studies showing no evidence of T-cell clonality argue against ALCL.

Peripheral T-Cell Lymphoma, Not Otherwise Specified (PTCL)

PTCL, like CHL, can have highly atypical large cells with RS-like features in a mixed inflammatory background. CD30 positivity can be seen in these cases, and even CD15 positivity can rarely be observed. Given that CHL is usually CD20 negative and CHL can aberrantly express T-cell antigens, a misdiagnosis of T-cell lymphoma may occur. However, most CHL cases will be dimly positive for PAX-5 and uniformly express CD30 (other than variable expression in PTCL). In addition, TCR gene rearrangement studies commonly show evidence of T-cell clonality in PTCL.

EBV+ Diffuse Large B-Cell Lymphoma (EBV+ DLBCL), NOS

This lymphoma shows clonal B cells that are positive for EBV but do not fall into one of the other named EBV-positive groups (such as lymphomatoid granulomatosis) in persons with no documented immunodeficiency. EBV should be demonstrated using EBER in situ hybridization stains, as LMP1 immunohistochemistry has a very low sensitivity compared to EBER. Morphologically, the polymorphic subtype shows a mixed proliferation of large, transformed cells, plasma cells, plasmablasts, lymphocytes, and, commonly, RS-like cells, whereas the monomorphic subtype reveals sheets of large cells. An additional characteristic feature is large areas of "geographic" necrosis. This lymphoma is often positive for CD30. Therefore, the most challenging differential diagnosis is EBV+ CHL. Strong, homogeneous expression of B-cell markers, including transcription factors OCT2 and BOB.1, and lack of CD15 support a diagnosis of EBV+ DLBCL, NOS.

Pulmonary Lymphomatoid Granulomatosis (PLG)

PLG has been well described in a separate chapter. In brief, PLG is a rare EBV+ B-cell lymphoproliferative disorder that predominantly affects the lung, which is characterized by a polymorphous lymphocytic infiltration containing EBV+, large, atypical B cells with morphology resembling immunoblasts and rarely HRS-like cells in a background with necrosis. Morphologic features with the presence of HRS-like cells, positivity for EBV, and necrosis in PLG can overlap with CHL. However, characteristic angioinvasion and angiodestruction of PLG is not seen in CHL. Although lesional cells are EBV+ and can express variable CD30, the cells in PLG commonly express CD45, CD19, CD79a, and CD20 without expression of CD15.

References

1. Radin AI. Primary pulmonary Hodgkin's disease. Cancer. 1990;65:550–63.
2. Cooksley N, Judge DJ, Brown J. Primary pulmonary Hodgkin's lymphoma and a review of the literature since. BMJ Case Rep. 2006;2014:2014–204020.
3. Nakachi S, Nagasaki A, Owen I, et al. Primary pulmonary Hodgkin lymphoma: two case reports and a review of the literature. Gan To Kagaku Ryoho. 2007;34:2279–82.
4. Connors JM, Ansell SM, Fanale M, Park SI, Younes A. Five-year follow-up of brentuximab vedotin combined with ABVD or AVD for advanced-stage classical Hodgkin lymphoma. Blood. 2017;130:1375–7.
5. Ansell SM, Lesokhin AM, Borrello I, et al. pd-1 blockade with nivolumab in relapsed or refractory Hodgkin's lymphoma. N Engl J Med. 2015;372:311–9.
6. Fromm JR, Thomas A, Wood BL. Flow cytometry can diagnose classical Hodgkin lymphoma in lymph nodes with high sensitivity and specificity. Am J Clin Pathol. 2009;131:322–32.
7. Stachura T, Malinowski E. Primary pulmonary Hodgkin's lymphoma with Epstein-Barr and cytomegaly virus infections. A case report and differential diagnosis. Pol J Pathol. 2003;54:79–83.
8. Yao D, Zhang L, Wu PL, Gu XL, Chen YF, Wang LX, Huang XY. Clinical and misdiagnosed analysis of primary pulmonary lymphoma: a retrospective study. BMC Cancer. 2018;18:281–5.
9. Jabbour MN, Nassif S, Chakhachiro Z. Undifferentiated nasopharyngeal carcinoma mimicking Hodgkin lymphoma with CD30 expression. Int J Surg Pathol. 2016;24:715–7.
10. Chen Y, Chen A, Jiang H, Zhang Y, Zhu L, Xia C, Yu H. HRCT in primary pulmonary lymphoma: can CT imaging phenotypes differentiate histological subtypes between mucosa-associated lymphoid tissue (MALT) lymphoma and non-MALT lymphoma? J Thorac Dis. 2018;10:6040–8.

37 Posttransplant Lymphoproliferative Disorders in Lung After Lung Transplantation Versus Infection and Inflammation

Paul D. Simonson and Zhao Ming (David) Dong

Case Presentation

A 59-year-old woman underwent bilateral lung transplant for overlapping chronic obstructive pulmonary disease and chronic bronchitis, in the setting of a 120-pack-year history of smoking cigarettes. Pretransplant evaluation demonstrated the presence of anti-EBV IgG but not IgM. After transplant, she had a prolonged hospital course that was complicated by acute respiratory distress syndrome, atrial fibrillation, acute renal failure, pneumonia, *Candida* wound infection, and rectal ulcer, necessitating a 4-month stay in the hospital. Immunosuppression was maintained using mycophenolate mofetil, tacrolimus, and steroids.

One month after discharge, the patient was readmitted after presentation at the pulmonary clinic with complaint of fevers and chills. A computed tomography (CT) scan demonstrated a 4.5 cm × 4.5 cm, well demarcated, central-enhancing, right upper lobe mass of the lung, as well as two 1–2 cm nodules in the left base and mediastinal adenopathy. A CT-guided needle biopsy of the right upper lobe mass demonstrated necrotic tissue and a proliferation of CD20-positive lymphocytes, some with large cell morphology and positive for EBV LMP1 immunostaining. The findings were consistent with posttransplant lymphoproliferative disorder (PTLD), suspicious for monomorphic diffuse large B-cell lymphoma (DLBCL) type. A bone marrow biopsy was negative for abnormal B-cell or plasma cell populations. Immunosuppression was decreased. A lung wedge resection was then performed. Grossly, the mass involved the visceral pleura. The cut surface was light pink and firm, with approximately 50% of the mass being necrotic. Microscopically, the specimen demonstrated the full range of CD20-positive B-cell maturation and polymorphism, from large immunoblasts to plasma cells, with small- and medium-sized lymphocytes in the background and multifocal necrosis (Fig. 37.1). Even though a kappa-light-chain-restricted clonal B-cell population was identified by flow cytometry, morphologic features of polymorphic lymphoplasmacytic proliferation argued against monomorphic DLBCL-type PTLD.

Weekly rituximab therapy (×4 weeks) was added in addition to the decrease in immunosuppression, her tacrolimus being decreased by 25% and her mycophenolate mofetil being decreased by 50%. Approximately 4 weeks after beginning treatment, the patient was feeling much better, with increased exercise tolerance. She denied any fevers, night sweats, bleeding, or bruising. Eight weeks after starting therapy for PTLD, there was no evidence of recurrence of the lung mass, no evidence of new or increased pulmonary nodules, and a decrease in mediastinal lymph nodes, consistent with remission. Four years later, the patient did not exhibit evidence of PTLD.

P. D. Simonson
Department of Pathology and Laboratory Medicine, Weill Cornell Medicine/New York-Presbyterian Hospital, New York, NY, USA

Z. Ming (David) Dong (✉)
Department of Laboratory Medicine and Pathology, Puget Sound VA Health Care System, University of Washington School of Medicine, Seattle, WA, USA
e-mail: Zhaoming.dong@va.gov

H. Xu et al. (eds.), *Practical Lung Pathology*, Practical Anatomic Pathology, https://doi.org/10.1007/978-3-031-14402-8_37

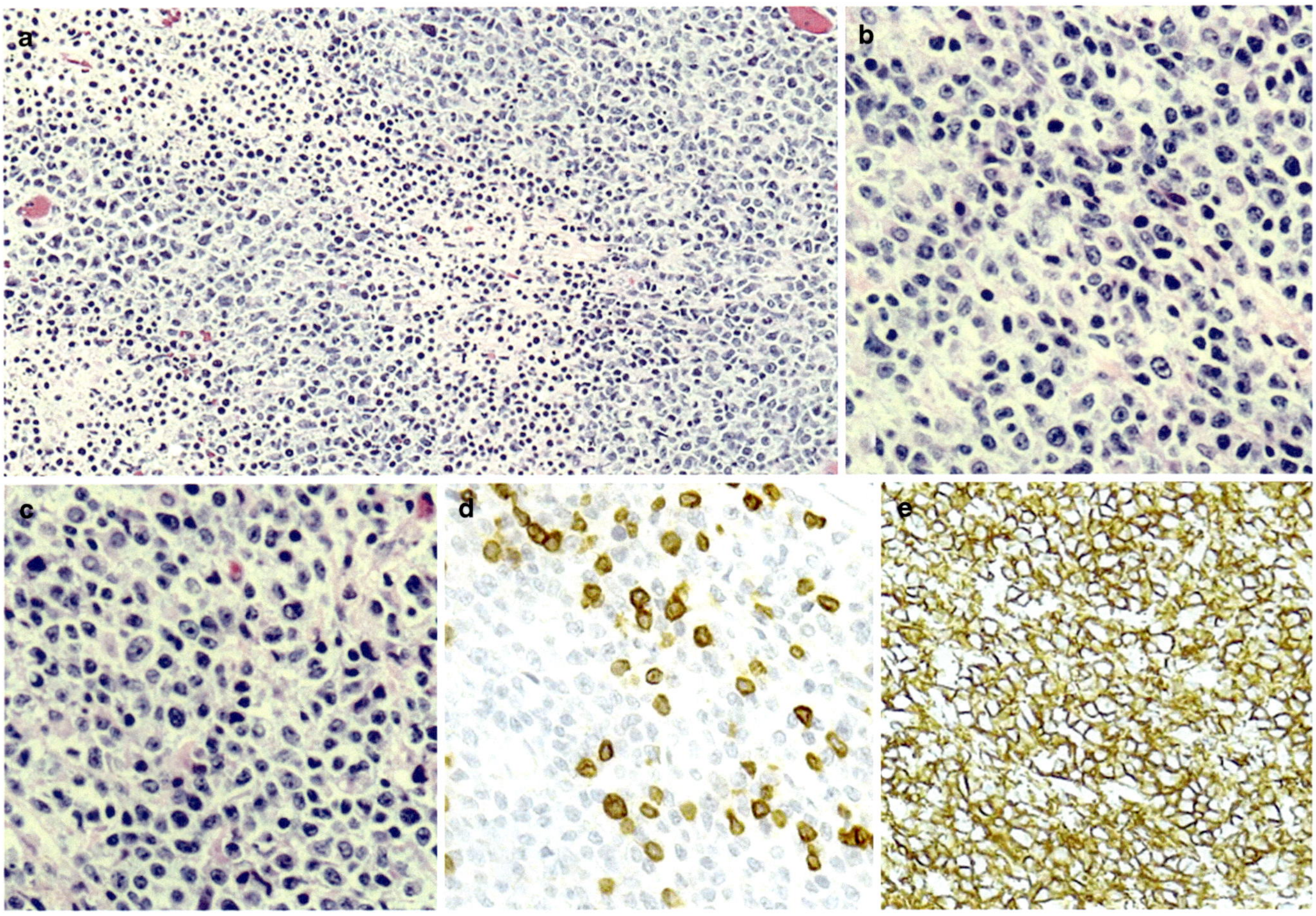

Fig. 37.1 Wedge resection of pulmonary mass, consistent with polymorphic PTLD. (**a**) Polymorphic infiltrate of lymphocytes effacing lung architecture with multifocal necrosis (large geographic areas of necrosis not shown, hematoxylin and eosin, 200×). (**b**, **c**) Polymorphic lymphocytes with atypical nuclei (hematoxylin and eosin, 200×). (**d**) CD3 immunostain (200×). (**e**) CD20 immunostain (100×)

Pathologic Diagnosis: EBV-Positive, Polymorphic Posttransplant Lymphoproliferative Disorder (PTLD) in the Lung After Transplantation

What Is the Definition of PTLD?

PTLD is defined in the current *World Health Organization (WHO) Classification of Tumors of Hematopoietic and Lymphoid Tissues* [1] as lymphoid or plasmacytic proliferations that develop as a consequence of immunosuppression in a recipient of a solid organ, bone marrow, or stem cell allograft. They constitute a spectrum that ranges from EBV-driven, polyclonal lymphoid proliferation to EBV-positive or EBV-negative proliferations indistinguishable from a subset of B-cell or, less often, T/NK-cell lymphomas that occur in immunocompetent individuals. The disorder is thought to be due to loss of control over EBV-immortalized B-cell lymphocytes as a result of loss of T-cell lymphocyte control, as a consequence of immunosuppression.

The highest risk of developing PTLDs exists in EBV-naïve patients who acquire the primary infection during solid organ transplantation. Risk of developing PTLD is highest in individuals receiving heart-lung, lung, or intestinal allografts, rather than stem cell transplant. Children have a much higher incidence than adults. Most solid organ-related PTLDs are of host origin, while most stem cell transplant-related PTLDs are of donor origin.

What Are the Clinical, Radiographic, Prognostic Features, and Treatment of PTLDs in the Lung After Lung Transplantation?

PTLDs in the setting of lung transplantation have some specificities [2]: a higher incidence (reportedly 2.5–8%) as compared with transplantation of most other organs (approximately 2× higher), frequent involvement of the engrafted lung, and the risk of dysfunction or loss of a vital graft if immunosuppression is reduced. Historically, most cases of PTLD among lung transplant recipients were reported to arise within the first year from transplantation (early-onset PTLD). However, more recent data suggest an increased incidence of PTLD cases beyond the first year from transplantation (late-onset PTLD). In a study that focused on differences between early and late appearing lung transplant PTLD [2], late appearing cases were less frequently positive for EBV with similar outcomes to early appearing cases. While early-onset PTLD nearly always involves the allograft lung, late appearing PTLD does so less frequently [3] with gastrointestinal tract involvement being more common [4]. Overall incidence of PTLD has decreased with time, presumably due to a combination of factors such as prolonged antiviral prophylaxis, improved detection assays, and anticipatory surveillance of EBV-negative patients.

Clinical presentation is variable, including fever and malaise, infectious mononucleosis-like disease, lymphadenopathy, mass lesions, viral septic shock-like presentations, and as an incidental finding [1].

Radiographically, lung findings may include isolated nodules or masses in the allograft, disseminated micronodules with an interstitial topography, or mediastinal lymphadenopathies [5]. In contrast, beyond the first year, intra-abdominal and disseminated forms of disease predominate [4].

Prognosis and management depend significantly on the category and subcategory of the identified PTLD. Nondestructive PTLDs often regress with reduction in immunosuppression (though graft rejection can limit the viability of this approach) and generally have an excellent prognosis. Many polymorphic PTLDs and some monomorphic PTLDs will also regress with decreased immunosuppression. Myelomatous lesions represent a group that generally is not expected to regress with decreased immunosuppression. When decreased immunosuppression fails to result in PTLD regression, other therapies may be tried, with varying results, including rituximab, brentuximab vedotin, chemotherapy, surgical excision, and local radiation. Classic Hodgkin lymphoma (CHL) PTLD is generally treated with conventional CHL therapy, with good results [1].

Serial monitoring of EBV DNA levels in peripheral blood is often used to help predict the risk and onset of PTLD and to guide preemptive therapy [4, 6]. Its use is likely most useful for seronegative solid organ transplant recipients, particularly children.

What Are the Pathologic Features of PTLDs in the Lung After Lung Transplantation?

There is tremendous heterogeneity in the histopathologic appearance of PTLDs. Currently, PTLDs are divided into four major categories based on the 2016 WHO classification [1]. Even though monomorphic PTLDs (M-PTLDs) are the most common subtype (60–80%), all other subtypes of PTLDs have been reported in the lung after lung transplantation, and their pathologic features are discussed as follows:

Nondestructive PTLDs

These PTLDs were formerly known as early lesions; however, this term has been deprecated due to confusion with the group of PTLDs that occur early after transplantation. By definition, these disorders are characterized by architectural preservation of the involved tissue and lack of features diagnostic of lymphoma. They can be subcategorized as plasmacytic hyperplasia, infectious mononucleosis-like, and florid follicular hyperplasia PTLDs. In plasmacytic hyperplasia, plasma cells are prominently admixed with small lymphocytes. In infectious mononucleosis-like lesions, there are numerous immunoblasts admixed with small lymphocytes and plasma cells. Florid follicular hyperplasia is a mass lesion with marked follicular hyperplasia. Immunophenotyping should demonstrate polytypic B cells, plasma cells, and T cells without immunophenotypic aberrancy. EBV is frequently present; great care should be taken in making this diagnosis if EBV is absent. This group of PTLDs commonly occurs at younger ages and generally involves lymph nodes or tonsils and adenoids. The involvement of extranodal sites such as lung is rare.

Polymorphic PTLDs (P-PTLDs)

These PTLDs form destructive lung masses. Unlike many lymphomas, they demonstrate the full range of B-cell maturation, from immunoblasts to plasma cells, with small- and medium-sized lymphocytes and irregular nuclear contours, some of which represent the typically prominent T-cell components. Numerous mitotic figures may be present, as well as areas of geographic necrosis. Scattered, large, bizarre cells that resemble Reed-Sternberg cells can also be present. As opposed to CHL, however, these Reed-Sternberg-like cells are typically CD30+, CD20+, and CD15-. Most cases have numerous EBER-positive cells. Some cases have areas that appear monomorphic within the same lesion; thus, there may be a continuous morphologic spectrum between these lesions and monomorphic PTLD (M-PTLD). Immunophenotypic studies demonstrate B cells and a variable proportion of heterogeneous T cells. Light chain restriction does not exclude the diagnosis, though clear-cut light chain restriction should be noted since some of these cases might represent M-PTLD DLBCL. P-PTLDs are expected to demonstrate clonally rearranged IG genes by molecular studies, though the clones are less dominant than in M-PTLDs. Distinction of P-PTLDs from M-PTLDs is understandably not always clear cut.

Monomorphic PTLDs (M-PTLDs

M-PTLDs fulfill criteria for one of the B- or NK/T-cell neoplasms, in the setting of prior transplant. The morphologic presentations are similar to the corresponding disorders in immunocompetent hosts, though there is usually associated EBV positivity and sometimes geographic necrosis. Monomorphic B-cell PTLDs most commonly resemble their counterparts diffuse large B-cell lymphoma, Burkitt lymphoma (less often), or a plasma cell neoplasm. Many are CD30+, and most are of non-germinal center type, based on immunohistochemistry. By contrast, cases that are EBV-negative tend to be of germinal center origin by immunohistochemistry. Burkitt lymphoma PTLDs tend to be CD10+. Among small B-cell lymphoid neoplasms, only EBV+ MALT lymphoma is also considered a type of M-PTLDs. Of the monomorphic T-cell PTLDs, the most common forms are peripheral T-cell lymphoma, NOS, and hepatosplenic T-cell lymphoma. About one third of cases are EBV-positive.

Classic Hodgkin Lymphoma (CHL) PTLDs

CHL PTLDs, least common of the PTLDs, are almost always EBV-positive and should fulfill the diagnostic criteria for CHL.

Patients may have more than one PTLD present, in single or separate sites. Due to the significant possibility of intralesional heterogeneity, excisional biopsy is preferred.

What Are the Differential Diagnoses for PTLDs in the Lung After Lung Transplantation?

Diagnosis of PTLD has significant treatment implications for the patient. Therefore, accurate diagnosis is critical. Since nondestructive PTLDs in lung are very rare and usually occur only in lymph nodes or tonsils, there is limited clinical utility for discussing their differential diagnosis from other lung diseases. M-PTLDs and CHL PTLDs present in lung as the corresponding disorders in immunocompetent hosts. Their differential diagnoses from other lung diseases have essentially been discussed in the other chapters. Therefore, the differential diagnosis of P-PTLDs in the lung after lung transplantation is the focus of this section. P-PTLDs commonly present as early-onset PTLDs, occurring a median of 4–11 months after lung transplantation. They rarely present in the first 2 months posttransplant but have been reported to present as early as posttransplant day 35 as a pulmonary parenchymal infiltrate [7].

The infiltrates of P-PTLDs often extend to involve bronchiolar epithelium and adjacent lung parenchyma. Therefore, the major differential diagnosis, based on morphology alone, includes acute cellular rejection, airway inflammation (lymphocytic bronchiolitis/bronchitis), infections, and EBV virus-associated smooth muscle tumors, which are further discussed as follows:

Acute Cellular Rejection Acute allograft rejection occurs in almost 30% of recipients, mostly during the first year following transplantation, and may occur as repetitive episodes. Typical CT signs are ground-glass opacities, pleural effusions, lung volume loss, and interlobular septal thickening [5, 7]. On histopathological examination, depending on the grade, findings can range from minimal, perivascular lymphoplasmacytic infiltrates to severe, diffuse, perivascular, and interstitial lymphoplasmacytic infiltrates associated with alveolar injury. Therefore, acute cellular rejection can display overlapping clinical, radiologic, and histologic features with P-PTLDs. However, necrosis associated with P-PTLDs is rarely seen in rejection. The large Reed-Sternberg-like cells and EBV positivity seen in P-PTLDs are also not identified in rejection.

Airway Inflammation (Lymphocytic Bronchiolitis/Bronchitis) This is defined as mononuclear cell infiltrates within the submucosa of the bronchioles. Depending on grading, findings range from rare, scattered mononuclear cells in the submucosa to dense lymphocytic infiltrates associated with damage to the overlying epithelium and lymphocytes within the epithelium. The significance of airway inflammation is controversial, but some think that it is likely to be as important as perivascular inflammation in acute rejection. In P-PTLDs, the lymphoid cells are predominantly B cells and are positive for EBV. However, airway inflammation is composed predominantly of T cells and EBV-negative.

Infections Lung-transplanted patients are at particular risk for allograft infections. The first postoperative month is the one most associated with bacterial and fungal pathogens. From the second to sixth month, long-term immunosuppression of T cells is responsible for viral pneumonias. After 6 months, the most commonly encountered pathogens are community-acquired viruses and bacteria or reactivated latent *Mycobacterium tuberculosis* and other mycobacteria [5]. Since mycobacterial infection can present with lung nodules in the context of fever and associate with infiltration of T cells and histiocytes and necrosis, they raise a challenging differential diagnosis with P-PTLDs. Careful evaluation for possible infection, including special stains, cultures, and molecular approaches, is therefore recommended.

EBV-Associated Smooth Muscle Tumors These tumors, including leiomyomas and leiomyosarcomas, are rare but positive for EBV and can happen in lung after solid organ (including lung) transplants [8]. Since the tumors contain varying proportions of CD3+ T cells and are positive for

EBV, they can be misdiagnosed as P-PTLDs. However, by histology, these tumors usually show prominent spindling. Immunohistochemical studies usually demonstrate smooth muscle differentiation (actin & desmin).

References

1. Swerdlow SH, Campo E, Harris NL, Jaffe ES, Pileri SA, Stein H, et al. WHO classification of tumours of haematopoietic and lymphoid tissues. Geneva: WHO Press; 2017.
2. Montpréville V, Pavec J, Ladurie F, Sacha A, Dominique M, Mercier F, et al. Lymphoproliferative disorders after lung transplantation: clinicopathological characterization of 16 cases with identification of very-late-onset forms. Respiration. 2015;90:451–9.
3. Muchtar E, Kramer MR, Vidal L, Ram R, Gurion R, Rosenblat Y, et al. Posttransplantation lymphoproliferative disorder in lung transplant recipients: a 15-year single institution experience. Transplantation. 2013;96:657–63.
4. Romero S, Montoro J, Guinot M, Almenar L, Andreu R, Balaguer A, et al. Post-transplant lymphoproliferative disorders after solid organ and hematopoietic stem cell transplantation. Leuk Lymphoma. 2019;60:142–50.
5. Habre C, Soccal PM, Triponez F, Aubert J, Krueger T, Martin SP, et al. Radiological findings of complications after lung transplantation. Insights Imaging. 2018;9:709–19.
6. Baldanti F, Rognoni V, Cascina A, Oggionni T, Tinelli C, Meloni F. Post-transplant lymphoproliferative disorders and Epstein-Barr virus DNAemia in a cohort of lung transplant recipients. Virol J. 2011;8:421–32.
7. Lewis AJ, Jagadeesh D, Mukhopadhyay S, Budev M, Mehta AC. Post-transplant lymphoproliferative disorder presenting on post-transplant day 35 as a pulmonary parenchymal infiltrate—a case report. Oxf Med Case Rep. 2018;8:237–9.
8. Hirama T, Tikkanen J, Pal P, Cleary S, Binnie M. Epstein-Barr virus-associated smooth muscle tumors after lung transplantation. Transpl Infect Dis. 2019;21(3):e13068. Epub 2019 Mar 27. https://doi.org/10.1111/tid.13068.

Part II

Non-neoplastic Lung Pathology

Usual Interstitial Pneumonia Versus Nonspecific Interstitial Pneumonia

38

L. Angelica Lerma, Christopher M. Chandler, and Haodong Xu

Case Presentation

A 58-year-old male, previous smoker presented with a 2-year history of slowly increasing dyspnea on exertion that was now preventing him from keeping up with his cycling team. He also had a 1-year history of nonproductive cough, which was worse in the morning and exacerbated by exercise. Over the preceding month, his shortness of breath prevented him from carrying 20-pound loads up the stairs in his home. He also endorsed snoring and non-radiating, non-positional back pain. He denied other symptoms, exposure to asbestos, or occupational dusts. He had no family history of lung disease.

Initial pulmonary function tests demonstrated a reduced FEV1 (67%) in proportion to FVC (59%) with a ratio of 88% and markedly decreased DLCO (35%), consistent with a restrictive pattern and reduced diffusion capacity. A high-resolution computed tomography (HRCT) of the chest showed peripheral basilar predominant reticulation and traction bronchiectasis, mild honeycombing at the left base, and no significant air trapping on expiratory views, read as "overall consistent with UIP pattern." The clinical differential at the time included hypersensitivity pneumonitis given exposure to down and elevated IgG levels to *Penicillium*, *Thermoactinomyces*, and *Aspergillus*. However, a differential cell count on a bronchoalveolar lavage (BAL) specimen did not show a lymphocytosis. Additional laboratory studies including serologic evaluation for collagen vascular disease were negative. The patient received a diagnosis of idiopathic pulmonary fibrosis (IPF) and started on nintedanib.

A repeat HRCT 3 months after initial presentation showed mild increase in the predominantly lower lobe lung fibrosis with honeycombing (Fig. 38.1). His functional status continued to decline over the next 3 months, and the patient started supplemental oxygen. He received a single lung transplant approximately 6 months after initial presentation.

On gross examination, the pleural surface of the explanted lung had cobblestoning (Fig. 38.2a); cut sections showed basilar fibrosis with subpleural accentuation. The upper lobe was less involved than the lower lobe, and focal bronchiectatic changes were present (Fig. 38.2b).

On microscopic examination, histologic sections from the explant showed subpleural and paraseptal severe interstitial fibrosis with an abrupt transition to zones of relatively normal alveoli, and subpleural honeycombing with bronchiolar metaplasia was present (Fig. 38.3a). Fibroblastic foci were present throughout (Fig. 38.3b, c). The pathologist diagnosed usual interstitial pneumonia (UIP) pattern, which, together with the clinical and radiographic features, supports the clinical diagnosis of IPF.

L. A. Lerma · C. M. Chandler · H. Xu (✉)
Department of Laboratory Medicine and Pathology, University of Washington Medical Center, Seattle, WA, USA
e-mail: xuh8@uw.edu

H. Xu et al. (eds.), *Practical Lung Pathology*, Practical Anatomic Pathology, https://doi.org/10.1007/978-3-031-14402-8_38

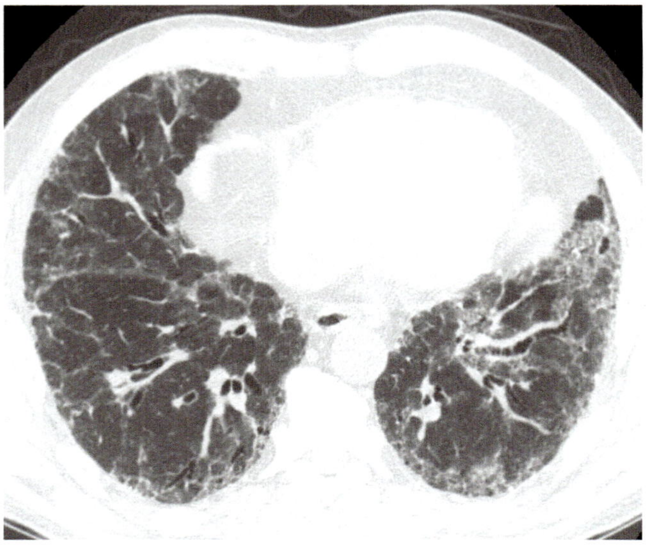

Fig. 38.1 High-resolution computed tomography (HRCT) of a patient with UIP pattern shows honeycombing and traction bronchiectasis with bibasilar predominance. The lung volumes are reduced

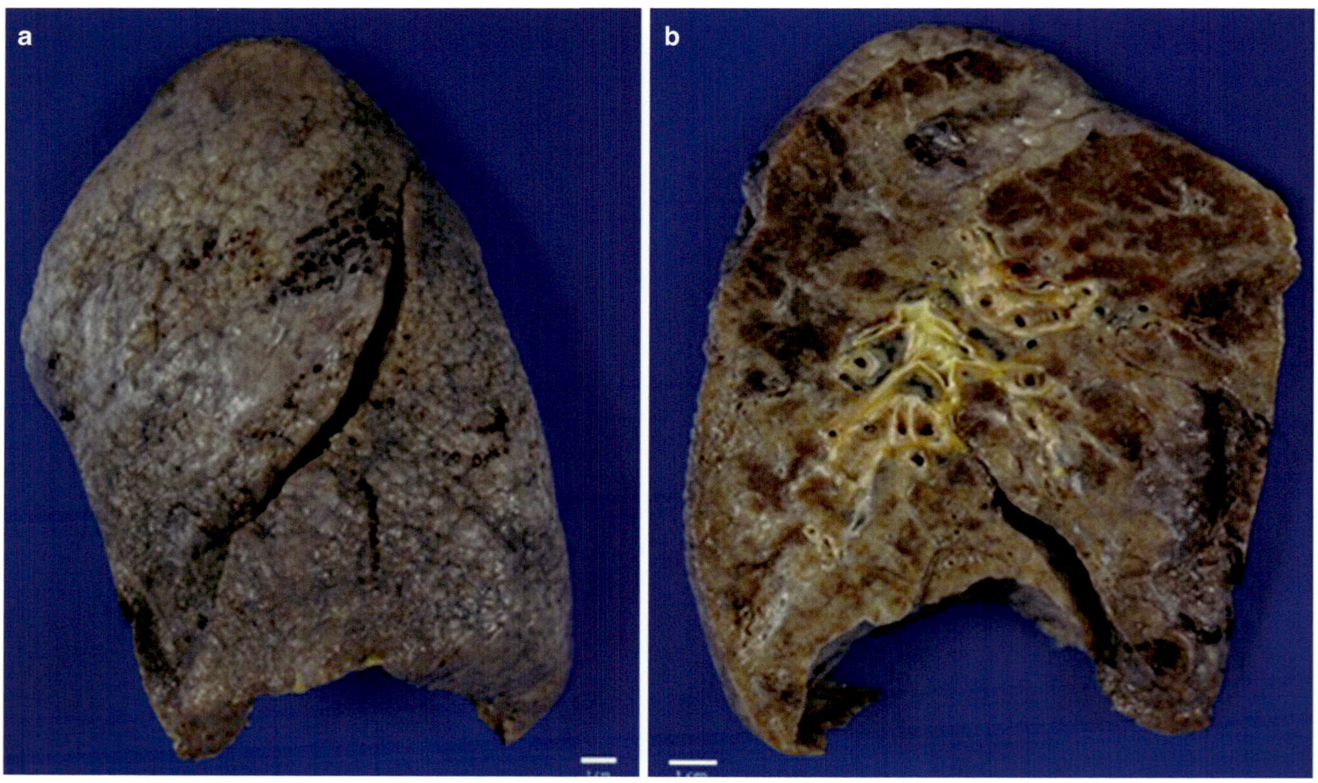

Fig. 38.2 Gross pathologic features of UIP. (**a**) Cobblestone appearance of the pleura. (**b**) Cut section in a parasagittal plane showing subpleural fibrosis, abrupt interface between affected and spared areas, lower lobe predominance, and focal honeycombing

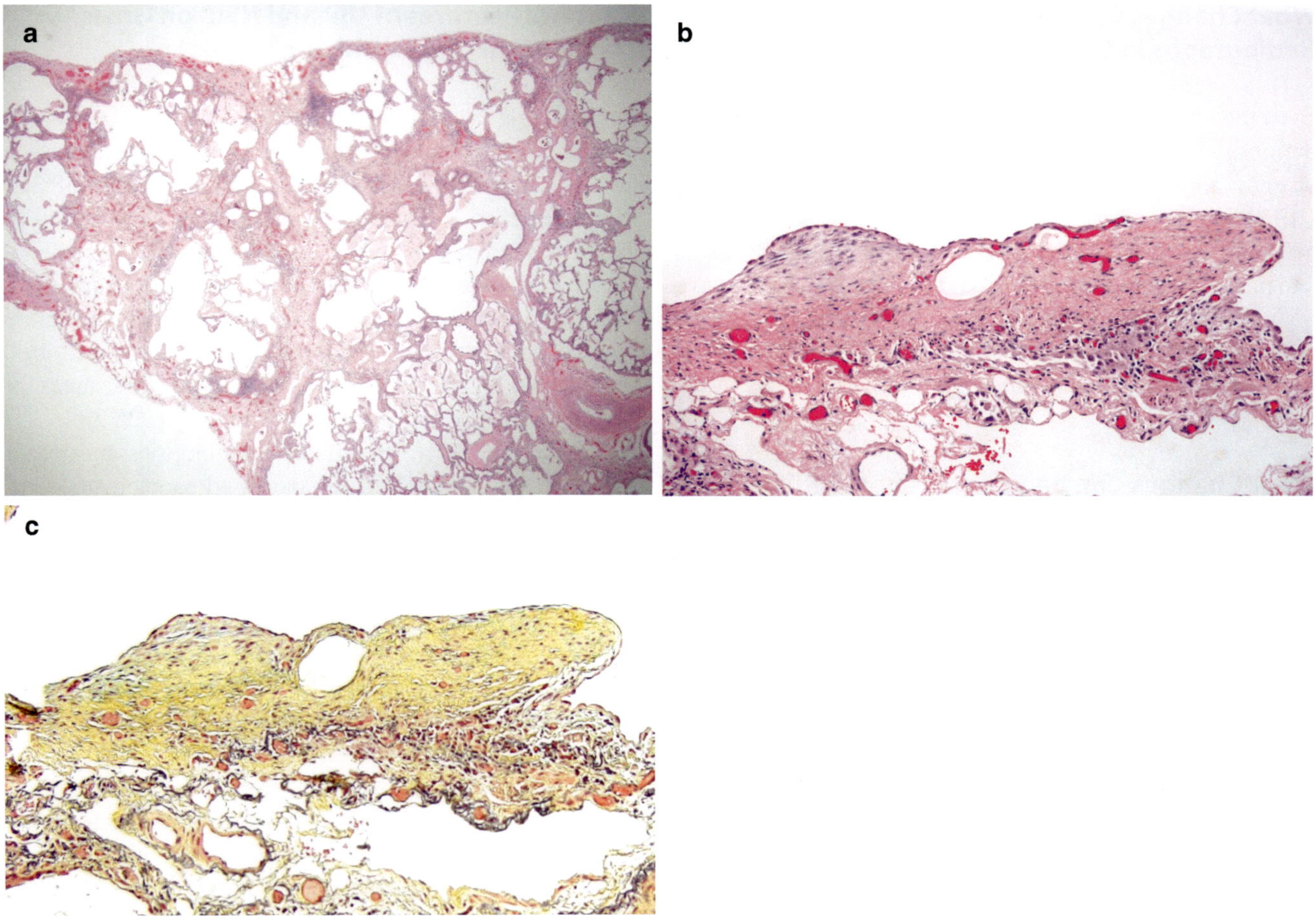

Fig. 38.3 (**a**) Subpleural cystic honeycombing typical of UIP (H&E, original magnification 40×). (**b**) Fibroblastic focus (H&E, original magnification 100×). (**c**) Fibroblastic focus (Movat pentachrome stain, original magnification 100×)

Final Pathological Diagnosis: Usual Interstitial Fibrosis (UIP)

What Are the Clinical Signs and Symptoms of NSIP and UIP?

Patients with UIP most commonly present in the sixth decade of life with years of stable nonproductive cough and dyspnea on exertion punctuated by episodes of functional decline. Although the presenting complaints are similar in duration, patients with NSIP often have an insidious decline and are a decade younger, or even children [1, 2].

Clinical examination of patients with UIP patients reveals tachypnea, bibasilar, and late inspiratory rales on chest auscultation (80%) [3]. Additional physical exam findings include clubbing of the fingernails (identified at presentation in 25–50% of patients) [4], and cardiac findings related to augmented P_2, a right-sided lift and S_3 gallop later in the course of UIP secondary to pulmonary hypertension. The physical exam findings are not distinct between either entity; however, fever and digital clubbing are uncommon in NSIP patients [5].

What Is the Clinical Course of These Diseases?

UIP's natural history varies between clinical stability and episodes of acute decompensation, with a mean survival of 32 months in idiopathic cases [1, 6]. In cases of known etiology, prognosis depends on the underlying cause and successful treatment of the primary disease process. The recently approved antifibrotic drugs, pirfenidone and nintedanib, have shown mortality reductions of over 40% in clinical trials, and thus patients with IPF are expected to survive longer as these medications become more widely utilized [7–9].

In contrast to UIP, NSIP is typically more indolent, with an overall 5-year survival rate of just over 80% which approaches 90% in idiopathic disease [2, 10]. Patients with mild disease, as defined by clinical symptoms and pulmonary function testing, can be followed at close intervals [11]. As the disease progresses, corticosteroids and additional immunosuppression are indicated [12, 13]. Within NSIP, the fibrosing variant is less common than the cellular variant, responds less well to treatment, and thus has a poorer prognosis [14].

What Changes Can be Seen on Chest Radiographs in UIP and NSIP?

Even though both entities have bibasilar, symmetrical distributions, UIP has a reticular pattern of fibrosis/opacification on chest X-ray (CXR) [15]. Fewer than 10% of patients with UIP have a normal CXR at presentation [16]. While a CXR may be part of the initial workup for cough and dyspnea, patients with suspected interstitial lung disease should have high-resolution computed tomography (HRCT) of their chest performed as it is an important part of initial evaluation and subsequent disease monitoring.

What Changes Can be Seen on Chest HRCT in UIP and NSIP?

Early manifestations of UIP on HRCT are fine irregular thickening of interfaces between secondary lobules, vasculature, and pleura [17]. An experienced thoracic radiologist can diagnose UIP on initial HRCT findings alone, provided there is honeycombing in a bibasilar and subpleural symmetric distribution, associated with bronchiectasis and/or bronchiolectasis [3, 17–20]. Honeycombing is defined as grouped air spaces with well-defined thick walls with the loss of lobular architecture, at least 0.5 cm in diameter. If the honeycombing pattern is not well-established ("reticular pattern") with the above distribution and/or ground-glass opacities are present, the designation of "probable UIP" is recommended [3, 4]. Less definite findings, such as subtle reticulation, mild ground-glass opacities or distribution of fibrosis which do not fit the prior categories, are classified as "indeterminate for UIP" [3]. A fourth category "alternative diagnosis" is used if the findings are most consistent with another entity. If the clinical presentation and HRCT findings are not definitive for UIP, then two site surgical lung biopsies (small wedge biopsies) from different lobes with bronchoalveolar lavage are the gold standard for diagnostic evaluation [3, 4, 16, 20]. The recent clinical validation of a molecular test based on gene expression profiles suggestive of UIP obtained from transbronchial biopsies (Envisia) may change the rate of surgical lung biopsy in the future [21].

NSIP shows variable and nonspecific findings on HRCT, commonly ground-glass opacities diffusely with bibasilar predominance [22]. In most cases, a reticular pattern is identified as at least a minor component [23]. Overlap with non-UIP diffuse parenchymal lung diseases is common; however, subpleural sparing, irregular linear opacities, patchy honeycombing, and nodular opacities should lead to careful consideration of diagnoses other than NSIP.

What Are Features of UIP and NSIP on Gross Examination of Surgical Specimens?

Surgical lung biopsies and resection specimens with UIP may have a cobblestone appearance to the pleural surface due to retraction and subpleural fibrosis (Fig. 38.2a). Sectioning shows subpleural, paraseptal, and/or peribronchiolar cystic changes, which coalesce into honeycombing and are surrounded by dense white fibrous bands. Both upper and lower lobes are typically involved bilaterally, but more severe fibrosis is evident in the periphery of the lower lobes. These changes are interspersed with tan-yellow areas of evolving fibrosis and grossly normal lung (Fig. 38.2b).

The changes in NSIP surgical lung biopsies and resections are more subtle. Initially, increased parenchymal density and decreased elasticity can be appreciated. The cut surfaces take on a yellow tint, which is more evenly distributed within the parenchyma in comparison to that of UIP; however, gross findings are not specific for either entity.

What Are the Histologic Features of the UIP Pattern?

Histologic sections of UIP surgical lung biopsies characteristically show a demarcated patchwork of three different histologic patterns: fibrosis and dense scarring, zones of injury, and relatively spared lung parenchyma. Areas of fibrosis have collapsed alveolar walls which form pleural based reticular spaces 1–3 mm in diameter. These spaces lack a central airway and are lined by either ciliated cuboidal, columnar, or metaplastic squamous epithelium. Smaller spaces coalesce along septa and subpleural spaces to form honeycombs, grouped air spaces with well-defined thick walls with loss of lobular architecture, at least 0.5 cm in diameter (Fig. 38.3a) [4]. As smooth muscle begins to proliferate (the so-called muscular cirrhosis of the lung), traction bronchiectasis can be appreciated. Some intraluminal mucus, variable amounts of neutrophils, and inflammatory debris are often present within small airways and honeycombs.

Zones of injury with the so-called fibroblastic foci are located at the interface between dense fibrosis and uninvolved lung [4]. Fibroblastic foci are crescent-shaped proliferations of myofibroblasts within myxoid appearing, immature collagen which expand the level of the basement membrane (Fig. 38.3b). Flattened epithelial cells line these proliferations and are associated with reactive type II macrophages. Cool et al. (2006) demonstrated that these areas are interconnected and nonneoplastic in nature [24]. As might be expected, progressive parenchymal changes cause remodeling of the associated vasculature, leading to intimal hyper-

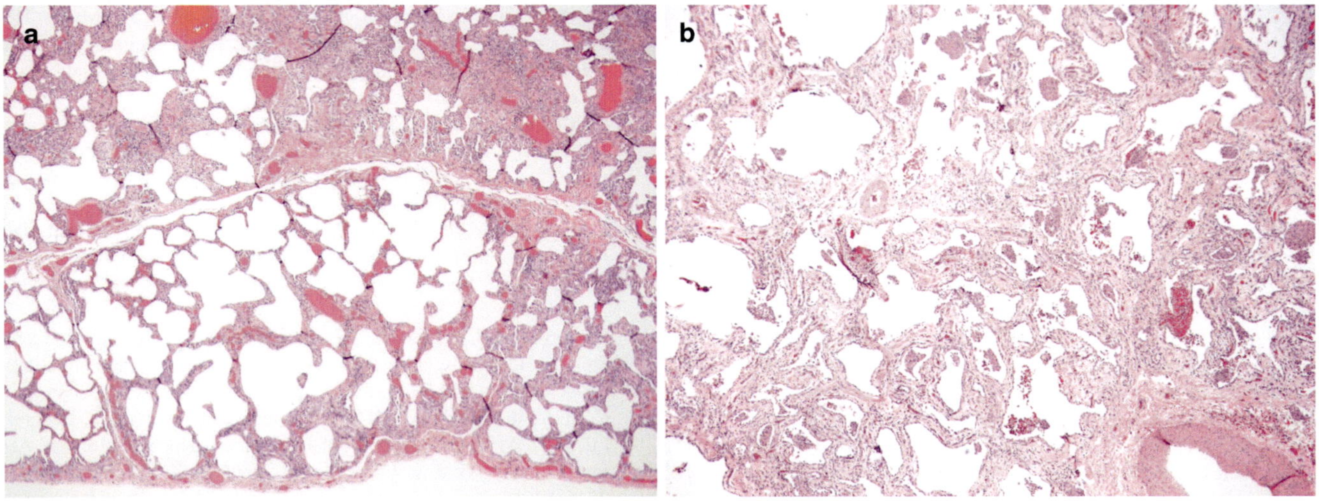

Fig. 38.4 NSIP with temporally homogenous fibrotic expansion of alveolar septa (H&E, original magnification (**a**) 40× and (**b**) 400×)

plasia and medial hypertrophy of the pulmonary arteries. Mild to moderate lymphoplasmacytic and sparse eosinophilic infiltrates are permissible. Alveolar macrophages with fine, brownish/yellowish cytoplasmic granules are frequently present in patients who are cigarette smokers [25]. Acute exacerbations of UIP may have features of acute lung injury, including diffuse alveolar damage [26].

Special stains are useful to highlight different zones of interest. The Masson trichrome stain (MT) highlights mature collagen in yellow, and fibroblastic foci appear light blue on a pentachrome Movat stain (Fig. 38.3c). Conveniently, elastic fibers are stained black on the pentachrome Movat stain which can be useful when evaluating the thickness of the intima or media of pulmonary arteries.

What Are the Histologic Features of NSIP?

NSIP is characterized by variable expansion, without destruction, of the alveolar septa by lymphoplasmacytic infiltrates with temporally homogenous fibrosis [4]. NSIP is subdivided into cellular and fibrosing variants depending on which component is more prominent. The cellular variant is characterized by uniform and dense mononuclear inflammation along alveolar walls, bronchovascular sheaths, and subpleural spaces [25]. The fibrosing variant is frequently associated with type II pneumocyte hyperplasia, vascular medial and intimal thickening, bronchiolar metaplasia, lymphoid aggregates, and pleural fibrosis [27]. Germinal centers may be observed. While there can be overlap in the histologic features of UIP and NSIP, the presence of any UIP-type pattern confers are worse prognosis, leading some to propose classifying any specimen with UIP and NSIP features as UIP [28–30]. As shown in Fig 38.4a, b, diffuse alveolar septa are thickened with fibrosis which is characteristic of fibrosing variant of NSIP.

References

1. Daniil ZD, Gilchrist FC, Nicholson AG, Hansell DM, Harris J, Colby TV, et al. A histologic pattern of nonspecific interstitial pneumonia is associated with a better prognosis than usual interstitial pneumonia in patients with cryptogenic fibrosing alveolitis. Am J Respir Crit Care Med. 1999;160(3):899–905.
2. Nagai S, Kitaichi M, Itoh H, Nishimura K, Izumi T, Colby TV. Idiopathic nonspecific interstitial pneumonia/fibrosis: comparison with idiopathic pulmonary fibrosis and BOOP. Eur Respir J. 1998;12(5):1010–9.
3. Raghu G, Remy-Jardin M, Myers JL, Richeldi L, Ryerson CJ, Lederer DJ, et al. American Thoracic Society, European Respiratory Society, Japanese respiratory society, and Latin American Thoracic Society diagnosis of idiopathic pulmonary fibrosis. An official ATS/ERS/JRS/ALAT clinical practice guideline. Am J Respir Crit Care Med. 2018;198(5):e44–68.
4. Leslie KO, Wick MR. Practical pulmonary pathology: a diagnostic approach. Philadelphia, PA: Elsevier; 2017.
5. Cottin V, Donsbeck AV, Revel D, Loire R, Cordier JF. Nonspecific interstitial pneumonia. Individualization of a clinicopathologic entity in a series of 12 patients. Am J Respir Crit Care Med. 1998;158(4):1286–93.
6. Akira M, Hamada H, Sakatani M, Kobayashi C, Nishioka M, Yamamoto S. CT findings during phase of accelerated deterioration in patients with idiopathic pulmonary fibrosis. AJR Am J Roentgenol. 1997;168(1):79–83.
7. King TE Jr, Brown KK, Raghu G, du Bois RM, Lynch DA, Martinez F, et al. BUILD-3: a randomized, controlled trial of bosentan in idiopathic pulmonary fibrosis. Am J Respir Crit Care Med. 2011;184(1):92–9.
8. King TE Jr, Bradford WZ, Castro-Bernardini S, Fagan EA, Glaspole I, Glassberg MK, et al. A phase 3 trial of pirfenidone in patients with idiopathic pulmonary fibrosis. N Engl J Med. 2014;370(22):2083–92.
9. Martinez FJ, Lederer DJ. Focus on idiopathic pulmonary fibrosis: advancing approaches to diagnosis, prognosis, and treatment. Chest. 2018;154(4):978–9.
10. Travis WD, Hunninghake G, King TE Jr, Lynch DA, Colby TV, Galvin JR, et al. Idiopathic nonspecific interstitial pneumonia: report of an American Thoracic Society project. Am J Respir Crit Care Med. 2008;177(12):1338–47.

11. Belloli EA, Beckford R, Hadley R, Flaherty KR. Idiopathic nonspecific interstitial pneumonia. Respirology. 2016;21(2):259–68.
12. Park IN, Jegal Y, Kim DS, Do KH, Yoo B, Shim TS, et al. Clinical course and lung function change of idiopathic nonspecific interstitial pneumonia. Eur Respir J. 2009;33(1):68–76.
13. Lee JY, Jin SM, Lee BJ, Chung DH, Jang BG, Park HS, et al. Treatment response and long term follow-up results of nonspecific interstitial pneumonia. J Korean Med Sci. 2012;27(6):661–7.
14. Katzenstein AL, Fiorelli RF. Nonspecific interstitial pneumonia/fibrosis. Histologic features and clinical significance. Am J Surg Pathol. 1994;18(2):136–47.
15. Grenier P, Chevret S, Belgelman C, Brauner MW, Chastang C, Valeyre D. Chronic diffuse infiltrative lung disease: determination of the diagnostic value of clinical data, chest radiography, and CT and Bayesian analysis. Radiology. 1994;191:383–90.
16. Travis WD. Non-neoplastic disorders of the lower respiratory tract. Washington, DC; Bethesda, MD: American Registry of Pathology; Armed Forces Institute of Pathology; Universities Associated for Research and Education in Pathology; 2002. p. 901–21.
17. Akira M, Sakatani M, Ueda E. Idiopathic pulmonary fibrosis: progression of honeycombing at thin-section CT. Radiology. 1993;189(3):687–91.
18. Lee JS, Im JG, Ahn JM, Kim YM, Han MC. Fibrosing alveolitis: prognostic implication of ground-glass attenuation at high-resolution CT. Radiology. 1992;184(2):451–4.
19. Lynch DA, Newell JD, Logan OM, King TE Jr, Muller NL. Can CT distinguish hypersensitivity pneumonitis from idiopathic pulmonary fibrosis? AJR Am J Roentgenol. 1995;165(4):807–11.
20. Humphries SM, Swigris JJ, Brown KK, Strand M, Gong Q, Sundy JS, et al. Quantitative high-resolution computed tomography fibrosis score: performance characteristics in idiopathic pulmonary fibrosis. Eur Respir J. 2018;52(3):1801384.
21. Raghu G, Flaherty KR, Lederer DJ, Lynch DA, Colby TV, Myers JL, et al. Use of a molecular classifier to identify usual interstitial pneumonia in conventional transbronchial lung biopsy samples: a prospective validation study. Lancet Respir Med. 2019;7(6):487–96.
22. Hartman TE, Swensen SJ, Hansell DM, Colby TV, Myers JL, Tazelaar HD, et al. Nonspecific interstitial pneumonia: variable appearance at high-resolution chest CT. Radiology. 2000;217(3):701–5.
23. Kim EY, Lee KS, Chung MP, Kwon OJ, Kim TS, Hwang JH. Nonspecific interstitial pneumonia with fibrosis: serial high-resolution CT findings with functional correlation. AJR Am J Roentgenol. 1999;173(4):949–53.
24. Cool CD, Groshong SD, Rai PR, Henson PM, Stewart JS, Brown KK. Fibroblast foci are not discrete sites of lung injury or repair: the fibroblast reticulum. Am J Respir Crit Care Med. 2006;174(6):654–8.
25. Katzenstein AL, Myers JL. Nonspecific interstitial pneumonia and the other idiopathic interstitial pneumonias: classification and diagnostic criteria. Am J Surg Pathol. 2000;24(1):1–3.
26. Collard HR, Ryerson CJ, Corte TJ, Jenkins G, Kondoh Y, Lederer DJ, et al. Acute exacerbation of idiopathic pulmonary fibrosis. An international working group report. Am J Respir Crit Care Med. 2016;194(3):265–75.
27. Travis WD, Matsui K, Moss J, Ferrans VJ. Idiopathic nonspecific interstitial pneumonia: prognostic significance of cellular and fibrosing patterns: survival comparison with usual interstitial pneumonia and desquamative interstitial pneumonia. Am J Surg Pathol. 2000;24(1):19–33.
28. Flaherty KR, Travis WD, Colby TV, Toews GB, Kazerooni EA, Gross BH, et al. Histopathologic variability in usual and nonspecific interstitial pneumonias. Am J Respir Crit Care Med. 2001;164(9):1722–7.
29. du Bois R, King TE. Challenges in pulmonary fibrosis x 5: the NSIP/UIP debate. Thorax. 2007;62(11):1008–12.
30. Kambouchner M, Levy P, Nicholson AG, Schubel K, Magois E, Feuillet S, et al. Prognostic relevance of histological variants in nonspecific interstitial pneumonia. Histopathology. 2014;65(4):549–60.

Hypersensitivity Pneumonitis Versus Usual Interstitial Pneumonia

39

Nicholas Stanzione and Gregory A. Fishbein

Case Presentation

A 65-year-old man is referred to a pulmonologist for longstanding cough and dyspnea. The patient has no significant medical or smoking history. Pulmonary function tests revealed somewhat reduced diffusion capacity for carbon monoxide (DLCO) and a mixed restrictive and obstructive pattern. Chest computed tomography (CT) demonstrated airway-centered interstitial fibrosis bilaterally, more prominent in the upper lobes, with areas of subpleural sparing and patchy ground-glass opacities (Fig. 39.1). Mosaic attenuation was noted on expiratory imaging. The clinical differential diagnosis included chronic hypersensitivity pneumonitis, usual interstitial pneumonia, and fibrotic nonspecific interstitial pneumonia. Diagnostic transbronchial cryobiopsies of the upper and lower lobes were performed, which demonstrated interstitial fibrosis that was predominantly located around bronchioles, with abundant peribronchiolar metaplasia, some associated chronic inflammation, and a focal poorly formed granuloma (Fig. 39.2). The patient's hobby of caring for various birds in his aviary was elucidated on further questioning following the biopsy.

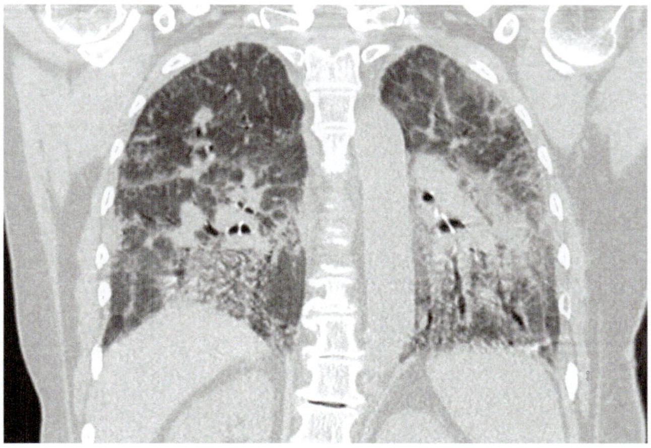

Fig. 39.1 HRCT showing diffuse bilateral diffuse coarse ground-glass opacities with thickened irregular interlobular septa, bronchiectasis and bronchiolectasis, architectural distortion, and inconspicuous honeycombing, consistent with hypersensitivity pneumonitis

N. Stanzione
VA Greater Los Angeles Healthcare System, Los Angeles, CA, USA

G. A. Fishbein (✉)
David Geffen School of Medicine, University of California, Los Angeles (UCLA), Los Angeles, CA, USA
e-mail: gfishbein@mednet.ucla.edu

H. Xu et al. (eds.), *Practical Lung Pathology*, Practical Anatomic Pathology, https://doi.org/10.1007/978-3-031-14402-8_39

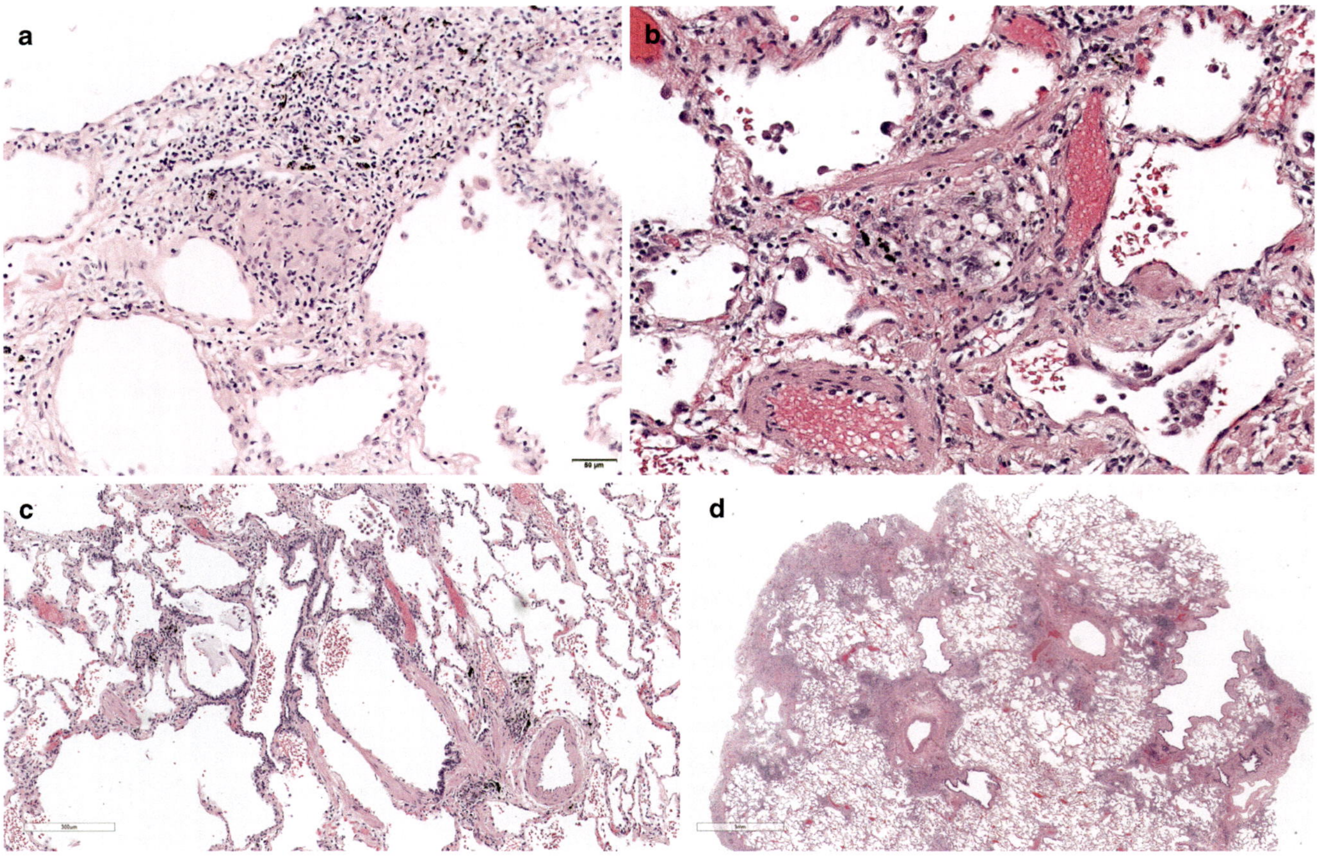

Fig. 39.2 (**a**) Non-necrotizing granuloma in a background of chronic mixed interstitial inflammation, (**b**) Poorly formed non-necrotizing granuloma, (**c**) Peribronchiolar alveolar spaces partially lined by metaplastic bronchiolar pseudostratified columnar ciliated epithelium, (**d**) Low power microscopic examination highlights the airway-centered interstitial fibrosis and inflammatory infiltrate

Pathologic Diagnosis: Chronic Hypersensitivity Pneumonitis

What Are some of the Differences in the Clinical Presentation of Patients with Hypersensitivity Pneumonitis (HP) Versus Usual Interstitial Pneumonia (UIP)?

When rendering a specific diagnosis of interstitial lung disease (ILD), it behooves the pathologist to investigate the clinical history of the patient. Knowledge of the tempo or progression of disease and the patient's symptoms will help determine the nature of the underlying disease and can help the pathologist determine where to focus the gross and microscopic examination [1]. In addition, understanding the pathophysiology of the ILD may help relate the clinical presentation to the pathologic findings.

In the case of HP, which encompasses a spectrum of immunologically mediated interstitial lung diseases secondary to exposure to a sensitizing antigen, the pathophysiology is related to abnormal and excessive reactivity to the causative antigen, ultimately resulting in fibrosis [2]. The implicated agents may include animal proteins, fungi, and bacteria (Table 39.1). As the sensitizing agent is introduced via inhalation, the result is airway-centered disease. As such, a diagnosis of HP signals clinicians to search and test for the source of exposure. Clinically, HP can be divided into acute, subacute, and chronic phases. While the exact definitions of these subgroups have not been clearly delineated, many studies have accepted that chronic HP is defined by the presence of fibrosis [3, 4]. Acute HP may present with recurring fevers, dyspnea, cough, and leukocytosis. The symptoms usually appear 4–6 h following exposure and may last for 12 h to several days, recurring with reexposure [2, 5]. Continuous or prolonged exposure to the inciting agent will lead to dyspnea, cyanosis, and respiratory failure with decreased total lung capacity and compliance [2].

UIP is a pattern of interstitial lung disease, first described by Liebow and Carrington in 1969 [7]. The UIP pattern may be seen with several underlying etiologies that include collagen vascular diseases, drug toxicity, environmental exposures, and certain genetic disorders (e.g., Hermansky-Pudlak syndrome, short telomere syndrome, etc.). In the absence of

Table 39.1 Various forms of hypersensitivity pneumonitis and their source/antigens [6]

Disease	Source	Antigen
Microorganisms		
Farmer's lung	Moldy hay, grain, silage	Saccharopolyspora (*Micropolyspora faeni*) Thermophilic actinomycetes
Ventilation pneumonitis	Contaminated forced-air systems	*Thermoactinomyces candidus*
Bagassosis	Moldy sugarcane (bagasse)	*Thermoactinomyces vulgaris*
Mushroom worker's lung	Moldy mushroom compost	*Thermoactinomyces sacchari*
Dry rot lung	Rotting wood decay	*Merulius lacrymans*
Suberosis	Moldy cork	*Thermoactinomyces viridis*
Detergent lung	Detergents	*Bacillus subtilis* enzymes
Malt worker's lung	Moldy barley	*Aspergillus fumigatus* *Aspergillus clavatus*
Sequoiosis	Moldy redwood dust	*Sequoia sempervirens*
Maple bark stripper's lung	Moldy maple bark	*Cryptostroma corticale*
Tobacco grower's lung	Tobacco mold	*Aspergillus* species
Winegrower's (Späetlase) lung	Grape mold	*Botrytis cinerea*
Cheese washer's lung	Moldy cheese	*Aspergillus clavatus* *Penicillium casei*
Woodworker's lung	Wood or wood pulp	*Alternaria* species
Paprika slicer's lung	Moldy paprika pods	*Mucor stolonifera*
Summer type pneumonitis	Contaminated old Japanese houses	*Trichosporon cutaneum*
Sewage worker's lung	Sewage	*Cephalosporium*
Sax lung	Saxophone mouthpiece	*Candida albicans*
Lycoperdonosis	Puffball spores	Puffball (*Lycoperdon perlatum*)
Dog house disease	Moldy animal bedding	*Aspergillus versicolor*
Sauna taker's lung	Contaminated sauna water	*Aureobasidium* species
Hot tub lung	Hot tub water	Nontuberculous mycobacteria
Animal protein		
Bird fancier's lung	Parakeets, pigeons, chickens, turkeys	Avian droppings, feathers, blood
Pituitary snuff taker's lung	Nasal inhalation of pituitary snuff	Bovine and porcine pituitary proteins
Fish meal worker's lung	Fish meal	Fish meal dust
Furrier's lung	Animal pelts	Animal fur dust
Bat lung	Bat droppings	Bat serum protein
Miller's lung	Insect infested grain	Wheat weevil (*Sitophilus granarius*)
Sericulturist's lung	Silk worm larvae	Silk worm larvae proteins
Unknown		
Coptic lung	Cloth mummy wrappings	
Grain measurer's lung	Cereal grain	
Coffee worker's lung	Coffee bean dust	
Thatched roof lung	Dead grass and leaves	
Tea grower's lung	Tea plants	
Tobacco grower's lung	Tobacco plants	

Adapted from Patel AM, Ryu JH, Reed CE. Hypersensitivity pneumonitis: Current concepts and future questions. J. Allergy Clin. Immunol. 2001;108:661–70

a known etiology, ILD with a UIP pattern is diagnostic of idiopathic pulmonary fibrosis (IPF) [7]. The pathophysiology of this pattern of interstitial lung disease is poorly understood but is believed to be related to environmental factors as well as genetic factors which lead to persistent epithelial injury and the release of pro-fibrotic factors, leading to abnormal proliferation and collagen production [2, 8]. Clinically, this is a disease of older individuals, and the diagnosis of UIP should be made cautiously in patients younger than 50 years old. Most patients present between 55 and 75 years old. UIP usually presents insidiously, with gradually increasing dyspnea on exertion and a dry cough, with hypoxemia, cyanosis, and clubbing occurring later in the course. Pulmonary function tests will show varying degrees of restrictive disease [9, 10].

How Do HP and UIP Differ on Radiographic Studies?

The most common radiographic chest study used today to evaluate patients with ILD is high-resolution computed tomography (HRCT). Since the clinical history and physical exam findings in HP and UIP are relatively nonspecific, an understanding of their imaging findings is important in making accurate diagnoses. In addition, in the setting of transplantation, HRCT images often recapitulate the gross appearance of the explanted lung.

In HP, since the pathophysiology is related to inhalation, the findings are present around bronchioles. Classic findings on HRCT include centrilobular ground-glass opacities (GGO) predominantly in the upper and mid-lung zones due to its distribution among regions with the most airflow, as well as mosaic attenuation, evidence of air trapping [5, 11].

The areas of architectural or parenchymal distortion (fibrosis) also follow this distribution. However, in cases of advanced CHP, the fibrosis may be more widespread, and the distribution may also involve the lower lung zones [1]. Additional findings seen in HP include reticulation, traction bronchiectasis, and bronchiolectasis [11]. The finding of patchy ground-glass opacities is suggestive of active (i.e., subacute) HP and helps distinguish CHP from UIP [4, 12]. Honeycombing, a radiographic finding often associated with UIP, has been reported in 16–69% of CHP cases; however, in CHP, there is seldom a basilar predominance [13]. Helpful HRCT findings favoring CHP include the presence of ill-defined centrilobular nodules in the mid- and upper lung zones [1].

HRCT in UIP patients is often helpful because interstitial fibrosis tends to involve the lower lobes more than upper lobes with a subpleural and paraseptal predilection and honeycombs (see Fig. 39.3) [1, 9, 10].

The fibrosis is often associated with peripherally located large, cystic spaces, also known as honeycombing, which indicate advanced fibrosis. Honeycombing is present in most patients and is highly suggestive of UIP [1, 9]. However, it may also be present in the end stage of fibrosing ILD of various etiologies and is therefore not entirely specific. Traction bronchiectasis and bronchiolectasis may also be seen. Classic UIP pattern fibrosis does not show ground-glass opacities unless there is superimposed lung injury (i.e., acute exacerbation) or pulmonary edema [9, 10]. Since UIP is more often seen in a patient who currently or previously smoke, emphysematous changes are often associated with UIP [4].

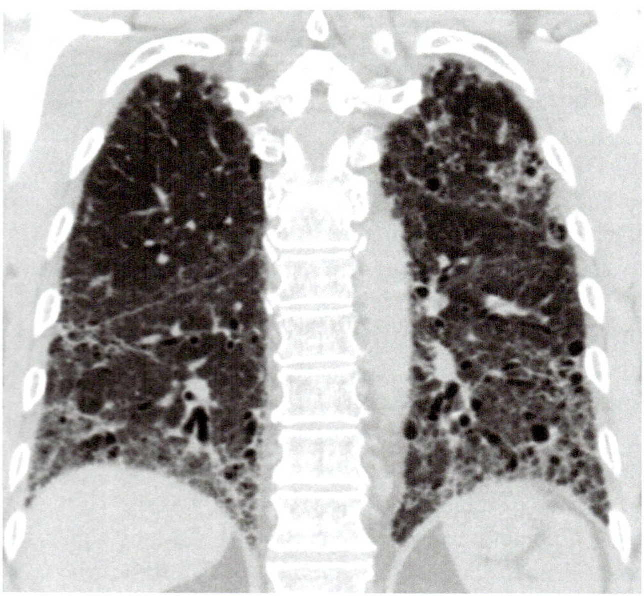

Fig. 39.3 HRCT showing peripheral greater than central, and lower greater than upper lobe thickened inter- and intralobular septa with subpleural reticulation, coarse ground-glass opacity, traction bronchiectasis and bronchiolectasis, and small cystic spaces/honeycombing changes

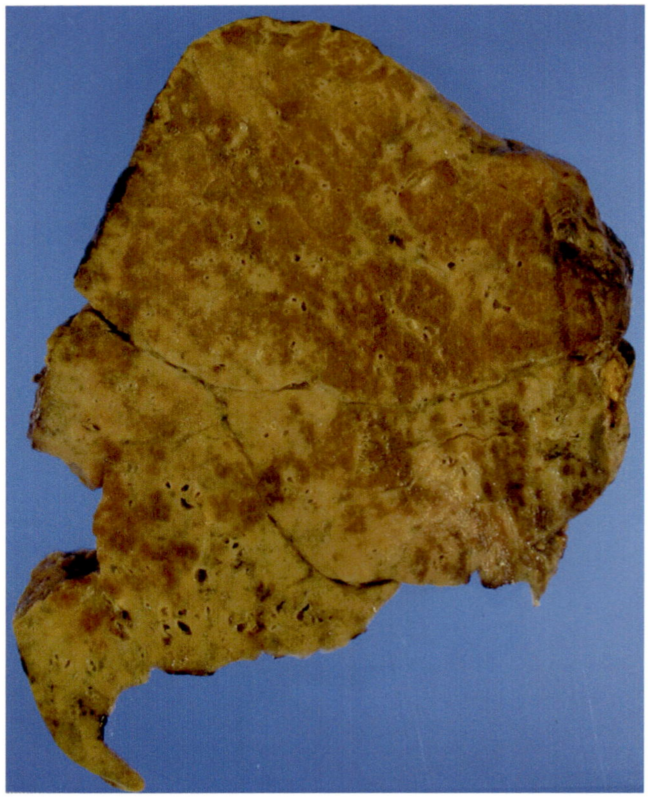

Fig. 39.4 Fibrosis predominantly involving the lower and middle lobes greater than the upper lobes with preferential involvement of the periphery lung fields, forming continuous block-like subpleural fibrosis of the lower lobes

What Are the Gross Pathologic Differences Between UIP and HP?

UIP demonstrates prominent fibrosis, with a predilection for the lower lung fields and lower portions of each lobe, as well as a subpleural and paraseptal distribution. The subpleural fibrosis and honeycomb changes result in a cobblestoned appearance to the visceral pleura. As the fibrosis in UIP is geographically heterogeneous, there is grossly patchy involvement, which is evidenced by fibrosis that may be prominent in the periphery of a lobule with sparing of the central portion (see Fig. 39.4) [8].

While CHP may show subpleural fibrosis as well, the fibrosis in UIP is usually more diffuse. The fibrosis in CHP is usually patchy and more centrally located (see Fig. 39.5).

How Can HP and UIP be Distinguished Histologically?

In HP, particularly in the subacute, or active, phase of disease, the histologic findings include peribronchiolar (airway-centric) interstitial chronic inflammatory infiltrates composed of lymphocytes, plasma cells, and, occasionally, a small

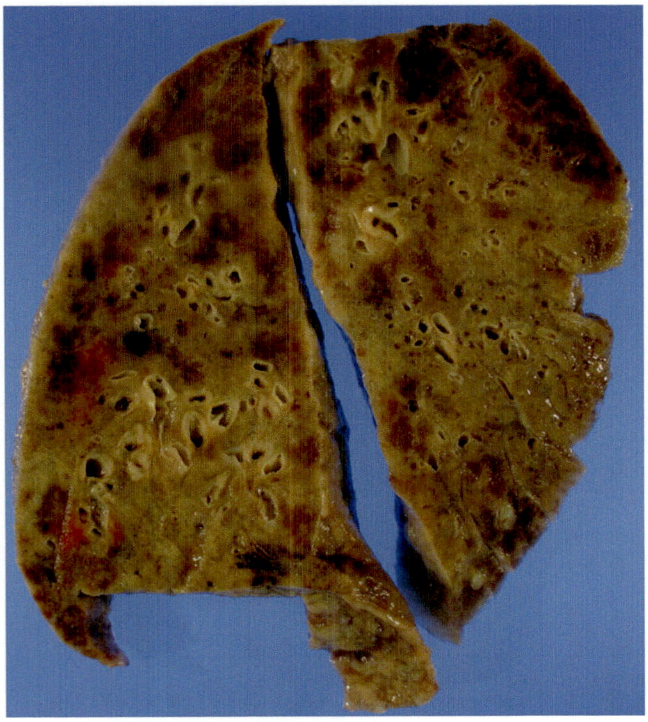

Fig. 39.5 Diffuse parenchymal fibrosis with patchy lower lobe involvement, radiating outward from the small airways with associated traction bronchiectasis, and areas of subpleural sparing

number of eosinophils [1, 3, 5]. Lymphoid aggregates may be present in HP with occasional lymphoid follicles [3, 4]. For the most part, the infiltrate resembles a cellular nonspecific interstitial pneumonia (NSIP) pattern, but in an airway-centered distribution. In addition, characteristic poorly formed non-necrotizing granulomas and giant cells are seen. Poorly formed non-necrotizing granulomas, while supportive of the diagnosis of CHP, are only found in up to 70% of cases [3].

Schaumann bodies, large concentrically lamellated, calcified structures present within the cytoplasm of giant cells, may be present [14]. In CHP, there is evidence of chronic parenchyma and small airway disease, such as organizing pneumonia, chronic airway inflammation (bronchiolitis), and peribronchiolar metaplasia (PBM) [3–5]. PBM, also called Lambertosis (named for its involvement of the channels of Lambert), is chronic change in which peribronchiolar alveolar walls are lined by metaplastic, ciliated bronchiolar epithelium.

PBM, chronic airway inflammation, and focal organizing pneumonia are all relatively nonspecific findings that may be seen incidentally in the lungs of patients without clinical interstitial lung disease. However, the presence of features of subacute HP, including peribronchiolar interstitial mixed chronic inflammation, is helpful to support a diagnosis of CHP, particularly in the end stage when fibrosis is the predominant finding. In late stages of CHP, interstitial fibrosis may be the predominant findings, particularly if patient has received immunosuppressive therapy. The fibrosis is typically airway-centered, surrounding the bronchovascular bundles.

Bridging fibrosis spreading from airway to airway, airway to interlobular septum, and/or airway to pleura, may be seen. As in UIP, subpleural fibrosis may be present in CHP. However, it is often much less marked than in classic UIP, and areas of subpleural sparing are typically present. Since CHP is a disease of ongoing inflammation and fibrosis, the quality of fibrosis may be quite heterogeneous, as seen in a UIP pattern. Dense pink collagen may be seen in proximity to loose collections of fibroblasts and myofibroblasts in myxoid stroma (i.e., fibroblastic foci). Therefore, identification of airway-centered inflammation and fibrosis, evidence of chronic airway injury (e.g., PBM), and characteristic poorly formed non-necrotizing granulomas are needed to confidently distinguish CHP from classic UIP.

UIP is characterized by spatially and temporally heterogeneous fibrosis with a lower lung zone and lower lobe predominant interstitial fibrosis and honeycombing. Spatially heterogeneous fibrosis refers to zones of normal lung tissue adjacent to zones of advanced fibrosis and remodeling with dense scarring of the alveolar parenchyma [1, 10]. Temporally heterogeneous fibrosis refers to the presence of young new scarring, in the form of fibroblastic foci, as well as advanced old scarring, in the form of dense, mature collagenized scar (Fig. 39.6) [10, 12].

The fibroblastic foci are composed of bulges of spindled fibroblasts within a slightly basophilic myxoid background. Fibroblastic foci are often seen at the intersection between advanced fibrosis and normal appearing lung parenchyma and may be the earliest histologic evidence of UIP [1, 8, 9]. In addition, there is often diffuse and continuous subpleural fibrosis forming large, solid blocks of fibrosis. Honeycomb change is commonly seen in the periphery, consisting of irregular respiratory epithelial-lined cysts containing mucus, mixed inflammation, and sometimes cholesterol-laden giant cells. Squamous metaplasia may be seen. As the cysts of honeycomb change may be lined by ciliated columnar epithelium, some experts require the presence of fibrosis on at least three sides of the cysts, to distinguish honeycombing from PBM [1]. Emphysematous changes may also be present in the background lung parenchyma. Cholesterol granulomas may be seen within the honeycombing as a post-obstructive phenomenon. However, if scattered interstitial non-necrotizing granulomas are present, one must consider CHP in the dif-

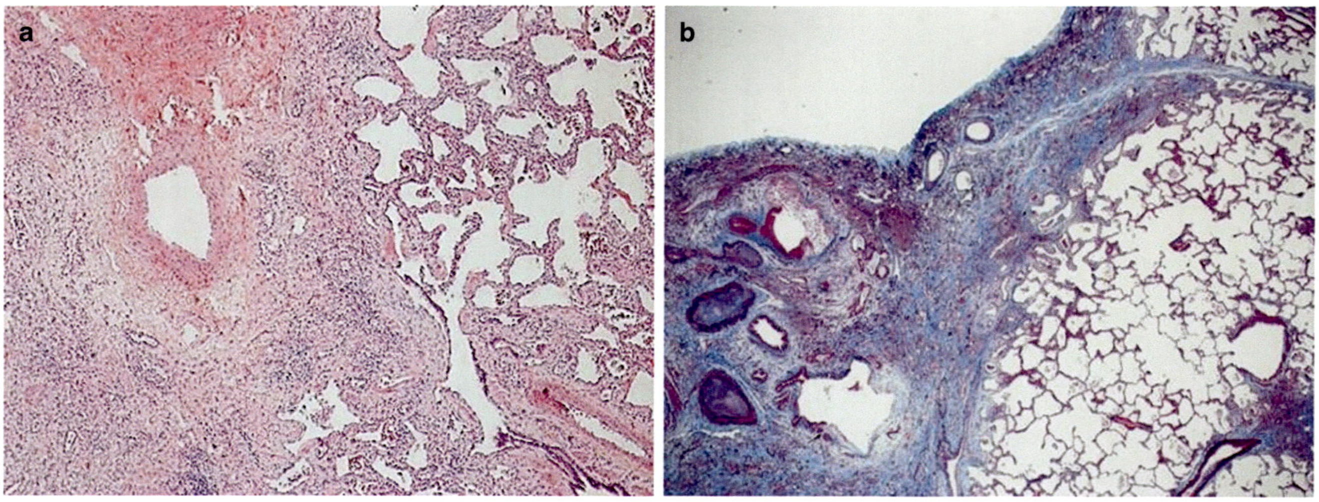

Fig. 39.6 (**a**) Spatial heterogeneity in UIP exhibited by adjacent alternating areas of interstitial fibrosis with dense scarring (*left*) and relatively preserved lung parenchyma (*right*); fibroblastic foci are often present at the advancing edge of the fibrosis (arrow), (**b**) trichrome stain highlights the interstitial fibrosis and fibroblast foci

ferential diagnosis. Similarly, evidence of chronic airway disease, such as PBM, should not be prominent in UIP. The presence of organizing pneumonia may also argue against a diagnosis of UIP. However, organizing pneumonia can be present in the setting of resolving acute exacerbation.

Are There Any Laboratory Tests That Can Aid in the Diagnosis of UIP or HP?

Idiopathic pulmonary fibrosis (IPF), which by definition shows a UIP pattern, has a strong genetic component. UIP/IPF patients have been shown to have increased expression of genes favoring tissue remodeling, epithelial genes, and myofibroblast genes [3]. Genetic alterations involving *TERT*, surfactant genes, and a single nucleotide polymorphism involving *MUC5B* have been implicated. In addition, patients with short telomeres have shorter survival times and are associated with faster disease progression [8, 11, 15, 16]. While the diagnosis of UIP is generally not made on transbronchial biopsies, there is however an increasing role for molecular testing in assisting to make this diagnosis, particularly on such small specimens, including next-generation sequencing panels and commercially available tests [17].

Patients with HP have been shown to demonstrate increased expression of genes favoring immune responses and T-cell activation [3]. There are also commercially available serologic panels that assess for the presence of immunoglobulins (IgGs) toward some of the most common antigens associated with HP, including *Aspergillus fumigatus*, *Aspergillus niger*, *Thermoactinomyces vulgaris*, and *pigeon serum*; however, these tests are often not comprehensive. In certain patients, these tests can provide supporting evidence for HP, but they are not diagnostic [18].

References

1. Leslie KO. My approach to interstitial lung disease using clinical, radiographic and histopathological patterns. J Clin Pathol. 2009;62:387–401.
2. Kumar V, Abbas AK, Aster JC. Robbins and Cotran pathologic basis of disease, vol. 684-685. 9th ed. Philadelphia, PA: Elsevier; 2015. p. 694–5.
3. Churg A, Bilawich A, Wright J. Pathology of chronic hypersensitivity pneumonitis. What is it? What are the diagnostic criteria? Why do we care? Arch Pathol Lab Med. 2018;142:109–19.
4. Takemura T, Akashi T, Kamiya H, et al. Pathological differentiation of chronic hypersensitivity pneumonitis from idiopathic pulmonary fibrosis/usual interstitial pneumonia. Histopathology. 2012;61:1026–35.
5. Miller R, Allen TC, Barrios RJ, et al. Hypersensitivity pneumonitis, a perspective from members of the pulmonary pathology society. Arch Pathol Lab Med. 2018;142:120–6.
6. Patel AM, Ryu JH, Reed CE. Hypersensitivity pneumonitis: current concepts and future questions. J Allergy Clin Immunol. 2001;108:661–70.
7. Liebow AA, Carrington CB. The interstitial pneumonias. In: Simon M, Potchen EJ, Lemay E, editors. Frontiers in pulmonary radiology. New York: Grune and Stratton; 1969. p. 102–41.
8. Wolters PJ, Collard HR, Jones KD. Pathogenesis of idiopathic pulmonary fibrosis. Annu Rev Pathol. 2014;9:157–79.
9. Chung J, Lynch D. The value of multidisciplinary approach to the diagnosis of usual interstitial pneumonitis and idiopathic pulmonary fibrosis: radiology, pathology and clinical correlation. Am J Roentgenol. 2016;206:463–71.
10. Smith ML. Update on pulmonary fibrosis. Arch Pathol Lab Med. 2016;140:221–9.
11. Travis WD, Costabel U, Hansell DM, et al. An official American Thoracic Society/European Respiratory Society statement: update of the international multidisciplinary classification of the idiopathic interstitial pneumonias. Am J Respir Crit Care Med. 2013;188:733–48.
12. Salvatore M, Smith M. Cross sectional imaging of pulmonary fibrosis translating pathology into radiology. Clin Imaging. 2018;51:332–6.
13. Cl S, Muller NL, Lynch DA, et al. Chronic hypersensitivity pneumonitis: differentiation from idiopathic pulmonary fibrosis and non-

specific interstitial pneumonia by using thin-section CT. Radiology. 2008;246:288–97.
14. Rosen Y. Pathology of sarcoidosis. Semin Respir Crit Care Med. 2007;28:36–52.
15. Cronkhite JT, Raghu G, Chin KM, et al. Telomere shortening in familial and sporadic pulmonary fibrosis. Am J Respir Crit Care Med. 2008;187:729–37.
16. Juge PA, Lee JS, Ebstein E, et al. *MUC5B* promoter variant and rheumatoid arthritis with interstitial lung disease. N Engl J Med. 2018;379(23):2209–19. https://doi.org/10.1056/NEJMoa1801562.s.
17. Lynch D, Colby T, Myers J, et al. Molecular diagnosis of usual interstitial pneumonia (UIP) from transbronchial biopsy is accurate in subjects without definite or probable UIP on CT. Chest. 2018;154:458A–9A.
18. Lacasse Y, Cormier Y. Hypersensitivity pneumonitis. Orphanet J Rare Dis. 2006;1:25. https://doi.org/10.1186/1750-1172-1-25.

Organizing Pneumonia Versus Usual Interstitial Pneumonia

40

Brian Mau, Lisa Noel Johnson, and Haodong Xu

Case Presentation

A 41-year-old man with a history of relapsed acute myeloid leukemia treated with multiple rounds of chemotherapy and allogeneic stem cell transplant 3 years prior, followed by double-cord stem cell transplant 1 month prior, presented with diffuse alveolar hemorrhage, CMV infection, volume overload, and worsening hypoxemic respiratory failure. A computerized tomography (CT) of the chest demonstrated bilateral lung consolidation and multiple nodular infiltrates (Fig. 40.1). A bronchoalveolar lavage was performed with laboratory studies suggestive of pulmonary hemorrhage and mixed bacterial pneumonia. He was started on broad spectrum antimicrobial therapy and was admitted to the intensive care unit. His respiratory status continued to worsen and was intubated. However, his condition continued to worsen despite therapy; he was ultimately transitioned to receiving comfort measures only and subsequently died.

An autopsy was performed. Postmortem examination of the lungs revealed heavy and diffusely consolidated lung parenchyma with several patchy areas of density in both upper lobes and the left lower lobe. There was patchy hemorrhage and bilateral pleural effusions. Postmortem viral, fungal, and bacterial cultures were negative. Histologic sections from the consolidated areas from the right lung demonstrated extensive organizing pneumonia (OP) with growth of immature fibroblastic cells filling the bronchiolar lumina and alveolar spaces (Fig. 40.2). Possible etiologies included infection, drug toxicity, and chronic graft-versus-host disease (CGVHD). Cryptogenic OP was considered in the differential; however, CGVHD was favored based on the correlation of the pathological findings with imaging studies, laboratory testing, and clinical history.

B. Mau · H. Xu (✉)
Department of Laboratory Medicine and Pathology, University of Washington Medical Center, Seattle, WA, USA
e-mail: brianmau@uw.edu; xuh8@uw.edu

L. N. Johnson
Department of Radiology, University of Washington Medical Center, Seattle, WA, USA
e-mail: lisanoel@uw.edu

H. Xu et al. (eds.), *Practical Lung Pathology*, Practical Anatomic Pathology, https://doi.org/10.1007/978-3-031-14402-8_40

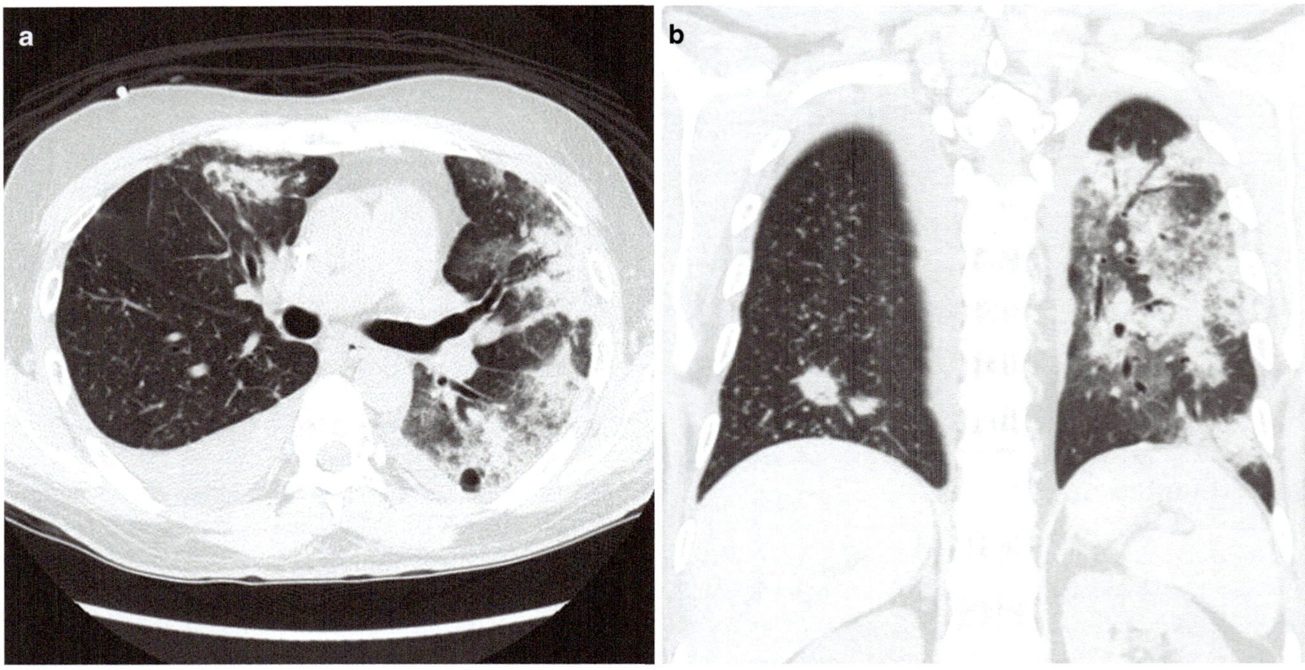

Fig. 40.1 (**a**) Axial noncontrast-enhanced CT chest through the mid-lungs (lung windowing) demonstrates left greater than right peripheral areas of nodular consolidation and ground glass. (**b**) Coronal CT chest redemonstrates multifocal areas of nodular consolidation with scattered areas of regional ground glass in both lungs (left greater than right)

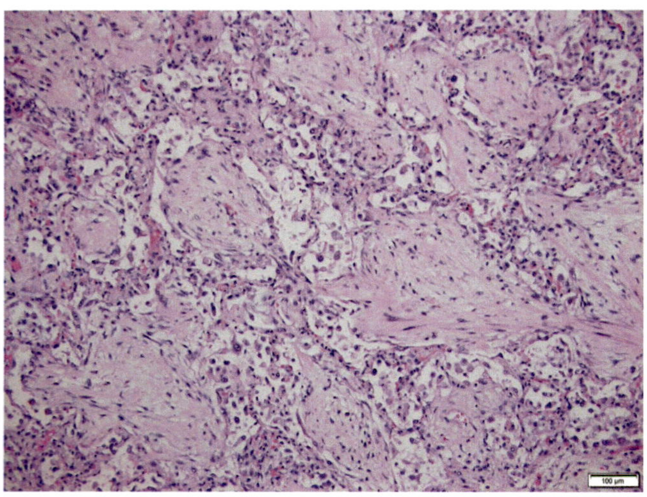

Fig. 40.2 Histological section showing lung parenchyma with foci of polypoid intraluminal plugs with fibroblasts embedded in a myxoid stroma involving alveolar spaces, or the so-called Masson bodies (H&E, 100×)

Final Pathologic Diagnosis: Organizing Pneumonia

What Are the Clinical and Prognostic Characteristics of Cryptogenic Organizing Pneumonia and How Do They Differ from Idiopathic Pulmonary Fibrosis?

Organizing pneumonia (OP) is one of the interstitial pneumonia patterns that can be seen in a variety of disease processes, such as malignancy, infection, graft-versus-host disease, and connective tissue disease [1–5]. If the causes for OP have been ruled out, a diagnosis of cryptogenic OP (COP) can be made. Patients with COP commonly present with cough and sometimes a flu-like illness [1]. Diagnosis of COP is made based on clinical presentation, radiologic imaging studies, lung biopsy, and excluding other potential causes for OP [3]. Most patients diagnosed with COP respond to corticosteroid therapy with resolution of symptoms, although some may relapse [1].

The typical prognosis of IPF is poorer than for COP. IPF is a type of progressive fibrosing interstitial pneumonia of unknown etiology. However, IPF is a known manifestation of, and frequently seen in, heritable telomere and telomerase disorders [6]. The radiologic and histopathologic correlate of IPF is usual interstitial pneumonia (UIP). The clinical diagnosis of IPF requires the exclusion of other known causes of interstitial lung disease, a pattern diagnostic of UIP on high-resolution CT (HRCT), or a combination of features of UIP on HRCT and histopathologic examination as described in the 2018 clinical practice guidelines established by the American Thoracic Society, European Respiratory Society, Japanese Respiratory Society, and Latin American Thoracic Society [7]. In cases of suspected IPF, serologic testing to aid in the exclusion of connective tissue diseases is also recommended [7]. Two drugs have been approved by the FDA for use in patients with IPF, the selective tyrosine kinase inhibitor nintedanib, and the synthetic pyridone antifibrotic agent pirfenidone. Both drugs have been shown to slow disease progression [8, 9]. However, lung transplantation is often necessary in patients with IPF.

Importantly, OP can be seen superimposed in the setting of UIP. This is especially significant in the setting of an acute exacerbation of IPF, which has significant prognostic implications [4, 10].

What Are the Radiologic Features of Organizing Pneumonia and How Do They Differ from Usual Interstitial Pneumonia?

Typical CT findings compatible with OP consist of patchy consolidation in a subpleural, peribronchial, and band-like pattern with ground-glass opacities in a perilobular pattern (Fig. 40.3). The reverse-halo sign (central ground glass opacity with peripheral consolidation), also called the atoll sign, was initially described in COP but has since been reported in association with invasive fungal infections such as pulmonary mucormycosis as well as other infections [11, 12].

Again, OP can be seen in addition to UIP. The criteria for UIP on radiologic imaging studies have been well established. For a definite radiologic diagnosis, there must be honeycombing, with or without peripheral traction bronchiectasis or bronchiolectasis, with a basal and subpleural predominance (Fig. 40.4). Radiologic criteria for probable and indeterminate for UIP have also been established [7].

What Histologic Features Can Be Used to Distinguish Organizing Pneumonia from Usual Interstitial Pneumonia?

OP can be seen on histopathologic examination as loose fibrocollagenous polypoid plugs that fill alveolar spaces, which may also extend into bronchiolar lumens. These collections of fibroblasts and myofibroblasts are called

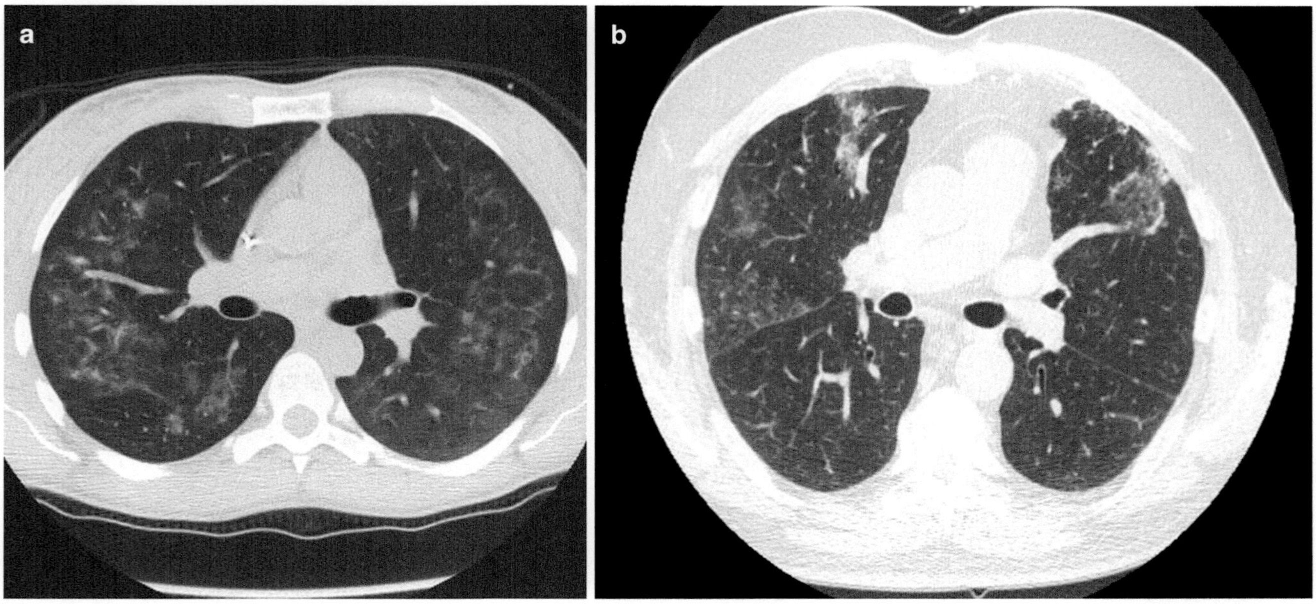

Fig. 40.3 CT demonstrating organizing pneumonia pattern. (**a**) Ground-glass opacities seen here are nonspecific but often represent an organizing pneumonia. (**b**) The opacity seen here in the left upper lobe with a ring of hyperattenuation can be described as a reverse halo sign, which can also be seen as a feature of organizing pneumonia

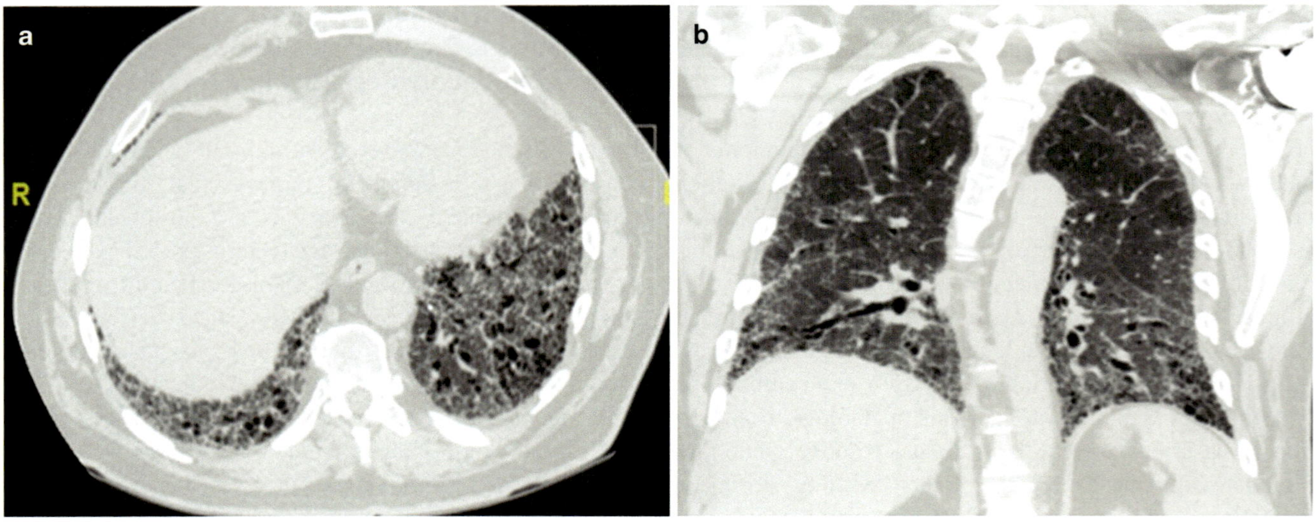

Fig. 40.4 CT demonstrating UIP pattern. (**a**, **b**) Features of interstitial fibrosis with honeycombing are seen with predominant involvement of lower lobes. These findings are consistent with a UIP pattern

Masson bodies [1, 2] (Fig. 40.5). Significant fibrosis and architectural distortion are not typical features of OP but can be seen in other interstitial lung diseases.

A diagnosis of UIP can be made if there is patchy fibrosis in a subpleural and paraseptal distribution involving the lower lobes more than the upper lobes. Classically the fibrosis is heterogeneous, with areas of lung parenchyma with significant fibrosis adjacent to areas that appear to be relatively unaffected [7, 10]. A commonly used descriptive term is "cystic/honeycomb change" which describes the architectural remodeling with characteristic features of cystic spaces and dense fibrosis (Fig. 40.6). At the "leading edges" of the fibrosis, fibroblastic foci may be seen. The fibroblastic foci seen in UIP are also well-defined areas of proliferation of fibroblasts and myofibroblasts in a myxoid background. However, compared to fibroblastic foci, Masson bodies of OP are localized in the alveolar spaces (Fig. 40.7a), whereas fibroblastic foci are loose organizing connective tissue juxtaposed with dense collagenous scar (Fig. 40.7b).

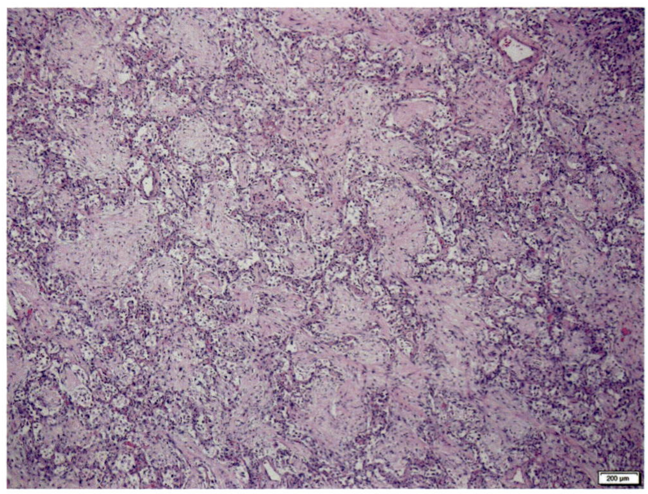

Fig. 40.5 Histologic section demonstrating organizing pneumonia. Masson bodies are seen filling the alveolar spaces (H&E, 40×)

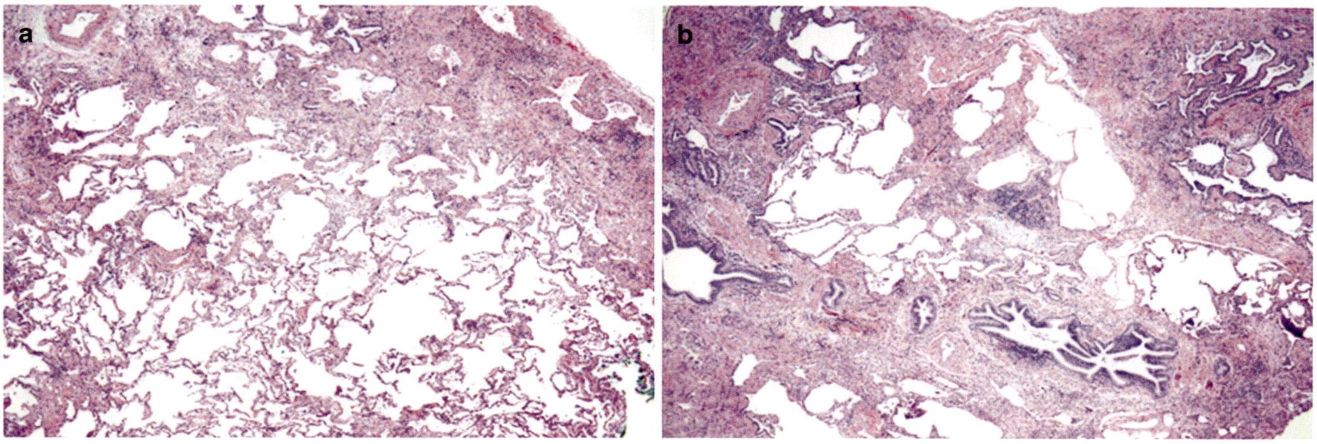

Fig. 40.6 H&E sections demonstrating UIP pattern. The subpleural and paraseptal interstitial fibrosis with cystic changes and fibroblast foci are seen more prominently in the right lower lobe (**b**, H&E, 100×) than in the upper lobe (**a**, H&E, 100×)

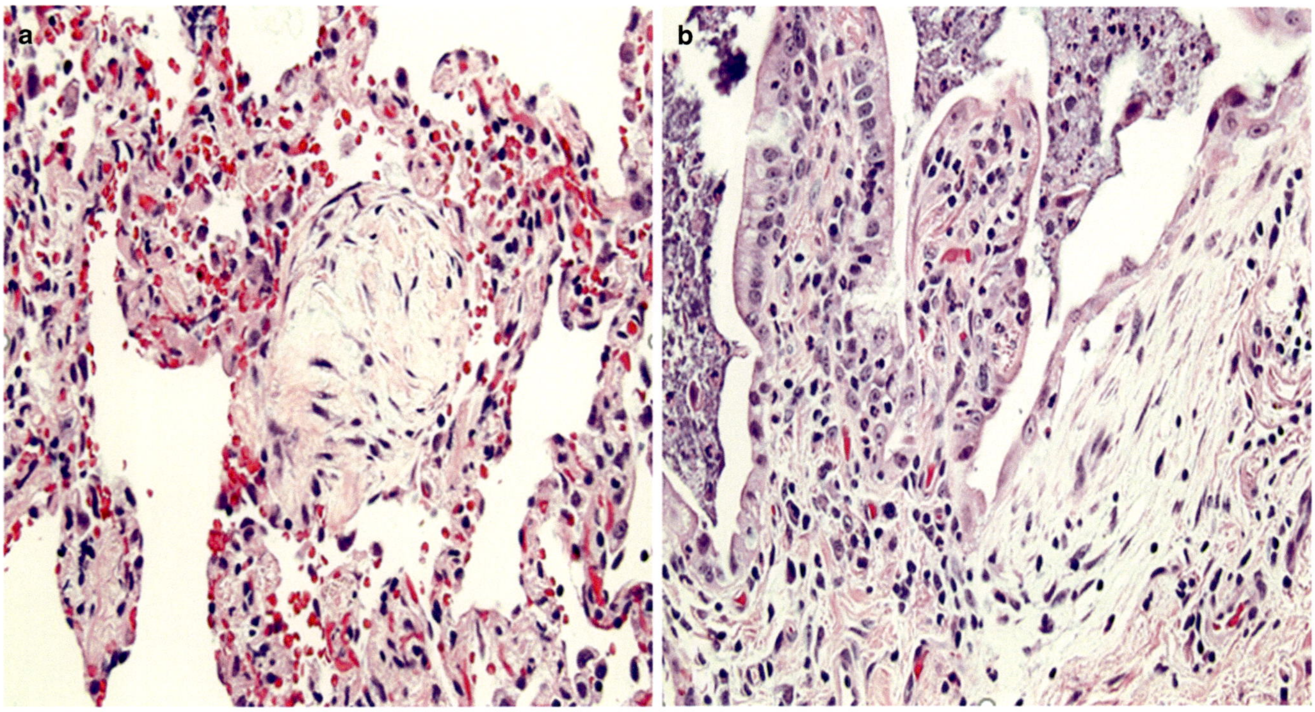

Fig. 40.7 Side-by-side comparison of a Masson body and a fibroblastic focus. (**a**) The Masson body is localized in the alveolar space (H&E, 400×). (**b**) This fibroblastic focus is juxtaposed to the dense collagenous scar (H&E, 400×)

References

1. Khan A, Al-Ghanem S, Al-Jahdali H, Bamefleh H. Bronchiolitis obliterans organizing pneumonia: pathogenesis, clinical features, imaging and therapy review. Ann Thorac Med. 2008;3(2):67.
2. Cordier J. Cryptogenic organising pneumonia. Eur Respir J. 2006;28(2):422–46.
3. King TE, Mortenson RL. Cryptogenic organizing pneumonitis. The North American experience. Chest. 1992;102(1):8S.
4. Travis W, Costabel U, Hansell D, King T, Lynch D, Nicholson A, et al. An official American Thoracic Society/European Respiratory Society statement: update of the international multidisciplinary classification of the idiopathic interstitial pneumonias. Am J Respir Crit Care Med. 2013;188(6):733–48.
5. Freudenberger T. Association between acute and chronic graft-versus-host disease and bronchiolitis obliterans organizing pneumonia in recipients of hematopoietic stem cell transplants. Blood. 2003;102(10):3822–8.
6. Armanios M. Telomerase and idiopathic pulmonary fibrosis. Mutat Res. 2012;730(1–2):52–8.
7. Raghu G, Remy-Jardin M, Myers J, Richeldi L, Ryerson C, Lederer D, et al. Diagnosis of idiopathic pulmonary fibrosis. An official

ATS/ERS/JRS/ALAT clinical practice guideline. Am J Respir Crit Care Med. 2018;198(5):e44–68.
8. King T, Bradford W, Castro-Bernardini S, Fagan E, Glaspole I, Glassberg M, et al. A phase 3 trial of pirfenidone in patients with idiopathic pulmonary fibrosis. N Engl J Med. 2014;370(22):2083–92.
9. Richeldi L, du Bois R, Raghu G, Azuma A, Brown K, Costabel U, et al. Efficacy and safety of Nintedanib in idiopathic pulmonary fibrosis. N Engl J Med. 2014;370(22):2071–82.
10. Cavazza A, Rossi G, Carbonelli C, Spaggiari L, Paci M, Roggeri A. The role of histology in idiopathic pulmonary fibrosis: an update. Respir Med. 2010;104:S11–22.
11. Kim SJ, Lee KS, Ryu YH, Yoon YC, Choe KO, Kim TS, et al. Reversed halo sign on high-resolution CT of cryptogenic organizing pneumonia: diagnostic implications. Am J Roentgenol. 2003;180(5):1251–4.
12. Maturu VN, Agarwal R. Reversed halo sign: a systematic review. Respir Care. 2014;59(9):1440–9.

41 Diffuse Alveolar Damage (Organizing Phase) Versus Nonspecific Interstitial Pneumonia

Nicholas Stanzione and Gregory A. Fishbein

Case Presentation

A 65-year-old previously healthy woman presented with a 10-day history of shortness of breath, fevers, and cough. She was initially treated with antibiotics for a presumed lower respiratory infection. The patient returned to the emergency department 2 days later with worsening respiratory symptoms, requiring intubation and ventilator support, as well as lower extremity edema. Chest X-rays demonstrated bilateral infiltrates with persistent ground-glass attenuation and airspace consolidations bilaterally, involving all lobes, with increased density of the right upper lobe consolidation (Fig. 41.1a). High-resolution computed tomography (HRCT) studies showed large areas of bilateral coalescent airspace consolidations (Fig. 41.1b).

Based on the imaging studies, the differential diagnosis included multifocal acute pneumonia, drug-related toxicity,

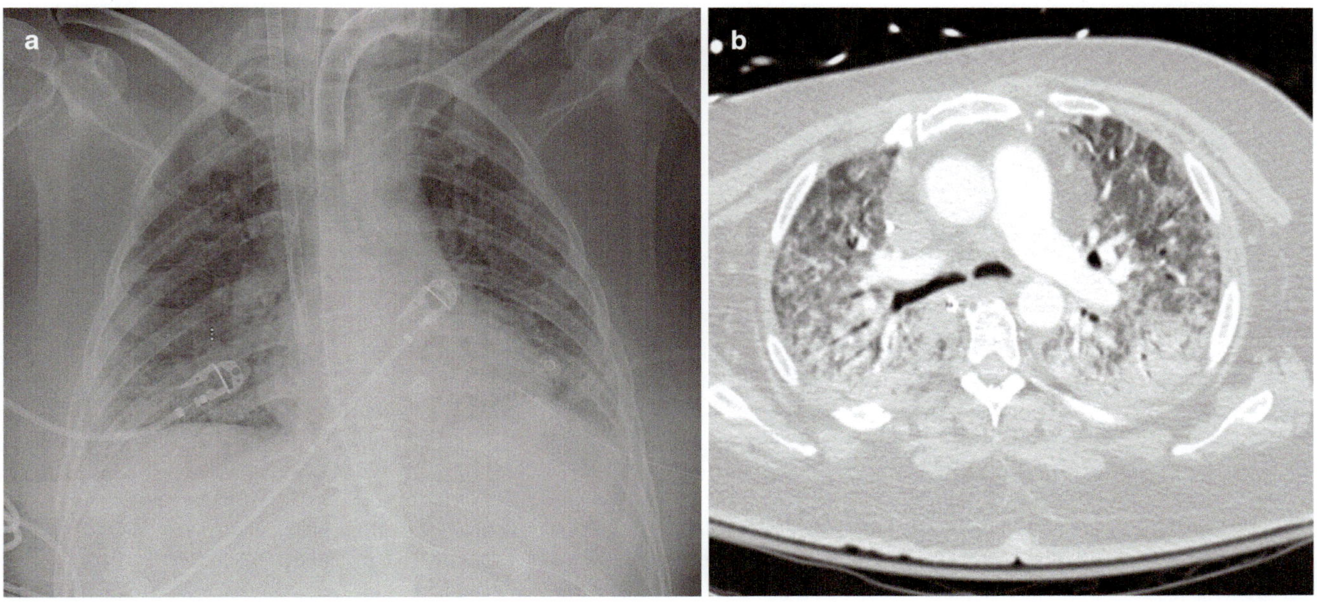

Fig. 41.1 (**a**) Chest X-ray showing bilateral diffuse hazy opacities ("whiteout"). (**b**) Post contrast CT scan of chest demonstrates bilateral upper lobe dominant course ground-glass opacity and lower lobe dominant consolidation without significant architectural distortion, suggestive of diffuse alveolar damage. Images contributed by Fereidoun Abtin, MD from UCLA Department of Radiology

N. Stanzione
VA Greater Los Angeles Healthcare System, Los Angeles, CA, USA

G. A. Fishbein (✉)
David Geffen School of Medicine, University of California, Los Angeles (UCLA), Los Angeles, CA, USA
e-mail: gfishbein@mednet.ucla.edu

H. Xu et al. (eds.), *Practical Lung Pathology*, Practical Anatomic Pathology, https://doi.org/10.1007/978-3-031-14402-8_41

and interstitial lung disease. The patient's white blood cell count was mildly elevated. Blood cultures were negative.

Bronchoscopy was performed which demonstrated patent airways with minimal secretions and no endobronchial lesion. The procedure was complicated by intermittent episodes of hypoxia. A transbronchial biopsy was performed, which showed uniform appearing areas of interstitial fibrosis with some alveolar sparing, prominent reactive pneumocyte II hyperplasia, and hyaline membranes (Fig. 41.2a, b); the interstitial fibrosis is highlighted by trichrome staining (Fig. 41.2c). These findings supported the diagnosis of diffuse alveolar damage (DAD), acute and organizing phases. With continued supportive care including high-flow oxygen therapy, the patient's respiratory status improved.

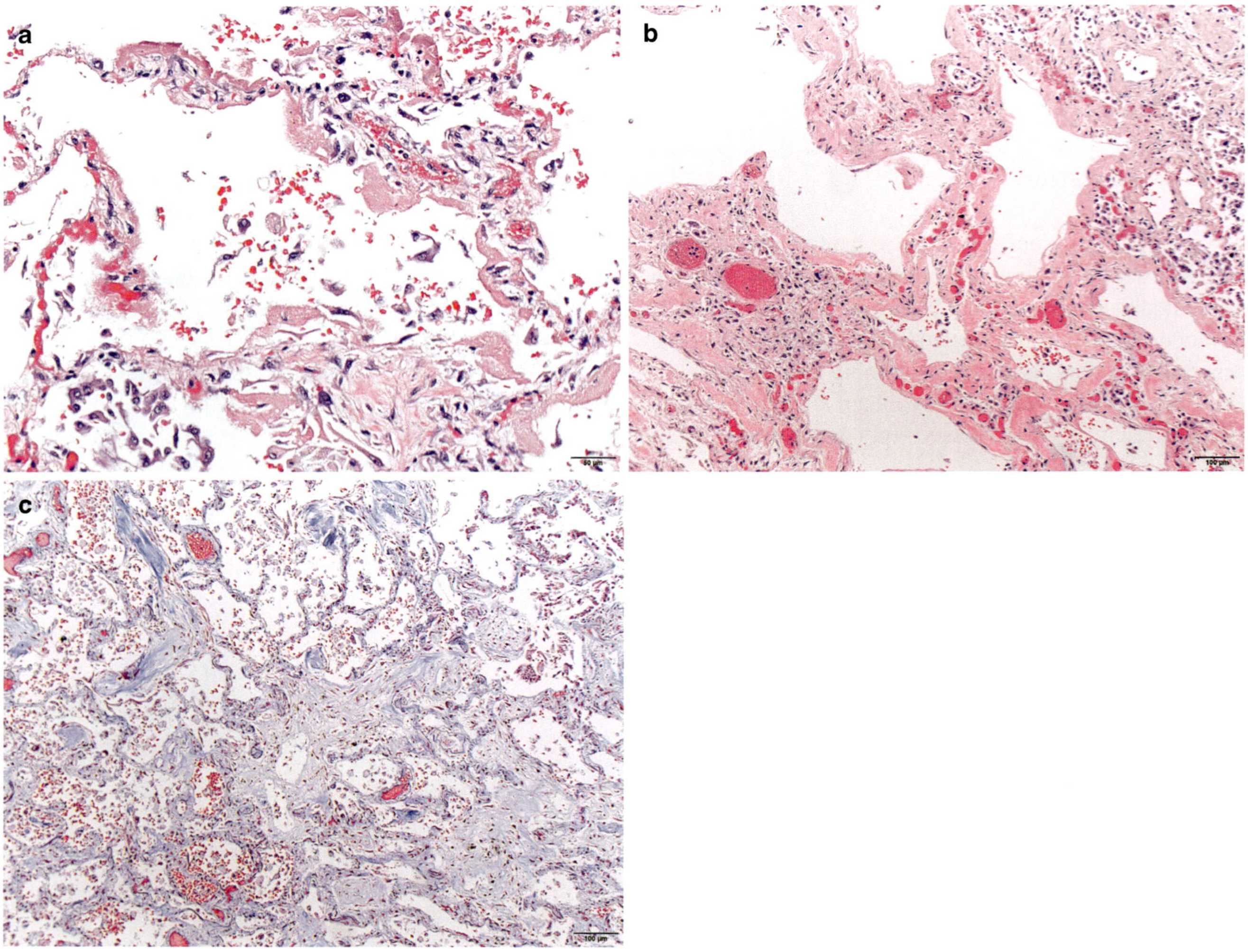

Fig. 41.2 (**a**) Acute phase of DAD with interstitial edema and prominent hyaline membranes lining the alveolar septa and focal organizing fibrosis. (**b**) Acute and organizing phases of DAD with hyaline membranes lining the alveolar septa interstitial fibrosis. (**c**) Organizing phase of DAD with trichrome stain highlighting the alveolar duct and interstitial fibrosis

Pathologic Diagnosis: Acute and Organizing Phases of Diffuse Alveolar Damage

What Is Diffuse Alveolar Damage?

Diffuse alveolar damage (DAD) is a histologic pattern of acute lung injury, seen as a pathologic manifestation of different clinical entities including acute lung injury (ALI), acute respiratory distress syndrome (ARDS), and acute interstitial pneumonitis (AIP, a.k.a. Hamman-Rich syndrome) [1, 2]. The DAD pattern of lung injury may also be secondary to infection, connective tissue disease, drug injury, ingestants, sepsis, shock, and radiation, among others. The pathophysiology of DAD is complex and not completely understood but is related to damage to pulmonary capillary endothelium and alveolar epithelium which leads to the leakage of fluid and cellular breakdown products, mediated by a complex network of inflammatory markers and genetic factors [1].

What Are the Phases of DAD?

Diffuse alveolar damage is histologically separated into three phases, which in reality represent an overlapping spectrum of findings: (1) acute/exudative phase; (2) organizing/proliferative phase, and (3) fibrotic phase [1, 3]. The acute phase usually occurs within the first week following pulmonary injury, and the most easily recognized histologically. Microscopic examination shows diffuse, uniform intra-alveolar and interstitial edema with the presence of hyaline membranes (Fig. 41.2a, b).

Hyaline membranes, the hallmark of DAD, are composed of cellular and proteinaceous debris, plasma proteins, and surfactant components, which appear as glossy, pink-eosinophilic membranes, lining the alveolar septa [1, 2]. The cellular debris is a result of endothelial cell and pneumocyte necrosis. Acute alveolar hemorrhage may also be present [3]. The organizing phase of DAD usually becomes more prominent 1 or more weeks following the injury and is characterized by fibroblast proliferation forming uniform interstitial fibrosis and granulation tissue in the alveolar spaces as the lung attempts to repair the damage (Fig. 41.2). Type 2 pneumocyte hyperplasia is often pronounced, demonstrating hobnail morphology. The pneumocytes may exhibit marked reactive cytologic atypia with scattered mitotic figures, and squamous metaplasia may be extensive; these findings should not be over interpreted as dysplasia or carcinoma in this clinical setting [1, 3]. The hyaline membranes characteristic of the acute phase gradually disappear and become incorporated into the alveolar septa, admixed with fibroblasts (Fig. 41.2a, b) [1]. In the fibrotic phase, the fibroblastic tissue becomes densely collagenous. End-stage honeycomb change may develop, as well as traction bronchiectasis and bronchiolectasis (Table 41.1).

Table 41.1 Gross and histologic features of diffuse alveolar damage

	Acute phase (early)	Organizing phase (late)	Fibrotic phase
Gross appearance	• Heavy and edematous	• Heavy	• Heavy, firm-rubbery
	• Firm, red-blue surfaces	• Less edematous, more firm	• Red-brown to gray
Histologic features	• Intra-alveolar edema	• Interstitial fibrosis	• Widened alveolar septa with collagenous fibrosis
	• Interstitial edema	• Pneumocyte hyperplasia	• Interstitial fibrosis
	• Hyaline membranes	• Pneumocyte atypia • Squamous metaplasia • Incorporation of hyaline membranes into septa	• ± Microscopic honeycomb changes

What Is Nonspecific Interstitial Pneumonia?

When initially introduced by Katzenstein and Fiorelli, nonspecific interstitial pneumonia (NSIP) was often used as a diagnosis whenever the pattern of disease could not be discretely classified into another more specific category of idiopathic interstitial pneumonia [2, 4]. NSIP was accepted as a specific pathologic entity in the 2013 American Thoracic Society/European Respiratory Society (ATS/ERS) [5]. Grossly, NSIP lungs often demonstrate firm parenchyma bilaterally, typically with subpleural sparing. The findings may be more prominent in the lower lobes (Fig. 41.3). Honeycomb changes may be seen, particularly in more advanced disease [2, 4]. Histologically, the classic NSIP pattern shows diffuse alveolar wall thickening with an even distribution and preservation of the alveolar architecture (Fig. 41.4) [2, 4, 5]. The changes are temporally homogeneous (i.e., normal alveolar tissue is generally not seen admixed within regions of advanced fibrosis) [6]. Honeycomb changes as well as fibroblastic foci should be inconspicuous or absent [4]. There are two major patterns observed in NSIP: cellular and fibrotic. The cellular pattern is characterized by the presence of a dense chronic lymphoid infiltrate within the alveolar septa, predominantly composed of lymphocytes and plasma cells.

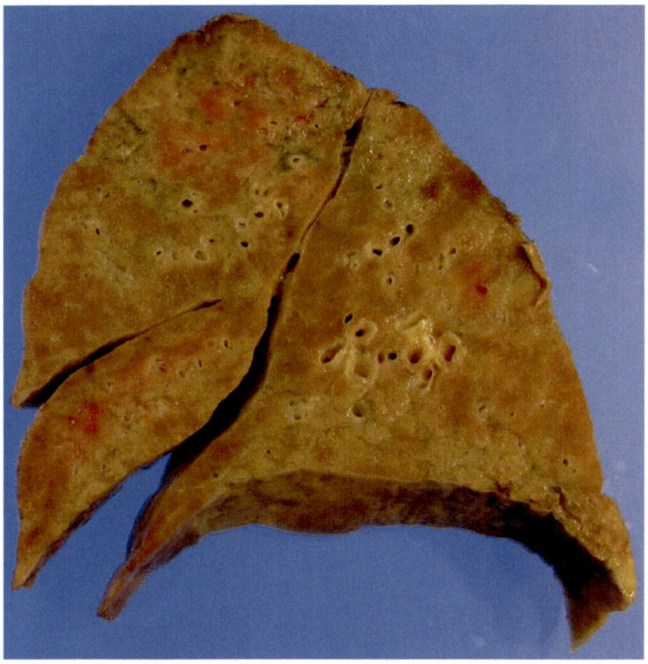

Fig. 41.3 Gross examination of NSIP lungs demonstrates diffusely firm, fibrotic parenchyma predominantly in the lower lung fields, with some subpleural sparing of the upper lobe

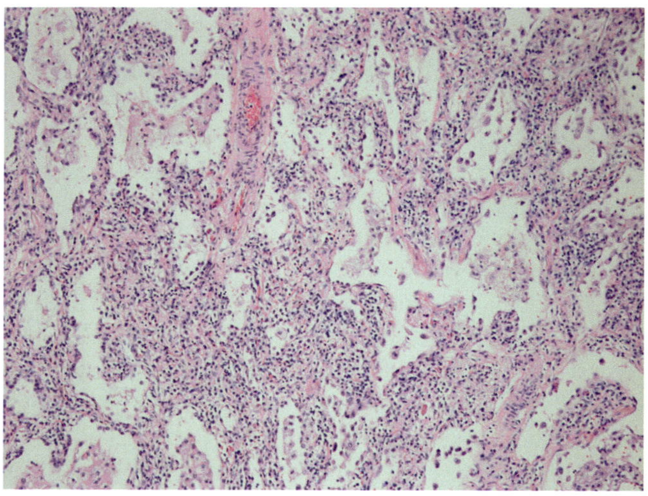

Fig. 41.4 Microscopic examination in fibrotic NSIP characterized by diffusely thickened and fibrotic alveolar walls with preservation of the alveolar architecture

The fibrotic pattern is more common and primarily characterized by the presence of dense uniform interstitial fibrosis without a significant inflammatory component and the absence of temporal or geographic heterogeneity. Cases may overlap, where both cellular and fibrotic patterns may be evident [2, 4].

How Do DAD and NSIP Overlap Histologically?

The diffuse and uniform interstitial widening that is seen in the organizing phase of DAD can be diagnostically challenging to separate from NSIP. Both can demonstrate diffusely thickened and fibrotic interstitium, with varying degrees of interstitial cellular infiltrates. Purely cellular NSIP will typically contain interstitial lymphocytic inflammation that far exceeds the inflammation seen in DAD. Distinguishing fibrosing NSIP from organizing DAD may present more of a challenge. The fibrosis in DAD has been described as loose and myxoid, appearing bluish-gray on routine sections, whereas the fibrosis in NSIP is more eosinophilic and densely collagenous [1, 7]. Residual hyaline membranes and alveolar duct fibrosis are indeed features of DAD. However, acute or organizing DAD in a background of fibrosing interstitial lung disease could represent an acute or subacute exacerbation of NSIP. In this setting, incorporation of clinical and radiographic information is critical, particularly when faced with small biopsies. Reactive pneumocyte hyperplasia tends to be more pronounced in organizing DAD. Fibrotic phase DAD can be indistinguishable from fibrotic NSIP.

How Can the Clinical History Help Distinguish DAD from NSIP?

The clinical counterpart of DAD is acute lung injury and ARDS. Most cases of ARDS develop within 2–5 days of hospitalization [3]. In 1994, the American-European Consensus Conference on ARDS formally defined ARDS as the presence of acute hypoxemia with (1) a ratio of partial pressure of arterial oxygen to the fraction of inspired oxygen (PaO_2:FIO_2) of 200 mm Hg or less, (2) bilateral infiltrates that are consistent with pulmonary edema radiographically, and (3) no clinical evidence of cardiac failure. The mortality rate for ARDS is very high, with historic rates of 50–60%, which increase with age, being highest in patients over 85 years old.

The clinical presentation of NSIP is dependent on the underlying etiology. Potential etiologies of NSIP pattern include connective tissues disease associated interstitial lung disease (CT-ILD), adverse drug reaction, infections, immunodeficiency diseases, familial pulmonary fibrosis, as well as idiopathic fibrosing NSIP. In the case of idiopathic NSIP, the patients are typically middle-aged women, in the fifth to sixth decades, who usually present with greater than 6 months of dyspnea and cough. It has been postulated that idiopathic NSIP may represent an unknown autoimmune disease. Pulmonary function testing typically demonstrates a restrictive physiology. Treatment of NSIP depends upon the underlying etiology; patients with CTD-associated NSIP often receive immunosuppression and immunomodulation. The prognosis of NSIP, regardless of etiology, is better than that of usual interstitial pneumonia (UIP) [2, 4]. However, disease evolution is very heterogeneous; a subset of patients progress to end-stage fibrosis [5]. When acute lung dysfunction occurs in the setting of chronic lung disease (i.e., acute exacerbation), the DAD pattern may be superimposed on a background of NSIP.

Can Radiographic Findings Help Distinguish DAD from NSIP?

Classically, patients with ARDS are described to have diffuse, bilateral "white out" pulmonary infiltrates on chest X-ray (see Fig. 41.1). However, on computed tomography (CT) scanning, the distribution is nonhomogeneous and is usually greater in the dependent portion of the lung [1]. In the appropriate clinical setting, diagnostic biopsies are generally not needed. However, a biopsy may be performed in cases with atypical presentations, to rule out an infectious etiology, or in cases where patients are not responding appropriately to therapeutic interventions [3].

The most common CT abnormality in NSIP is bilateral ground-glass opacities. About 75% of cases show reticular opacities, traction bronchiectasis, and bronchiolectasis (Fig. 41.5) [4–6]. Subpleural sparing is a helpful feature to distinguish NSIP from UIP [5]. Honeycombing may occur; however, it should not be a dominant feature, particularly at the time of presentation; the prevalence and extent of honeycombing increase as the disease progresses [4, 5].

Are There Any Ancillary Studies That Can Be Used to Distinguish DAD from NSIP?

There are no ancillary studies that can definitively differentiate DAD and NSIP. Clinical, radiographic, and histologic correlation is the mainstay of diagnosis.

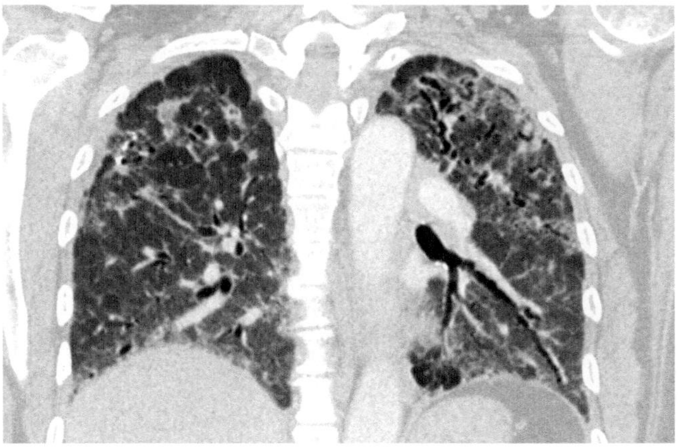

Fig. 41.5 Coronal CT of NSIP showing bilateral, lower and upper lobe, symmetric ground-glass opacities with marked traction bronchiectasis

References

1. Beasley MB. The pathologist's approach to acute lung injury. Arch Pathol Lab Med. 2010;134(5):719–27.
2. Leslie KO. My approach to interstitial lung disease using clinical, radiological and histopathological patterns. J Clin Pathol. 2009;62(5):387–401.
3. Butt Y, Kurdowska A, Allen TC. Acute lung injury: a clinical and molecular review. Arch Pathol Lab Med. 2016;140(4):345–50.
4. Smith ML. Update on pulmonary fibrosis: not all fibrosis is created equally. Arch Pathol Lab Med. 2016;140(3):221–9.
5. Travis WD, Costabel U, Hansell DM, King TE Jr, Lynch DA, Nicholson AG, et al. ATS/ERS Committee on Idiopathic Interstitial Pneumonias. An official American Thoracic Society/European Respiratory Society statement: update of the international multidisciplinary classification of the idiopathic interstitial pneumonias. Am J Respir Crit Care Med. 2013;188(6):733–48.
6. Salvatore M, Smith ML. Cross sectional imaging of pulmonary fibrosis translating pathology into radiology. Clin Imaging. 2018;51:332–6.
7. Hughes KT, Beasley MB. Pulmonary manifestations of acute lung injury: more than just diffuse alveolar damage. Arch Pathol Lab Med. 2017;141(7):916–22.

Chronic Eosinophilic Pneumonia Versus Organizing Pneumonia

42

Lisa Han and Haodong Xu

Case Presentation

A 64-year-old woman with a recent history of profound peripheral eosinophilia (>1000/mm^3), bronchospasm, and waxing and waning bilateral peripheral ground-glass infiltrates on chest computed tomography (CT) (Fig. 42.1). The patient has a long history of seasonal allergies. Two years prior to current presentation, she experienced her first episode of serious bronchospasm with pulmonary infiltrates associated with peripheral eosinophilia. She also had at least two hospitalizations of pneumonia and bronchospasm, treated with antibiotics and steroids. The patient was on steroids at the time of the current wedge biopsies of the right upper, middle, and lower lobes of the lung. There was no etiology clinically identified to explain the histological findings. Histology showed numerous eosinophils, both as sheets filling airspaces and admixed with alveolar macrophages and lymphocytes, with interstitial eosinophilic infiltration and reactive type II pneumocytes. The findings were most prominent in the lower and upper lobes close to the fissure. There were foci of organizing pneumonia (OP) with focal alveolar fibrin and focal subpleural osseous metaplasia. Eosinophil necrosis, granulomas, and inflammatory infiltration of vessels in uninvolved areas were not identified in the biopsies. A GMS stain was negative for fungal organisms (Fig. 42.2).

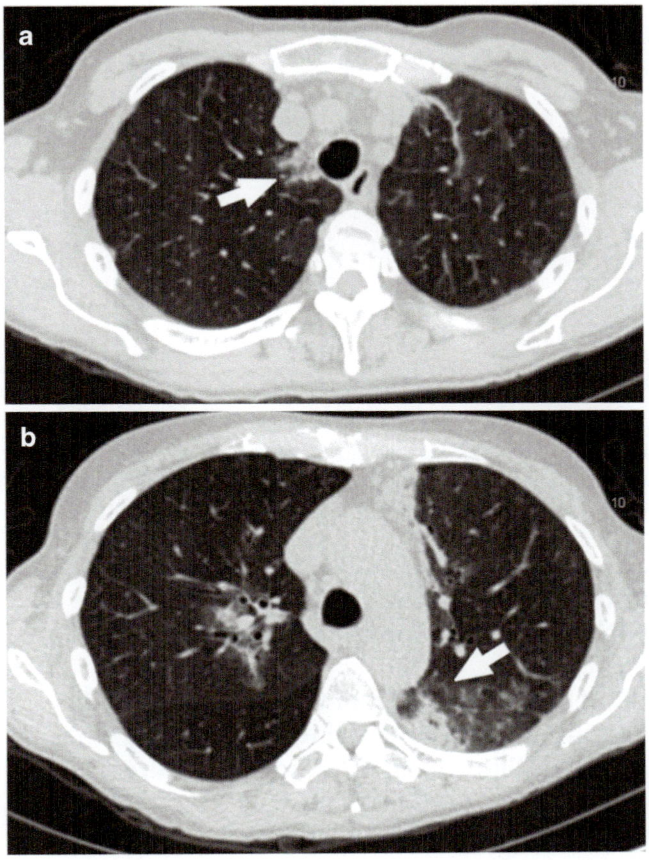

Fig. 42.1 Conventional CT image shows bilateral areas of peripheral reticulation, clustered nodular opacities, and ground-glass attenuation in the right upper lobe (**a**) and left lower lobe (**b**). Central airways are patent without suspicious filling obstruction. No significant pleural effusion or pneumothorax is appreciated

L. Han (✉)
Department of Laboratory Medicine and Pathology, University of Washington Medical Center, Seattle, WA, USA

Department of Pathology, University of Chicago Medical Center, Chicago, IL, USA

H. Xu
Department of Laboratory Medicine and Pathology, University of Washington Medical Center, Seattle, WA, USA
e-mail: xu8@uw.edu

H. Xu et al. (eds.), *Practical Lung Pathology*, Practical Anatomic Pathology, https://doi.org/10.1007/978-3-031-14402-8_42

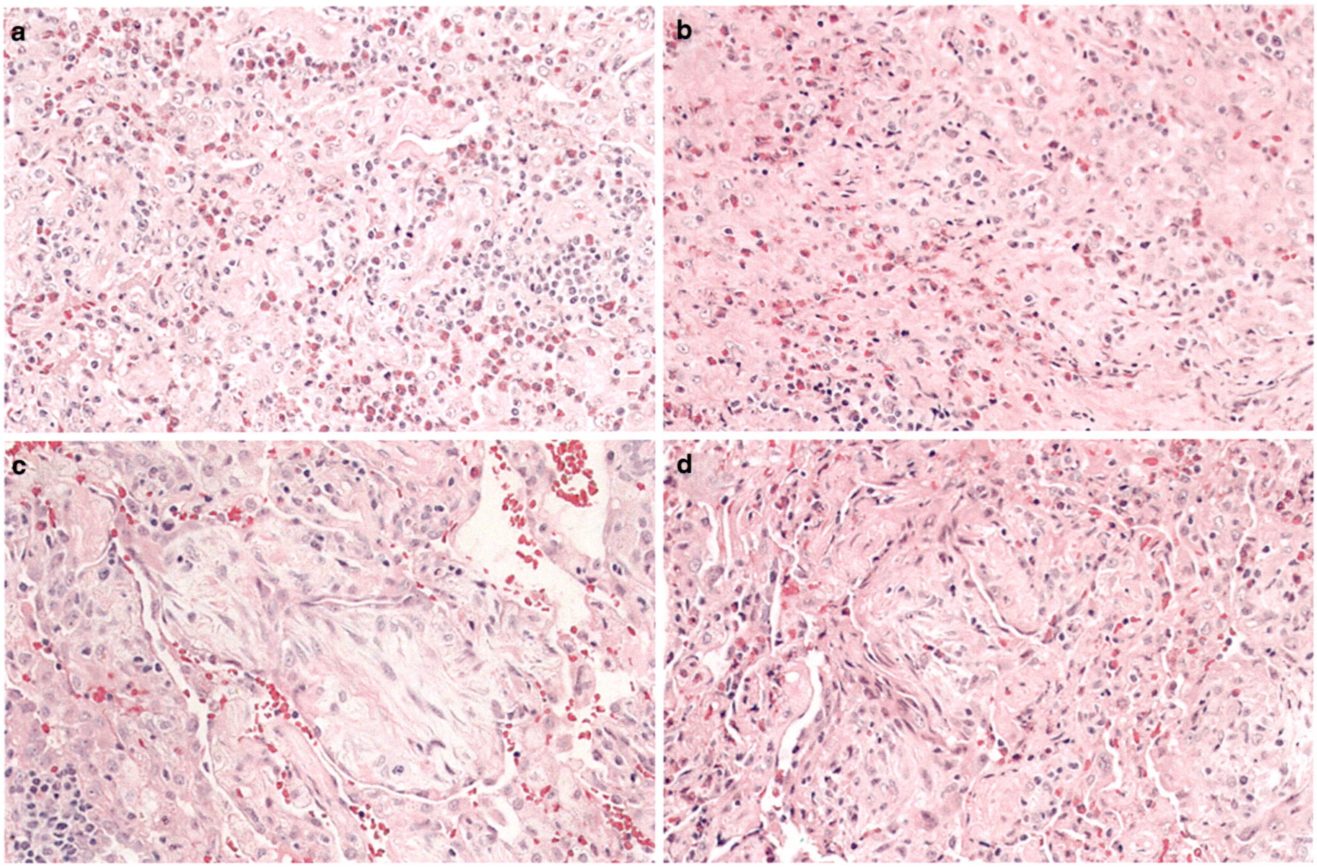

Fig. 42.2 Histologic sections show intra-alveolar eosinophils admixed with macrophages and lymphocytes and with reactive type II pneumocytes (**a**), abundant eosinophilic infiltrate within interstitium (**b**), scattered foci of organizing pneumonia without (**c**) and with eosinophils (**d**). (**a**)–(**d**), H&E 400× magnification

Pathologic Diagnosis: Consistent with Chronic Eosinophilic Pneumonia

What Is the Definition of Chronic Eosinophilic Pneumonia and Organizing Pneumonia? What Are Their Clinical and Prognostic Features?

Chronic eosinophilic pneumonia (CEP) is characterized by abundant eosinophils in the airspaces often accompanied by interstitial inflammation. This rare disorder with idiopathic etiology can develop at any age, although the age of onset is between 30–50 years. Unlike acute eosinophilic pneumonia, women are twice as likely affected, and more than half of cases are associated with atopy and allergic disease such as bronchial asthma. Most patients (>60%) with CEP are non-smokers. Patients most frequently present with cough and dyspnea and, rarely, with respiratory failure and chest pain. Peripheral blood eosinophilia (mean >30%) and elevated IgE levels (mean >500 IU) are also characteristically associated with CEP [1, 2]. The current diagnosis of CEP is outlined in Table 42.1 and typically does not necessitate a lung biopsy.

Table 42.1 Diagnostic criteria for CEP

Features	Specifics
Respiratory symptoms	Lasting at least 2 weeks
Abnormal chest radiology	Diffuse pulmonary alveolar consolidation with air bronchogram and/or ground-glass opacities, especially with peripheral predominance
Bronchoalveolar lavage (BAL) or lung biopsy demonstrating eosinophilia	Differential cell count >40% or peripheral blood eosinophils >1000/mm^3
Exclusion of other pneumonias with eosinophilic features	Examples include drug reaction, parasitic infection, eosinophilic granulomatosis with polyangiitis (EGPA), and allergic bronchopulmonary aspergillosis (ABPA), see below

The prognosis of CEP is favorable as patients dramatically improve with corticosteroid treatment at initial presentation as well as relapse; however, recurrences are common, occurring in more than half of the patients after stopping treatment [3, 4].

In contrast to CEP, which is viewed as an idiopathic diagnosis of exclusion, OP is a histologic pattern for airspace-predominant pathology, which is often a component of another disease or, less frequently, idiopathic/cryptogenic OP. Although eosinophils are not a prominent feature of OP, they may be slightly increased in the BAL of patients with cryptogenic OP. In the vast majority of cases, the increase in eosinophils is slight and less than the increase in lymphocytes. The prognosis of OP mirrors that of its primary etiology. In the case of cryptogenic OP, treatment with corticosteroids leads to recovery in up to 85% of patients [5].

What Are the Radiographic Features of Chronic Eosinophilic Pneumonia?

CEP has classically been described on chest X-ray as having "photographically negative shadow of pulmonary edema," characterized by peripheral airspace consolidation involving mainly the upper lobes. This finding, however, is not specific for CEP and is present in only a quarter of patients [3, 6]. High-resolution CT (HRCT) typically demonstrates bilateral peripheral subpleural airspace consolidation (found in up to 85%), septal thickening, and ground-glass attenuations and is helpful in separating CEP from other eosinophilic lung diseases such as acute eosinophilic pneumonia, ABPA, and EGPA. Organizing pneumonia (OP) can share similar HRCT findings in that it can present with bilateral peripheral subpleural consolidations. However, these are more often perilobular and peribronchiolar, sometimes creating a polygonal appearance. Consolidations are also often accompanied by non-septal linear or reticular opacities and bronchial dilation [7, 8]. In both types of pneumonia, imaging abnormalities rapidly regress after corticosteroid therapy.

What Are the Pathogenesis and Pathologic Features of Chronic Eosinophilic Pneumonia, and How Does That Differ from Organizing Pneumonia?

The pathogenesis of CEP has been theorized to be directly due to eosinophilic release of pro-inflammatory molecules and activation markers. Recent studies to clarify the etiology of CEP through T-cell receptor gene rearrangement analysis in BAL show oligoclonal expansion of T cells, suggesting antigen-driven stimulation and an important interaction between T cells and eosinophils [9, 10].

The main pathologic finding of CEP is abundant eosinophils admixed with a variable number of macrophages within intact airspaces. Occasionally, eosinophilic breakdown products such as Charcot-Leyden crystals are found in the cytoplasm of macrophages. Accompanying interstitial lymphoplasmacytic inflammation is variable, and there should be an absence of significant fibrosis and tissue necrosis. A fibrinous intra-alveolar exudate similar to that found in acute fibrinous and organizing pneumonia (AFOP), although usually mixed with eosinophils, may be present. This exudate may undergo organization creating fibroblastic plugs that resemble OP, except for the abundant eosinophils. Cryptogenic OP, with its characteristic intra-alveolar fibroblastic tissue plugs, tends to center on and around bronchioles with mild to moderate lymphoplasmacytic interstitial inflammatory infiltrates with eosinophils as a minor component. One study quantifying the number of eosinophils per ×160 microscopic fields found a median of 221 eosinophils in CEP versus 7 in cryptogenic OP [11]. However, the distinction between CEP and OP may be impossible after corticosteroid treatment which may result in rapidly depletion of eosinophils from the airspaces but preservation of some fibroblastic plugs. In this case, clinical history, particularly pretreatment peripheral eosinophilic count, as well as waxing and waning peripheral consolidation on imaging are crucial in making the correct diagnosis. Table 42.2 further contrasts the pathologic findings between CEP and OP. Non-necrotizing granulomas are identified in 10–20% of CEP cases, which may be a histiocytic response to eosinophil necrosis. In this case, the absence of destructive vasculitis rules out Churg-Strauss Syndrome (CSS) [12].

Table 42.2 Pathologic findings of CEP and OP

Feature	Chronic eosinophilic pneumonia	Organizing pneumonia
Location of eosinophils	Intra-alveolar collections	Scattered in interstitium[a]
Amount of eosinophils	Abundant[a]	Focal[a]
Fibrous intra-alveolar fibroblastic plugs	Few to abundant	Characteristic finding
Composition of intra-alveolar components	Predominantly eosinophils, some macrophages and fibroblasts, Charcot-Leyden crystals/eosinophil granules within the cytoplasm of macrophages	Fibroblasts, neutrophils, macrophages, and lymphocytes

[a] Prior to corticosteroid treatment

What Are Other Differential Diagnoses for Chronic Eosinophilic Pneumonia?

The differential diagnosis for CEP includes CSS, pulmonary Langerhans cell histiocytosis (PLCH), parasitic infections, and reactive eosinophilic pleuritis.

CSS may morphologically be very similar to CEP with the presence of intra-alveolar eosinophils, clinical history of asthma, and peripheral blood eosinophilia. However, CSS shows necrotizing vasculitis, granulomatous inflammation, and positive serum perinuclear-anti-neutrophils cytoplasmic antibodies (P-ANCA) [13].

PLCH may present with patchy peribronchiolar distribution of eosinophils. However, they are typically found in the interstitium rather than intra-alveolar and are diagnostically characterized by associated CD1a-, S100-, and langerin-positive Langerhans cells and pigmented macrophages related to cigarette smoking [14, 15].

Increased eosinophils may or may not be a feature in parasitic infections such as dirofilariasis; however, these usually present with necrotizing intrapulmonary nodules within which the parasite is identified.

Reactive eosinophilic pleuritis is an incidental histological finding associated with pneumothorax due to virtually any cause, such as apical blebs, and shows mesothelial cell hyperplasia with a large number of eosinophils mixed with histiocytes and lymphocytes [16].

References

1. Sveinsson OA, Isaksson HJ, Gudmundsson G. [Chronic eosinophilic pneumonia in Iceland: clinical features, epidemiology and review]. Laeknabladid 2007;93(2):111–6.
2. Suzuki Y, Oyama Y, Hozumi H, Imokawa S, Toyoshima M, Yokomura K, et al. Persistent impairment on spirometry in chronic eosinophilic pneumonia: a longitudinal observation study (Shizuoka-CEP study). Ann Allergy Asthma Immunol. 2017;119(5):422–428.e2.
3. Cottin V. Eosinophilic lung diseases. Clin Chest Med. 2016;37(3):535–56.
4. Suzuki Y, Suda T. Eosinophilic pneumonia: a review of the previous literature, causes, diagnosis, and management. Allergol Int. 2019;68(4):413–9.
5. Costabel U, Teschler H, Guzman J. Bronchiolitis obliterans organizing pneumonia (BOOP): the cytological and immunocytological profile of bronchoalveolar lavage. Eur Respir J. 1992;5(7):791–7.
6. Jeong YJ, Kim K-I, Seo IJ, Lee CH, Lee KM, Kim KN, et al. Eosinophilic lung diseases: a clinical, radiologic, and pathologic overview. Radiographics. 2007;27(3):617–37; discussion 637–639.
7. Johkoh T, Müller NL, Akira M, Ichikado K, Suga M, Ando M, et al. Eosinophilic lung diseases: diagnostic accuracy of thin-section CT in 111 patients. Radiology. 2000;216(3):773–80.
8. Arakawa H, Kurihara Y, Niimi H, Nakajima Y, Johkoh T, Nakamura H. Bronchiolitis obliterans with organizing pneumonia versus chronic eosinophilic pneumonia: high-resolution CT findings in 81 patients. AJR Am J Roentgenol. 2001;176(4):1053–8.
9. Shimizudani N, Murata H, Kojo S, Adachi Y, Keino H, Tsuchida F, et al. Analysis of T cell receptor V(beta) gene expression and clonality in bronchoalveolar fluid lymphocytes from a patient with chronic eosinophilic pneumonitis. Lung. 2001;179(1):31–41.
10. Freymond N, Kahn J-E, Legrand F, Renneville A, Cordier J-F, Cottin V. Clonal expansion of T cells in patients with eosinophilic lung disease. Allergy. 2011;66(11):1506–8.
11. Olopade CO, Crotty TB, Douglas WW, Colby TV, Sur S. Chronic eosinophilic pneumonia and idiopathic bronchiolitis obliterans organizing pneumonia: comparison of eosinophil number and degranulation by immunofluorescence staining for eosinophil-derived major basic protein. Mayo Clin Proc. 1995;70(2):137–42.
12. Churg A, Muller N. Atlas of interstitial lung disease pathology. Philadelphia, PA: Lippincott Williams & Wilkins; 2014.
13. Greco A, Rizzo MI, De Virgilio A, Gallo A, Fusconi M, Ruoppolo G, et al. Churg-Strauss syndrome. Autoimmun Rev. 2015;14(4):341–8.
14. Berres M-L, Merad M, Allen CE. Progress in understanding the pathogenesis of Langerhans cell histiocytosis: back to Histiocytosis X? Br J Haematol. 2015;169(1):3–13.
15. El Demellawy D, Young JL, de Nanassy J, Chernetsova E, Nasr A. Langerhans cell histiocytosis: a comprehensive review. Pathology. 2015;47(4):294–301.
16. McDonnell TJ, Crouch EC, Gonzalez JG. Reactive eosinophilic pleuritis. A sequela of pneumothorax in pulmonary eosinophilic granuloma. Am J Clin Pathol. 1989;91(1):107–11.

Pulmonary Langerhans Cell Histiocytosis with Fibrosis Versus Organizing Pneumonia

43

Thomas H. Long and Haodong Xu

Case Presentation

A 68-year-old man with a 50 pack-year smoking history fell from a ladder. Computed tomography (CT) imaging for the chest demonstrated innumerable bilateral pulmonary nodules ranging from several millimeters to several centimeters in size, showing a bronchovascular distribution (Fig. 43.1) with relative peripheral sparing and background centrilobular emphysema. The patient was noted to meet clinical criteria for chronic obstructive pulmonary disease (COPD) with an obstructive pattern and bronchodilator response. Due to the concern for neoplastic as well as infectious/inflammatory etiologies, wedge biopsy of the left upper lung lobe was performed. Flow cytometry and microbiological cultures from the tissue were unrevealing. Gross examination demonstrated multiple white-tan ill-defined nodules. On histopathologic examination, the nodules contained radiating fibrotic lung parenchyma (Fig. 43.2a) associated with a mixed inflammatory infiltrate including abundant eosinophils. Areas of airspace organization (fibroblastic proliferation filling airspaces) and increased pigmented alveolar macrophages were present (Fig. 43.2b). Notably, there were frequent clusters and aggregates of atypical cells with admixed lymphocytes, plasma cells, and eosinophils forming a nodular aggregate (Fig. 43.3a), and these cells had eosinophilic, variably pigmented cytoplasm and mildly atypical ovoid nuclei with membrane irregularities, including prominent grooves (Fig. 43.3b). These cells were positive for CD1a and S100 by immunohistochemistry (Fig. 43.3c, d). GMS and AFB stains for fungal and acid-fast organisms were negative (not shown).

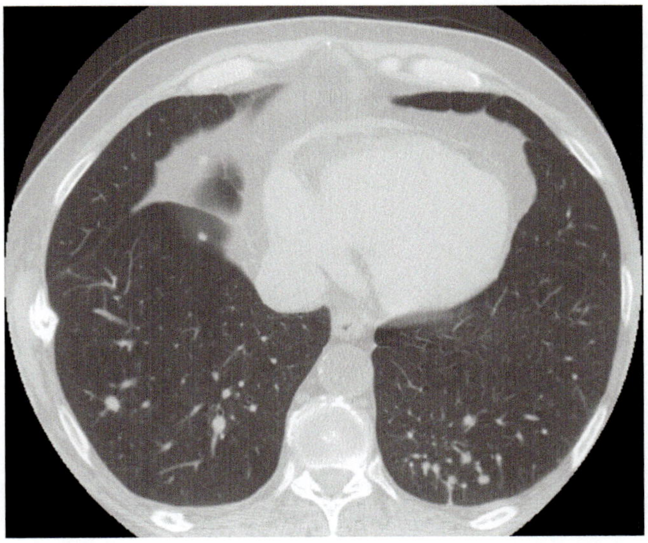

Fig. 43.1 Numerous bilateral bronchiolar centric pulmonary nodules on CT. Cysts were absent in this case

T. H. Long · H. Xu (✉)
Department of Laboratory Medicine and Pathology, University of Washington Medical Center, Seattle, WA, USA
e-mail: thomlo@uw.edu; xuh8@uw.edu

H. Xu et al. (eds.), *Practical Lung Pathology*, Practical Anatomic Pathology, https://doi.org/10.1007/978-3-031-14402-8_43

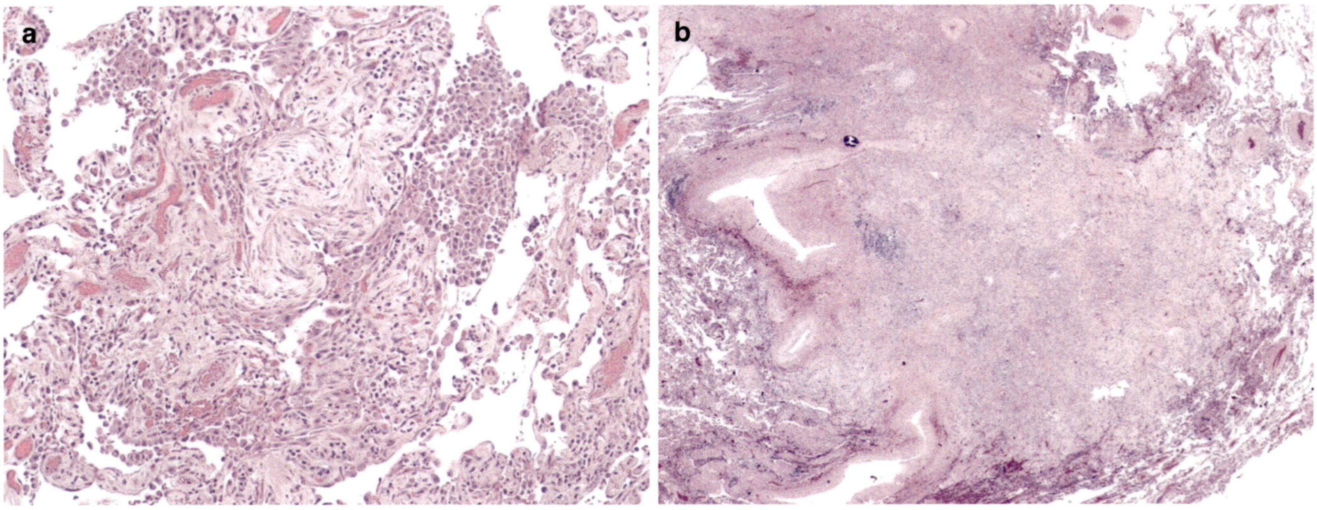

Fig. 43.2 H&E section shows PLCH with stellate nodule from low power (**a**, H&E: 40×). Airspace organization is present forming Masson bodies composed of spindled myofibroblasts in a loose myxoid matrix at peripheral areas, and numerous alveolar cigarette smoking macrophages are present in airspaces (**b**, H&E: 100×)

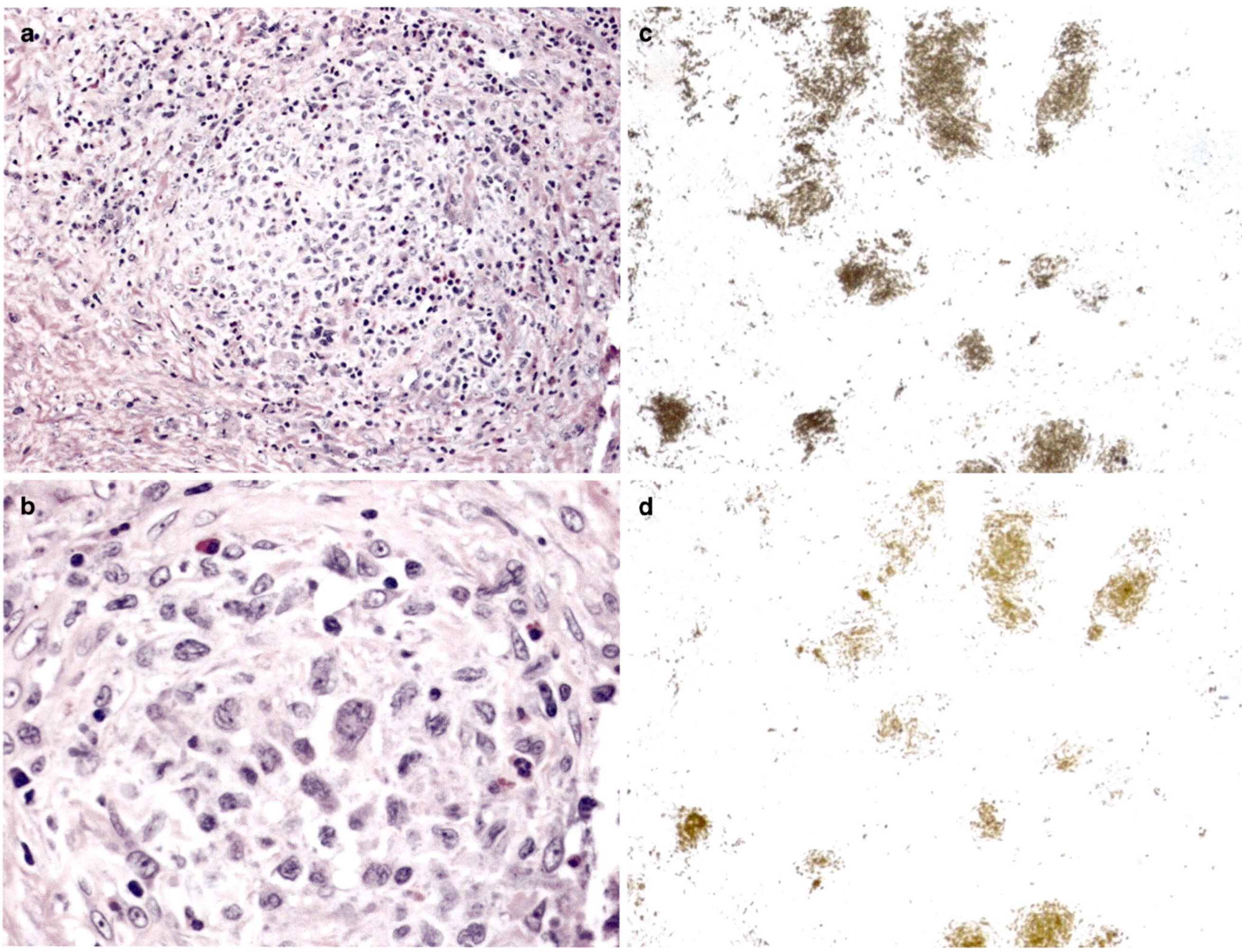

Fig. 43.3 (**a**) Langerhans cells with admixed lymphocytes, plasma cells, and eosinophils form a nodular aggregate. (**b**) A high-power view shows the classic folded/grooved nuclei of the Langerhans cells. (**c**) CD1a immunohistochemical staining of Langerhans cell aggregates. (**d**) S100 immunohistochemical staining of Langerhans cell aggregates. H&E: (**a**) 40× and (**b**) 200×; IHC: (**c**) and (**d**), 40×

Pathologic Diagnosis: Pulmonary Langerhans Cell Histiocytosis

What Is Pulmonary Langerhans Cell Histiocytosis?

Pulmonary Langerhans cell histiocytosis (PLCH) is a histiocytic disorder caused by abnormal proliferation of myeloid-derived dendritic cells that can act clinically as a form of interstitial lung disease. Histiocytic disorders in general are poorly understood and represent a collection of related but distinct diseases ranging from localized to systemic and indolent to aggressive. Langerhans cell histiocytosis (LCH) in general follows this same pattern. It can be localized or systemic and behaves very differently in different body sites and patient populations. Classic PLCH is localized to the lung and is primarily seen in adult smokers, with greater than 90% of patients having a history of smoking [1]. Extrapulmonary involvement occurs in 10–15% of patients and predominantly affects skin, lymph nodes, hypothalamus, and bone [1]. Extrapulmonary forms of LCH are more likely to show clonal genetic alterations, most commonly BRAF V600E mutation, and therefore are considered to represent a neoplastic process. In contrast, PLCH has a variable rate of reported clonal alterations (28–89% for *BRAF* and 11–19% for *MAP2K1* mutations), and it is controversial whether these lesions represent a true neoplasm, a reactive process, or a mixture of both [1, 2]. Clinically, PLCH is often asymptomatic; however, cough, dyspnea on exertion, fatigue, and spontaneous pneumothorax (10–20%) can be associated with PLCH [1].

What Are the Typical Imaging Findings of Pulmonary Langerhans Cell Histiocytosis?

Imaging findings in PLCH tend to vary depending on the disease stage; however, they typically involve the upper and middle lobes, while the lower lobe is commonly spared. Early PLCH usually demonstrates multiple nodules, ranging from 1 to 10 mm in size, sometimes surrounded by ground-glass opacities with a variably irregular or stellate border. Some lesions may show central lucency or cavitation, which may progress into cystic lesions. Lesions may also regress or progress to extensive fibrosis associated with cystic spaces (paracicatricial emphysema). Findings in advanced disease usually reflect extensive scarring/fibrosis and can include reticular and nodular opacities, fibrocystic changes, and honeycombing. Costophrenic angle sparing can be seen [3, 4]. These findings can mimic other forms of interstitial lung disease.

What Are the Pathologic Features of Pulmonary Langerhans Cell Histiocytosis?

Much like the radiographic findings, the histopathologic features depend on whether tissue is obtained in an early or advanced stage of PLCH. Gross examination can show small bronchiolocentric irregular nodules in the early stages and fibrotic/cystic changes in advanced disease. Microscopic features of nodules include stellate lesions centered on bronchioles and alveolar ducts composed of varying proportions of fibrosis, mixed inflammatory infiltrates including lymphocytes, plasma cells, macrophages, eosinophils, and Langerhans cells. The latter are characterized by eosinophilic cytoplasm and prominent nuclear grooves. Langerhans cells are present in early lesions but can be sparse or absent in late or "burnt-out" PLCH [4]. Organizing pneumonia, prominent cigarette-related smoking alveolar macrophages, and interstitial inflammation can be seen in association with these nodules, particularly at the periphery of the lesions [4, 5]. As the disease progresses, there is destruction of bronchiolar walls and adjacent alveolar parenchyma. This process produces the scarring and cystic changes seen in advanced disease, which can be patchy, geographic, or diffuse in severe cases. Langerhans cells characteristically express a combination of CD1a and S100 by immunohistochemistry. It should be noted that S100 is nonspecific in isolation and may stain other lung cell types, including macrophages [4]. Langerin (CD207) appears to be exclusively expressed by Langerhans cells, owing to its involvement in the formation of Birbeck granules. These are cytoplasmic organelles characteristic of Langerhans cells, and seen on electron microscopy [4, 6]. It is important to note that the presence of scattered Langerhans cells is not sufficient for the diagnosis, as they can be seen in numerous other conditions. PLCH typically has more obvious clustering and aggregation of the abnormal Langerhans cells, but in difficult cases, clinical and radiographic correlation may be helpful.

What Is the Differential Diagnosis of Pulmonary Langerhans Cell Histiocytosis?

The differential diagnosis of PLCH includes infection, reactive changes adjacent to unsampled neoplasm, respiratory bronchiolitis (RB)/desquamative interstitial pneumonia (DIP), Erdheim-Chester disease, hypersensitivity pneumonitis, eosinophilic pneumonia, and idiopathic organizing pneumonia, among others. In all cases, a significant Langerhans cell infiltrate is the primary distinguishing finding. In late stage PLCH, the findings may be nonspecific and overlap with other causes of interstitial lung disease patterns such as usual interstitial pneumonia (UIP).

What Is Organizing Pneumonia?

Organizing pneumonia (OP) is a pattern of injury rather than a specific disease entity, which can be secondary to multiple etiologies, including infection, drug toxicity, radiation, collagen vascular disease, other interstitial lung diseases, adjacent neoplasm, or any prior lung insult, such as diffuse alveolar damage. Thus, this finding generally prompts a search for the inciting lung injury/process. Cryptogenic OP is a diagnosis of exclusion, representing an idiopathic form of OP [3, 5, 7]. Characteristic findings on histopathology include filing of alveolar spaces, respiratory bronchioles, and small airways with myofibroblasts ("organization") which form nodules of these "Masson bodies" [3, 8, 9].

What Differentiates Pulmonary Langerhans Cell Histiocytosis from Organizing Pneumonia Clinically?

In contrast to PLCH, cryptogenic OP, when described as a clinical syndrome, can present with shortness of breath, fever, malaise, and weight loss, sometimes following a respiratory tract infection [3, 7]. Studies have shown no convincing association between cryptogenic OP and cigarette smoking, in contrast to PLCH.

What Differentiates Pulmonary Langerhans Cell Histiocytosis from Organizing Pneumonia on Imaging?

Cryptogenic OP predominantly affects the subpleural and lower lung zones [3], in contrast to PLCH, which relatively spares the lower lobes. On CT imaging, bronchovascular and subpleural ground-glass opacities are seen in approximately 90% of cryptogenic OP patients [7]. These can be surrounded by dense airway consolidation, which has been referred to as the "reverse halo sign." Cysts are not a common feature of cryptogenic OP. Overlapping with PLCH can occur; however, subcentimeter nodules are a feature of both entities [3, 7].

What Differentiates Pulmonary Langerhans Cell Histiocytosis from Organizing Pneumonia on Histopathology?

Airspace organization can be seen in PLCH and cryptogenic OP. However, OP is a nonspecific pattern of injury, and care must be taken to exclude other findings that would render a specific diagnosis. In the case of PLCH, a stellate pattern of fibrosis and frequent eosinophils may be helpful clues. Ultimately, the most important diagnostic criterion to distinguish between OP and PLCH is the identification of abnormal Langerhans cell proliferation. Confirmation can be aided by immunohistochemistry (S100, CD1a and langerin). After careful exclusion of clinical or pathologic findings to suggest a specific etiology, a diagnosis of cryptogenic organizing pneumonia may be appropriate.

References

1. Demartino E, Go RS, Vassallo R. Langerhans cell histiocytosis and other histiocytic diseases of the lung. Clin Chest Med. 2016;37(3):421–30.
2. Pierry C, Caumont C, Blanchard E, Brochet C, Doumes G, Gros A, et al. Assessment of BRAF mutation in pulmonary Langerhans cell histiocytosis in tissue biopsies and bronchoalveolar lavages by droplet digital polymerase chain reaction. Virchows Arch. 2018;472(2):247–58.
3. Pfeifer K, Mian A, Adebowale A, Alomari A, Kalra V, Krejci E, et al. Radiographic and pathologic manifestations of uncommon and rare pulmonary lesions. Can Assoc Radiol J. 2016;67(2):179–89.
4. Roden AC, Yi ES. Pulmonary langerhans cell histiocytosis: an update from the pathologists' perspective. Arch Pathol Lab Med. 2016;140(3):230–40.
5. Ling CH, Ji C, Raymond DP, Bourne PA, Xu HD. Uncommon features of pulmonary Langerhans' cell histiocytosis: analysis of 11 cases and a review of the literature. Chin Med J. 2010;123(4):498–501.
6. Valladeau J, Ravel O, Dezutter-dambuyant C, Moore K, Kleijmeer M, Liu Y, et al. Langerin, a novel C-type lectin specific to Langerhans cells, is an endocytic receptor that induces the formation of Birbeck granules. Immunity. 2000;12(1):71–81.
7. Lee JW, Lee KS, Lee HY, Chung MP, Yi CA, Kim TS, et al. Cryptogenic organizing pneumonia: serial high-resolution CT findings in 22 patients. AJR Am J Roentgenol. 2010;195(4):916–22.
8. Larsen BT, Colby TV. Update for pathologists on idiopathic interstitial pneumonias. Arch Pathol Lab Med. 2012;136(10):1234–41.
9. Demedts M, Costabel U. ATS/ERS international multidisciplinary consensus classification of the idiopathic interstitial pneumonias. Eur Respir J. 2002;19(5):794–6.

IgG4-Related Lung Disease Versus Other Fibroinflammatory Processes

44

Jennifer J. Chia and Gregory A. Fishbein

Case Presentation

A previously healthy 68-year-old male presented to his primary care physician with fatigue, episodic dizziness, and rapid heartbeat when exercising. The symptoms were attributed to anemia, likely secondary to bleeding internal hemorrhoids. On follow-up, he endorsed 25 lb of unintentional weight loss and was found to have severe thrombocytopenia. Serologic studies showed elevated serum IgG; serum protein electrophoresis (SPEP) showed polyclonal hypergammaglobulinemia. Computed tomography (CT) of the chest showed hilar adenopathy and multifocal peripheral pulmonary opacities (Fig. 44.1). A segmentectomy was performed.

On gross examination, the specimen demonstrated a 4.3 cm, tan-gray, ill-defined mass interdigitating with the surrounding lung parenchyma near the periphery. There was pleural thickening overlying the mass. No cystic spaces, hemorrhage, or necrosis was noted. Histologic sections demonstrated a fibroinflammatory infiltrate in an exquisitely perivascular distribution (Fig. 44.2).

The infiltrate consisted primarily of plasma cells but also included lymphocytes and numerous eosinophils. Transmural vascular involvement and stenosis were seen. Immunohistochemistry for IgG4, IgG, and CD138 were performed and demonstrated >50 IgG4-positive plasma cells per high-power field (Fig. 44.3).

Approximately 70% of the IgG-positive plasma cells were also positive for IgG4. The findings were reported as *highly suggestive of IgG4-related disease*. Further clinical workup revealed markedly elevated serum IgG4, and a clinical diagnosis of IgG4-related disease was made.

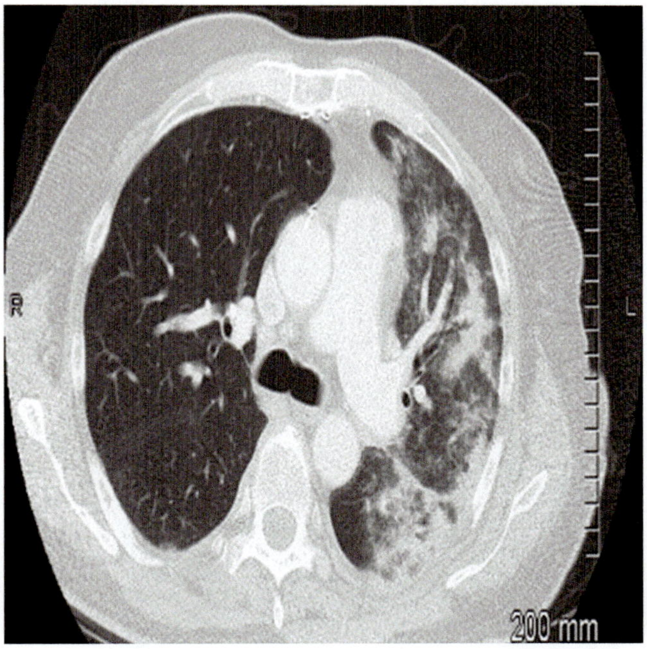

Fig. 44.1 Chest CT demonstrating patchy, bilateral ground-glass opacities, consolidation, and nodules in the upper lobe

J. J. Chia · G. A. Fishbein (✉)
Department of Pathology and Laboratory Medicine, David Geffen School of Medicine at UCLA, Los Angeles, CA, USA
e-mail: jchia@mednet.ucla.edu; gfishbein@mednet.ucla.edu

H. Xu et al. (eds.), *Practical Lung Pathology*, Practical Anatomic Pathology, https://doi.org/10.1007/978-3-031-14402-8_44

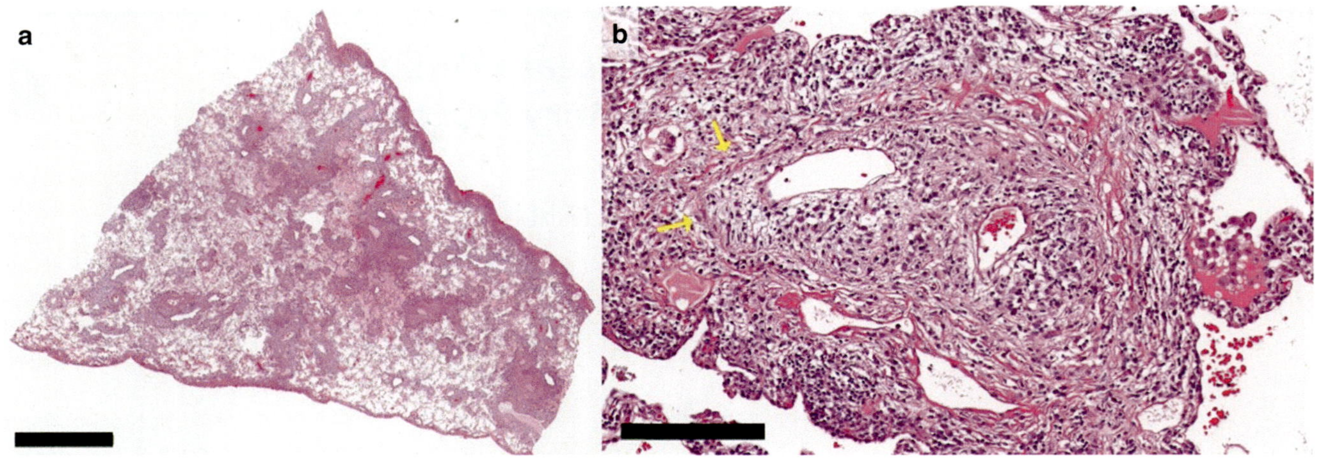

Fig. 44.2 (**a**) At low power, the lesion consists of multiple coalescing areas of dense immune infiltrate around peripheral bronchovascular structures and along the pleura; there is no solid component identified. Storiform fibrosis is not appreciated. Scale bar represents 5 mm. (**b**) At high power, the immune infiltrate is revealed to be rich in plasma cells, eosinophils, and lymphocytes. A vein is obliterated by the lymphoplasmacytic infiltrate (arrows) and partially recanalized. Scale bar represents 200 μm

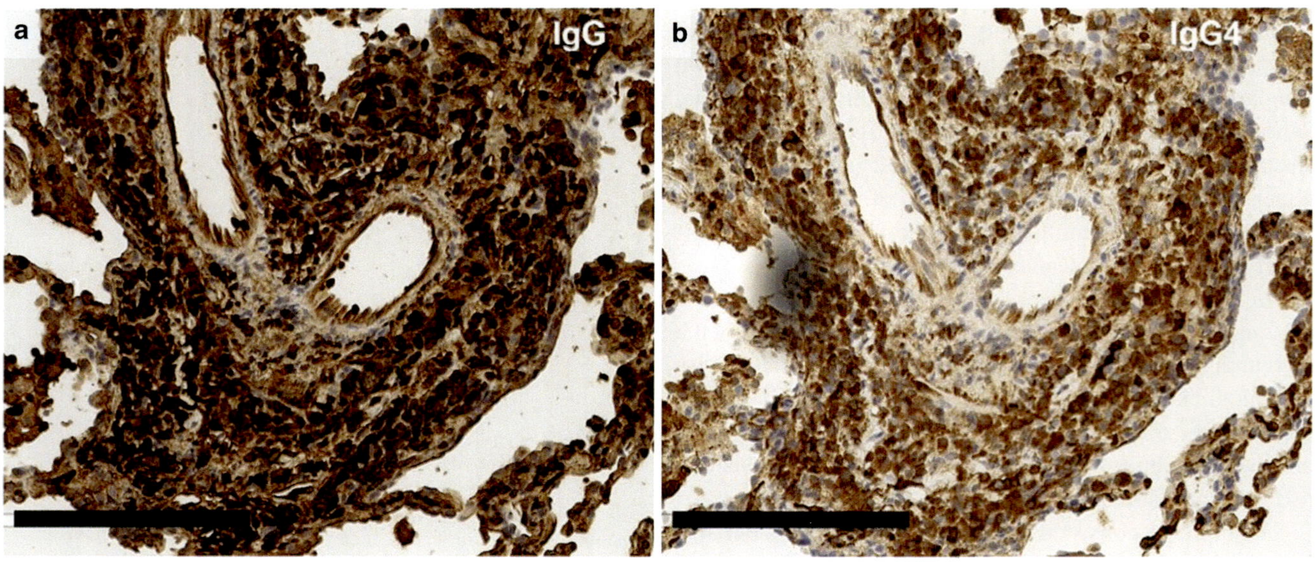

Fig. 44.3 IgG4 (**a**) and IgG (**b**) immunostains. IgG4 stain highlighting >50 plasma cells per high-powered field. IgG4-positive plasma cells represented ~70% of the total number of IgG-positive plasma cells. Scale bar represents 200 μm

Final Diagnosis: Pulmonary IgG4-Related Disease

What Are the Histologic and Immunohistochemical Criteria for Diagnosing IgG4-Related Lung Disease?

The histologic criteria for IgG-related disease in the lung are based on the same findings as IgG4-related disease in other organ systems and include dense lymphoplasmacytic inflammation, fibrosis, and obliterative phlebitis (Table 44.1).

Table 44.1 Histologic criteria for IgG4-related disease in the lung

Histologic criteria for IgG4-related disease in the lung
1. Dense lymphoplasmacytic infiltrate
2. Fibrosis, often storiform[a]
3. Obliterative phlebitis[b]

[a] In the lung, fibrosis may not be storiform in the context of a nonsolid lesion (Fig. 44.1)

[b] Obliterative arteritis rather than phlebitis can been seen in solid lung lesions [1, 2]

Storiform-type fibrosis is less frequently seen in nonsolid lesions. Furthermore, obliterative arteritis, rather than phlebitis, may be present [1, 2]. Immunohistochemical criteria differ between small biopsies and excisional specimens and are based on (1) the quantity of IgG4-positive plasma cells per high-power field and (2) the percentage of plasma cells that are IgG4-positive (Table 44.2).

Can a Definitive Diagnosis of IgG4-Related Disease Be Given Based on Histopathology and Immunohistochemistry Alone?

No. A definitive diagnosis of IgG4-related disease requires clinical correlation; thus, cases should be signed out according to the level of histopathologic suspicion. Resection specimens can be termed "highly histologically suggestive of IgG4-related disease" or "probable histologic features of IgG4-related disease" [1].

For small biopsy specimens, even identification of all histologic features should be termed "probable histologic features of IgG4-related disease" due to the possibility of sampling error [1].

How Do We Know If a Resection Specimen Meets "Highly Histologically Suggestive" or "Probable Histologic Features" Criteria?

If, in a resection specimen, immunohistochemistry demonstrates IgG4 positivity in greater than 40% of plasma cells and the number of IgG4-positive plasma cells is greater than 50 per high-power field, the level of suspicion depends on the number of histologic features identified (Fig. 44.4). These features include (1) dense lymphoplasmacytic infiltrate, (2) fibrosis, and (3) obliterative phlebitis.

How Do We Determine the IgG4 Plasma Cell Ratio?

The IgG4 plasma cell ratio can be determined by comparing IgG4+ cells to the total number of plasma cells. This can be done using immunohistochemistry with IgG4 and IgG antibodies. In practice, CD138 may be a useful substitute for IgG, as the latter is frequently laden with high background staining.

Table 44.2 Immunohistologic criteria for IgG4-related disease in the lung [1]

Biopsy	Excision
1. >20 IgG4+ plasma cells (/hpf)	1. >50 IgG4+ plasma cells (/hpf)
2. IgG4+ plasma cells constitute > 40% of all plasma cells	2. IgG4+ plasma cells constitute > 40% of all plasma cells

What Else Should We Include in the Differential When Considering a Diagnosis of IgG4-Related Lung Disease?

Inflammatory myofibroblastic tumor (IMT), pulmonary nodular sclerosis classic Hodgkin lymphoma (NSCHL), organizing abscess, and pulmonary Langerhans cell histiocytosis (PLCH) are fibroinflammatory lesions that may histologically resemble IgG4-related disease.

Are Clinical and Imaging Findings Helpful to Distinguish IgG4-Related Disease from Other Fibroinflammatory Conditions Such as IMT and NSCHL?

Tables 44.3 and 44.4 enumerate the clinical and radiographic (Fig. 44.5) features of IgG4-related disease, IMT, and pulmonary NSCHL.

What Are the Main Histologic Differences Between IgG4-Related Disease, IMT, and Pulmonary NSCHL?

Histologic features that help distinguish IgG4-related disease from IMT and pulmonary NSCHL are listed in Table 44.5 and shown in Fig. 44.6.

How Do We Distinguish IgG4-Related Disease from an Organizing Abscess?

An organizing abscess may mimic a solid pattern of IgG4-related disease; however, it is unlikely to meet the numerical or ratio criteria for IgG4+ plasma cells (Fig. 44.7).

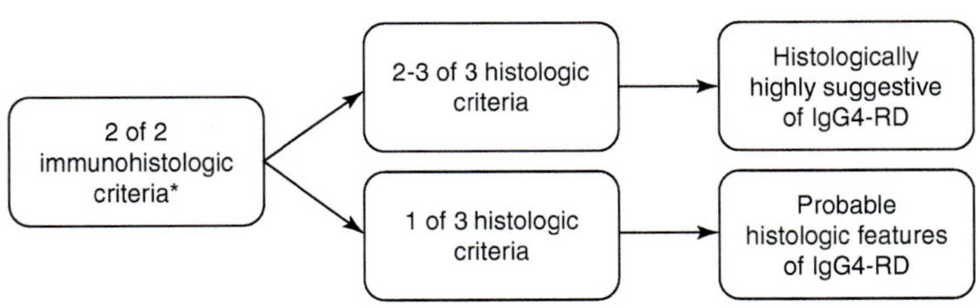

Fig. 44.4 Necessary steps for a diagnosis of IgG4-related lung disease of a resection specimen and the qualitative strength with which it can be rendered. *Note that biopsy specimens have different numerical criteria for IgG4+ plasma cells (Table 44.2) and should at the most be qualitatively designated as "probable histologic features of IgG4-related disease" [1]

Table 44.3 Clinical features of IgG4-related disease and other fibroinflammatory lesions of the lung [1–5]

Clinical features	IGG4-related disease	Inflammatory myofibroblastic tumor	Pulmonary NSCHL
Sex	Male > female	Male = female	Male = female
Average age (range)	60 years (40–80)	Bi-modal: 8 years, 44 years	15–34 years
Key signs and symptoms	Half are incidental, half nonspecific pulmonary symptoms	50–60% asymptomatic; fevers, nonspecific pulmonary symptoms	B-symptoms in 40% of patients
Laboratory findings	Often but not always elevated serum IgG4	Elevated erythrocyte sedimentation rate (ESR), thrombocytosis, hypergammaglobulinemia	Nonspecific

NSCHL nodular sclerosing classical Hodgkin lymphoma

Table 44.4 Imaging features of IgG4-related disease, inflammatory myofibroblastic tumor, and pulmonary NSCHL [4, 6, 7]

Imaging features	IGG4-related disease	Inflammatory myofibroblastic tumor	Pulmonary NSCHL
Localization	Usually peripheral	80% peripheral; 20% central (bronchial or tracheal possible)	Subpleural and peripheral
Focality	Multiple or single foci	Single foci ≫ multiple	Multiple foci ≫ single
Patterns	Solid nodular, round ground glass, alveolar interstitial, or bronchovascular patterns	Well-circumscribed; rarely irregular nodules	Numerous cavitary lung lesions
Radiographic mimics	Malignancy, nonspecific interstitial pneumonia, lymphoproliferative disorder, sarcoidosis	Primary malignancy, single metastasis, rarely pneumonia-like	Infection

NSCHL nodular sclerosing classical Hodgkin lymphoma

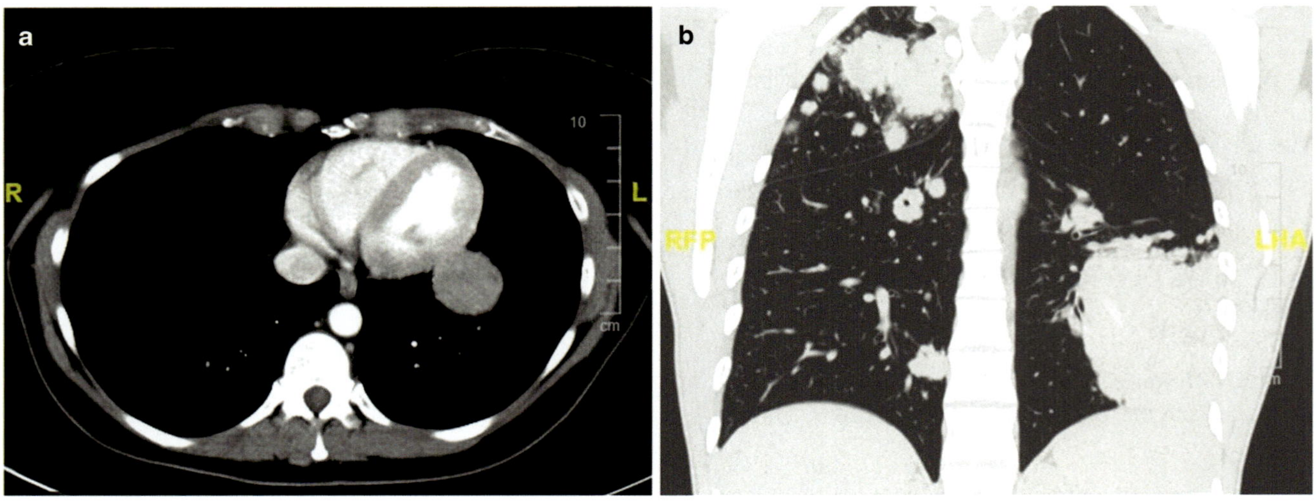

Fig. 44.5 CT imaging of the chest for (**a**) inflammatory myofibroblastic tumor (IMT) demonstrating a single, well-circumscribed lesion and (**b**) pulmonary nodular sclerosis classic Hodgkin lymphoma (NSCHL) with numerous, ill-defined peripheral lesions

Table 44.5 Histologic features of IgG4-related disease, inflammatory myofibroblastic tumor, and pulmonary sclerosing classical non-Hodgkin's lymphoma (NSCHL)

Histologic features	IGG4-related disease	Inflammatory myofibroblastic tumor	Pulmonary NSCHL
Fibrosis pattern	Storiform[a]	Rarely fibrosis	Concentric around lymphoid aggregates
Infiltrate	Lymphoplasmacytic, plasma cells predominate, eosinophils are frequently increased	Fibrohistiocytic, plasma cells can be numerous	Mixed inflammation including neutrophils and eosinophils
Tissue distribution	Bronchovascular, intraparenchymal, subpleural	Parenchymal	Lymphatic and subpleural
Focality	Multiple or single foci	Single foci ≫ multiple	Multiple foci ≫ single
Other	Obliterative phlebitis or arteritis[b] within dense immune infiltrate	Orderly, fascicular arrangement of myofibroblasts	Lacunar-type Hodgkin/Reed-Sternberg cells; necrosis

[a] In the lung, fibrosis may not be storiform in the context of a nonsolid lesion
[b] Obliterative arteritis can been seen in solid lung lesions [1, 2, 4, 5]

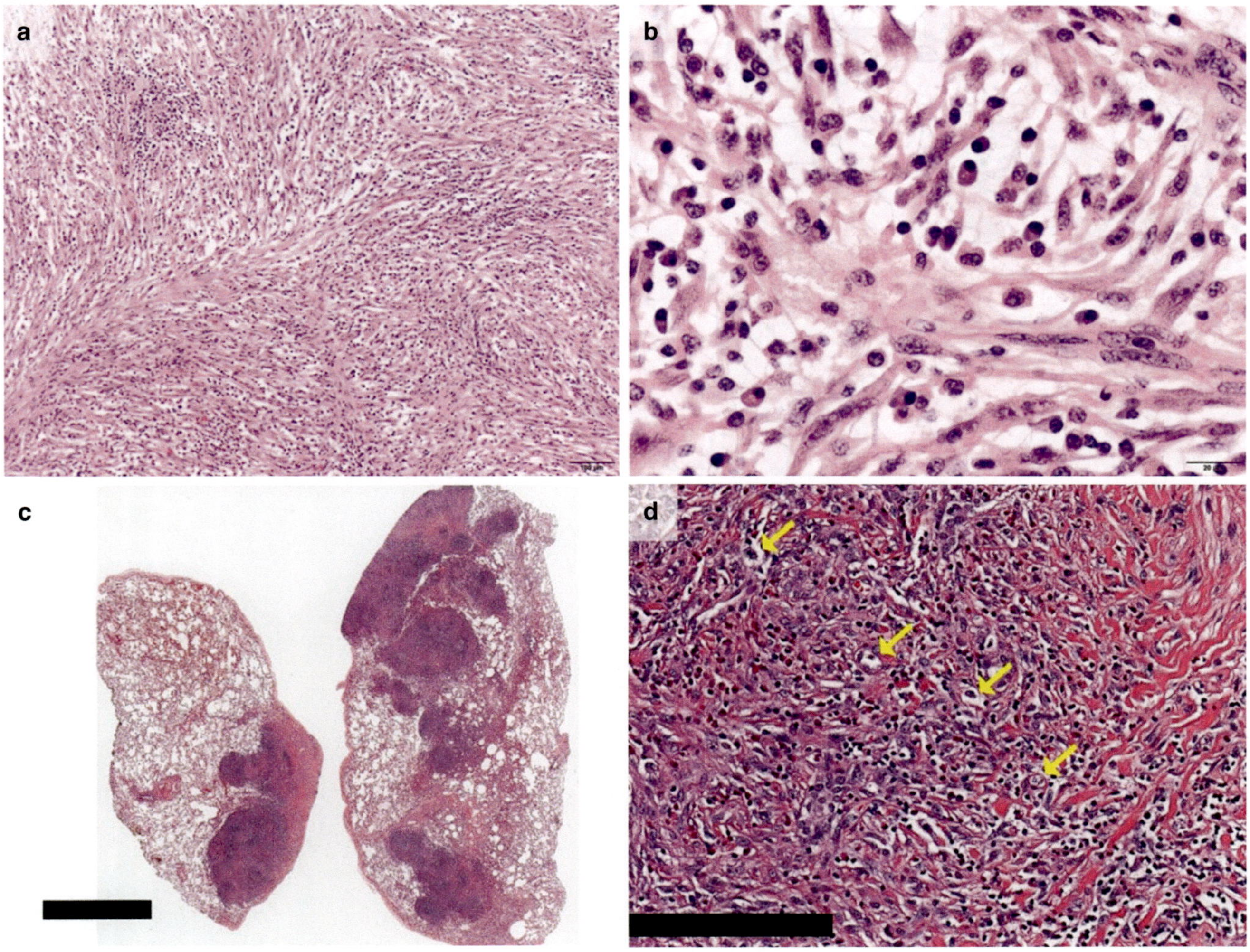

Fig. 44.6 Histologic findings in inflammatory myofibroblastic tumor and nodular sclerosing classical Hodgkin lymphoma (NSCHL). (**a**) Medium power view of inflammatory myofibroblastic tumor demonstrates well-organized fascicles of stromal cells with admixed inflammatory cells; (**b**) high power demonstrates the plasma cell preponderance of the inflammatory infiltrate. (**c**) Low-power view of pulmonary NSCHL demonstrates its subpleural and lymphatic distribution, as well as concentric fibrosis surrounding round, follicle-like inflammatory deposits; scale bar represents 4 mm; (**d**) high power demonstrates a mixed inflammatory infiltrate with many eosinophils and scattered Hodgkin/Reed-Sternberg cells (arrows); scale bar represents 200 μm

Furthermore, the presence of necrosis is incompatible with IgG4-related disease and may suggest either an infectious etiology or nodular sclerosing classical Hodgkin lymphoma [1].

What Is the Difference Between IgG4-Related Disease and Plasma Cell Granuloma?

The term plasma cell granuloma (a.k.a. inflammatory pseudotumor) is out of date. Most entities previously designated as plasma cell granulomas would now be reclassified as IMT. However, a subset of cases of plasma cell granuloma likely did represent IgG4-related disease [8].

How Do We Distinguish IgG4-Related Disease from Pulmonary Langerhans Cell Histiocytosis?

Pulmonary Langerhans cell histiocytosis (PLCH) is a relatively common fibroinflammatory lesion that temporally evolves from a Langerhans cell-rich lesion to a stellate scar. These lesions can be single or multiple and are eosinophil-rich, and thus intermediate-stage lesions with peribronchovascular fibrosis, chronic inflammation, and eosinophils may resemble IgG4-related disease. However, PLCH is not plasma cell rich and occurs in patients with significant cigarette smoke exposure, which, if active, will likely be reflected

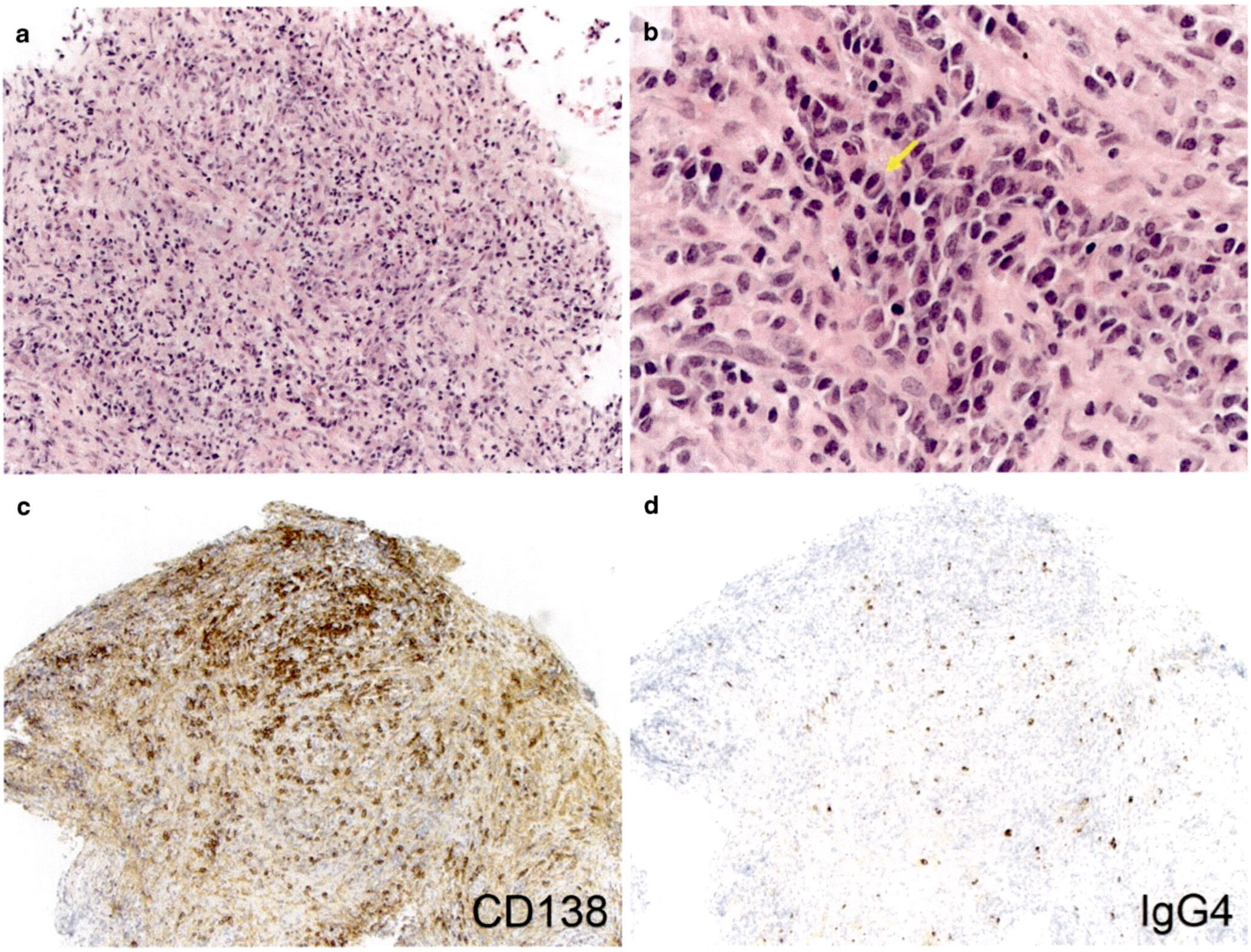

Fig. 44.7 Histology and immunohistochemistry of an organizing abscess. (**a**, **b**) Medium- and high-power views demonstrating plasma cell-rich inflammation (arrow). No obliterative vasculitis or storiform fibrosis are seen. (**c**) CD138 immunostain highlights plasma cells. (**d**) IgG4 immunostain highlights only a small subset of plasma cells

in background lung parenchyma. PLCH has a predilection for the upper lobes. The hallmark of PLCH is the presence of Langerhans cells that are immunoreactive to S100, CD1a, and Langerin.

Is Elevated Serum IgG4 a Necessary Criterion for IgG4-Related Disease?

No. Up to 40% of patients with biopsy-proven IgG4-related disease of the pancreas have normal serum IgG4 levels [9]. There are fewer reports of pulmonary IgG4-related disease, all of whom in a small study had elevated serum IgG4; only 50% of patients with pleural-based IgG4-related disease had elevated serum IgG4 [2].

Are Distinct or Distant Foci of IgG4+ Plasma Cells and Obliterative Vasculitis Supportive of a Diagnosis of IgG4-Related Disease?

No, the obliterative phlebitis must be within a dense lymphoplasmacytic lesion with IgG4+ plasma cells [1].

Is the Vasculitis Found in IgG4-Related Disease Necrotizing or Non-necrotizing?

Non-necrotizing or necrotizing vasculitis suggests an alternative diagnosis [1].

Can IgG4-Related Disease Affect the Pleura?

Yes, the pleura can be affected with or without involvement of the lung parenchyma; the diagnostic criteria are the same as the lung (Tables 44.1 and 44.2; Fig. 44.2) [2].

References

1. Deshpande V, Zen Y, Chan JKC, Yi EE, Sato Y, Yoshino T, et al. Consensus statement on the pathology of IgG4-related disease. Mod Pathol. 2012;25(9):1181–92.
2. Zen Y, Inoue D, Kitao A, Onodera M, Abo H, Miyayama S, et al. IgG4-related lung and pleural disease: a clinicopathologic study of 21 cases. Am J Surg Pathol. 2009;33(12):1886–93.
3. Chun YS, Wang L, Nascimento AG, Moir CR, Rodeberg DA. Pediatric inflammatory myofibroblastic tumor: anaplastic lymphoma kinase (ALK) expression and prognosis. Pediatr Blood Cancer. 2005;45(6):796–801.
4. Mani H, Jaffe ES. Hodgkin lymphoma: an update on its biology with new insights into classification. Clin Lymphoma Myeloma. 2009;9(3):206–16.
5. Panagiotopoulos N, Patrini D, Gvinianidze L, Woo WL, Borg E, Lawrence D. Inflammatory myofibroblastic tumour of the lung: a reactive lesion or a true neoplasm? J Thorac Dis. 2015;7(5):908–11.
6. Inoue D, Zen Y, Abo H, Gabata T, Demachi H, Kobayashi T, et al. Immunoglobulin G4–related lung disease: CT findings with pathologic correlations. Radiology. 2009;251(1):260–70.
7. Guermazi A, Brice P, de Kerviler E, Fermé C, Hennequin C, Meignin V, et al. Extranodal Hodgkin disease: spectrum of disease. Radiographics. 2001;21(1):161–79.
8. Zen Y, Kitagawa S, Minato H, Kurumaya H, Katayanagi K, Masuda S, et al. IgG4-positive plasma cells in inflammatory pseudotumor (plasma cell granuloma) of the lung. Hum Pathol. 2005;36(7):710–7.
9. Sah RP, Chari ST. Serologic issues in IgG4-related systemic disease and autoimmune pancreatitis. Curr Opin Rheumatol. 2011;23(1):108–13.

Pulmonary Alveolar Proteinosis Versus Pulmonary Edema

45

Karen E. Trevino and Chen Zhang

Case Presentation

A 43-year-old male smoker presents to his primary care physician with a 1-week history of nonproductive cough and shortness of breath with activity. On physical examination, the patient is afebrile, and lungs are clear to auscultation. The patient is sent home with supportive care measures as a viral respiratory infection is suspected.

The patient then returns to his physician a week later with worsening symptoms including worsening cough and shortness of breath. He remains afebrile, but pulse oximetry demonstrates an oxygen saturation of 88% on room air. A chest X-ray (Fig. 45.1) is performed and demonstrates bilateral hazy opacities in a "bat wing" distribution. Due to the presence of opacities in a nonspecific pattern, a high-resolution chest computed tomography (CT) is ordered that demonstrates bilateral ground-glass opacities with thickened intralobular septa in a "crazy paving pattern" (Fig. 45.2).

A bronchoalveolar lavage (BAL) specimen is obtained to rule out infection. The specimen is sent for culture and for cytologic examination. The cultures are all negative. A Papanicolaou stain of the cytospin slide prepared from the BAL fluid shows scattered alveolar macrophages with abundant amorphous material in the background (Fig. 45.3a). A periodic acid-Schiff (PAS) stain demonstrates strong positive staining of the amorphous material (Fig. 45.3b).

The H&E-stained slide prepared from the transbronchial biopsy shows intact alveolar lung architecture. However, the alveolar spaces are filled with a granular and frothy proteinaceous material that contains cholesterol clefts and alveolar macrophages (Figs. 45.4a, b). The proteinaceous material stains positively with PAS (Fig. 45.4c). A Gomori's methenamine silver (GMS) stain is negative for fungal organisms or *Pneumocystis* (Fig. 45.4d).

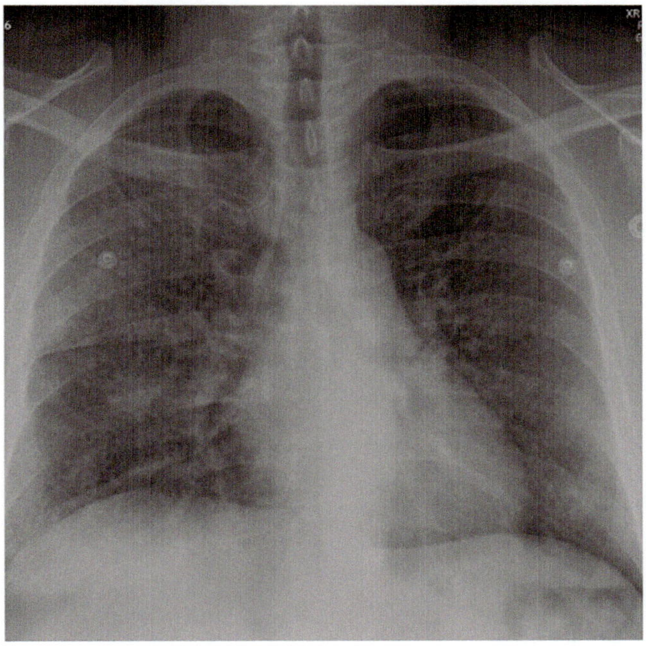

Fig. 45.1 Chest X-ray features of PAP. The Chest X-ray of a patient with PAP demonstrates bilateral hilar based hazy opacities in a "bat wing" distribution. Similar changes can be seen in patients with pulmonary edema

K. E. Trevino
Department of Pathology and Laboratory Medicine, Indiana University School of Medicine, Indianapolis, IN, USA
e-mail: schellek@iupui.edu

C. Zhang (✉)
Weill Cornell Medicine, Department of Pathology and Laboratory Medicine, New York, NY, USA
e-mail: fjr9007@med.cornell.edu

H. Xu et al. (eds.), *Practical Lung Pathology*, Practical Anatomic Pathology, https://doi.org/10.1007/978-3-031-14402-8_45

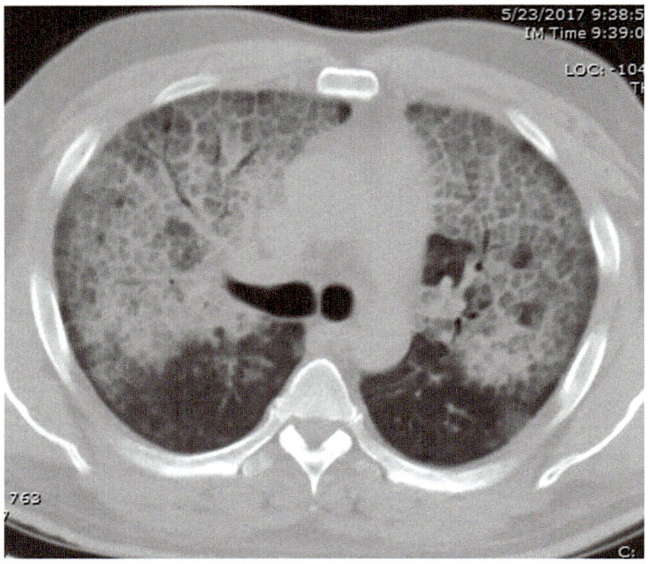

Fig. 45.2 Chest CT features of PAP. PAP demonstrates bilateral ground-glass opacities and thickened inter- and intralobular septa in a "crazy paving" pattern. Pulmonary edema can also present with this pattern, especially in cases of pulmonary edema due to acute respiratory distress syndrome

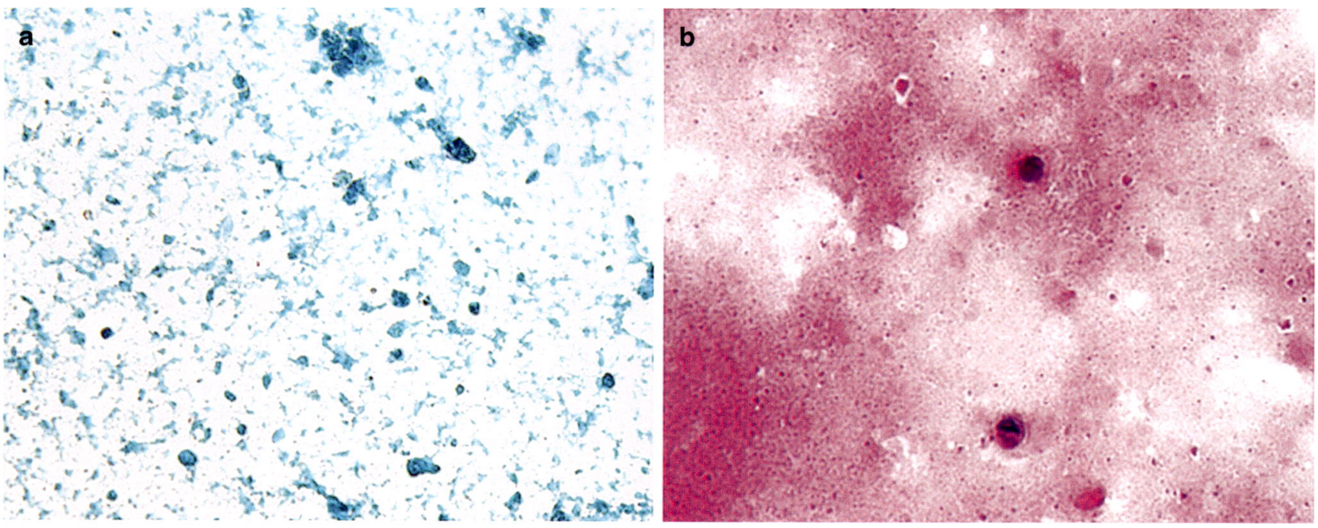

Fig. 45.3 Cytological features of PAP. A cytospin preparation of the bronchoalveolar lavage fluid from a patient with PAP demonstrates scattered alveolar macrophages and abundant amorphous proteinaceous material which shows up as green granules or globules on Papanicolaou stain (**a**) The amorphous material stains positive with PAS stain (**b**)

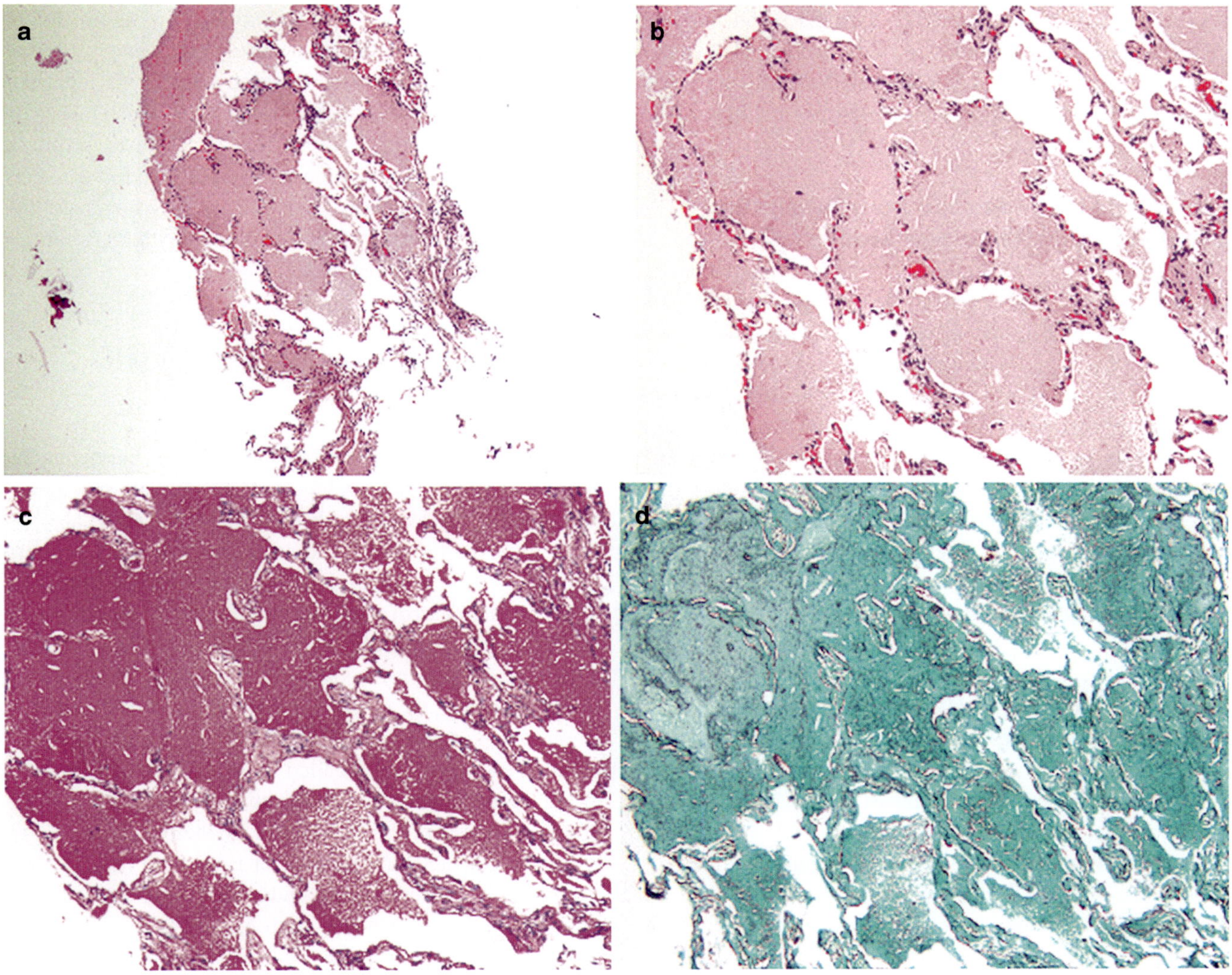

Fig. 45.4 Histologic features of PAP. (**a**) Low magnification view of the transbronchial biopsy demonstrates preserved alveolar architecture, lack of inflammatory infiltrate, and filling of alveolar spaces with eosinophilic, proteinaceous material. H&E, 40× magnification. (**b**) Higher magnification photomicrograph shows that the intra-alveolar proteinaceous material is slightly granular with occasional cholesterol clefts. H&E, 200× magnification. (**c**) This proteinaceous material stains positively with PAS stain. (**d**) GMS stain is negative for fungal organisms or *Pneumocystis*

Pathologic Diagnosis: Pulmonary Alveolar Proteinosis (PAP)

How Does the Demographics and Clinical Symptoms Differ Between PAP and Pulmonary Edema?

PAP usually occurs in patients aged 20–60, with peak incidence in the third and fourth decades and has a 2:1 male predilection [1, 2]. Clinically, PAP typically presents as a subacute respiratory illness causing dyspnea and decreased oxygen saturation that worsens over a period of weeks to months. Many patients present with nonproductive cough. Fever is less common, unless secondary infection has developed. However, symptoms vary widely, and approximately 1/3 of patients are asymptomatic [1, 3]. Underlying illness can be related to the development of PAP, but greater than 90% of adult cases are autoimmune in origin.

On the other hand, pulmonary edema is inherently linked to underlying disease, such as congestive heart failure or acute respiratory distress syndrome. As such, the patient population with pulmonary edema fits within the demographics of the underlying causes and is more likely to be older than those with PAP. Pulmonary edema tends to occur more acutely over a period of hours to days, comparing with the more subacute onset of PAP and usually presents as dyspnea and hypoxemia.

Can PAP Be Distinguished from Pulmonary Edema Through Radiologic Studies?

On chest X-rays, PAP appears similar to pulmonary edema with bilateral, hilar-based, hazy opacities, often described as having a "bat wing" distribution. On high-resolution CT, PAP appears as bilateral ground-glass opacities. Additional imaging support for PAP includes thickened intralobular septa overlying the ground-glass opacities, resulting in a cobblestone or "crazy paving" pattern. However, this pattern (Figs. 45.1 and 45.2) is not specific for PAP, since other entities, such as pulmonary edema, acute respiratory distress syndrome, organizing pneumonia, and lipoid pneumonia can have similar imaging features [4, 5].

What Cytological and Histological Findings Are Indicative of a Diagnosis of PAP?

PAP is often definitively diagnosed on BAL specimen or transbronchial lung biopsy (Figs. 45.3 and 45.4). Characteristic features on BAL include a milky white gross appearance and PAS-positive material on cytology. On Papanicolaou stain, this material appears as orange or green globules inside and outside of macrophages [6]. On surgical biopsy, the alveolar structures should remain preserved. The most prominent feature is PAS-positive frothy proteinaceous material filling the alveolar spaces, and often cholesterol clefts are present. There is typically little or no inflammatory infiltrate accompanying this material [7, 8]. Lung fibrosis is uncommon but can be present in cases of PAP and does not necessarily signify a second diagnosis. The differential diagnosis for PAP on cytology or lung biopsy includes infection (often atypical infections such as *Pneumocystis jirovecii*), lipoid pneumonia, pulmonary edema, and diffuse alveolar damage [9, 10]. The distinction can be made with PAS staining of amorphous material and is additionally supported by negative microbiology studies.

Can Any Laboratory Tests Outside of Tissue Biopsy Be Useful in Establishing a Diagnosis of PAP?

Additional laboratory studies that can assist with the diagnosis of PAP include granulocyte-macrophage colony-stimulating factor (GM-CSF) antibodies in serum and/or BAL fluid and lactate dehydrogenase levels. The presence of GM-CSF antibody is highly sensitive and specific (approximately 100%) in cases of autoimmune PAP, which makes up a great majority of adult cases [11, 12]. However, serum or fluid levels of GM-CSF antibody have not been found to correlate with disease severity [13]. Lactate dehydrogenase levels are elevated serum of 80% of patients with PAP, but this finding is highly nonspecific [2].

What Are the Causes of PAP, and How Is It Treated?

PAP is a disease of decreased clearance of surfactant by alveolar macrophages, leading to its accumulation in alveolar spaces. It was first described in 1958 by Rosen et al. [14]. PAP can be both primary and secondary in origin. Primary causes of PAP are based on the role of GM-CSF in regulation of clearance of surfactant by alveolar macrophages [15]. Rarely, defects in GM-CSF signaling or surfactant production can result in hereditary or congenital PAP (<1% of cases). However, the more common cause of primary PAP is the presence of antibodies to GM-CSF, also known as autoimmune PAP (previously called idiopathic PAP). This is the most common cause of PAP in adults, representing 90–95% of adult cases, and can be verified by the presence of antibodies to GM-CSF in serum or in BAL fluid [11, 12, 16]. Additionally, PAP can be secondary in origin and is linked to environmental exposures such as high-level dust exposures, hematologic dyscrasias, and allogeneic stem cell transplant. The pathogenesis of secondary PAP is thought to be due to relative GM-CSF deficiency and/or macrophage dysfunction [17].

Treatment for PAP depends on the severity of symptoms. In mild cases, the process can be self-limited and requires only supportive therapy. In more symptomatic patients, the most effective method of treatment is whole lung lavage. Patients who fail treatment with whole lung lavage can be trialed on inhaled GM-CSF, rituximab, or plasmapheresis [18]. Patients who do respond to whole lung lavage can have recurrence of symptoms and on average require repeat lavage in 15 months, with an average of 2.5 procedures required per patient in 5 years [2, 19]. There are few studies on the success of transplant in patients with PAP. A major concern, which has been reported in multiple case studies, is the recurrence of PAP in the transplanted lung [20, 21]. Additionally, PAP has been found to occur secondarily in lung transplants in some patients that originally suffered from other pulmonary diseases due to presumed immune dysregulation due to immunosuppression [22, 23].

Are Patients with PAP More Prone to Any Specific Secondary Infections?

Yes, patients are more prone to develop atypical infections, theorized to be due to impaired macrophage function. In particular, patients have a higher rate of infection with mycobacteria and *Nocardia* spp. Additionally, decreased GM-CSF has been linked to a higher rate of disseminated *Nocardia* infections, even in patients without PAP [12, 24].

What Is the Prognosis for Patients with PAP?

Prognosis in patients with PAP is seldom reported as the underlying cause (such as hematologic malignancy), or complications (such as secondary infection) can greatly influence outcomes. Likewise, the prognosis tends to range widely, from spontaneous resolution to multiple recurrences, to even death. However, the most important prognostic factor described is the development of fibrosis, which is a poor prognostic factor [25, 26].

References

1. Inoue Y, Trapnell BC, Tazawa R, Arai T, Takada T, Hizawa N, et al. Characteristics of a large cohort of patients with autoimmune pulmonary alveolar proteinosis in Japan. Am J Respir Crit Care Med. 2008;177(7):752–62.
2. Seymour JF, Presneill JJ. Pulmonary alveolar proteinosis: progress in the first 44 years. Am J Respir Crit Care Med. 2002;166(2):215–35.
3. Shah PL, Hansell D, Lawson PR, Reid KB, Morgan C. Pulmonary alveolar proteinosis: clinical aspects and current concepts on pathogenesis. Thorax. 2000;55(1):67–77.
4. Holbert JM, Costello P, Li W, Hoffman RM, Rogers RM. CT features of pulmonary alveolar proteinosis. AJR Am J Roentgenol. 2001;176(5):1287–94.
5. Johkoh T, Itoh H, Muller NL, Ichikado K, Nakamura H, Ikezoe J, et al. Crazy-paving appearance at thin-section CT: spectrum of disease and pathologic findings. Radiology. 1999;211(1):155–60.
6. Chou CW, Lin FC, Tung SM, Liou RD, Chang SC. Diagnosis of pulmonary alveolar proteinosis: usefulness of papanicolaou-stained smears of bronchoalveolar lavage fluid. Arch Intern Med. 2001;161(4):562–6.
7. Prakash UB, Barham SS, Carpenter HA, Dines DE, Marsh HM. Pulmonary alveolar phospholipoproteinosis: experience with 34 cases and a review. Mayo Clin Proc. 1987;62(6):499–518.
8. Wang BM, Stern EJ, Schmidt RA, Pierson DJ. Diagnosing pulmonary alveolar proteinosis. A review and an update. Chest. 1997;111(2):460–6.
9. Alberti A, Luisetti M, Braschi A, Rodi G, Iotti G, Sella D, et al. Bronchoalveolar lavage fluid composition in alveolar proteinosis. Early changes after therapeutic lavage. Am J Respir Crit Care Med. 1996;154(3 Pt 1):817–20.
10. Poletti V, Costabel U, Casoni GL, Bigliazzi C, Drent M, Olivieri D. Rare infiltrative lung diseases: a challenge for clinicians. Respiration. 2004;71(5):431–43.
11. Uchida K, Nakata K, Trapnell BC, Terakawa T, Hamano E, Mikami A, et al. High-affinity autoantibodies specifically eliminate granulocyte-macrophage colony-stimulating factor activity in the lungs of patients with idiopathic pulmonary alveolar proteinosis. Blood. 2004;103(3):1089–98.
12. Kumar A, Abdelmalak B, Inoue Y, Culver DA. Pulmonary alveolar proteinosis in adults: pathophysiology and clinical approach. Lancet Respir Med. 2018;6(7):554–65.
13. Lin FC, Chang GD, Chern MS, Chen YC, Chang SC. Clinical significance of anti-GM-CSF antibodies in idiopathic pulmonary alveolar proteinosis. Thorax. 2006;61(6):528–34.
14. Rosen SH, Castleman B, Liebow AA. Pulmonary alveolar proteinosis. N Engl J Med. 1958;258(23):1123–42.
15. Dranoff G, Crawford AD, Sadelain M, Ream B, Rashid A, Bronson RT, et al. Involvement of granulocyte-macrophage colony-stimulating factor in pulmonary homeostasis. Science. 1994;264(5159):713–6.
16. Kitamura T, Tanaka N, Watanabe J, Uchida, Kanegasaki S, Yamada Y, et al. Idiopathic pulmonary alveolar proteinosis as an autoimmune disease with neutralizing antibody against granulocyte/macrophage colony-stimulating factor. J Exp Med. 1999;190(6):875–80.
17. Chaulagain CP, Pilichowska M, Brinckerhoff L, Tabba M, Erban JK. Secondary pulmonary alveolar proteinosis in hematologic malignancies. Hematol Oncol Stem Cell Ther. 2014;7(4):127–35.
18. Leth S, Bendstrup E, Vestergaard H, Hilberg O. Autoimmune pulmonary alveolar proteinosis: treatment options in year 2013. Respirology. 2013;18(1):82–91.
19. Campo I, Luisetti M, Griese M, Trapnell BC, Bonella F, Grutters J, et al. Whole lung lavage therapy for pulmonary alveolar proteinosis: a global survey of current practices and procedures. Orphanet J Rare Dis. 2016;11(1):115.
20. Takaki M, Tanaka T, Komohara Y, Tsuchihashi Y, Mori D, Hayashi K, et al. Recurrence of pulmonary alveolar proteinosis after bilateral lung transplantation in a patient with a nonsense mutation in CSF2RB. Respir Med Case Rep. 2016;19:89–93.
21. Santamaria F, Brancaccio G, Parenti G, Francalanci P, Squitieri C, Sebastio G, et al. Recurrent fatal pulmonary alveolar proteinosis after heart-lung transplantation in a child with lysinuric protein intolerance. J Pediatr. 2004;145(2):268–72.
22. Philippot Q, Cazes A, Borie R, Debray MP, Danel C, Hurtado Nedelec M, et al. Secondary pulmonary alveolar proteinosis after lung transplantation: a single-centre series. Eur Respir J. 2017;49(2):1601369.
23. Albores J, Seki A, Fishbein MC, Abtin F, Lynch JP III, Wang T, et al. A rare occurrence of pulmonary alveolar proteinosis after lung transplantation. Semin Respir Crit Care Med. 2013;34(3):431–8.
24. Rosen LB, Rocha Pereira N, Figueiredo C, Fiske LC, Ressner RA, Hong JC, et al. Nocardia-induced granulocyte macrophage colony-stimulating factor is neutralized by autoantibodies in disseminated/extrapulmonary nocardiosis. Clin Infect Dis. 2015;60(7):1017–25.
25. Akira M, Inoue Y, Arai T, Sugimoto C, Tokura S, Nakata K, et al. Pulmonary fibrosis on high-resolution CT of patients with pulmonary alveolar proteinosis. AJR Am J Roentgenol. 2016;207(3):544–51.
26. Goldstein LS, Kavuru MS, Curtis-McCarthy P, Christie HA, Farver C, Stoller JK. Pulmonary alveolar proteinosis: clinical features and outcomes. Chest. 1998;114(5):1357–62.

Nonspecific Interstitial Pneumonia Versus Lymphoid Interstitial Pneumonia Versus Follicular Bronchiolitis

46

Brian D. Cone and Gregory A. Fishbein

Clinical Presentation and Imaging

A 47-year-old man presented with a history of cough and progressive dyspnea. The cough started roughly 10 months prior and was nonproductive. The patient was a former smoker, though he quit over 25 years ago. During that time, he experienced a single episode of community-acquired pneumonia, from which he recovered fully. His past medical history also includes benign prostatic hyperplasia and persistent low-grade arthralgia, primarily affecting his lower extremities and hands, for which he has taken over-the-counter nonsteroidal anti-inflammatory drugs. He does not take any other medications. He has no known organic dust or occupational exposures, nor does he own birds. He has worked in the same office for greater than 20 years as an insurance adjuster.

Physical examination was mostly unremarkable. There was no digital clubbing or other signs of peripheral cyanosis. However, mild but symmetrical swelling of the proximal interphalangeal joints was seen. Spirometry demonstrated impaired total lung capacity (TLC) and decreased forced vital capacity (FVC). Diffusion capacity for carbon monoxide (DLCO) was also less than predicted. Overall pulmonary functional testing (PFT) was compatible with restrictive physiology.

A high-resolution computed tomography (HRCT) scan was obtained and demonstrated a relatively symmetric distribution of reticular and ground-glass opacities, primarily affecting the left lower lobe and the basilar aspects of the right middle and right lower lobes (Fig. 46.1). Traction bronchiectasis was noted in one lung field. There were no cystic or honeycomb changes seen. An open lung wedge biopsy was subsequently ordered.

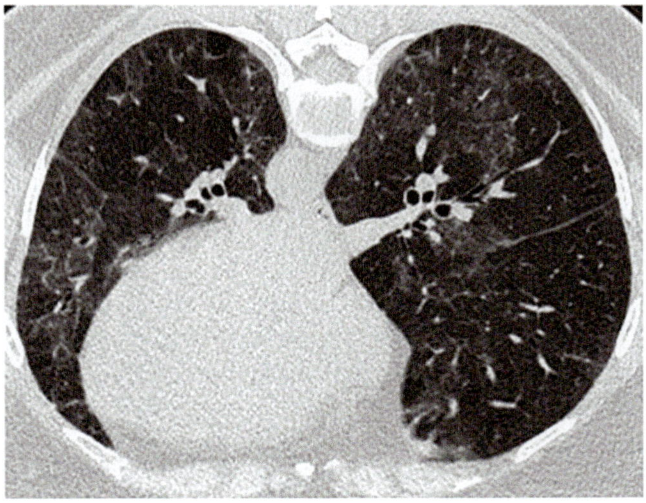

Fig. 46.1 Chest HRCT. Axial high-resolution CT of the chest showing diffuse, ground-glass opacities that were present in all lobes

Histologic sections of the wedge biopsy appeared diffusely abnormal. Low magnification shows uniform expansion of the interstitium by small mature lymphocytes and plasma cells. The infiltrate has moderate cellularity throughout the biopsy (Fig. 46.2). Aside from moderate expansion of the alveolar walls, the lung architecture is otherwise intact. The bronchovascular bundles and pleura were uninvolved. No organizing pneumonia, fibroblastic foci, granulomas, or microcystic honeycomb changes were identified.

B. D. Cone · G. A. Fishbein (✉)
Department of Pathology and Laboratory Medicine, David Geffen School of Medicine at UCLA, Los Angeles, CA, USA
e-mail: gfishbein@mednet.ucla.edu

H. Xu et al. (eds.), *Practical Lung Pathology*, Practical Anatomic Pathology, https://doi.org/10.1007/978-3-031-14402-8_46

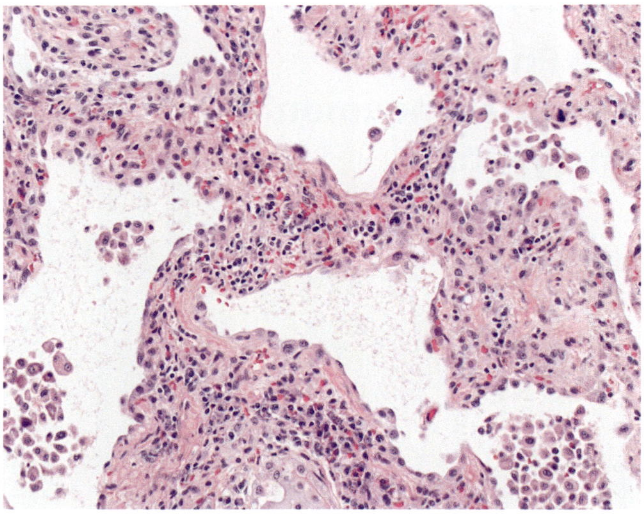

Fig. 46.2 NSIP, cellular variant. Histologic section shows a diffuse process that uniformly affects the alveolar septa. At medium power, the cellular lymphoid infiltrate can be readily appreciated. Microscopic honeycombing and fibroblastic foci are absent [H&E stain; 200× magnification]

The Final Pathologic Diagnosis Rendered: Nonspecific Interstitial Pneumonia, Cellular Pattern

What Is the Differential Diagnosis of Interstitial Lymphoid Infiltrates in the Lung?

For cases in which a diagnostic lung biopsy reveals a prominent lymphoplasmacytic infiltrate, whether focal or diffuse, there are several diagnoses that should always be considered in the differential. Primarily, these include lymphoid interstitial pneumonia, follicular bronchiolitis, nodular lymphoid hyperplasia, cellular variant of nonspecific interstitial pneumonia, intraparenchymal lymph node sampling, and lastly, lymphoma. By evaluating the location and extent of the cellular infiltrates, one can readily narrow the differential diagnosis. It can then be further refined by examining whether other key features are present, such as well-formed lymphoid follicles, interstitial fibrosis, or peribronchiolar granulomas.

What Is NSIP?

NSIP is a histologic pattern of interstitial lung disease characterized by a diffuse and homogenous expansion of the alveolar septa by inflammatory cells and/or fibrosis. The term NSIP was proposed by Katzenstein and Fiorelli in 1994 to characterize certain cases of idiopathic interstitial pneumonia (IIP) that did not histologically or prognostically conform to the major categories of that time: usual interstitial pneumonia (UIP), desquamative interstitial pneumonia, and acute interstitial pneumonia. Although historically NSIP has sometimes been considered a "wastebasket" term, it has evolved to refer to a specific pattern of interstitial lung disease that may be primary (idiopathic) or secondary. The NSIP pattern can be seen in numerous clinical situations and is the most common pattern of ILD associated with connective tissue disease, such as systemic lupus erythematosus, scleroderma, rheumatoid arthritis, and Sjogren's syndrome. ILD with an NSIP pattern may even be the first presentation of said diseases. Prior acute lung injury or drug reaction may also cause an NSIP pattern [1–3].

What Is the Typical Clinical Presentation for NSIP?

Due to the various clinical associations, the presenting symptoms of NSIP are nonspecific and are commonly seen with other chronic diffuse lung diseases. These symptoms include dry cough, progressive shortness of breath, and fatigue. Less commonly, weight loss, fever, and digital clubbing may be seen. When secondary to a connective tissue disease, such as rheumatoid arthritis, Sjögren's syndrome, or polymyositis, extrapulmonary symptoms like polyarthritis or *sicca* syndrome may dominate the clinical picture [1, 3, 4]. Pulmonary function testing will typically reveal a restrictive defect, with reduced TLC, FVC, and DLCO [2].

What Is the Typical Clinical Presentation of LIP?

The clinical features of LIP overlap with cellular NSIP. The most common LIP-associated diseases include rheumatoid arthritis, Sjögren's syndrome, other collagen vascular diseases, HIV/AIDS, and other states of aberrant immune status. Whether LIP can be truly idiopathic is controversial [4]. The presenting symptoms include cough and progressive dyspnea. Fever, fatigue, and weight loss are less common. Just as with NSIP, patients may present with extrapulmonary symptoms related to underlying systemic disease [5–7]. PFTs are unlikely to be discriminatory between NSIP and LIP, as both conditions usually demonstrate restrictive physiology. The most common PFT results in LIP are reduced FVC, FEV1, TLC, and decreased DLCO [7].

What Is FB and How Does It Typically Present Clinically?

Follicular bronchiolitis is a reactive/nonneoplastic pulmonary lymphoproliferative disease that consists of hyperplastic bronchial-associated lymphoid tissue (BALT). By definition, FB primarily affects the airways and spares the alveolated parenchyma. In all cases, discrete peribronchiolar lymphoid follicles should be readily apparent and will often contain well-formed germinal centers [8, 9].

There is considerable overlapping symptomatology between NSIP and FB. Patients diagnosed with either NSIP or FB may have nearly identical presentations along with nonspecific imaging findings. Both entities are commonly diagnosed in patients with the same underlying conditions, most notably CVD. Both NSIP and FB are commonly associated with Sjögren's syndrome and rheumatoid arthritis [10, 11]. Identification of FB or NSIP in a biopsy specimen should raise suspicion for occult CVD. Peripheral eosinophilia is seen in those with hypersensitivity syndromes. Primary or idiopathic cases of FB are rare, although a familial form is described [12]. Pulmonary function tests in FB produce inconsistent results, often revealing restrictive, obstructive, or normal ventilation patterns [8, 13, 14].

What Are Radiographic Findings That Support a Diagnosis of NSIP?

Radiographic imaging studies are important elements in the diagnosis of all interstitial lung diseases. Although there is considerable overlap among the various entities, a concise differential diagnosis can often be rendered based on imaging alone. Chest X-rays in patients with NSIP show increased interstitial markings primarily involving the lower lung fields, bilaterally [15]. NSIP characteristically has a homogenous and symmetrical appearance on HRCT. The scans most often show extensive and bilateral reticular infiltrates and ground-glass opacities, affecting nearly 50% of the lung fields. Lobar volume loss can sometimes be appreciated. Sparing of the subpleural parenchyma may be seen and is an important finding that distinguishes NSIP from UIP. In cases of NSIP with appreciable interstitial fibrosis (NSIP-F), traction bronchiectasis occur secondary to scarring. Honeycomb change is usually minimal or absent [15–17].

What Are Radiographic Findings That Support a Diagnosis of LIP or FB?

The main HRCT findings in LIP are similar to those seen in NSIP. Bilateral ground-glass opacities mainly affecting the basilar aspect of lungs should be identifiable in all cases. A distinguishing feature in most cases is the presence of thin-walled peribronchovascular cysts, which can have a striking appearance. Other findings include reticular opacities, patchy airspace consolidation, interlobular septal thickening, subpleural nodules, and occasional centrilobular nodules [18].

In FB, chest X-rays may demonstrate reticular or reticulonodular opacities, and in the majority of patients, bilateral centrilobular nodules measuring 1–3 mm in diameter may be seen on HRCT. In cases with post-obstructive changes, such as obstructive pneumonia with intraluminal exudates, a more distinctive finding can emerge and is referred to as "tree/cotton-in-bud" pattern [8, 9, 14].

Are Gross Pathology Findings Useful in Distinguishing NSIP, LIP, and FB?

With advanced chest imaging, the radiographic findings effectively recapitulate the gross appearance of the lung. The presence and/or distribution of fibrosis and honeycomb change may be helpful to distinguish NSIP from UIP. However, there are no specific gross features that help distinguish NSIP from LIP or FB. Interestingly, the unique radiographic finding of peribronchovascular cysts in LIP is unlikely to be identified grossly.

What Are the Histologic Features of NSIP? What Histologic Subtypes/Patterns of NSIP Are Important in the Context of This Patient?

There are two widely recognized histologic patterns of NSIP, a cellular pattern, NSIP-C, and a fibrotic pattern, NSIP-F [19]. In NSIP-C, there is a diffuse but uniform appearing infiltration of alveolar septa by small, mature lymphocytes and plasma cells (Fig. 46.2). While the septa may widen due to the infiltrates, there should be no architectural distortion. Often, the subpleural region is spared, which is a distinguishing feature of NSIP. The lining alveolar epithelium can exhibit type II pneumocyte hyperplasia. This makes the pneumocytes appear more prominent or hobnailed. Peribronchiolar accentuation of the lymphoid infiltrates can also be seen but should not overshadow the interstitial process. Alveolar airspace organization may be focally present. Other nonspecific findings, such as peribronchiolar metaplasia, scattered lymphoid aggregates with or without germinal centers, focal accumulation of intra-alveolar macrophages, and cholesterol clefts, may be present [1, 2, 4]. In the cellular pattern, interstitial fibrosis is inconspicuous or absent.

NSIP-F shows the uniform architectural pattern of NSIP but is a predominantly fibrosing process rather than an inflammatory process. In NSIP-F, the interstitial compartment is widened as collagen bundles accrue within the alveolar walls. Lymphoid infiltrates are mild or absent. Uniform and diffuse involvement is the hallmark feature of NSIP. In NSIP-F, there should be no variation in the age of the fibrosis from field to field. Foci of loose fibroblasts actively elaborating collagen in a myxoid stroma (i.e., fibroblastic foci), if present, should not accompany dense interstitial fibrosis or honeycomb change in NSIP [1, 2].

What Are the Histologic Features of LIP?

On low magnification, histologic sections reveal an interstitial pneumonia composed of diffusely infiltrative lymphoid cells, largely confined to the alveolated pulmonary parenchyma. The airways are, for the most part, spared. The increased cellularity from infiltrating lymphocytes imparts an overall low-power blue appearance that more closely resembles lymphoma than other interstitial pneumonias (Fig. 46.3).

The lymphoid tissue is primarily composed of small mature lymphocytes, with varying amounts of plasma cells and histiocytes. Atypia or intranuclear inclusions in the lymphocytes should not be seen. This interstitial infiltrate may be more pronounced in the parenchyma along the bronchovascular bundles, adjacent to interlobular septa, and in the subpleural parenchyma. Other nonspecific findings can be encountered and include type II pneumocyte hyperplasia; hyperplastic lymphoid aggregates with germinal centers; scattered, poorly formed, non-necrotizing granulomas; and multinucleated giant cells [6, 7, 13].

The lymphoid population in LIP is, by definition, polytypic. Immunohistochemistry staining with CD3 can be used to highlight the T-cell preponderance along with CD20 and CD138 to highlight the admixed B lymphocytes and plasma cells, respectively [20].

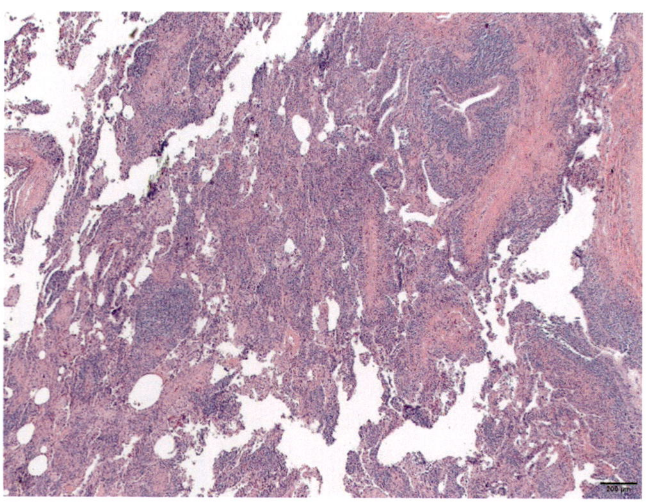

Fig. 46.3 Lymphoid interstitial pneumonia. A representative image of LIP showing a diffuse lymphoid infiltration of the alveolar septa. The diagnosis of LIP can only be made once lymphoma is excluded [H&E stain; 40× magnification]

How Do the Histologic Features of NSIP and LIP Overlap?

The fibrotic pattern of NSIP is unlikely to be confused with LIP, as it characteristically shows a uniform expansion of the alveolar septa by dense collagen, without abundant interstitial inflammation. However, the cellular pattern of NSIP may boast exuberant interstitial lymphoid infiltrate and can be difficult to distinguish from LIP. In fact, many cases that were regarded as LIP in the past would now be considered cellular NSIP [21].

What Are the Histologic Features of FB?

The cardinal histopathologic feature of FB is small airway inflammation arranged in follicles with well-formed germinal centers. This characteristic lesion should be identified in all cases of FB and can usually be seen at low magnification. FB is thought to develop from a polyclonal hyperplasia of existing bronchus-associated lymphoid tissue (BALT). The normal anatomic distribution of BALT primarily includes sites along the bronchial tree, interlobular septa, and subpleural lymph nodes. Some peribronchial nodules may be small and solitary and are situated between the affected bronchiole and its accompanying pulmonary artery. Other foci may contain larger, more expansive follicles that coalesce and subsequently obscure or even obliterate the bronchiolar lumen (Fig. 46.4). In these more exuberant cases, a reticulin or trichrome stain may be helpful to highlight distorted airways. In general, the follicles are confined to the peribronchiolar interstitium and interlobular septa. While the lymphocytic infiltrate spares adjacent airspaces and alveolar septa, foamy macrophages and other associated post-obstructive changes are common. Likewise, affected airways may also contain mucus plugs and a neutrophilic exudate secondary to obstruction. Severe damage to the bronchiolar epithelium or fibrinoid necrosis of the vascular walls should not be present [8, 9, 14].

The immunophenotype of lymphoid tissue in FB is consistent with that of reactive germinal centers forming elsewhere in the body. Immunohistochemical staining with CD20 or CD79a will highlight germinal center B cells, while staining with CD3 will highlight T cells more in the peripheral interfollicular areas.

Do the Histologic Features of NSIP and FB Overlap?

For the most part, no. The inflammation and subsequent fibrosis affect different compartments. While NSIP may affect the bronchovascular interstitium, its uniform alveolar septal involvement should dominate the histologic picture.

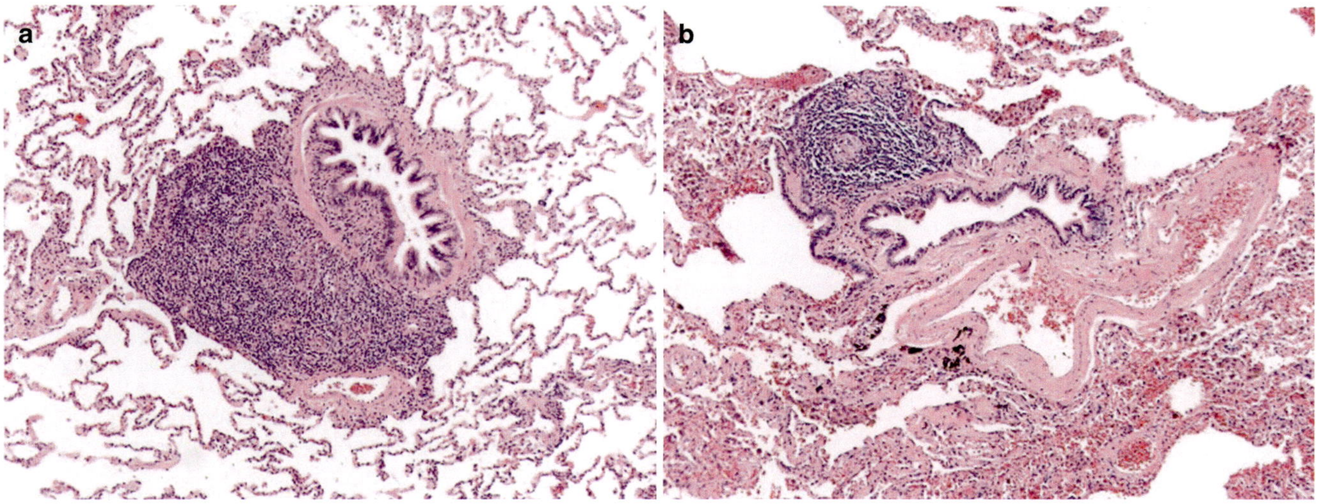

Fig. 46.4 Follicular bronchiolitis. (**a**) On slightly higher magnification, this lymphoid follicle is classically situated between the bronchial and the pulmonary artery. Slight compression of the bronchiolar lumen is seen. Both findings are classic features of FB. (**b**) In this example, the adjacent lung tissue is completely normal, with no extension of the lymphoid cells [H&E stains; 100× magnification]

FB can, and often does, track along interlobular septa and involve the subpleural parenchyma, although it should not extend into the adjacent alveolar airspaces and septa [9]. Although NSIP and FB occur in distinct patterns, they may occur together and frequently do in patients with CVD, such as Sjogren's syndrome and rheumatoid arthritis.

What Are the Recommended Ancillary Studies Needed for This Case?

The histopathologic workup of a case of NSIP does not usually require ancillary studies or special stains. In the absence of clinical or radiographic features suggestive of a low-grade lymphoma, careful evaluation of H&E stained sections is sufficient. In some cases of NSIP, particularly when there is both fibrosis and inflammation, a trichrome or other collagen stain may be used to better assess the degree of architectural remodeling. Robust interstitial collagen staining would favor NSIP over LIP.

In highly cellular cases possibly representing LIP, an Epstein-Barr encoding region (EBER) in situ hybridization study may be useful to exclude EBV infection as a possible cause for the lymphoid proliferation [22]. There are no reported cases of NSIP secondary to EBV infection.

There are no recommended or highly useful ancillary studies available to help differentiate NSIP and FB, as they can reliably be distinguished by H&E alone.

What Are Key Features That Can Distinguish NSIP from LIP and FB?

The distinction between cellular NSIP and LIP can be challenging in some situations, especially if the inflammatory infiltrate in NSIP-C is prominent and fibrosis is absent. When evaluating interstitial lung diseases, low-magnification assessment of diagnostic challenging cases is most helpful. At low power, LIP will take on a bluer appearance than cellular NSIP. The lymphocytic infiltrate in LIP is sufficiently robust that immunohistochemistry to rule out lymphoma must be performed in essentially all cases. The inflammation in NSIP can be extensive. However, it usually does not rise to the level at which lymphoma is high on the differential diagnosis. Architecturally, NSIP will have a more uniform appearance with better preservation of the alveolar structures. While not entirely effaced, the alveolar architecture in LIP will be somewhat distorted, in contrast. Radiographic findings may aid the distinction. The finding of thin-walled peribronchovascular cysts would favor LIP [9, 12].

The key takeaway points for distinguishing NSIP from FB again harken back to evaluating the tissue at low power. FB will appear as small to large nodules of lymphoid follicles distributed along airways, with compression of the lumens and preservation of adjacent alveolar tissue. It is again, however, noted that in some patients, NSIP and FB will both be present.

What Is the Prognosis for NSIP? How Does This Differ from LIP and FB?

In NSIP-C, the 5- and 10-year survival rates have been reported to be as high as 100% in some studies, particularly when no significant fibrosis is present. These patients have an excellent response to corticosteroid and/or immunosuppressive treatment [1, 2]. While still favorable when compared to UIP, which carries a dismal prognosis, patients with NSIP-F may be less responsive to these treatments [19, 23, 24]. Some even progress to a more severe interstitial pneumonia, clinically appearing as an overt idiopathic pulmonary fibrosis [4, 17, 18].

The prognosis for patients with LIP is quite variable. In certain cases, such as with HIV+ patients, treatment can be focused on the underlying disease with initiation of antiretroviral therapy. In this setting, complete resolution of pulmonary disease can be seen, and this can hold true when LIP is found secondary to other treatable underlying diseases [25]. Otherwise, symptomatic treatment with corticosteroids, or immunosuppressive and cytotoxic medications can be used [18]. Progression of LIP to end-stage lung disease requiring transplantation or causing death can occur [26]. Whether LIP can evolve into lymphoma is somewhat controversial. Case studies and review of literature indicate that the risk of LIP transforming into a pulmonary lymphoma is low [7].

The prognosis for FB is usually good. Though some studies have shown that when FB is diagnosed in patients less 30 years of age, their disease course may be more progressive [8, 9]. In many cases, immunosuppressants or other biologics are used to treat FB, reflecting the need to treat the underlying disease rather than the just the pulmonary disorder. In the rare cases of primary or familial FB, macrolide antibiotics have been used and have shown symptomatic improvement [14].

References

1. Katzenstein AL, Fiorelli RF. Nonspecific interstitial pneumonia/fibrosis. Histologic features and clinical significance. Am J Surg Pathol. 1994;18(2):136–47.
2. Cottin V, Donsbeck AV, Revel D, Loire R, Cordier JF. Nonspecific interstitial pneumonia. Individualization of a clinicopathologic entity in a series of 12 patients. Am J Respir Crit Care Med. 1998;158(4):1286–93.
3. Katzenstein AL, Myers JL. Nonspecific interstitial pneumonia and the other idiopathic interstitial pneumonias: classification and diagnostic criteria. Am J Surg Pathol. 2000;24(1):1–3.
4. Palmucci S, Roccasalva F, Puglisi S, Torrisi SE, Vindigni V, Mauro LA, et al. Clinical and radiological features of idiopathic interstitial pneumonias (IIPs): a pictorial review. Insights Imaging. 2014;5(3):347–64.
5. Carrington BC, Liebow AA. Lymphocytic interstitial pneumonia (abstract). Am J Pathol. 1966;48:36.
6. Liebow AA, Carrington CB. Diffuse pulmonary lymphoreticular infiltrations associated with dysproteinemia. Med Clin North Am. 1973;57(3):809–43.
7. Cha SI, Fessler MB, Cool CD, Schwarz MI, Brown KK. Lymphoid interstitial pneumonia: clinical features, associations and prognosis. Eur Respir J. 2006;28(2):364–9.
8. Yousem SA, Colby TV, Carrington CB. Follicular bronchitis/bronchiolitis. Hum Pathol. 1985;16:700.
9. Travis WD, Galvin JR. Non-neoplastic pulmonary lymphoid lesions. Thorax. 2001;56(12):964–71.
10. Capobianco J, Grimberg A, Thompson BM, Antunes VB, Jasinowodolinski D, Meirelles GSP. Thoracic manifestations of collagen vascular diseases. Radiographics. 2012;32(1):33–50.
11. Stojan G, Baer AN, Danoff SK. Pulmonary manifestations of Sjögren's syndrome. Curr Allergy Asthma Rep. 2013;13(4):354–60.
12. Franchi LM, Chin TW, Nussbaum E, Riker J, Robert M, Talbert WM. Familial pulmonary nodular lymphoid hyperplasia. J Pediatr. 1992;121(1):89–92.
13. Flaherty KR, Martinez FJ, Travis W, Lynch JP. Nonspecific Interstitial Pneumonia (NSIP). Semin Respir Crit Care Med. 2001;22(4):423–34.
14. Tashtoush B, Okafor NC, Ramirez JF, Smolley L. Follicular bronchiolitis: a literature review. J Clin Diagn Res. 2015;9(9):OE01–5.
15. Belloli EA, Beckford R, Hadley R, Flaherty KR. Idiopathic nonspecific interstitial pneumonia. Respirology. 2016;21(2):259–68.
16. Hartman TE, Swensen SJ, Hansell DM, Colby TV, Myers JL, Tazelaar HD, et al. Nonspecific interstitial pneumonia: variable appearance at high-resolution chest CT. Radiology. 2000;217(3):701–5.
17. Park JS, Lee KS, Kim JS, Park CS, Suh YL, Choi DL, et al. Nonspecific interstitial pneumonia with fibrosis: radiographic and CT findings in seven patients. Radiology. 1995;195(3):645–8.
18. Johkoh T, Ichikado K, Akira M, Honda O, Tomiyama N, Mihara N, et al. Lymphocytic interstitial pneumonia: follow-up CT findings in 14 patients. J Thorac Imaging. 2000;15(3):162–7.
19. Travis WD, Matsui K, Moss J, Ferrans VJ. Idiopathic nonspecific interstitial pneumonia: prognostic significance of cellular and fibrosing patterns: survival comparison with usual interstitial pneumonia and desquamative interstitial pneumonia. Am J Surg Pathol. 2000;24(1):19–33.
20. Sirajuddin A, Raparia K, Lewis VA, Franks TJ, Dhand S, Galvin JR, et al. Primary pulmonary lymphoid lesions: radiologic and pathologic findings. Radiographics. 2016;36(1):53–70.
21. Tanaka T, Ishida K. Update on rare idiopathic interstitial pneumonias and rare histologic patterns. Arch Pathol Lab Med. 2018;142(9):1069–79.
22. van Zyl-Smit RN, Naidoo J, Wainwright H, Said-Hartley Q, Davids M, Goodman H, et al. HIV associated Lymphocytic Interstitial Pneumonia: a clinical, histological and radiographic study from an HIV endemic resource-poor setting. BMC Pulm Med. 2015;15:38.
23. Tomassetti S, Ryu JH, Piciucchi S, Chilosi M, Poletti V. Nonspecific interstitial pneumonia: what is the optimal approach to management? Semin Respir Crit Care Med. 2016;37(3):378–94.
24. Schneider F, Hwang DM, Gibson K, Yousem SA. Nonspecific interstitial pneumonia: a study of 6 patients with progressive disease. Am J Surg Pathol. 2012;36(1):89–93.
25. Dufour V, Wislez M, Bergot E, Mayaud C, Cadranel J. Improvement of symptomatic human immunodeficiency virus-related lymphoid interstitial pneumonia in patients receiving highly active antiretroviral therapy. Clin Infect Dis. 2003;36(10):e127–30.
26. Koss MN, Hochholzer L, Langloss JM, Wehunt WD, Lazarus AA. Lymphoid interstitial pneumonia: clinicopathological and immunopathological findings in 18 cases. Pathology. 1987;19(2):178–85.

Respiratory Bronchiolitis Versus Desquamative Interstitial Pneumonia

47

Brian D. Cone and Gregory A. Fishbein

Clinical Presentation and Imaging

A 43-year-old man presented with chronic cough and progressive dyspnea. He has no other significant past medical history. The cough was occasionally productive, with yellow to white thick mucus. His social history was significant for moderate alcohol use and a 30-pack-year history of smoking. He works as a circuit court judge and has no known environmental exposures. His family history is significant for lung cancer, with his father and grandmother both dying of squamous cell carcinoma. His mother is alive, with no history of cancer or lung disease.

Physical exam findings included digital clubbing and discoloration of the skin on the second and third fingers of his dominant hand. Chest auscultation demonstrated prominent crackles that persisted following forced cough. There were no other significant exam findings. Pulmonary function testing was performed and demonstrated an overall restrictive ventilatory defect and diminished diffusion capacity for carbon monoxide.

A chest X-ray showed patchy bibasilar opacities, with relatively normal upper lung fields. A high-resolution chest CT was obtained and reinforced the X-ray findings. There were diffuse ground-glass opacities present, predominantly in the lower lobes, including the subpleural parenchyma (see Fig. 47.1). The upper lung zones were relatively spared.

Following thoracoscopic diagnostic wedge biopsy from the right lower lobe, histologic examination revealed diffusely abnormal lung with nearly all the airspaces containing sheets of histiocytes with a glassy, eosinophilic appearance (see Fig. 47.2). The pneumocytes lining the airspaces were flat or inconspicuous in most areas. Alveolar walls were significantly widened by bands of fibrosis intermixed with bundles of hyperplastic smooth muscle. The interstitium was largely hypocellular. No fibroblastic foci were seen. Inspection of the intra-alveolar histiocytes on higher power demonstrated finely granular golden-tinged pigment. Sporadic lymphoid aggregates were present along the airways. No granulomas were seen. Overall, the changes were uniform and were present in all fields examined.

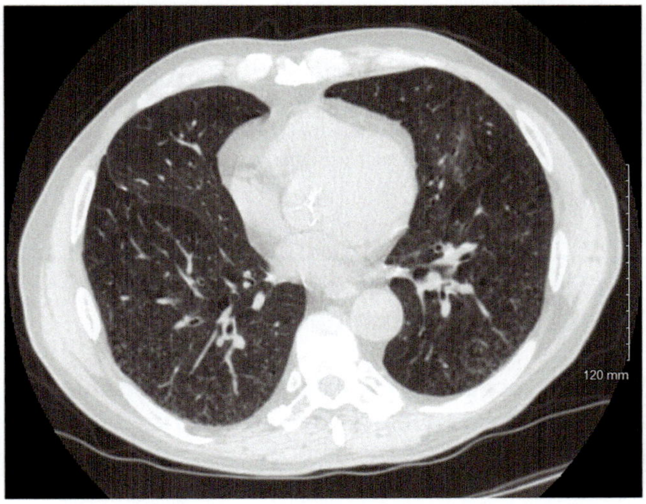

Fig. 47.1 HRCT of patient. An axial high-resolution CT scan of the chest shows basilar centrilobular nodules and small cysts, present bilaterally. (Figure courtesy of Travis Kauffman, DO, University of Missouri Kansas City, Kansas City, MO)

B. D. Cone · G. A. Fishbein (✉)
Department of Pathology and Laboratory Medicine, David Geffen School of Medicine at UCLA, Los Angeles, CA, USA
e-mail: gfishbein@mednet.ucla.edu

H. Xu et al. (eds.), *Practical Lung Pathology*, Practical Anatomic Pathology, https://doi.org/10.1007/978-3-031-14402-8_47

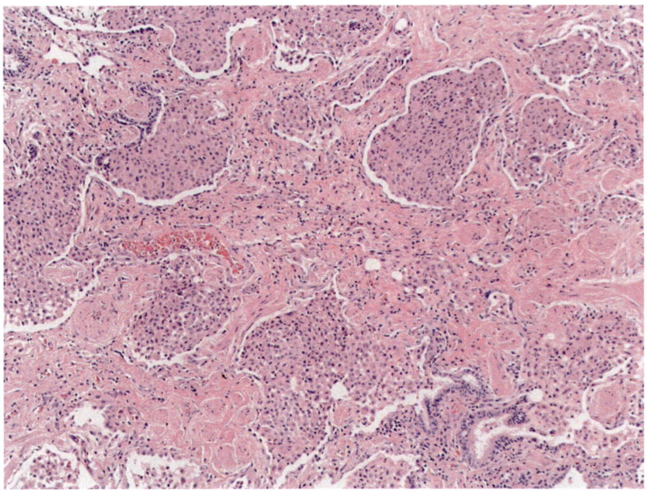

Fig. 47.2 Desquamative interstitial pneumonia (DIP). In DIP, the majority of airspaces are filled with compact sheets of glassy eosinophilic histiocytes. The surrounding interstitial space contains a mixture of collagen deposition (fibrosis) and smooth muscle hypertrophy [H&E stain; 100× magnification]

The Final Pathologic Diagnosis Rendered: Desquamative Interstitial Pneumonia

What Is Desquamative Interstitial Pneumonia and How Does It Relate to Respiratory Bronchiolitis?

Desquamative interstitial pneumonia (DIP) is a pulmonary disease characterized by the accumulation of macrophages within the alveoli, which form sheets of glassy eosinophilic cells that can distend the airspaces. According to the ATS/ERS 2013 consensus, smoking-related interstitial pneumonias (IIP) include respiratory bronchiolitis-associated interstitial lung disease (RB-ILD) and desquamative interstitial pneumonia (DIP) [1, 2]. Together, they represent a spectrum of pulmonary disease, largely characterized by macrophage accumulation of varying degree and distribution. Unfortunately, the literature regarding the clinical features, histologic characteristics, and even the nomenclature is both confusing and inconsistent.

What Is the Typical Clinical Presentation for RB?

By definition, RB is asymptomatic and is more a histologic biomarker of smoking than a clinical disease. The lesion is often incidentally seen in lung specimens sampled from smoking patients. In isolation, the finding is of little to no clinical significance and merely confirms the patient's history of smoking [3, 4].

What Is the Distinction Between RB and RB-ILD? What Is the Typical Clinical Presentation of RB-ILD?

In essence, respiratory bronchiolitis-associated interstitial lung disease (RB-ILD) is the clinical correlate of the RB histomorphology when identified in patients that also have clinical manifestations of interstitial lung disease [5]. However, the use and distinction of these terms are not consistent throughout the literature.

RB-ILD is a rare disorder that usually occurs in heavy smokers, with equal sex incidence. Patients diagnosed with RB-ILD tend to be younger, typically ranging from 30 to 60 years of age at time of diagnosis. Symptoms include chronic cough and shortness of breath. Subjective wheezing and inspiratory crackles are reported in a minority of patients. If there is progressive exertional dyspnea or other, more severe complaints, such as hemoptysis or peripheral cyanosis, then other diagnoses should be strongly considered [6, 7].

Limited data suggests that pulmonary function testing can show various patterns, including normal, mixed obstructive and restrictive, or purely restrictive impairment. A reduction in diffusion capacity for carbon monoxide (DLCO) can also be seen and may be disproportionate to the relatively mild symptoms. Patients diagnosed with RB-ILD typically do not go on to experience chronic, progressive interstitial lung disease. Even patients who continue smoking tend to have a stable course [3, 6–8].

What Are the Typical Radiographic Findings in RB-ILD?

In contrast to pulmonary function tests, RB-ILD often demonstrates characteristic radiographic findings. Although chest X-rays are often normal, HRCT scans often show ground-glass opacities or centrilobular nodules that are upper lobe predominant. The bronchi can appear thickened, and emphysema may be present [2, 7].

What Is the Typical Clinical Presentation of DIP?

DIP can affect both men and women and almost always occurs in heavy smokers. Affected individuals tend to be older than those with RB-ILD, but about 10 years younger than those diagnosed with UIP. Not all cases of DIP are seen in smokers. A variety of other conditions may very rarely demonstrate a reactive, DIP-like histologic picture. These include drug reaction, asbestosis, and collagen vascular diseases such as systemic lupus erythematosus or rheumatoid arthritis [7, 9].

Symptoms include dry cough and slow onset dyspnea. In contrast to RB-ILD, as many as 50% of patients with DIP have digital clubbing. Pulmonary function testing shows mild to moderate restriction and decreased diffusion capacity for carbon monoxide. The degree of impairment often is less pronounced than with other interstitial lung diseases [7, 10].

What Are the Typical Radiographic Findings in DIP?

Chest X-rays can show bibasilar ground-glass opacities in about one quarter of patients with DIP, although they can be normal in some patients. On HRCT, ground-glass attenuation is nearly always identified and is lower lobe predominant, which distinguishes DIP from most other pulmonary diseases that are related to particulate inhalation [7]. Subpleural distribution of the opacities is also present. Bronchial dilation, or pseudobronchiectasis, can be seen and is a form of reversible airway dilation, distinguished from traction bronchiectasis by its lack of tortuosity or string of beads appearance. Oftentimes, small cystic changes can be present and are worrisome for honeycombing; however, these too are known to be reversible. Overall, the pulmonary parenchymal architecture is more or less preserved, in contrast to UIP [10, 11].

What Are the Histologic Features of RB/RB-ILD?

The preponderance of literature state that the histologic differences between RB and RB-ILD are indistinguishable [3, 7, 8]. In RB/RB-ILD, low magnification of histologic sections shows focal bronchiolocentric accumulation of glassy, eosinophilic appearing macrophages. Mild to moderate distortion of the bronchioles can be seen, appearing dilated or irregularly shaped. Mild fibrotic changes can thicken the walls of the involved bronchioles. Chronic inflammation can be present within the bronchial interstitium. The accumulation of macrophages can extend to adjacent alveolar ducts and peribronchiolar airspaces. On higher power, the luminal macrophages show very fine, gold-to-brown granular cytoplasmic pigmentation [5, 6, 10, 12] (see Fig. 47.3).

What Are the Histologic Features of DIP?

Histologic sections from patients with DIP will appear pink or eosinophilic on low magnification on account of the diffuse filling of airspaces by pigmented macrophages. The alveolar walls become widened by interstitial fibrosis, which should be mild to moderate and uniform throughout. Higher magnification will highlight the airspaces filled with sheets

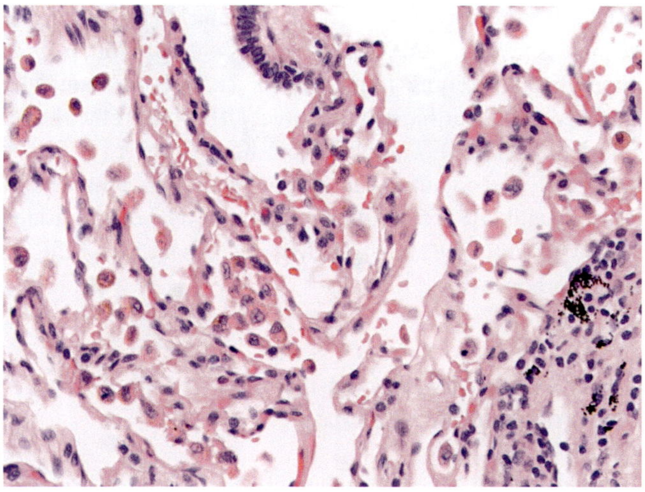

Fig. 47.3 Respiratory bronchiolitis (RB). Loose collections of finely pigmented alveolar smokers' macrophages accumulate in airspaces surrounding a respiratory bronchiole [H&E stain; 400× magnification]

of macrophages, which contain the same finely granular, gold-brown pigment (smoker's pigment). While the majority of the accumulated cells are mononuclear, scattered multinucleated giant cells can be seen [10]. Chronic inflammatory infiltrates can be present and are most often centered around the respiratory bronchioles. Interstitial plasma cells and rare eosinophils can also be seen.

Airspace enlargement and interstitial widening of the alveolar septa can be seen in DIP. The septa are widened secondary to collagen deposition and scant inflammatory cell infiltrates. Smooth muscle hypertrophy is also common. Pneumocyte hyperplasia can be focally present. The collagen should be mature, and fibroblastic foci should not be seen [1, 10].

How Are DIP and RB/RB-ILD Distinguished Radiographically?

The HRCT can help distinguish RB-ILD from DIP as there should be apparent differences in distribution of the opacities and centrilobular nodules. In RB-ILD, they should be found predominantly in the upper lobes, whereas in DIP, they are lower lobe predominant and subpleural. The presence of lower zone cystic lesions also favors DIP [7].

How Are DIP and RB/RB-ILD Distinguished Histologically?

Both RB and DIP are characterized by accumulations of intra-alveolar, finely pigmented macrophages. In DIP, the accumulations form dense uniform aggregates and diffusely involve the airspaces. In RB/RB-ILD, the accumulations are more sparse and bronchiolocentric [7]. Sparing of distal airspaces would be more consistent with RB-ILD. If interstitial thickening is present in RB-ILD, it should be confined to the peribronchiolar area. DIP, on the other hand, can demonstrate more distal interstitial fibrosis [10]. It is important to recognize that the histopathologic changes of RB-ILD and DIP exist along a spectrum. The distinction is somewhat arbitrary and arguably unnecessary, according to some authors [10].

Can the Diagnoses of RB-ILD and/or DIP Be Made on a Small Biopsy?

The presence of RB is a common incidental finding in smokers. In addition, focal areas showing DIP-like changes are sometimes encountered in resection specimens from patients without DIP. Therefore, while it is appropriate to comment on the presence, quantity, and quality (e.g., pigmented, hemosiderin-laden, foamy, etc.) of alveolar macrophages, small transbronchial biopsies are insufficient to render the diagnoses of RB-ILD or DIP.

What Is the Prognosis for RB, RB-ILD, and DIP?

As all three entities are smoking-related, smoking cessation is a first-line recommendation regardless of its effectiveness in disease management. RB will likely be present histologically as long as the patient continues smoking and may even remain in up to half of ex-smokers [3]. As mentioned, RB-ILD does not typically progress and has an excellent prognosis, as many patients tend to stabilize even without cessation. That said, the symptoms and physiologic defects can persist, even with smoking cessation. Corticosteroid use is controversial, as there is no clear evidence of its efficacy beyond some transient symptomatic improvement [6]. The 10-year survival rate for DIP is about 70% [9]. Overall, smoking cessation, with or without treatment, gives an excellent prognosis when compared to other interstitial lung diseases.

What Other Diagnoses Can Be Considered in This Case?

Pulmonary Langerhans cell histiocytosis (PLCH) is almost exclusively seen in cigarette smokers and frequently coexists with RB and DIP. The hallmark finding of PLCH is a reactive proliferation of Langerhans cells that form nodules along small airways with a stellate appearance. In its active phase, Langerhans cells will be seen accompanied by eosinophils. Organizing pneumonia may surround the nodules. In the "burnt-out" phase, the inflammatory cells may no longer be present; only acellular stellate scars remain. Radiographically, PLCH demonstrates small cysts in the upper lobes, predominantly around the periphery. Because PLCH, RB, and DIP are all associated with smoking, it is not surprising that they may all be seen in the same patient. Therefore, these entities are often grouped together into what is commonly called smoking-related interstitial lung disease (SR-ILD). In one review of PLCH cases, all contained RB/DIP-like changes [6, 13].

What Ancillary Studies Can Be Used in the Pathologic Workup of This Patient?

As with many interstitial lung diseases, immunohistochemical stains are of limited utility in the workup of RB, RB-ILD, and DIP. Immunostains are helpful, however, to demonstrate the Langerhans cells of PLCH. These cells are immunoreactive to CD1a, S100, and Langerin. Special stains, such as trichrome or elastin stains, may be helpful in some cases to highlight the small airways and vasculature. Iron stains may or may not highlight the pigmented intra-alveolar macrophages depending on the content of the particulate matter.

References

1. Liebow AA, Steer A, Billingsley JG. Desquamative interstitial pneumonia. Am J Med. 1965;39:369–404.
2. Travis WD, Costabel U, Hansell DM, King TE, Lynch DA, Nicholson AG, et al. An official American Thoracic Society/ European Respiratory Society statement: update of the international multidisciplinary classification of the idiopathic interstitial pneumonias. Am J Respir Crit Care Med. 2013;188(6):733–48.
3. Konopka KE, Myers JL. A review of smoking-related interstitial fibrosis, respiratory bronchiolitis, and desquamative interstitial pneumonia: overlapping histology and confusing terminology. Arch Pathol Lab Med. 2018;142(10):1177–81.
4. Niewoehner DE, Jerome K, Rice DB. Pathologic changes in the peripheral airways of young cigarette smokers. N Engl J Med. 1974;291(15):755–8.
5. Craig PJ, Wells AU, Doffman S, Rassl D, Colby TV, Hansell DM, et al. Desquamative interstitial pneumonia, respiratory bronchiolitis and their relationship to smoking. Histopathology. 2004;45(3):275–82.
6. Portnoy J, Veraldi KL, Schwarz MI, Cool CD, Curran-Everett D, Cherniack RM, et al. Respiratory bronchiolitis-interstitial lung disease. Chest. 2007;131(3):664–71.
7. Bak SH, Lee HY. Overlaps and uncertainties of smoking-related idiopathic interstitial pneumonias. Int J Chron Obstruct Pulm Dis. 2017;12:3221–9.

8. Reddy TL, Mayo J, Churg A. Respiratory bronchiolitis with fibrosis. High-resolution computed tomography findings and correlation with pathology. Ann Am Thorac Soc. 2013;10(6):590–601.
9. Carrington CB, Gaensler EA, Coutu RE, FitzGerald MX, Gupta RG. Natural history and treated course of usual and desquamative interstitial pneumonia. N Engl J Med. 1978;298(15):801–9.
10. Katzenstein AL, Myers JL. Idiopathic pulmonary fibrosis: clinical relevance of pathologic classification. Am J Respir Crit Care Med. 1998;157(4):1301–15.
11. Akira M, Yamamoto S, Hara H, Sakatani M, Ueda E. Serial computed tomographic evaluation in desquamative interstitial pneumonia. Thorax. 1997;52(4):333–7.
12. Katzenstein A-LA, Mukhopadhyay S, Zanardi C, Dexter E. Clinically occult interstitial fibrosis in smokers: classification and significance of a surprisingly common finding in lobectomy specimens. Hum Pathol. 2010;41(3):316–25.
13. Vassallo R, Jensen EA, Colby TV, Ryu JH, Douglas WW, Hartman TE, et al. The overlap between respiratory bronchiolitis and desquamative interstitial pneumonia in pulmonary Langerhans cell histiocytosis: high-resolution CT, histologic, and functional correlations. Chest. 2003;124(4):1199–205.

Constrictive Bronchiolitis

48

Chen Zhang

Clinical History

A 58-year-old female former smoker presents with worsening shortness of breath for 6 months which began as "flu"-like symptoms. A cardiac review is negative for ischemic heart disease. She is currently on no medications. She has a history of sleep apnea and uses a continuous positive airway pressure (CPAP) at night. She states that she feels fine when sleeping with the CPAP on but gets shortness of breath as she gets out of bed with a few steps. Her pulmonary function testing reveals a moderately obstructive ventilatory defect, with FVC 2.47 L (64% predicted), FEV1 1.21 L (41% predicted), TLC 5.75 L (101% predicted), and diffusion capacity 48% predicted. There is no response to bronchodilators. A high-resolution chest computed tomography (CT) scan shows bilateral mosaic attenuation and air trapping of the lungs, most prominent in the lower lobes (Fig. 48.1).

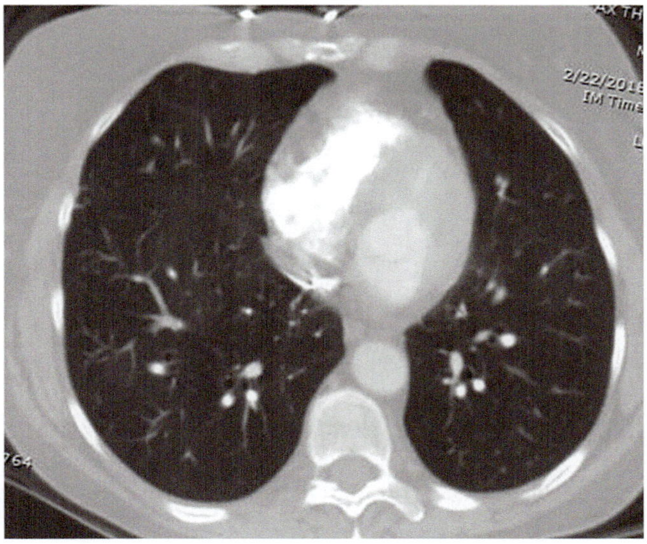

Fig. 48.1 Constrictive bronchiolitis. Chest CT scan demonstrating bilateral mosaic attenuation and air trapping

Pathologic Findings

Video-assisted thoracoscopic surgery (VATS) wedge biopsies from the right upper, middle, and lower lobes were performed. The histologic findings from the three lobes are similar and show near normal alveolar lung parenchyma under low magnification (Fig. 48.2). However, closer examination under higher magnification (Fig. 48.3a, b) reveals show luminal narrowing of some bronchioles, associated with subepithelial fibroblast proliferation. An elastic stain (Fig. 48.3c) demonstrates that the fibroblast proliferation occurs between the respiratory epithelium and the elastic layer. Some bronchioles are even completed obliterated with fibrosis and chronic inflammation (Fig. 48.4a, b). The bronchiole remnants are considerably smaller than the adjacent pulmonary arteries. An elastic stain highlights the residual bronchial elastic layer surrounding the obliterated lumina (Fig. 48.4c).

C. Zhang (✉)
Weill Cornell Medicine, Department of Pathology and Laboratory Medicine, New York, NY, USA
e-mail: fjr9007@med.cornell.edu

H. Xu et al. (eds.), *Practical Lung Pathology*, Practical Anatomic Pathology, https://doi.org/10.1007/978-3-031-14402-8_48

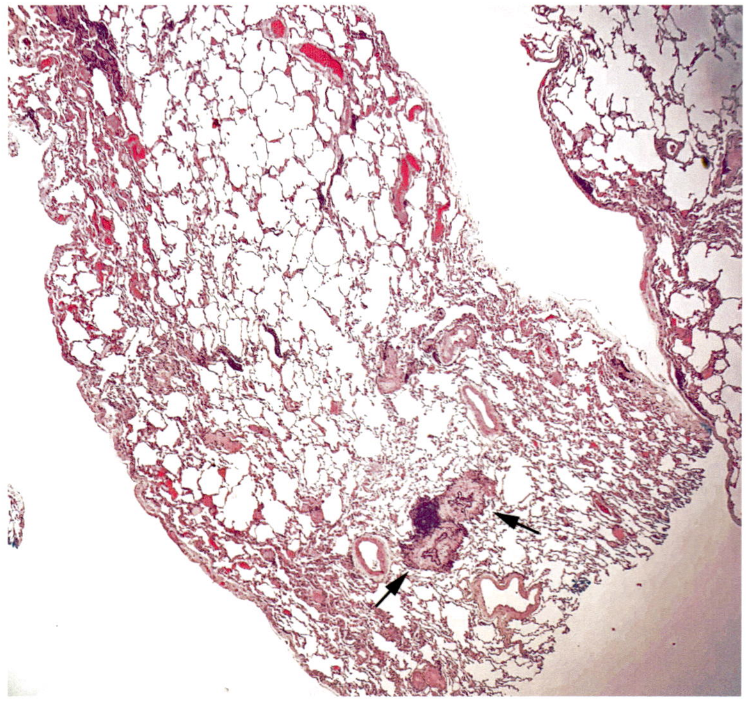

Fig. 48.2 Constrictive bronchiolitis. Low-magnification photomicrograph of a lung wedge biopsy showing largely unremarkable alveolar lung parenchyma. A few bronchioles (arrows) have thickened walls, a feature that is inconspicuous and easily overlooked at this magnification. H&E, 20×

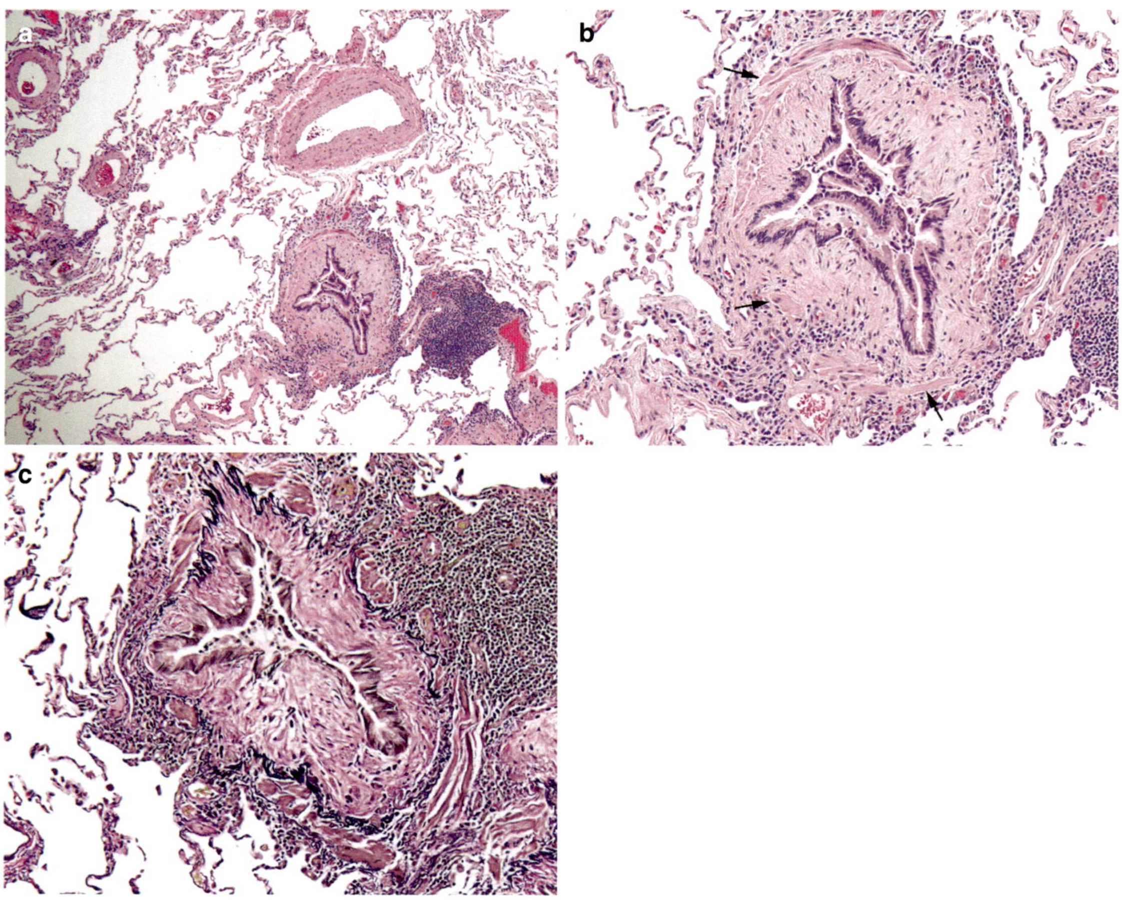

Fig. 48.3 Constrictive bronchiolitis. (**a**) Intermediate magnification showing narrowed small airway lumina due to subepithelial fibrosis. H&E, 100× (**b**) High-magnification photomicrograph illustrating prominent fibroblast proliferation in a collagenous and myxoid stroma situated between the respiratory epithelium and the smooth muscle layer (arrows). H&E, 200× (**c**) High-magnification photomicrograph of an elastic tissue stain highlights the fibrosis that separates respiratory epithelium from the elastic layer. 200×

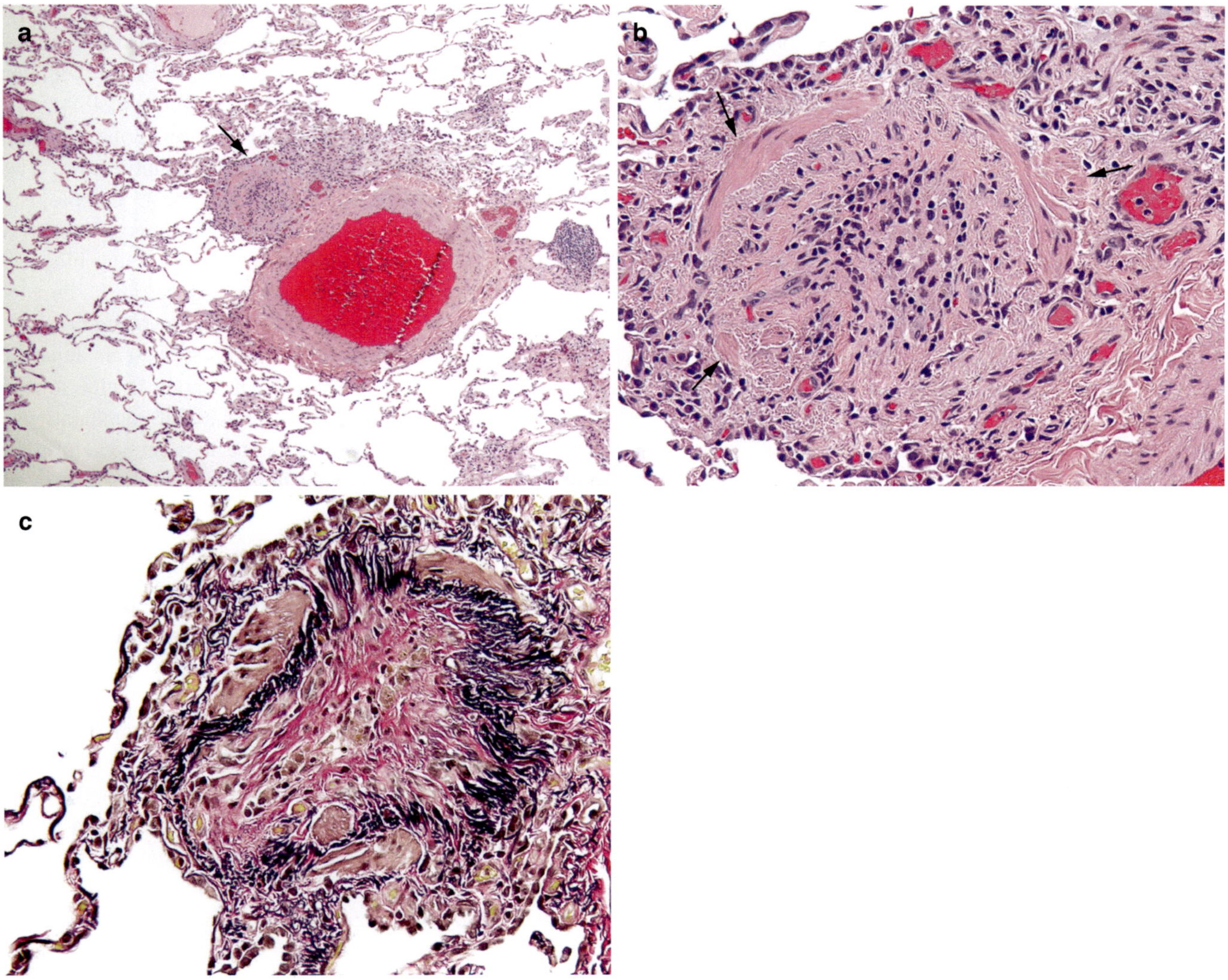

Fig. 48.4 Constrictive bronchiolitis. (**a**) Low-magnification photomicrograph of constrictive bronchiolitis at a later stage. A completely obliterated bronchiole (arrow) is significantly smaller than the adjacent pulmonary artery. H&E, 20× (**b**) Higher magnification showing that the lumen of the bronchiole is completely obliterated by fibrosis with a scant infiltrate of inflammatory cells. The bronchiole is recognizable by its residual smooth muscle layer (arrows). H&E, 200× (**c**) An elastic stain highlights the residual elastic layer (arrows) of the obliterated bronchiole. 200×

Diagnosis: Constrictive Bronchiolitis (CB)

What Are the Etiologies and Clinical Presentations of Constrictive Bronchiolitis?

CB, also known as obliterative bronchiolitis, is a rare small airway disease that is most commonly encountered in lung or stem cell transplant recipients in whom it is a manifestation of chronic rejection [1] or graft-versus-host disease [2, 3], respectively. Other less common causes include infection, drug toxicity, connective tissue disease (rheumatoid arthritis), and toxic inhalation [4–7]. In rare patients, it may be a form of idiopathic small airway disease (Table 48.1) [8, 9].

Table 48.1 Etiologies of constrictive bronchiolitis

Chronic rejection in recipients of lung transplantation
GVHD in recipients of bone marrow transplantation
Systemic collagen vascular diseases (such as rheumatoid arthritis)
Infections (such as RSV, CMV, adenovirus, influenza virus, and mycoplasma)
Toxic fumes (ammonia, nitrogen dioxide) or ingestions (*Sauropus androgynus* juice)
Drug toxicities (penicillamine, gold)
Skin diseases (paraneoplastic pemphigus, Stevens-Johnson syndrome, toxic epidermal necrolysis)
Idiopathic

CMV cytomegalovirus, *GVHD* graft-versus-host disease, *RSV* respiratory syncytial virus

The clinical term "bronchiolitis obliterans syndrome (BOS)" refers to the clinical syndrome caused by constrictive bronchiolitis during chronic rejection in lung transplant recipients [1, 10]. It is unrelated to and should not be confused with "bronchiolitis obliterans organizing pneumonia (BOOP)."

Clinically, patients usually present with progressive cough and dyspnea. Pulmonary function tests usually show obstructive changes but may also show variable degrees of restrictive defects. Chest X-ray typically shows overinflation without significant infiltrates. High-resolution chest CT scan demonstrates air trapping (Fig. 48.1), sometimes associated with ground-glass opacities [11].

What Are the Histologic Features of Constrictive Bronchiolitis? What Are the Key Features to Differentiate Constrictive Bronchiolitis from Normal Lung?

Histologically, the most striking feature of CB is that the pathologic changes seem to be disproportionately "mild" compared to the severe clinical symptoms. The distal alveolar parenchyma in constrictive bronchiolitis appears normal. Hyperinflation can usually be appreciated radiologically but is not evident under the microscope, especially when the specimen is artificially collapsed during surgery and/or histologic processing. Mild chronic inflammatory infiltrates surrounding the bronchioles may be seen; however, significant inflammation or fibrosis are almost never present in constrictive bronchiolitis. The diagnostic lesions involve small bronchioles and can be scattered or focal, and some small bronchioles can be entirely normal. The involved bronchioles typically have narrowed or obliterated lumina, and the diameter of the involved bronchiole is considerably smaller than that of the accompanying artery. Luminal narrowing of the bronchioles is due to fibroblast proliferation and/or collagen deposition within the subepithelial stroma [12, 13]. An elastic stain is helpful in revealing the elastic layer of the airway and the fibrosis that occurs between the bronchiolar epithelium and elastic layer (Figs. 48.2, 48.3, and 48.4).

The lung biopsy with constrictive bronchiolitis can be pretty much unremarkable under low magnification. The diagnostic lesions can be subtle and focal. Pathologists should pay extra attention searching for features of constrictive bronchiolitis in the seemingly "normal" lung biopsies from patients with significant clinical respiratory impairment. At the later stage of the disease, the involved bronchioles can be entirely replaced by small fibrous scars adjacent to a pulmonary artery. At low magnification, a clue to this situation is seeing "naked" arteries without accompanying bronchioles. An elastic stain can be extremely helpful in highlighting the residual elastic tissue of the destroyed bronchioles.

What Are the Key Features to Differentiate Constrictive Bronchiolitis from Organizing Pneumonia?

Constrictive bronchiolitis needs to be differentiated from organizing pneumonia (previous termed bronchiolitis obliterans-organizing pneumonia, BOOP), which typically has a better prognosis. Organizing pneumonia is a nonspecific reaction of bronchioles to acute/subacute lung injury caused by various etiologies, most commonly infectious. Microscopically, organizing pneumonia is characterized by replacement of the proximal airspaces with fibroblastic plugs within a loose myxoedematous stroma. Differentiation between organizing pneumonia/BOOP and constrictive bronchiolitis is usually not challenging, especially when evaluated in combination with clinical and radiological information (Table 48.2). However, confusion may be caused by the similar names of these two entities.

Table 48.2 Features useful to differentiate constrictive bronchiolitis from organizing pneumonia (previously BOOP)

Features		Constrictive bronchiolitis	Organizing pneumonia/BOOP
Clinical presentation		Chronic severe dyspnea, cough	Subacute onset, commonly with antecedent upper respiratory tract infection or pneumonia
Radiological findings		Mosaic attenuation, air trapping, hyperinflation	Ground-glass opacities
Microscopic features	Bronchiolar fibrosis	Subepithelial fibrosis with luminal narrowing and/or obliteration	Polypoid intraluminal fibroblast plugs; normal-sized bronchiolar lumen
	Entirely scarred bronchioles	Characteristic in later stage	No
	Associated interstitial pneumonia	No	Usually present
	Accumulation of foamy alveolar macrophages	No	Usually present

BOOP bronchiolitis obliterans-organizing pneumonia

What Are the Treatment Options and Prognosis of Constrictive Bronchiolitis?

The prognosis of constrictive bronchiolitis, irrespective of etiology, is poor. Most patients deteriorate and die of respiratory failure within months to years after the initial diagnosis, although the rate of decline is variable. Secondary bacterial infections may accelerate the disease course. Most patients do not respond to corticosteroids or cytotoxic medication, which have significant potential toxicity. Macrolide antibiotics with immunomodulatory effects have been used, with some anecdotal successes, to treat and/or prevent BOS in lung transplant recipients [14, 15]. However, additional studies are required to determine the role and benefit of macrolide therapy in CB. Lung transplantation is currently the only viable treatment option in patients with severe disease.

References

1. Belperio JA, Weigt SS, Fishbein MC, Lynch JP III. Chronic lung allograft rejection: mechanisms and therapy. Proc Am Thorac Soc. 2009;6(1):108–21.
2. Chien JW, Martin PJ, Gooley TA, Flowers ME, Heckbert SR, Nichols WG, et al. Airflow obstruction after myeloablative allogeneic hematopoietic stem cell transplantation. Am J Respir Crit Care Med. 2003;168(2):208–14.
3. Kotloff RM, Ahya VN, Crawford SW. Pulmonary complications of solid organ and hematopoietic stem cell transplantation. Am J Respir Crit Care Med. 2004;170(1):22–48.
4. King TE Jr. Miscellaneous causes of bronchiolitis: inhalational, infectious, drug-induced, and idiopathic. Semin Respir Crit Care Med. 2003;24(5):567–76.
5. Akpinar-Elci M, Travis WD, Lynch DA, Kreiss K. Bronchiolitis obliterans syndrome in popcorn production plant workers. Eur Respir J. 2004;24(2):298–302.
6. Chang H, Wang JS, Tseng HH, Lai RS, Su JM. Histopathological study of Sauropus androgynus-associated constrictive bronchiolitis obliterans: a new cause of constrictive bronchiolitis obliterans. Am J Surg Pathol. 1997;21(1):35–42.
7. Schwarz MI, Lynch DA, Tuder R. Bronchiolitis obliterans: the lone manifestation of rheumatoid arthritis? Eur Respir J. 1994;7(4):817–20.
8. Kraft M, Mortenson RL, Colby TV, Newman L, Waldron JA Jr, King TE Jr. Cryptogenic constrictive bronchiolitis. A clinicopathologic study. Am Rev Respir Dis. 1993;148(4 Pt 1):1093–101.
9. Lynch JP III, Weigt SS, DerHovanessian A, Fishbein MC, Gutierrez A, Belperio JA. Obliterative (constrictive) bronchiolitis. Semin Respir Crit Care Med. 2012;33(5):509–32.
10. Weigt SS, Wallace WD, Derhovanessian A, Saggar R, Saggar R, Lynch JP, et al. Chronic allograft rejection: epidemiology, diagnosis, pathogenesis, and treatment. Semin Respir Crit Care Med. 2010;31(2):189–207.
11. Gunn ML, Godwin JD, Kanne JP, Flowers ME, Chien JW. High-resolution CT findings of bronchiolitis obliterans syndrome after hematopoietic stem cell transplantation. J Thorac Imaging. 2008;23(4):244–50.
12. Markopoulo KD, Cool CD, Elliot TL, Lync DA, Newell JD Jr, Hale VA, et al. Obliterative bronchiolitis: varying presentations and clinicopathological correlation. Eur Respir J. 2002;19(1):20–30.
13. Couture C, Colby TV. Histopathology of bronchiolar disorders. Semin Respir Crit Care Med. 2003;24(5):489–98.
14. Shitrit D, Bendayan D, Gidon S, Saute M, Bakal I, Kramer MR. Long-term azithromycin use for treatment of bronchiolitis obliterans syndrome in lung transplant recipients. J Heart Lung Transplant. 2005;24(9):1440–3.
15. Yates B, Murphy DM, Forrest IA, Ward C, Rutherford RM, Fisher AJ, et al. Azithromycin reverses airflow obstruction in established bronchiolitis obliterans syndrome. Am J Respir Crit Care Med. 2005;172(6):772–5.

49 Granulomatosis with Polyangiitis Versus Mycobacterial/Fungal Infection

Jason V. Scapa and Gregory A. Fishbein

Case Presentation

A 55-year-old Caucasian man presents with a 3-week history of fever and malaise along with hemoptysis and dyspnea that have developed within the past 5 days. He has a productive cough with blood-tinged sputum. His speech suggests shortness of breath. Over the past month, he has noticed weight loss and general fatigue. His past medical history is notable for several bouts of rhinosinusitis requiring prolonged antibiotic courses, in addition to a referral to an otolaryngologist. Additionally, he states that he has suffered from joint pain over the past year. Physical exam is notable for a low-grade fever, decreased oxygen saturation, focally decreased breath sounds, and dullness to percussion at the lung bases. A chest X-ray shows a solid nodular lesion at the base of the right lung. A computed tomography (CT) scan reveals a 2.1 cm cavitary lesion at the base of the right lung, corresponding to the chest X-ray abnormality (Fig. 49.1a). Initial laboratory

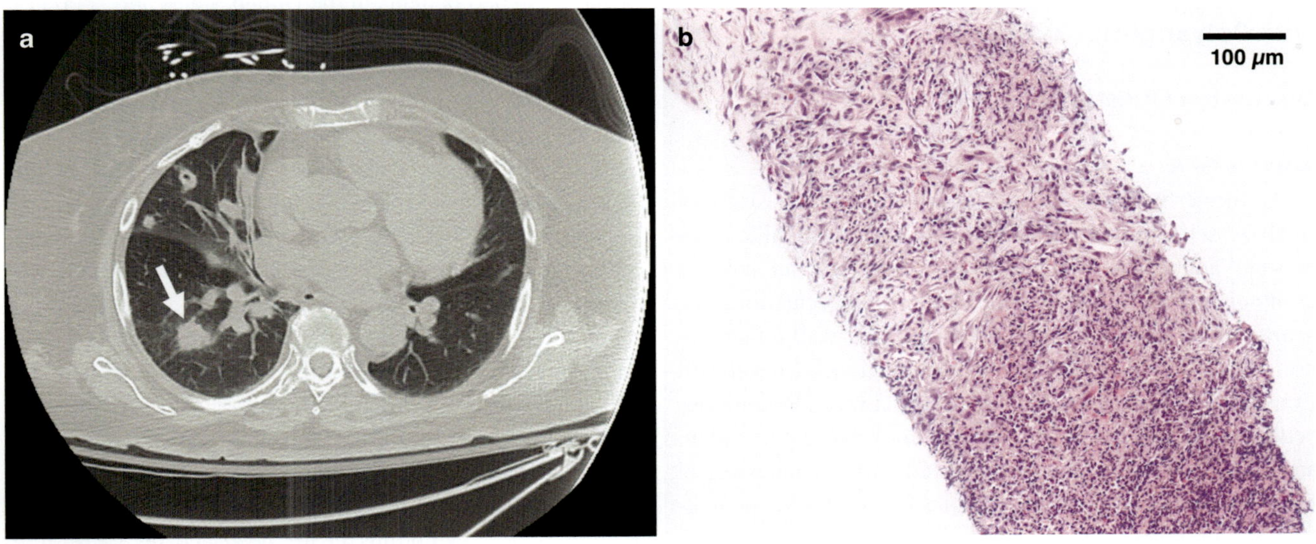

Fig. 49.1 Radiographic and biopsy findings from case presentation. (**a**) Computed tomography (CT) scan demonstrating a 2.1-cm cavitary lesion in lower lobe of the right lung (arrow). (**b**) Core needle biopsy showing vasculitis with granulomatous inflammation and "blue necrosis" (hematoxylin and eosin stain [H&E], 140×)

J. V. Scapa
Department of Pathology, Kaiser Permanente - Orange County, Anaheim, CA, USA
e-mail: jason.v.scapa@kp.org

G. A. Fishbein (✉)
Department of Pathology and Laboratory Medicine, David Geffen School of Medicine at UCLA, Los Angeles, CA, USA
e-mail: gfishbein@mednet.ucla.edu

H. Xu et al. (eds.), *Practical Lung Pathology*, Practical Anatomic Pathology, https://doi.org/10.1007/978-3-031-14402-8_49

results are remarkable for a slightly elevated white blood cell count and mild normocytic anemia. A urinalysis shows 3+ blood and 2+ protein. Blood cultures and serologies are sent, and antibiotics are started. Initial serologic testing demonstrates the presence of antibodies against cytoplasmic proteinase-3 (PR-3), also referred to as c-ANCA. Following the result, a lung biopsy is scheduled for the next day.

Permanent section of the needle core lung biopsy (Fig. 49.1b) illustrates granulomatous inflammation with parenchymal necrosis, particularly in the centrilobular zones. At low power, there are areas of geographic necrosis that appear basophilic with high power showing neutrophilic and karyorrhectic debris. There are histiocytes palisading and surrounding the necrosis. Occasional small giant cells are seen within the granulomatous inflammation. Pulmonary vessels may occasionally show perivascular chronic inflammation composed predominately of lymphocytes and plasma cells. A Ziehl-Neelsen tissue stain for acid fast bacilli (AFB), Grocott's methenamine silver (GMS), and periodic acid-Schiff (PAS) stain for fungal elements are negative. A tissue elastin stain demonstrates disruption of the elastic lamina in the vessels.

Pathologic Diagnosis: Granulomatosis with Polyangiitis (GPA)

Discussion Questions

What Is GPA?

GPA, formerly known as Wegener's granulomatosis, is a small vessel vasculitis associated with antineutrophilic cytoplasmic antibodies (ANCA). Vasculitides are an eclectic group of diseases that have diverse clinical presentations, but nearly all have some component of vascular wall inflammation [1, 2]. In 2012, the Revised International Chapel Hill Consensus Conference (CHCC) Nomenclature of Vasculitides better categorized noninfectious vasculitis and defined them according to the type of vessel involved—this includes vessel size, function, and structural attributes [3]. Table 49.1 demonstrates the recent classification developed by the 2012 CHCC. Pulmonary vasculitides encompass mainly small vessels and capillaries, although medium and large vessels can be involved in certain conditions [4]. The 2012 CHCC defined small vessel vasculitides as those impacting "small intraparenchymal arteries, arterioles, capillaries, and venules." The consensus group further organized the small vessel vasculitides by their pathophysiologic origin—those marked by immune-complex formation and those associated with ANCAs. ANCA-associated vasculitides (AAVs) comprise a trio of small vessel vasculitides: granulomatosis with polyangiitis (GPA), eosinophilic granulomatosis with polyangiitis (EGPA), and microscopic polyangiitis (MPA).

Table 49.1 Vasculitides classified by vessel size [3]

Large vessels
Giant cell (temporal) arteritis
Takayasu arteritis[a]
Medium vessels
Kawasaki disease
Polyarteritis nodosa[a]
Small vessels
ANCA-associated vasculitis
Granulomatosis with polyangiitis (Wegener's granulomatosis)[a]
Microscopic polyangiitis[a]
Eosinophilic granulomatosis with polyangiitis (Churg-Strauss syndrome)[a]
Immune complex small vessel vasculitis
IgA vasculitis (Henöch-Schonlein purpura)[a]
Anti-glomerular basement membrane disease (Goodpasture syndrome)[a]
Cryoglobulinemic vasculitis[a]
Anti-C1q vasculitis
Variable-sized vessels
Behçet's disease[a]
Cogan syndrome

[a]Indicates pulmonary involvement

How Does a Patient with GPA Present Clinically?

GPA is the most common pulmonary vasculitis, with a prevalence of 30,000 patients in the United States and 2600 new cases a year [5]. GPA is more typically seen in older adults, although cases have been reported in all ages [6]. While there is no gender predilection, GPA is seen predominately in Caucasian individuals [7]. Constitutional symptoms stem from the inflammatory nature of the disease and include fatigue and malaise, anorexia, fever, and weight loss [8]. Nonspecific localized symptoms comprise rhinosinusitis, cough, dyspnea, urinary abnormalities, arthralgias, and neurologic dysfunction. Prodromal systemic symptoms can begin and last for months before organ-specific manifestations appear. Therefore, given the nonspecific findings, it is difficult to distinguish clinical symptoms from infection since both can present with "B-symptoms" such as fever, fatigue, night sweats, and weight loss.

Because GPA affects the upper and lower respiratory tract, signs and symptoms in the head and neck are often seen. Persistent rhinosinusitis, rhinorrhea, nasal discharge, oral ulcers, and conductive and sensorineural hearing loss have been seen in patients with GPA. Ophthalmic symptoms such as conjunctivitis, corneal ulceration, scleritis, optic neuropathy, uveitis, and retinal vasculitis can also be seen. Lower airway manifestations include hoarseness, cough, dyspnea, stridor, and pleural pain. Hemoptysis may represent alveolar hemorrhage, which can be life threatening. In the lungs, pulmonary consolidations, nodules, atelectasis, and pleural effusion may also be present. Although only 18% of patients have renal involvement at time of initial presentation, about 80% will go on to develop glomerulonephritis within the first 2 years of disease onset [9]. Glomerulonephritis can present as asymptomatic hematuria, rising creatinine, proteinuria, and rapid progressive glomerulonephritis with crescent formation. Less frequently involved sites include the skin, nervous, and gastrointestinal systems.

What Are the Diagnostic Features of GPA?

GPA is a small vessel vasculitis marked by granulomatous inflammation. While multiple clinicopathologic criteria have been described by the CHCC, the American College of Rheumatology [10], and the European Medicine Agency [11], the main features of GPA include radiographic evidence of pulmonary nodules or fixed infiltrates, nasal or oral inflammation, microscopic hematuria, and granulomatous inflammation on biopsy.

ANCAs are antibodies that target one of two antigens found in neutrophils: the cytoplasmic proteinase-3 (PR-3), which is termed c-ANCA, and the perinuclear myeloperoxidase (MPO), also known as p-ANCA [12]. ANCA are tested by two laboratory methods: screening with indirect immunofluorescence (IFF) and more specific enzyme-linked immunosorbent assays (ELISA). Serologically, GPA typically shows c-ANCA positivity with 90% specificity. Seven percent of GPA will show p-ANCA and 3% will be negative for ANCA [13]. The sensitivity of ANCA for the diagnosis of GPA and MPA is 81–85% [14]. The diagnosis of any vasculitis, including GPA, relies on compilation of the clinical, radiographic, laboratory, and histopathologic findings.

What Are the Imaging Findings of GPA and Mycobacterial/Fungal Infection?

In GPA, imaging studies primarily focus on lung manifestations. Computed tomography (CT) and chest radiographs can show bilateral lung nodules, infiltrates, cavitary lesions, ground-glass opacities, and pleural opacities. CT scans of the head and neck may reveal lesions in the sinuses, orbits, and mastoids, particularly in patients displaying upper airway symptoms [15].

Radiography of tuberculous processes will often show the presence of one or more Ghon foci, where the initial host response occurs and appears as small nodules. Calcified lymph nodes may be seen in combination with these, constituting the Ghon complex. When the host response is not sufficient, large mass-like lesions can form. Endobronchial spread is possible giving rise to patchy consolidations with tree-in-bud opacities and additional adjacent nodules. Cavitary lesions can form when the lesion undergoes central necrosis and cystic change. Lobar or segmental infiltration can be seen in addition to abundant small nodules (miliary disease) [16]. Fungal and nontuberculous mycobacterial infections can show similar findings to tuberculous processes, including nodules and cavitary lesions.

What Are the Gross Findings in GPA?

As the radiographic findings would suggest, gross examination of the lungs will often demonstrate bilateral nodules, approximately 2–3 cm in greatest dimension with or without cavitation. The nodules frequently display irregular borders with dark yellow to red areas of central necrosis. Consolidation and hemorrhage may be visually present, but the intervening parenchyma usually appears normal. When nodules are absent, the gross lungs may show features of diffuse alveolar hemorrhage (DAH) or interstitial fibrosis.

What Are the Histopathologic Findings in GPA?

The staple microscopic features of GPA are a triad of parenchymal necrosis, vasculitis, and granulomatous inflammation (Fig. 49.2) [17, 18]. Low-power magnification shows large areas with geographic necrosis that appears basophilic and termed "blue necrosis." Higher magnification illustrates that these necrotic zones contain microabscesses with neutrophilic and nuclear debris. Peripherally located histiocytes and multinucleated giant cells are seen surrounding the necrosis in what is described as a so-called cartwheel pattern. The giant cells often appear paradoxically small with dark cytoplasm.

The vasculitis of GPA impacts small vessels (under 5 mm in diameter) and includes arterioles, venules, and capillaries. The regions of vessel wall inflammation are typically next to larger areas of geographic necrosis. The vessel walls commonly have chronic inflammatory infiltrates along with neutrophils, fibrinoid and transmural necrosis, and granulomas. Disruption of the internal and external elastic lamina in these vessels can be demonstrated using a tissue elastin stain. Scarring of the vessels, showing intimal proliferation and medial changes, is frequently seen. In cases of DAH, hemosiderin-laden macrophages with neutrophilic capillaritis are present.

The extravascular granulomas are composed of multinucleated giant cells that evince angulated cytoplasmic edges and peripherally located hyperchromatic, syncytially arranged nuclei in a ring or horseshoe pattern. There is a tendency for the granulomas to be located in the centrilobular zones and are typically accompanied by mixed inflammation including lymphocytes, neutrophils, eosinophils, histiocytes, and plasma cells.

There are other nonspecific histologic findings of GPA, which may be present at the periphery of the necrotic zones. Organizing pneumonia can be observed in areas adjacent to granulomatous inflammation or hemorrhage. If prominent, these findings could represent bronchiolitis obliterans organizing pneumonia (BOOP)—like variant of GPA. This uncommon histologic pattern has been described in a 16-patient case series [19]. Other findings include lymphoid aggregates, bronchiolitis, bronchocentric granulomatosis,

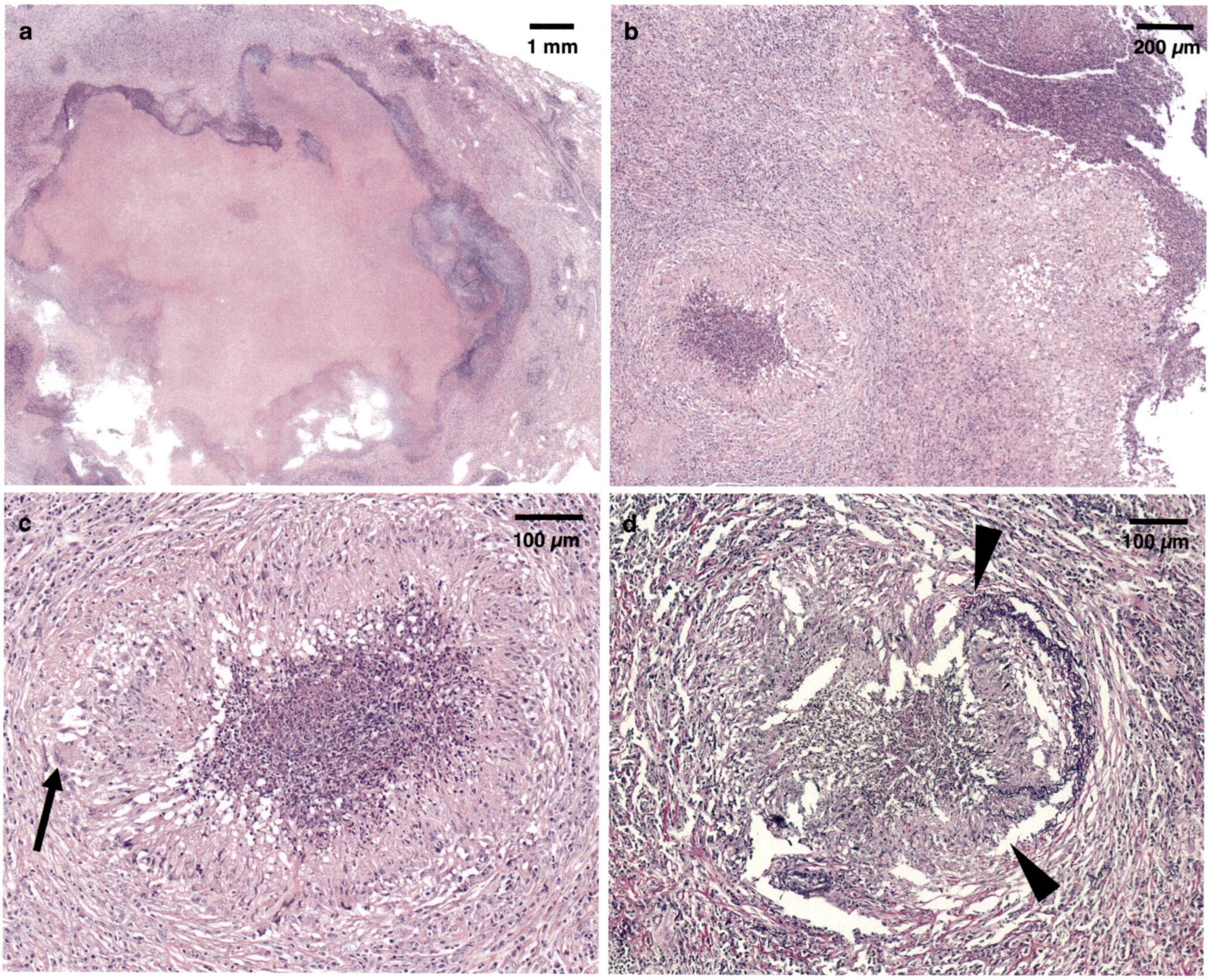

Fig. 49.2 Granulomatosis with polyangiitis (GPA) with a variety of parenchymal and vascular lesions. (**a**) Low-magnification architectural view demonstrating geographic "blue necrosis" with adjacent areas of granulomatosis inflammation (hematoxylin and eosin stain [H&E], 10×). (**b**) Section demonstrating blue necrosis with adjacent palisading granulomatous inflammation and a medium-sized artery with vasculitis (H&E, 50×). (**c**) Vasculitis with multinucleated giant cell (arrow) within vessel wall in GPA (H&E, 140×). (**d**) Elastin stain of vessel showing disruption of the elastic lamina by diffuse chronic and granulomatous inflammation in GPA (H&E, 140×)

interstitial fibrosis, and foamy macrophages, similar to lipoid pneumonia. Xanthogranulomatous lesions can be seen with cholesterol clefts [20]. Eosinophils can be present; however, if these are prominent, they should raise the consideration of EGPA, eosinophilic pneumonia, drug toxicity, or infection.

How Does GPA Differ Histologically from Pulmonary Infections Such as Mycobacterial or Fungal Infection?

The major differential consideration in GPA is infection given the presence of necrotizing granulomatous inflammation. Clinically, infection and GPA can present with systemic symptoms of fever, fatigue, and weight loss, along with pulmonary nodules and cavitary lesions on imaging. The histologic appearance of pulmonary infections usually shows more eosinophilic central necrosis with a marked lymphoplasmacytic infiltrate that typically has pink zones of necrosis with a blue peripheral rim (Fig. 49.3). This is in contrast to the blue central necrosis due to neutrophil and karyorrhectic debris of GPA. The multinucleated giant cells are more epithelioid in nature and are often numerous in infectious processes. Infectious processes may have necrotizing and/or well-formed non-necrotizing granulomas. In contrast, well-formed non-necrotizing granulomas are not a feature of GPA.

Despite these subtle histologic differences, special stains for microorganisms such as Ziehl-Neelsen tissue stain for acid fast bacilli (AFB) and Grocott's methenamine silver (GMS) and periodic acid-Schiff (PAS) stain for fungal elements should be performed if there is even remote consider-

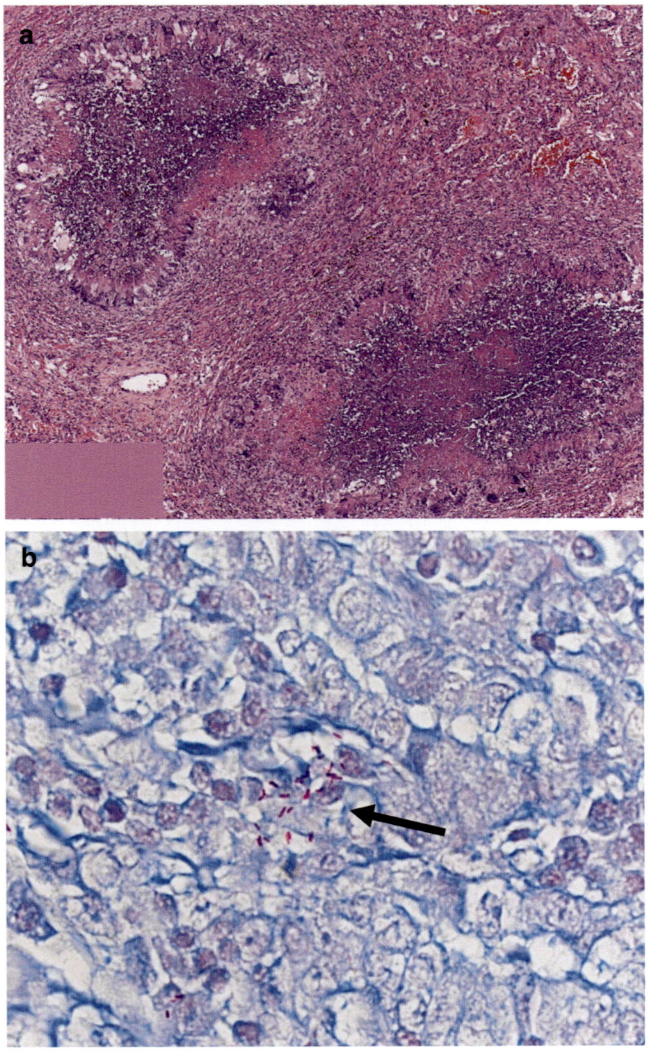

Fig. 49.3 Necrotizing granulomas and infection. (**a**) Pulmonary necrotizing granulomas of the lung showing pink, caseating necrosis with peripherally oriented epithelioid histiocytes and multinucleated giant cells (hematoxylin and eosin stain [H&E], 40×). (**b**) Aggregate of mycobacteria within center of necrotizing granuloma (arrow) (Ziehl-Neelsen stain, 600×)

ation for infection. Typically, the infectious elements will be at the center of the granulomatous inflammation. GMS may show yeast (e.g., *Blastomycosis*, *Cryptococcus*, *Histoplasmosis*, *Coccidioides*), hyphae (e.g., *Aspergillus* species, *mucormycosis*), or both (i.e., *Candida* species) [21]. Tuberculous and nontuberculous mycobacteria appear as straight or slightly curved rods, 0.2–0.6 μm wide and 1.0–10 μm long, on the AFB stain. Common nontuberculous mycobacteria include *Mycobacterium avium* complex (MAC), *M. kansasii*, *M. abscessus*, and *M. chelonae*. If infection is high on the differential diagnosis, it may be prudent to evaluate multiple deeper levels with special stains. Additionally, auramine-rhodamine stain by fluorescent microscopy can be more sensitive for the detection of mycobacterium than Ziehl-Neelsen [22]. Molecular testing by polymerase chain reaction or next-generation sequencing can also be performed on formalin-fixed paraffin-embedded sections for identification and speciation of fungal and mycobacterial organisms.

References

1. Lanham J, Elkon K, Pusey C, Hughes G. Systemic vasculitis with asthma and eosinophilia: a clinical approach to the Churg-Strauss syndrome. Medicine. 1984;63(2):65–81.
2. Mark E, Flieder D, Matsubara O. Treated Wegener's granulomatosis: distinctive pathological findings in the lungs of 20 patients and what they tell us about the natural history of the disease. Hum Pathol. 1997;28(4):450–8.
3. Jennette JC, Falk RJ, Bacon PA, Basu N, Cid MC, Ferrario F, et al. 2012 Revised International Chapel Hill Consensus Conference Nomenclature of Vasculitides. Arthritis Rheum. 2013;65(1):1–11.
4. Travis WD, Colby TV, Lombard C, Carpenter HA. A clinicopathologic study of 34 cases of diffuse pulmonary hemorrhage with lung biopsy confirmation. Am J Surg Pathol. 1990;14(12):1112–25.
5. Mahr AD. Epidemiological features of Wegener's granulomatosis and microscopic polyangiitis: two diseases or one "anti-neutrophil cytoplasm antibodies-associated vasculitis" entity? APMIS Suppl. 2009;117(s127):41–7.
6. Jennette JC, Falk RJ. Small-vessel vasculitis. N Engl J Med. 1997;337(21):1512–23.
7. Falk RJ, Hogan S, Carey TS, Jennette JC. Clinical course of anti-neutrophil cytoplasmic autoantibody-associated glomerulonephritis and systemic vasculitis. The Glomerular Disease Collaborative Network. Ann Intern Med. 1990;113(9):656–63.
8. Hoffman GS, Kerr GS, Leavitt RY, Hallahan CW, Lebovics RS, Travis WD, et al. Wegener granulomatosis: an analysis of 158 patients. Ann Intern Med. 1992;116(6):488–98.
9. Fauci AS, Haynes BF, Katz P, Wolff SM. Wegener's granulomatosis: prospective clinical and therapeutic experience with 85 patients for 21 years. Ann Intern Med. 1983;98(1):76–85.
10. Roa JK, Allen NB, Pincus T. Limitations of the 1990 American College of Rheumatology classification criteria in the diagnosis of vasculitis. Ann Intern Med. 1998;129(5):345–52.
11. Watts R, Lane S, Hanslik T, Hauser T, Hellmich B, Koldingsnes W, et al. Development and validation of a consensus methodology for the classification of the ANCA-associated vasculitides and polyarteritis nodosa for epidemiological studies. Ann Rheum Dis. 2007;66(2):222–7.
12. Rao DA, Wei K, Merola JF, O'Brien WR, Takvorian SU, Dellaripa PF, et al. Myeloperoxidase-antineutrophil cytoplasmic antibodies (MPO-ANCA) and proteinase 3-ANCA without immunofluorescent ANCA found by routine clinical testing. J Rheumatol. 2015;42(5):847–52.
13. Kallenberg CG. Key advances in the clinical approach to ANCA-associated vasculitis. Nat Rev Rheumatol. 2014;10(8):484–93.
14. Hagen EC, Daha MR, Hermans J, Andrassy K, Csernok E, Gaskin G, et al. Diagnostic value of standardized assays for anti-neutrophil cytoplasmic antibodies in idiopathic systemic vasculitis. EC/BCR Project for ANCA Assay Standardization. Kidney Int. 1998;53(3):743–53.
15. Cordier JF, Valeyre D, Guillevin L, Loire R, Brechot JM. Pulmonary Wegener's granulomatosis. A clinical and imaging study of 77 cases. Chest. 1990;97(4):906–12.
16. Bomanji JB, Gupta N, Gulati P, Das CJ. Imaging in tuberculosis. Cold Spring Harb Perspect Med. 2015;5(6):5.
17. Travis WD, Hoffman GS, Leavitt RY, Pass HI, Fauci AS. Surgical pathology of the lung in Wegener's granulomatosis. Review

of 87 open lung biopsies from 67 patients. Am J Surg Pathol. 1991;15(4):315–33.
18. Lombard CM, Duncan SR, Rizk NW, Colby TV. The diagnosis of Wegener's granulomatosis from transbronchial biopsy specimens. Hum Pathol. 1990;21(8):838–42.
19. Uner A, Rozum-Slota B, Katzenstein A. Bronchiolitis obliterans-organizing pneumonia (BOOP)-like variant of Wegener's granulomatosis: a clinicopathologic study of 16 cases. Am J Surg Pathol. 1996;20(7):794–801.
20. Travis WD. Common and uncommon manifestations of Wegener's granulomatosis. Cardiovasc Pathol. 1994;3(3):217–25.
21. Gaurner J, Brandt ME. Histopathologic diagnosis of fungal infections in the 21st century. Clin Microbiol Rev. 2011;24(2):247–80.
22. Kommareddi S, Abramowsky C, Swinehart G, Hrabak L. Nontuberculous mycobacterial infections: comparison of the fluorescent auramine-O and Ziehl-Neelsen techniques in tissue diagnosis. Hum Pathol. 1984;15(11):1085–9.

50 Eosinophilic Granulomatosis with Polyangiitis Versus Eosinophilic Pneumonia

Jason V. Scapa and Gregory A. Fishbein

Case Presentation

A 40-year-old Caucasian woman presents with a 2-month history of fever and fatigue with occasional dyspnea. Her past medical history is remarkable for poorly controlled asthma for the past 10 years that required robust regimens of glucocorticoids. She has a long history of atopy, including scattered rashes and allergic rhinitis since childhood. Physical exam is notable for low-grade fever, decreased oxygen saturation, wheezing, and dullness to percussion at the lung bases. There are tender subcutaneous skin nodules over her extensor surfaces of the arms and legs. A chest X-ray shows ill-defined nodular lesions bilaterally. A computed tomography (CT) scan shows bilateral nodules with bronchiectasis, small- and medium-sized airway thickening, and subpleural scars. Initial laboratory results are notable for a leukocytosis with increased eosinophils (7500 eosinophils per microliter). Initial serologic testing demonstrates the presence of p-ANCA as well as increased immunoglobulin E (IgE). An open lung biopsy is performed.

Microscopic examination of the lung biopsy demonstrates diffuse eosinophilic pneumonia, with eosinophils and histiocytes present in the alveolar spaces and interstitial compartment (Fig. 50.1). Eosinophils are present within the lumens and walls of small bronchi, which also show subepithelial basement membrane thickening and smooth muscle hypertrophy, consistent with asthmatic bronchitis. Small vessels show perivascular and transmural collections of infiltrating eosinophils with fibrinoid necrosis and rare thrombosis. Eosinophilic microabscesses and eosinophilic necrosis surrounded by palisading histiocytes and multinucleated giant cells are also seen. A Ziehl-Neelsen tissue stain for acid fast bacilli (AFB) and Grocott-Gomori methenamine silver (GMS) stain for fungal elements are negative.

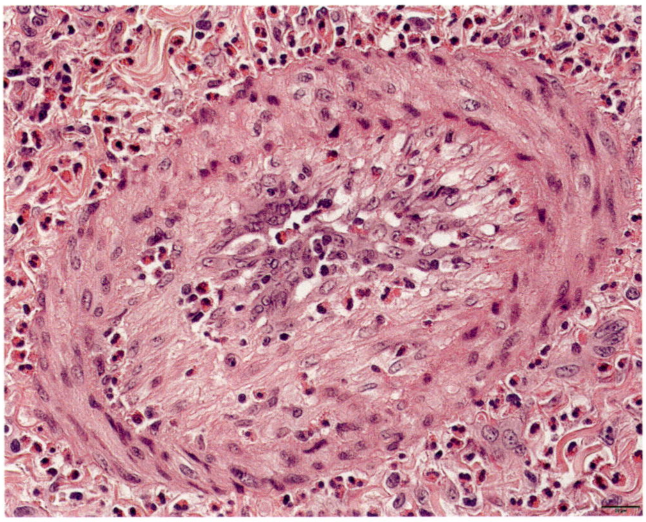

Fig. 50.1 Patient lung wedge biopsy showing eosinophilic inflammation and vasculitis (hematoxylin and eosin stain [H&E], 400×)

Pathologic Diagnosis

The constellation of asthma, eosinophilic pneumonia, and pulmonary vasculitis in the setting of peripheral hypereosinophilia, p-ANCA positivity, and childhood atopy is diagnostic of eosinophilic granulomatosis with polyangiitis (EGPA, formerly Churg-Strauss syndrome).

Discussion Questions

What Is Eosinophilic Pneumonia?

Eosinophilic pneumonia (EP) is a histologic pattern of lung disease characterized by infiltration of the pulmonary alveo-

J. V. Scapa
Department of Pathology, Kaiser Permanente - Orange County, Anaheim, CA, USA
e-mail: jason.v.scapa@kp.org

G. A. Fishbein (✉)
Department of Pathology and Laboratory Medicine, David Geffen School of Medicine at UCLA, Los Angeles, CA, USA
e-mail: gfishbein@mednet.ucla.edu

H. Xu et al. (eds.), *Practical Lung Pathology*, Practical Anatomic Pathology, https://doi.org/10.1007/978-3-031-14402-8_50

Table 50.1 Differential diagnosis for pulmonary eosinophilia

Infections
• Transpulmonary larvae passage helminths
– *Ascaris lumbricoides*
– *Strongyloides stercoralis*
– Hookworm (*Ancylostoma duodenale*, *Necator americanus*)
• Invasive pulmonary helminths
– *Echinococcus*
– *Paragonimus*
– *Taenia solium*
• Fungal infections
– *Coccidioides*
– Allergic bronchopulmonary aspergillosis (ABPA)
Drugs and toxins
• Medications
– Nonsteroidal anti-inflammatory drugs (NSAIDs)
– Antimicrobials (ampicillin, minocycline, nitrofurantoin, sulfonamides, daptomycin)
– Anticonvulsants
– Diuretics
– Sulfa drugs
– Amiodarone
– Methotrexate
• Toxins
– Aluminum silicate
– Scorpion stings
– Inhaled heroin
– Marijuana
– Dust
– Tobacco
– Smoke
– Scotchgard
Idiopathic eosinophilic pneumonias
• Acute
• Chronic
Other causes
• Eosinophilic granulomatosis with polyangiitis (a.k.a. Churg-Strauss disease)
• Granulomatosis with polyangiitis (a.k.a. Wegener's granulomatosis)
• IgG4-related disease
• Histiocytoses (e.g., Langerhans cell histiocytosis)
• Hypereosinophilic syndrome
• Sarcoidosis
• Neoplasms

lar and interstitial compartments by eosinophils. EP may occur in isolation or as a manifestation of a larger disease process. Such disorders include infection, hypersensitivity reactions to drugs or toxins, tumors, and rheumatologic disease (Table 50.1). The etiology is often not apparent from the histopathology alone. Cases in which no pathologic or clinical etiology is identified are termed idiopathic EP.

What Is the Differential Diagnosis of Eosinophilic Pneumonia?

Infection should always be considered in the setting of eosinophilia. Since the life cycle of many helminths involves the passage of larvae through the lungs before migrating to the gastrointestinal tract, pulmonary eosinophilia may indicate parasitic infection. These organisms include *Strongyloides stercoralis*, *Ascaris* sp. (*A. lumbricoides*, *A. suum*), and hookworms (*Ancylostoma duodenale*, *Necator americanus*) [1]. Other helminths such as *Echinococcus*, *Paragonimus*, and *Taenia solium* can directly invade the pulmonary parenchyma and cause EP. Fungal infections, particularly *Coccidioides*, can present with EP [2]. EP is also present in allergic bronchopulmonary aspergillosis, which is a hypersensitivity reaction in the setting of airway colonization by *Aspergillus* species [3].

EP may also be seen in the setting of hypersensitivity reaction to toxins or medications. These can present as eosinophilic pneumonia alone or multiorgan dysfunction, such as drug reaction with eosinophilia and systemic symptoms (DRESS) syndrome [4]. Common medications associated with EP include nonsteroidal anti-inflammatory drugs (NSAIDs), antimicrobials (such as nitrofurantoin, minocycline, ampicillin, sulfonamides, and daptomycin), anticonvulsants, beta blockers, diuretics, methotrexate, amiodarone, and other sulfa drugs [5]. A variety of toxins may also cause pulmonary eosinophilia, including Scotchgard, aluminum silicate, scorpion venom, heroin, dust, tobacco, and other chemicals used in manufacturing.

EP may be seen in setting of peripheral hypereosinophilia of any etiology as part of the so-called hypereosinophilic syndrome (HES). HES may be idiopathic or secondary to a number of disorders, including eosinophilic granulomatosis with polyangiitis (EGPA, a.k.a. Churg-Strauss syndrome). Pulmonary eosinophilia is a feature of a variety of uncommon disease processes, such as histiocytoses, IgG4-related disease, granulomatosis with polyangiitis (a.k.a. Wegener's granulomatosis), and lymphoma (e.g., classic Hodgkin lymphoma). In the absence of an identifiable clinical or pathologic etiology, EP may be deemed idiopathic. Idiopathic EP may be acute or chronic. Idiopathic acute EP and chronic EP are distinct clinical entities both characterized by eosinophilic infiltrates in the lung.

What Is Meant by Acute and Chronic Eosinophilic Pneumonia?

Idiopathic acute eosinophilic pneumonia (AEP) clinically presents as acute respiratory failure in an otherwise healthy patient. It has been suggested that AEP may represent a hypersensitivity reaction to an unidentified inhalant [6]. These patients will display acute onset (less than 4 weeks duration) of nonproductive cough, dyspnea, fever with malaise, night sweats, chest pain, and myalgia [7]. Physical exam shows high fever with inspiratory crackles and expiratory rhonchi on auscultation of the thorax. Peripheral eosinophilia is usually absent, but increased eosinophils are seen in bronchoalveolar lavage (BAL) cytology. Chest radiographs demonstrate mixed ground-glass and reticular opacities ranging from patchy to diffuse. Typical histologic features of AEP include intra-alveolar fibrin with varying degrees of organization, admixed with degranulating eosinophils and macrophages. Acute lung injury with hyaline membranes may be present. Eosinophils can be seen in both the interstitial and alveolar compartments. The process may be focal. AEP is exquisitely steroid responsive. If sampling is performed following administration of corticosteroids, only scant eosinophils may be seen.

Chronic eosinophilic pneumonia (CEP) is a progressive illness that can present with fever, cough, progressive dyspnea, wheezing, and night sweats [8]. Patients with CEP may have preexisting atopic conditions such as asthma or allergic rhinitis. The disease usually has a gradual onset over several months. Peripheral eosinophilia is usually present. BAL cytology shows marked increase in eosinophils. Radiographically, CEP tends to display bilateral peripheral or pleural-based opacities. Biopsy is usually not necessary to establish the diagnosis if clinical, radiographic, and BAL features are present. Microscopic examination will show intra-alveolar and interstitial eosinophils and macrophages, similar to AEP. Eosinophilic necrosis with giant cells, airway eosinophilia, and perivascular eosinophilic infiltrates may be present, which may lead to a misdiagnosis of EGPA. In contrast to EGPA, necrotizing vasculitis is not a feature of CEP. Furthermore, EGPA is a systemic syndrome affecting multiple organ systems. The diagnosis of EGPA requires clinical correlation and cannot be made based on pathology alone.

What Is Eosinophilic Granulomatosis with Polyangiitis (EGPA)?

EGPA, also called Churg-Strauss syndrome or allergic granulomatous angiitis, is a systemic disorder characterized by atopic disease (e.g., asthma, allergic rhinitis), peripheral eosinophilia, tissue eosinophilia with granulomas, and small vessel vasculitis. EGPA is often associated with antineutrophil cytoplasmic antibodies (ANCA), usually directed against myeloperoxidase (anti-MPO) with a perinuclear staining pattern (p-ANCA). Pulmonary involvement is common, but EGPA may also affect the skin, heart, peripheral nervous system, gastrointestinal tract, and kidney.

What Are the Clinical Features of EGPA?

EGPA presents as a clinical constellation of allergic rhinitis, asthma, peripheral eosinophilia, multi-organ tissue eosinophilia, and small vessel necrotizing vasculitis. EGPA mainly affects the upper and lower respiratory tracts. The lung is involved in 70% of cases [9]. Asthma is a hallmark clinical feature of EGPA and is usually present in 90% of patients with the disease [10]. EGPA typically also involves the peripheral nervous system, heart, skin, gastrointestinal tract, upper respiratory tract, and/or musculoskeletal system. Skin lesions include tender subcutaneous nodules on the extensor surfaces, especially the elbows. Macular and papular erythematous rashes may also be present. Peripheral neuropathy can be seen in 75% of patients with EGPA. Cardiomyopathy and pericarditis occur in a subset of individuals. However, cardiac involvement represents a significant cause of death in patients with EGPA.

What Laboratory Findings Support the Diagnosis of EGPA?

Laboratory testing in patients with EGPA reveals marked increase in blood eosinophils, usually 5000–9000 eosinophils per microliter. ANCA positivity is seen in about 31% of cases. Of these, p-ANCA and c-ANCA are present in 64% and 36% of cases, respectively [11]. Immunoglobulin E (IgE) levels are often increased. Other nonspecific laboratory findings include leukocytosis, normocytic anemia, positive low-titer rheumatoid factor, and hypergammaglobulinemia.

How Does EGPA Affect the Lung?

EGPA typically presents in three phases—the prodromal phase, eosinophilic phase, and vasculitic phase. In the prodromal phase, the characteristic finding in the lung is asthma. In the eosinophilic phase, the lungs develop eosinophilic pneumonia. Finally, in the vasculitic phase, necrotizing small vessel vasculitis composed of a primarily eosinophilic infiltrate is present. Like all vasculitides, EGPA does not always progress as described in the textbooks. The three phases usually but not necessarily occur sequentially in the order described above.

What Are the Histopathologic Findings in EGPA?

The hallmark histopathologic pulmonary features of EGPA are asthmatic bronchitis, eosinophilic pneumonia (EP), extravascular granulomatous inflammation, and necrotizing vasculitis of small-to-medium-sized vessels (Fig. 50.2). These histologic findings may not all be present since the disease often progresses in stages. Asthmatic bronchitis presents microscopically as eosinophilic airway inflammation, subepithelial basement membrane thickening, smooth muscle hypertrophy, tissue edema, and mucous plugging. EP is accompanied by varying degrees of intra-alveolar fibrin deposition, organizing pneumonia, and reactive type II pneumocytes. Also present are the unique extravascular "allergic granulomas" of EGPA, composed of eosinophilic necrosis surrounded by palisading histiocytes and multinucleated giant cells. The granulomas can become fibrotic and calcified as they heal and scar. Arteries and sometimes veins demonstrate perivascular and transmural eosinophilic inflammation with fibrinoid necrosis and thrombosis. Diffuse alveolar hemorrhage with eosinophilic capillaritis has also been described.

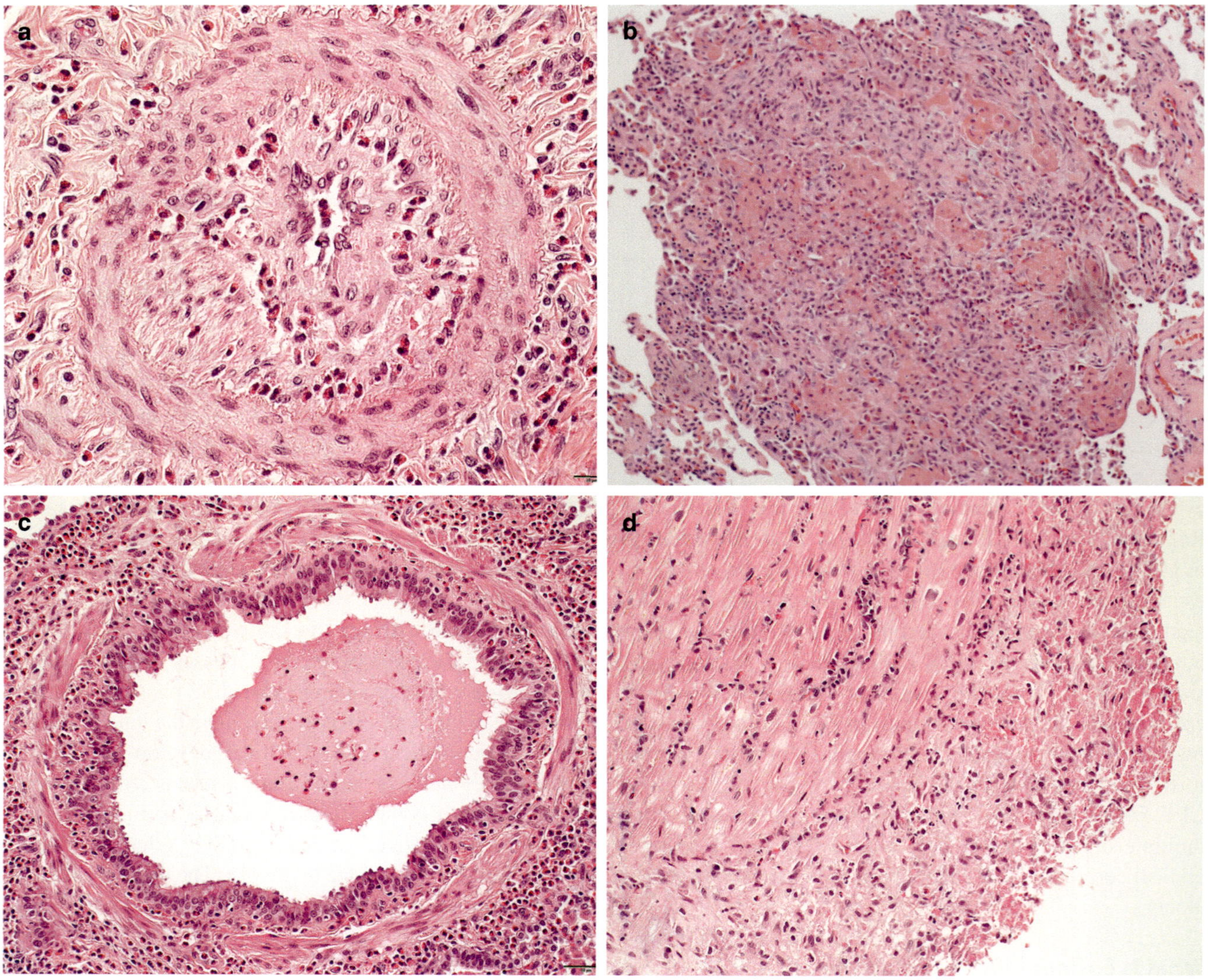

Fig. 50.2 Pulmonary and cardiac involvement by eosinophilic granulomatosis with polyangiitis (EGPA). (**a**) Pulmonary parenchyma with small-sized vessel infiltrated by eosinophils (hematoxylin and eosin stain [H&E], 400×). (**b**) Lung parenchyma with eosinophilic granuloma (H&E, 200×). (**c**) Pulmonary involvement by EGPA demonstrating asthmatic bronchiolitis with eosinophils within the airway wall (hematoxylin and eosin stain [H&E], 200×). (**d**) Heart biopsy displaying eosinophilic endomyocarditis in the setting of EGPA (H&E, 200×)

How Is EGPA Histologically Distinguished from Acute (AEP) and Chronic (CEP) Eosinophilic Pneumonia?

Eosinophilic pneumonia (EP) is a pattern of lung injury in which eosinophils infiltrate the alveolar and interstitial compartments of the lung parenchyma (Fig. 50.3). EGPA, AEP, and CEP are distinct clinical entities in which EP is a characteristic histologic feature. Although there is substantial morphologic overlap between these entities, one defining feature of EGPA that is not seen in AEP or CEP is necrotizing vasculitis. The diagnoses of EGPA, AEP, and CEP can only be established with clinical and radiographic correlation.

What Are the Radiographic Findings in EGPA and How Do They Differ from Acute and Chronic Eosinophilic Pneumonia?

Radiographic imaging in EGPA can demonstrate the presence of transient bilateral pulmonary infiltrates that are migratory or non-fixed in size and location over time. High-resolution computed tomography (HRCT) can show peribronchial thickening, septal thickening, and indistinct opacities [12].

At the onset of acute eosinophilic pneumonia (AEP), chest X-ray findings may be subtle reticular or ground-glass opacities with "Kerley B" lines—short parallel lines at the

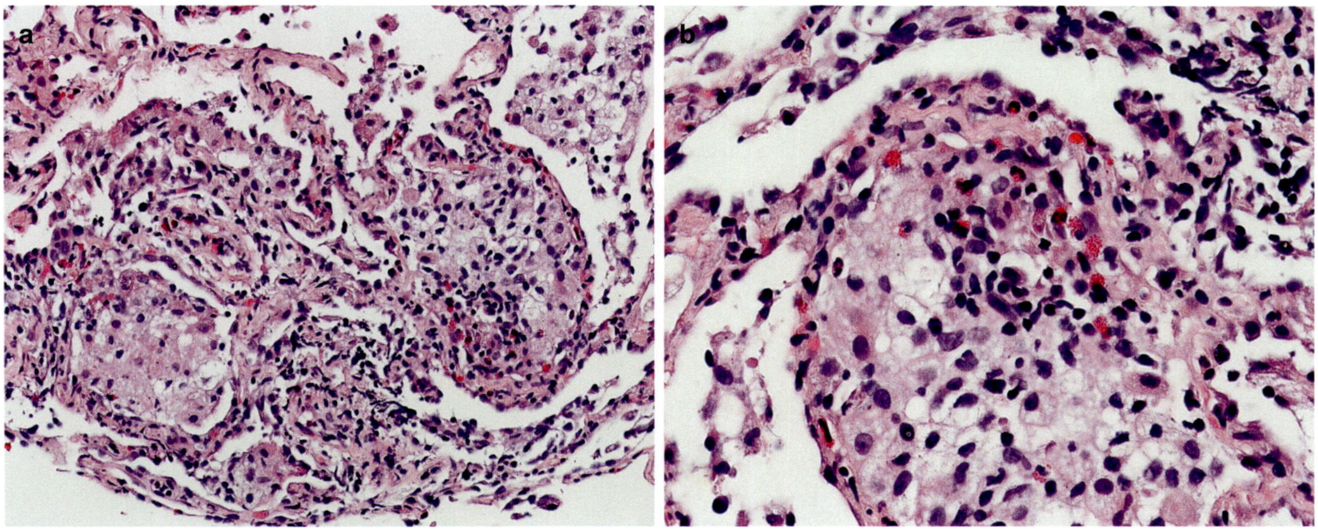

Fig. 50.3 Eosinophilic pneumonia. (**a**) Pulmonary parenchyma with interstitial and alveolar eosinophilic inflammation (hematoxylin and eosin stain [H&E], 200×). (**b**) Higher magnification showing interstitial and alveolar eosinophils (hematoxylin and eosin stain [H&E], 400×)

lung periphery that represent interlobular septa. Diffuse mixed ground-glass opacities develop as the disease progresses. HRCT usually shows bilateral patchy ground-glass or reticular opacities in a random distribution. Pleural effusion may be noted [13]. Chronic eosinophilic pneumonia (CEP), on the other hand, typically demonstrates bilateral peripheral or subpleural non-segmental, consolidative opacities, sometimes described as the "photographic negative" of pulmonary edema [14]. These consolidations are typically more prominent in the upper lobes.

How Does EGPA Differ from GPA?

Granulomatosis with polyangiitis (GPA), formerly called Wegener's granulomatosis, is an entity entirely distinct from EGPA. The hallmark histologic features of GPA are geographic basophilic ("blue") necrosis, neutrophilic microabscesses, necrotizing granulomatous inflammation, vasculitis of small arteries and veins, and neutrophilic capillaritis with diffuse alveolar hemorrhage. The inflammation in GPA is often rich in eosinophils. However, the necrosis in GPA is blue, owing to the nuclear dust of karyorrhectic neutrophils. In EGPA, the necrosis is brightly pink, as it is mainly composed of degranulated eosinophils. Both are associated with ANCA positivity. However, the ANCA generally associated with GPA is anti-PR3 (C-ANCA), whereas the ANCA generally associated with EGPA is anti-MPO (P-ANCA). Be forewarned, however, while usually true this is not always the case.

An eosinophilic variant of this disease, perhaps better designated EV-GPA, has been described in multiple case reports [15–17]. This variant is accepted as a mimic of EGPA, as its distinguishing feature is a prominent tissue infiltrate composed predominantly of eosinophils. However, unlike EGPA, the classic features of GPA, such as geographic blue necrosis and neutrophilic microabscesses, remain present. In addition, the key clinical features of EGPA, such as asthma, atopy, and peripheral eosinophilia, are absent.

References

1. Wilson ME, Weller PF. Eosinophilia. In: Tropical infectious diseases: principles, pathogens and practice, 2 Guerrant RL, Walker DH, Weller PF (Eds), Philadelphia, PA: Elsevier 2006. p. 1478.
2. Saubolle MA, McKellar PP, Sussland D. Epidemiologic, clinical, and diagnostic aspects of coccidioidomycosis. J Clin Microbiol. 2007;45(1):26–30.
3. Gibson PG. Allergic bronchopulmonary aspergillosis. Semin Respir Crit Care Med. 2006;27(2):185–91.
4. Soloman J, Schwartz M. Drug-, toxin-, and radiation therapy-induced eosinophilic pneumonia. Semin Respir Crit Care Med. 2006;27(2):192–7.
5. Camus P. The Drug-induced respiratory disease website. Eosinophilic pneumonia (pulmonary infiltrates and eosinophilia). https://www.pneumotox.com/pattern/view/4/I.c/eosinophilic-pneumonia-pulmonary-infiltrates-and-eosinophilia. Accessed 8 Nov 2018.
6. Badesch DB, King TE, Schwarz MI. Acute eosinophilic pneumonia: a hypersensitivity phenomenon? Am Rev Respir Dis. 1989;139(1):249–52.
7. Rhee CK, Min KH, Yim NY, Lee JE, Lee NR, Chung MP. Clinical characteristics and corticosteroid treatment of acute eosinophilic pneumonia. Eur Respir J. 2013;41(2):402–9.
8. Jederlinic PJ, Sicilian L, Gaensler EA. Chronic eosinophilic pneumonia. A report of 19 cases and a review of the literature. Medicine. 1988;67(3):154–62.
9. Seo P, Stone JH. The antineutrophil cytoplasmic antibody-associated vasculitides. Am J Med. 2004;117(1):39–50.
10. Comarmond C, Pagnoux C, Khellaf M, Cordier JF, Hamidou M, Viallard JF, et al. Eosinophilic granulomatosis with polyangiitis (Churg-Strauss): clinical characteristics and long-term follow-up of the 383 patients enrolled in the French Vasculitis Study Group cohort. Arthritis Rheum. 2013;65(1):270–81.

11. Cottin V, Bel E, Bottero P, Dalhoff K, Humbert M, Lazor R, et al. Revisiting the systemic vasculitis in eosinophilic granulomatosis with polyangiitis (Churg-Strauss): a study of 157 patients by the Groupe d'Etudes et de Recherche sur les Maladies Orphelines Pulmonaires and the European Respiratory Society Taskforce on eosinophilic granulomatosis with polyangiitis (Churg-Strauss). Autoimmun Rev. 2017;16(1):1–9.
12. Worthy SA, Müller NL, Hansell DM, Flower CD. Churg-Strauss syndrome: the spectrum of pulmonary CT findings in 17 patients. AJR Am J Roentgenol. 1998;170(2):297–300.
13. Daimon T, Johkoh T, Sumikawa H, Honda O, Fujimoto K, Koga T. Acute eosinophilic pneumonia: thin-section CT findings in 29 patients. Eur J Radiol. 2008;65(3):462–7.
14. Gaensler EA, Carrington CB. Peripheral opacities in chronic eosinophilic pneumonia: the photographic negative of pulmonary edema. AJR Am J Roentgenol. 1977;128(1):1–13.
15. Al-Hakami H, Al-Arfaj AS, Al-Sohaibani M, Khalil NA. An eosinophilic variant granulomatosis with polyangiitis involving the dura, bilateral orbits, and mastoids. Saudi Med J. 2016;37(6):690–3.
16. Henochowicz S, Eggensperger D, Pierce L, Barth WF. Necrotizing systemic vasculitis with features of both Wegener's granulomatosis and Churg-Strauss vasculitis. Arthritis Rheum. 1986;29:565–9.
17. Yousem SA, Lombard CM. The eosinophilic variant of Wegener's granulomatosis. Hum Pathol. 1988;19(6):682–8.

Pulmonary Sarcoidosis Versus Mycobacterial/Fungal Disease in the Lung

51

James A. Mays, Joshua A. Lieberman, and Haodong Xu

Case Presentation

A 53-year-old man with a past medical history of steroid-responsive restrictive lung disease and asbestos exposure presented to clinic with increased dyspnea on exertion. He has had a longstanding history of presumptive sarcoidosis based on prior chest radiograph findings that has been stable for several years, but recently he has shown increasing dyspnea, chronic cough, and congestion along with a chest computed tomography (CT) scan that showed concern for increased interstitial fibrosis that is most prominent in the upper lobes. Multiple transbronchial biopsies have been attempted, but no definitive etiology has been found either for an infectious etiology or for evidence of sarcoidosis. A repeat chest CT shows upper lobe-predominant reticulonodularity in a perilymphatic distribution with areas of subpleural sparing; it also showed a few mildly enlarged mediastinal lymph nodes, some of which showed peripheral calcification (Fig. 51.1). An interferon-gamma release assay for tuberculosis (TB) infection is equivocal. Because of the lack of treatment response and concern for possible atypical infection or interstitial lung disease, he underwent wedge biopsy of the left upper lobe.

The left upper lobe showed numerous, well-formed, conglomerated non-necrotizing granulomas primarily in a lymphatic distribution including localizations in the bronchiovascular bundles and visceral pleural areas (Fig. 51.2). It also showed organizing pneumonia with intermixed areas of intra-alveolar fibrin aggregates with acute inflammatory infiltrates, characteristic of acute fibrinous and organizing pneumonia (AFOP, not shown). Overall, the granulomatous component was held to be morphologically compatible with the patient's clinical history of sarcoidosis. The patient's AFOP was due to a lung injury; neither microbiologic culture nor special stains for organisms identified an infectious etiology. The patient's oral steroid dose was increased, and he was slowly tapered with symptom resolution over the next 3 months, remaining stable at 5 mg of prednisone daily.

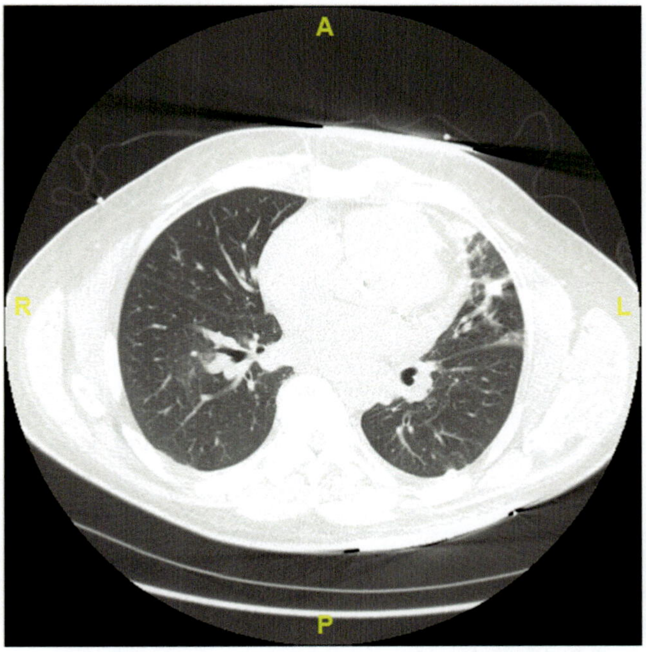

Fig. 51.1 Chest CT showing mediastinal lymphadenopathy, left upper lone consolidation, and perilymphatic nodules in the right upper and lower lobes

J. A. Mays
Department of Laboratory Medicine and Pathology, University of Washington Medical Center, Seattle, WA, USA

Department of Pathology, Massachusetts General Hospital, Boston, MA, USA
e-mail: jamays@mgh.harvard.edu

J. A. Lieberman · H. Xu (✉)
Department of Laboratory Medicine and Pathology, University of Washington Medical Center, Seattle, WA, USA
e-mail: joshuaal@uw.edu; xu8@uw.edu

H. Xu et al. (eds.), *Practical Lung Pathology*, Practical Anatomic Pathology, https://doi.org/10.1007/978-3-031-14402-8_51

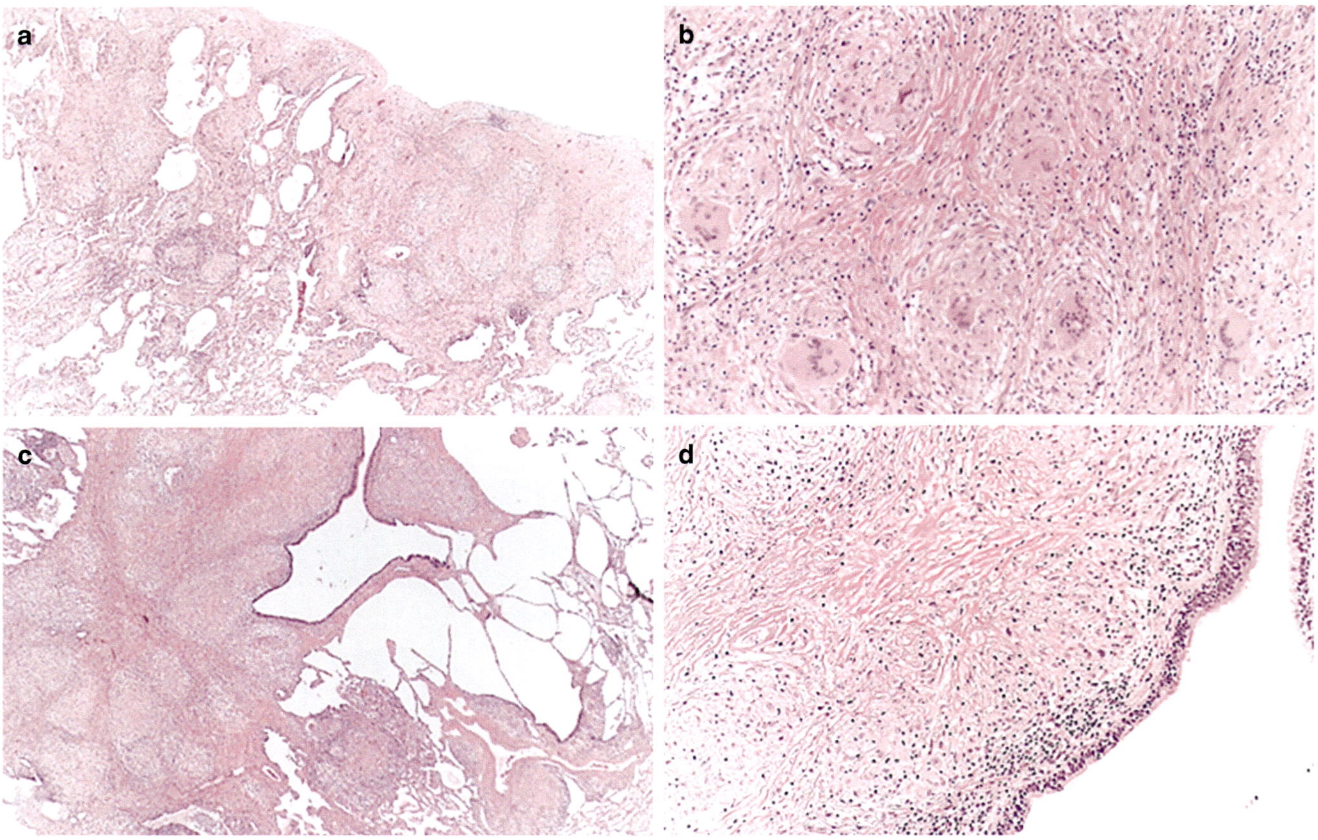

Fig. 51.2 Lung wedge resection showing tightly clustered, well-formed non-necrotizing granulomas localized in the bronchovascular bundles (**a**, **b**) and visceral pleural areas (**c**, **d**). H&E: (**a**, **c**) 40×; (**b**, **d**) 200×

Final Diagnosis: Non-necrotizing Granulomas, Consistent with Sarcoidosis, in a Background of Acute Fibrinous and Organizing Pneumonitis

Comment: The lymphatic distribution of non-necrotizing granulomas and negative stains for AFB and fungi supports a diagnosis of sarcoidosis. Clinical, radiographic, and microbiologic correlation is necessary to make the clinical diagnosis of sarcoidosis.

Clinical Considerations

Sarcoidosis is a chronic granulomatous disease of unknown etiology that involves the lung in a large majority of cases. Most patients present with systemic symptoms including fatigue, weight loss, fever, and malaise; in cases that involve the lung, frequent symptoms include dyspnea and dry cough. Sarcoidosis can markedly vary in its severity and symptoms, with some patients having essentially normal pulmonary function tests and others having severe dysfunction. Severe sarcoidosis can mimic other fibrotic lung diseases or chronic infectious processes in both the degree of lung fibrosis and its impairment of pulmonary function. Because of its poorly characterized etiology, sarcoidosis is to some degree a diagnosis of exclusion and should only be put forward when other causes of chronic granulomatous disease (e.g., mycobacterial and fungal infection, berylliosis) have been sufficiently ruled out [1].

Among other causes of granulomatous disease in the lung, *Mycobacterium tuberculosis* stands out as among the most important [2–4]. Although it is frequently recognized as a source of chronic lung infection and pulmonary nodules, no screening test for infection is definitive, and surgical pathology will sometimes be the initial point of diagnosis for an otherwise unexpected infection. As such, it is essential to rule it out when entertaining a diagnosis of sarcoidosis. In addition to *Mycobacterium tuberculosis*, nontuberculous mycobacteria (NTM) are also important infectious agents in the lung. The prevalence and incidence of NTM incidence are increasing, particularly among patients over age 65, in whom NTM prevalence in the United States may now exceed that of TB by tenfold or more [3, 4]. These nontuberculous mycobacteria are essentially ubiquitous environmental organisms, and patients who become infected with them usually have either preexisting immunosuppression or chronic lung disease. On occasion, microbiologic cultures will show nontuberculous mycobacteria of uncertain clinical significance; histologic examination to assess the host response can be helpful in determining whether these findings represent true infection in these cases.

Radiologic Features

Pulmonary imaging is an important part of the diagnosis of sarcoidosis, because staging is heavily based upon radiographic findings. The most classic finding is bilateral hilar adenopathy; however, the lung parenchyma can have a variety of findings, including diffuse reticular opacities, ground-glass opacities, nodules, or nothing at all. Radiologic staging of sarcoidosis is performed as follows: Stage 0: normal radiographic findings; Stage I: bilateral hilar adenopathy; Stage II: bilateral hilar adenopathy along with reticular opacities, more frequently in the upper lung fields; Stage III: reticular opacities without hilar adenopathy; Stage IV: extensive fibrosis with reticular opacities and volume loss, often in association with traction bronchiectasis and cavitation [5].

High-resolution CT scans are more sensitive than chest radiographs in detecting lung abnormalities, but since they frequently detect abnormalities in otherwise asymptomatic people, they do not play a central role in staging. Other ancillary tests to support a diagnosis of sarcoidosis include gallium-67 scintigraphy, which can show increased uptake in the parotid and lacrimal glands, creating a so-called panda bear pattern, which increases suspicion for sarcoidosis [6].

Histologic Features

The sine qua non of sarcoidosis is granuloma formation. These non-necrotizing granulomas are typically clustered in a lymphatic distribution and most commonly identified in the subpleural region, interlobular septa, and bronchovascular tree. In particular, the subpleural area is a characteristic site that is not commonly seen in mycobacterial infection [7]. The granulomas of sarcoidosis tend to be small, well-formed, tightly clustered, and embedded in a surrounding area of collagen fibrosis (Fig. 51.2). Giant cells are often plentiful. These areas can sometimes have a rim of lymphocytic inflammation. Pulmonary vessels can also frequently be involved by granulomas or giant cells and can be often appreciated on transbronchial biopsy [8]. Concordant with the high prevalence of hilar lymphadenopathy in sarcoidosis, granulomas nearly always involve the peribronchial or mediastinal lymph nodes [9]. While several different inclusion bodies (e.g., Schaumann bodies or asteroid bodies) may be seen in up to 10% of cases, these findings are neither necessary nor pathognomonic for sarcoidosis [10].

The histologic features of sarcoidosis have some differences from tuberculosis and other granulomatous diseases, which may allow the pathologist to favor one over the others even in the absence of microbiologic data. One feature is the tendency of sarcoidosis to involve the lung in a lymphatic distribution, as opposed to the airway distribution that is more common in mycobacterial disease. This feature is most easily appreciated in the subpleural region, where tightly clustered, well-formed granulomas would be much less indicative of mycobacterial infection (Fig. 51.2). However, as with much in these entities, this feature is not a rule, and pleural involvement by tuberculosis is estimated to occur in about 30% of patients [11]. Another feature that favors sarcoidosis is the nature of the granulomatous inflammation. Sarcoid granulomas are usually tightly clustered, well-formed, and non-necrotizing, as compared to the much more frequently necrotizing granulomatous inflammation of both TB and NTM or fungal infection (Fig. 51.3). Tuberculosis and NTM infections have similar histologic patterns, and acid-fast bacilli are often not visible [12, 13]. Multiple other histologic patterns can be produced by mycobacteria or fungi, including nodules, cavitation, and interstitial pneumonitis. In aggregate, an understanding of the characteristic histologic findings of sarcoidosis can lead one to favor it as the most likely diagnosis, but this finding must be interpreted in light of the patient's other clinical and radiographic findings.

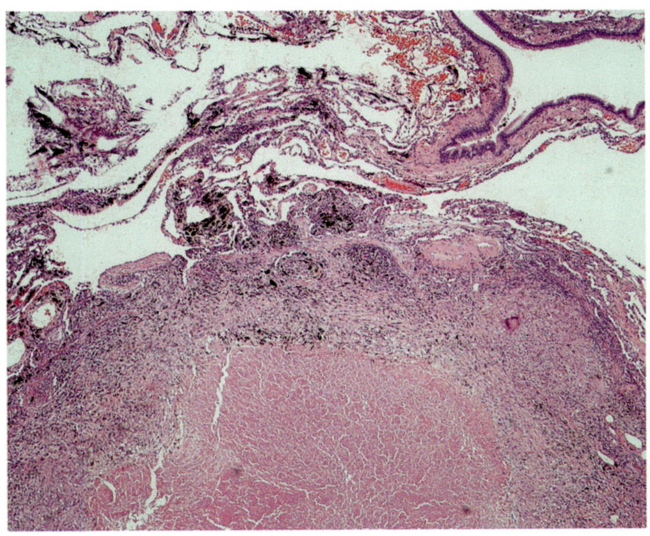

Fig. 51.3 Histologic section showing a necrotizing granuloma (H&E 200×)

Special Stains and Microbiologic Features

Both acid-fast stains and microbiologic testing are indicated in all lung specimens with granulomatous disease, regardless of whether the granulomas are necrotizing or not. Silver stains to assess for fungal disease are also recommended. Given the importance of antimicrobial susceptibility data, culture is also necessary in cases of suspected tuberculosis. Although negative microbiologic testing for tuberculosis is reassuring when making a diagnosis of sarcoidosis, some caution is warranted because no single negative result definitively rules out tuberculosis. For instance, approximately 20% of patients with pleural tuberculosis do not have definitive evidence of mycobacteria by histopathologic examination or mycobacterial culture [11, 14]. Newer PCR-based methods have similar sensitivity to culture with high positive and negative predictive values. However, as with other methods, false negative results are known, and at least one study of pleural biopsies has found a 10% false negative rate for specimens ultimately found to contain tuberculosis [15].

Key Points for Distinguishing Sarcoidosis from Mycobacterial and Other Infections

What Are Three Key Histopathologic Features That Favor a Diagnosis of Sarcoidosis Over Mycobacterial Infection? Are These Findings Specific?

Several features favor sarcoid over infection: distribution of the lesion(s), types of granulomas, and the presence of inclusion bodies and/or absence of microorganisms.

Distribution Unlike mycobacterial infections that tend to distribute along the airways, sarcoidosis tends to follow a lymphatic distribution pattern. Also different from mycobacterial infections, which tend to spare the pleura, sarcoidosis is more likely to involve the pleura and subpleural space. In addition, the lesions in sarcoidosis may involve peribronchial and mediastinal lymph nodes as well as pulmonary vasculature.

Granulomas and surrounding inflammation Sarcoidosis typically presents with tight, epithelioid, granulomas that are (almost) entirely non-necrotizing. These may be associated with lymphocytic inflammation and surrounding collagen fibrosis. In contrast, both NTM and TB infections classically have necrotizing granulomas. Neutrophilic inflammation is also an important clue suggesting an infectious etiology.

Additional features The presence of Schaumann or asteroid bodies suggests but is not specific for sarcoid; many TB and NTM cases have very few visible microorganisms. Nonetheless, these findings are not very specific. For example, up to 30% of TB cases involve the pleura. Taken together with clinical history and ancillary studies, such as interferon release assays for TB, culture, and PCR, these features help rule in sarcoidosis and help exclude infection. A diagnosis of pulmonary sarcoidosis is most secure when there is agreement between clinical presentation, radiographic imaging, and histological findings. Disagreement between any of the three should cause the diagnosis to be treated as preliminary.

Other than *Mycobacterium tuberculosis*, What Infections Should Be Considered in a Patient with Granulomatous Pulmonary Inflammation?

In addition to TB, nontuberculous mycobacterial infections are an important and potentially overlooked cause of granulomatous inflammation. NTM infections in particular should be suspected in older or immunocompromised patients with consistent histopathology findings, particularly if concurrent testing for tuberculosis is negative. NTM can be quite difficult to treat and, if suspected, should be followed up with culture and/or PCR to identify the pathogen. Fungal infections may also present with a similar pattern of inflammation. Filamentous bacterial species such as *Nocardia* spp., *Aggregatibacter* spp., and *Actinomyces* spp. are also worth considering. Special stains for acid-fast bacilli and silver stains for fungus often aid in the evaluation.

Other than Infections, What Other Diseases Should Be Considered in a Patient with Granulomatous Pulmonary Inflammation?

Several other noninfectious entities can present with similar tissue reaction patterns. Pneumoconioses, particularly berylliosis, are an important consideration as is hypersensitivity pneumonitis which may be caused by a variety of environmental or occupational exposures. Rheumatoid arthritis and other autoimmune diseases should also be considered but are beyond the scope of this chapter.

References

1. Hunninghake GW, Costabel U, Ando M, Baughman R, Cordier JF, du Bois R, et al. ATS/ERS/WASOG statement on sarcoidosis. American Thoracic Society/European Respiratory Society/World Association of Sarcoidosis and other Granulomatous Disorders. Sarcoidosis Vasc Diffuse Lung Dis. 1999;16(2):149–73.
2. Blackmon GM, Raghu G. Pulmonary sarcoidosis: a mimic of respiratory infection. Semin Respir Infect. 1995;10(3):176–86.

3. Winthrop KL, Marras TK, Adjemian J, Zhang H, Wang P, Zhang Q. Incidence and prevalence of nontuberculous mycobacterial lung disease in a large United States managed care health plan, 2008-2015. Ann Am Thorac Soc. 2020;17(2):178–85.
4. Abubakar I, Gupta RK, Rangaka MX, Lipman M. Update in tuberculosis and nontuberculous mycobacteria 2017. Am J Respir Crit Care Med. 2018;197(10):1248–53.
5. Baughman RP, Culver DA, Judson MA. A concise review of pulmonary sarcoidosis. Am J Respir Crit Care Med. 2011;183(5):573–81.
6. Brantley SD, Orzel JA, Weiland FL, Bower JH. Parotid gland biopsy and 67Ga imaging correlation in systemic sarcoidosis. Chest. 1987;91(3):403–7.
7. Wilen SB, Rabinowitz JG, Ulreich S, Lyons HA. Pleural involvement in sarcoidosis. Am J Med. 1974;57(2):200–9.
8. Takemura T, Matsui Y, Oritsu M, Akiyama O, Hiraga Y, Omichi M, et al. Pulmonary vascular involvement in sarcoidosis: granulomatous angiitis and microangiopathy in transbronchial lung biopsies. Virchows Arch A Pathol Anat Histopathol. 1991;418(4):361–8.
9. Iwai K, Takemura T, Kitaichi M, Kawabata Y, Matsui Y. Pathological studies on sarcoidosis autopsy. II. Early change, mode of progression and death pattern. Acta Pathol Jpn. 1993;43(7–8):377–85.
10. Rosen Y, Vuletin JC, Pertschuk LP, Silverstein E. Sarcoidosis: from the pathologist's vantage point. Pathol Annu. 1979;14(Pt 1):405–39.
11. Ferrer JS. Pleural tuberculosis: incidence, pathogenesis, diagnosis, and treatment. Curr Opin Pulm Med. 1996;2(4):327–34.
12. Fowler J, Mahlen SD. Localized cutaneous infections in immunocompetent individuals due to rapidly growing mycobacteria. Arch Pathol Lab Med. 2014;138(8):1106–9.
13. Jarzembowski JA, Young MB. Nontuberculous mycobacterial infections. Arch Pathol Lab Med. 2008;132(8):1333–41.
14. Scharer L, McClement JH. Isolation of tubercle bacilli from needle biopsy specimens of parietal pleura. Am Rev Respir Dis. 1968;97(3):466–8.
15. Hasaneen NA, Zaki ME, Shalaby HM, El-Morsi AS. Polymerase chain reaction of pleural biopsy is a rapid and sensitive method for the diagnosis of tuberculous pleural effusion. Chest. 2003;124(6):2105–11.

52 Histoplasmosis, Blastomycosis, Coccidioidomycosis, and Cryptococcosis in the Lung

James A. Mays, Joshua A. Lieberman, and Haodong Xu

Case Presentation

A 62-year-old man presents to clinic with a 4-month history of persistent malaise, shortness of breath, and nonproductive cough. He has a past medical history of psoriatic arthritis for which he is taking a monoclonal antibody immunosuppressive medication. He states that he has felt this way since an extended trip that included visits to Arizona, Mississippi, and Texas. A CT scan shows a 2.2 cm peripheral lung nodule in the right upper lung that has been slowly increasing in size over the past 3 months (Fig. 52.1). Serologic tests are equivocal, and he agrees to a biopsy of the pulmonary nodule. Histologic sections show a nodule consisting predominantly of caseating necrosis with rare scattered poorly staining spherules and degenerated forms that are highlighted by a GMS stain (Fig. 52.2). These forms appear to range markedly in size from <10 μm to approximately 100 μm. Rare spherules contain many small endospores, while smaller spherules do not contain these structures (Fig. 52.2). A histologic diagnosis of coccidioidomycosis is made, and the patient is prescribed a 3-month course of fluconazole.

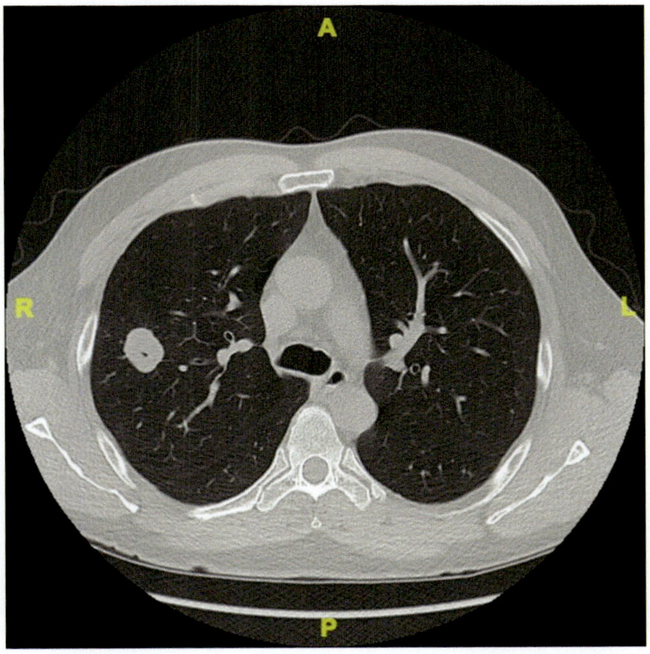

Fig. 52.1 2.2 cm lung nodule with 0.3 cm of cavitation and bronchiectasis in the right upper lobe. Focal hilar lymphadenopathy was also identified; no other masses or consolidations were noted

J. A. Mays
Department of Laboratory Medicine and Pathology, University of Washington Medical Center, Seattle, WA, USA

Department of Pathology, Massachusetts General Hospital, Boston, MA, USA
e-mail: jamays@mgh.harvard.edu

J. A. Lieberman · H. Xu (✉)
Department of Laboratory Medicine and Pathology, University of Washington Medical Center, Seattle, WA, USA
e-mail: joshuaal@uw.edu; xu8@uw.edu

H. Xu et al. (eds.), *Practical Lung Pathology*, Practical Anatomic Pathology, https://doi.org/10.1007/978-3-031-14402-8_52

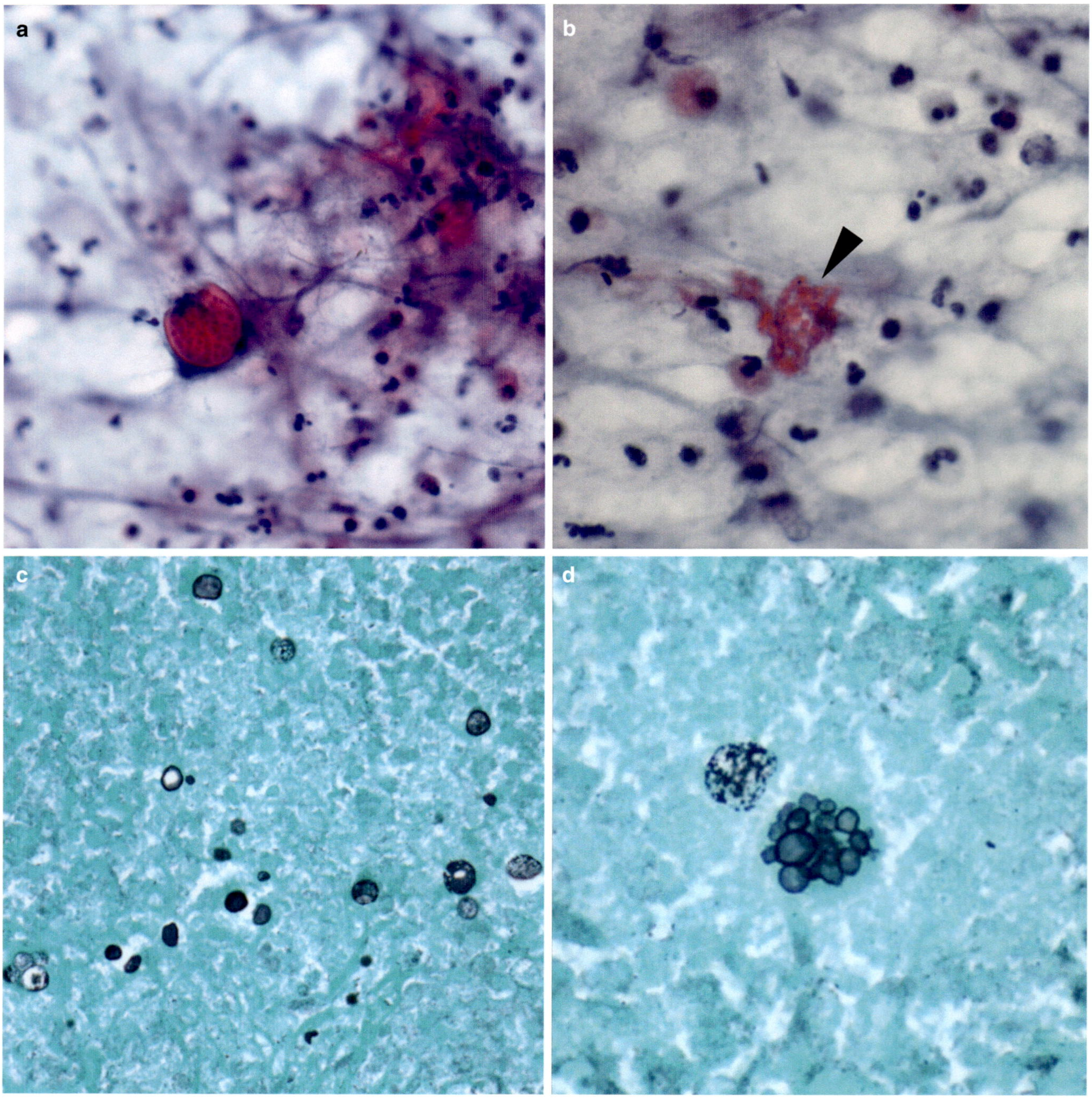

Fig. 52.2 Morphologic variation in coccidioidomycosis. (**a**) Mature spherules of *Coccidioides* spp. containing visible endospores from a Papanicolaou-stained FNA aspirate (400×). (**b**) Free endospores (arrowhead) remain after spherule rupture (Papanicolaou-stained, 400×). (**c**) Immature *Coccidioides* spp. spherules stained with GMS have variable size and shape; endospores are not observed (200×). (**d**) Maturing *Coccidioides* spp. spherules stained by GMS with a degrading spherule in the background (400×)

Final Pathologic Diagnosis: Coccidioidomycosis of the Lung

Clinical Considerations

Histoplasma capsulatum, *Blastomyces dermatitidis*, and *Coccidioides immitis/posadasii* are frequently encountered pulmonary pathogens in immunocompetent hosts. *Cryptococcus neoformans* is more frequently encountered in immunocompromised patients such as those with HIV/AIDS, organ transplant, and prolonged courses of immunosuppressive medications. However, *C. gattii* has been shown to cause clinically severe infections in immunocompetent hosts [1, 2]. While all are environmental soil fungi, the geographic distribution varies. *Histoplasma* is most frequently found in the distribution of the Ohio and Mississippi rivers [3]; *Blastomyces* shares these river valleys but also extends throughout the Great Lakes, St. Lawrence River, and parts of Canada [4]. *Coccidioides* is an endemic pathogen in the southwestern United States, Mexico, parts of Central and South America [5], and arid regions of the northwestern United States [6]. *Cryptococcus neoformans* has a global distribution [7], while *C. gattii* has a more limited distribution with outbreak- [1] and non-outbreak-related infections occurring in the Western and Northwestern regions of North America [2], as well as tropical and subtropical regions [8].

These mycoses all have a wide range of associated clinical severity. Histoplasmosis is most frequently asymptomatic and self-limiting [9] but can produce an acute presentation, a chronic infection akin to mycobacterial disease, or disseminated disease. A similar range of severity and time course exists for blastomycosis, which can have a varied clinical presentation and frequently presents with concurrent skin involvement [10, 11]. *Coccidioides* most frequently presents as a flu-like illness but, like the others, can present with more chronic, fibrocavitary, or disseminated disease [12]. Unlike *Blastomyces* which produces disseminated disease in 20–50% of patients [13, 14], dissemination occurs in ~1% of cases of coccidioidomycosis, and patients of African and Pacific Islander descent are at increased risk [15, 16]. *Cryptococcus* most frequently has a subacute or chronic clinical presentation but has been shown to asymptomatically colonize the respiratory tract in hosts with prior pulmonary disease [17] and can present as disseminated disease in profoundly immunocompromised patients. The most common and feared clinical complication of cryptococcosis is cerebromeningitis. In all of these mycoses, the manner of clinical presentation alone is generally insufficient to rule out any given fungus. However, an appropriate travel history, immunocompetency status, and certain symptoms (e.g., neurological involvement for *Cryptococcus* and skin involvement for *Blastomycosis*) can markedly influence the differential diagnosis.

Serologic testing for *Coccidioides* usually begins with enzyme immunoassays and are confirmed by immunodiffusion and complement fixation, titers of which track with disease states [18]. Antigenic testing for *Cryptococcus* is available in serum and CSF and is an important adjuvant test, particularly to evaluate for cryptococcal cerebromeningitis [19]. Antigenic tests are available for *Coccidioides*, *Blastomyces*, and *Histoplasma*, but antigens are cross-reactive across these and other yeasts [20, 21].

Radiologic Features

Because these different mycoses can have varied clinical presentations and distributions, radiographic findings can vary and overlap. However, there are still characteristic findings in typical presentations of disease. In acute histoplasmosis, radiographs most often show patchy pneumonia in one or more lobes with frequently noted hilar or mediastinal lymph nodes [22]. Severe disease can show diffuse pulmonary reticulonodular pulmonary infiltrates. In blastomycosis, acute presentations are more likely to present with airspace consolidation, and chronic presentations are more likely to present with mass-forming lesions [23]. In coccidioidomycosis, many patients have generally unremarkable radiographic findings; less than half show patchy areas of consolidation, and a minority show hilar lymph node enlargement [12]. In an immunocompetent patient, *Cryptococcus* can show multiple small well-defined nodules or focal areas of consolidation with an upper lobe predominance [24, 25].

Histologic and Immunophenotypic Features

In invasive disease, the shared morphology of these four mycoses is that of yeast or yeast-like forms; it is this feature that groups them as a common differential diagnosis. Upon the detection of candidate yeast forms in a biopsy or surgical specimen, delineation between the different mycoses can be made by several features, including size, shape (oval, round, or pleomorphic), pattern of budding (narrow, broad, or varied), and certain characteristic morphologic or staining features. A summary table of morphologic features is presented in Table 52.1.

Table 52.1 Morphologic differential of endemic mycoses

	Histoplasma	*Blastomycosis*	*Coccidioides*	*Cryptococcus*
Size	2–5 μm	8–20 μm	20–100 μm	5–15 μm
Shape	Round	Varied	Round	Varied
Budding	Narrow-based	Broad-based	None	Narrow-based
Other features	Intracellular pathogen within histiocytes; may be seen extracellularly	Double-contoured and refractile wall	Mature spherules with endospores (2–5 μm), occasionally hyphae	Mucicarmine-staining capsule, acapsular forms exist

Histoplasma spp. infects alveolar macrophages and is predominantly seen as an intracellular pathogen within phagocytic cells [26] with small, ovoid yeast forms (2–5 μm) that are the smallest of the yeasts forms discussed in this chapter (Fig. 52.3a). These typically stain poorly in routine preparations but can be observed as phagocytosed forms in the cytoplasm of macrophages. While other yeasts such as *Cryptococcus* can overlap in size with *Histoplasma*, the overall population of other yeasts is typically pleomorphic with larger forms present. *Histoplasma* shows narrow-based budding that contrasts with *Blastomyces*' broad-based budding.

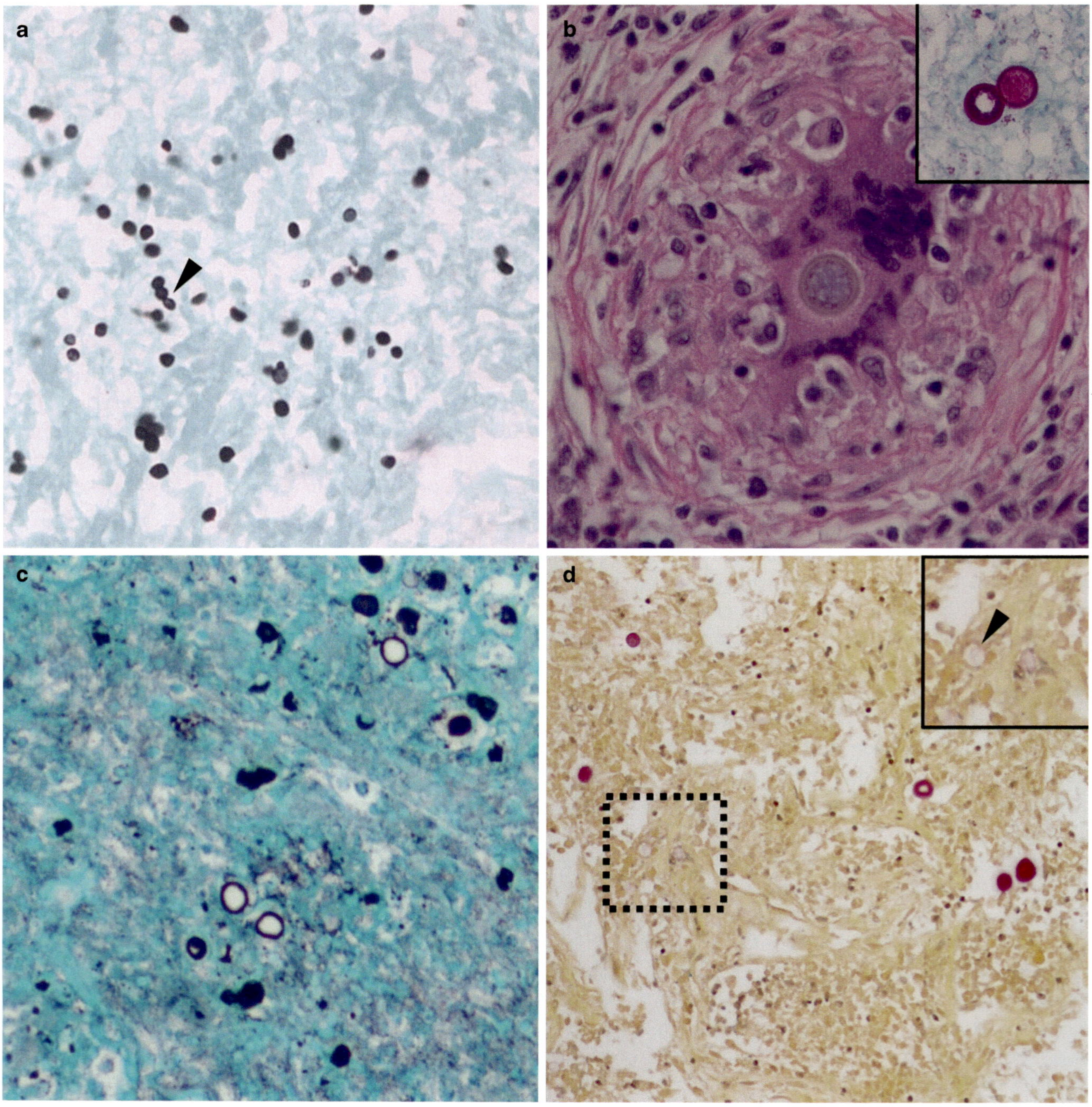

Fig. 52.3 Representative morphology of *Histoplasma*, *Blastomyces*, and *Cryptococcus*. (**a**) Histoplasmosis with small, ovoid yeast forms with narrow-based budding. (**b**) Blastomycosis with a range of intermediate-sized (12–23 μm) spherical yeasts. These are larger than *Histoplasma* and have broad-based budding with double-contoured cell walls (inset: PAS stain). (**c**) GMS stain of *Cryptococcus* with variably shaped and sized spherules without budding. (**d**) Mucicarmine stain highlighting mucoid capsule of *Cryptococcus*. Occasional possible capsule-deficient forms are present (inset)

Blastomyces are double-contoured, refractile, and typically 8–15 μm in size, creating morphologic overlap with either *Cryptococcus* (smaller forms) or *Coccidioides* (larger forms). Occasionally, very small forms mimicking *Histoplasma* in size can occur, but, as with *Cryptococcus*, these will typically exist in a continuum of size, including forms with more classic morphology [27]. The broad-based attachment of blastoconidia to their parent cells is the most reliable feature to distinguish *Blastomyces* from similar sized mimics (Fig. 52.3b, inset). *Blastomyces* (Fig 52.3b) will also be larger than *Histoplasma* (Fig 52.3a) if measurements with a calibrated micrometer can be made. The double cell wall is also a helpful finding (Fig. 52.3b).

The most characteristic finding of *Coccidioides* is that of a large, mature spherule greater than 30 μm containing multiple endospores (Fig. 52.2a). Smaller, immature spherules can be seen, which are generally ovoid and varied in size (Fig. 52.2c, d); these spherules can be confused with the yeast forms of other mycoses. Endospores are small (2–5 μm) (Fig. 52.2b) and may be difficult to identify in the absence of spherules [28]. Unlike other invasive yeasts, occasional hyphae and arthroconidia can occasionally be seen. When mature endospore-laden spherules are present, a confident diagnosis can be made, but if only immature spherules or degenerated forms are present, then a diagnosis is less certain and should be correlated with serology, immunofluorescence, or fungal culture.

Cryptococcus has intermediate-sized (most typically 4–7 μm) yeast forms with narrow budding (Fig. 52.3c), surrounded by a mucoid capsule that characteristically stains with a Mucicarmine stain (Fig. 52.3d). These yeasts may be pleomorphic, ranging up to 15 μm. Capsule-deficient forms can be present. Particularly in caseous or necrotic nodules, cryptococcal cells may be small, nonviable, distorted, and acapsular, becoming potentially confused with *Histoplasma*. Cryptococcal forms are typically not easily seen in an H&E stain, especially in the case of degenerated cells or resolving/resolved infections. In the case of unsuccessful fungal culture, immunofluorescence or molecular studies may be undertaken in order to make a histologic diagnosis.

Molecular Testing

Fungal culture should be performed in all clinical scenarios where invasive fungal disease is suspected. However, invasive fungal disease is often an unexpected finding, and fungal culture can sometimes produce isolates that are of uncertain clinical significance. Histologic evaluation, including assessment of host response, adds valuable information in these cases [28]. There are, however, cases where morphologic findings are not entirely specific for an etiology, and fungal culture has either failed or was not performed. In these cases, PCR-based methods performed on the formalin-fixed, paraffin-embedded tissue are becoming increasingly common and useful diagnostic tools [29, 30]. While molecular-based methods are largely more sensitive than histologic ones, a negative result does not definitively rule out invasive fungal disease in cases with strong histologic evidence or clinical suspicion. Degradation of DNA in nonviable organisms or after formalin fixation can cause a sample's total fungal DNA content to be below the threshold of detection for that assay, and caution in such cases is warranted. For cultured isolates of *Coccidioides*, DNA hybridization probes are available.

Key Points for Differentiating Coccidioides, Cryptococcus, Blastomyces, and Histoplasma

Each of These Pathogens Has Yeast or Yeast-Like Forms in Tissue: What Morphologic Features Distinguish Them?

Size is an important feature distinguishing these organisms (see Table 52.1), but other key morphologic features are often visible. A unique feature of *Coccidioides* distinct from *Histoplasma*, *Blastomyces*, and *Cryptococcus* is the formation of spherules, generally greater than 30 μm diameter; mature spherules are laden with endospores (2–5 μm). *Cryptococcus* spp. usually have a capsule that stains with mucicarmine. *Blastomyces* has a thick, double-contoured cell wall and divides by broad-based budding, whereas *Histoplasma* lacks the double-contoured wall and divides by narrow-based budding.

What Are Important Pitfalls in the Identification of These Organisms?

The pathologist should be aware of capsule-deficient *Cryptococcus*, small-variant *Blastomyces*, and the presence of free *Coccidioides* endospores in the absence of spherules. Free endospores are small and may hide in the background. Small-variant *Blastomyces* typically has a range of sizes, helping to distinguish from *Histoplasma capsulatum*. Serologic tests such as cryptococcal antigen may help diagnose capsule-deficient *Cryptococcus*. Other yeasts, such as *Candida* spp. and *Sporothrix* spp. may appear similar in histologic section.

What Additional Diagnostic Testing Is Important/Should Be Recommended?

Fungal culture and molecular microbiologic testing are far more specific than histologic assessment for species identification. Culture should be taken in lesions with a high suspicion, and the laboratory should be alerted to concern for *Coccidioides* or *Histoplasma* due to the significant risk of occupational exposure. Fungal PCR can be performed on the paraffin block in cases without a microbiologic diagnosis. Serologic testing for either antibodies or antigens is often helpful, but cross-reactivity among these and other yeasts is an important concern.

References

1. Kidd SE, Hagen F, Tscharke RL, Huynh M, Bartlett KH, Fyfe M, et al. A rare genotype of Cryptococcus gattii caused the cryptococcosis outbreak on Vancouver Island (British Columbia, Canada). Proc Natl Acad Sci. 2004;101(49):17258–63.
2. Harris JR, Lockhart SR, Sondermeyer G, Vugia DJ, Crist MB, D'Angelo MT, et al. Cryptococcus gattii infections in multiple states outside the US Pacific Northwest. Emerg Infect Dis. 2013;19(10):1620–6.
3. Manos NE, Ferebee SH, Kerschbaum WF. Geographic variation in the prevalence of histoplasmin sensitivity. Dis Chest. 1956;29(6):649–68.
4. Bradsher RW, Chapman SW, Pappas PG. Blastomycosis. Infect Dis Clin N Am. 2003;17(1):21–40, vii.
5. Edwards PQ, Palmer CE. Prevalence of sensitivity to Coccidioidin, with special reference to specific and nonspecific reactions to Coccidioidin and to Histoplasmin. Dis Chest. 1957;31(1):35–60.
6. Litvintseva AP, Marsden-Haug N, Hurst S, Hill H, Gade L, Driebe EM, et al. Valley fever: finding new places for an old disease: Coccidioides immitis found in Washington State soil associated with recent human infection. Clin Infect Dis. 2015;60(1):e1–3.
7. Levitz SM. The ecology of Cryptococcus neoformans and the epidemiology of Cryptococcosis. Rev Infect Dis. 1991;13(6):1163–9.
8. Kwon-Chung KJ, Bennett JE. High prevalence of Cryptococcus neoformans var. gattii in tropical and subtropical regions. Zentralbl Bakteriol Mikrobiol Hyg [A]. 1984;257(2):213–8.
9. Goodwin RA, Loyd JE, Des Prez RM. Histoplasmosis in normal hosts. Medicine (Baltimore). 1981;60(4):231.
10. Sarosi GA, Davies SF. Blastomycosis. Am Rev Respir Dis. 1979;120(4):911–38.
11. Vanek J, Schwarz J, Hakim S. North American blastomycosis: a study of ten cases. Am J Clin Pathol. 1970;54(3):384–400.
12. Kim K-I, Leung AN, Flint JD, Muller NL. Chronic pulmonary coccidioidomycosis: computed tomographic and pathologic findings in 18 patients. Can Assoc Radiol J. 1998;49(6):401–7.
13. Anderson JL, Meece JK, Hall MC, Frost HM. Evidence of delayed dissemination or re-infection with Blastomyces in two immunocompetent hosts. Med Mycol Case Rep. 2016;13:9–11.
14. Saccente M, Woods GL. Clinical and laboratory update on blastomycosis. Clin Microbiol Rev. 2010;23(2):367–81.
15. Brown J, Benedict K, Park BJ, Thompson GR. Coccidioidomycosis: epidemiology. Clin Epidemiol. 2013;5:185–97.
16. Mease L. Pulmonary and extrapulmonary coccidioidomycosis, active component, U.S. Armed Forces, 1999-2011. MSMR. 2012;19(12):2–4.
17. Pappas PG. Cryptococcal infections in non-HIV-infected patients. Trans Am Clin Climatol Assoc. 2013;124:61–79.
18. McHardy IH, Dinh B-TN, Waldman S, Stewart E, Bays D, Pappagianis D, et al. Coccidioidomycosis complement fixation titer trends in the age of antifungals. J Clin Microbiol. 2018;56(12):e01318-18.
19. Rajasingham R, Wake RM, Beyene T, Katende A, Letang E, Boulware DR. Cryptococcal meningitis diagnostics and screening in the era of point-of-care laboratory testing. J Clin Microbiol. 2019;57(1):e01238–18.
20. Frost HM, Novicki TJ. Blastomyces antigen detection for diagnosis and management of blastomycosis. J Clin Microbiol. 2015;53(11):3660–2.
21. Theel ES, Jespersen DJ, Harring J, Mandrekar J, Binnicker MJ. Evaluation of an enzyme immunoassay for detection of Histoplasma capsulatum antigen from urine specimens. J Clin Microbiol. 2013;51(11):3555–9.
22. Gurney JW, Conces DJ. Pulmonary histoplasmosis. Radiology. 1996;199(2):297–306.
23. Fang W, Washington L, Kumar N. Imaging manifestations of blastomycosis: a pulmonary infection with potential dissemination. Radiographics. 2007;27(3):641–55.
24. Lindell RM, Hartman TE, Nadrous HF, Ryu JH. Pulmonary Cryptococcosis: CT findings in immunocompetent patients. Radiology. 2005;236(1):326–31.
25. Fox DL, Müller NL. Pulmonary Cryptococcosis in immunocompetent patients: CT findings in 12 patients. Am J Roentgenol. 2005;185(3):622–6.
26. Garfoot AL, Rappleye CA. Histoplasma capsulatum surmounts obstacles to intracellular pathogenesis. FEBS J. 2016;283(4):619–33.
27. Tuttle JG, Lightwaedt HE, Altshuler CH. Systemic North American blastomycosis. Report of a case with small forms of blastomycetes. Am J Clin Pathol. 1953;23(9):890–7.
28. Guarner J, Brandt ME. Histopathologic diagnosis of fungal infections in the 21st century. Clin Microbiol Rev. 2011;24(2):247–80.
29. Lass-Flörl C, Mutschlechner W, Aigner M, Grif K, Marth C, Girschikofsky M, et al. Utility of PCR in diagnosis of invasive fungal infections: real-life data from a multicenter study. J Clin Microbiol. 2013;51(3):863–8.
30. McCarthy MW, Walsh TJ. PCR methodology and applications for the detection of human fungal pathogens. Expert Rev Mol Diagn. 2016;16(9):1025–36.

Pneumocystis jirovecii Pneumonia Versus Histoplasmosis

53

James A. Mays, Joshua A. Lieberman, and Haodong Xu

Case Presentation

A 57-year-old man with a past medical history of bilateral lung transplant presented with increasing shortness of breath to his outpatient pulmonologist. Chest computed tomography (CT) showed diffuse patchy infiltrates, most prominent in the para-hilar region, with associated lymphadenopathy (Fig. 53.1). The patient underwent bronchoscopy and transbronchial biopsy, which showed granulomatous inflammation with few associated organisms, thought to be consistent with *P. jirovecii*. Prolonged treatment for pneumocystis pneumonia was not effective, and the patient eventually underwent wedge biopsy, which showed necrotizing granulomas and small, narrow-based budding yeasts, morphologically most consistent with *H. capsulatum* (Fig. 53.2). Fungal cultures obtained from fresh tissue confirmed the diagnosis.

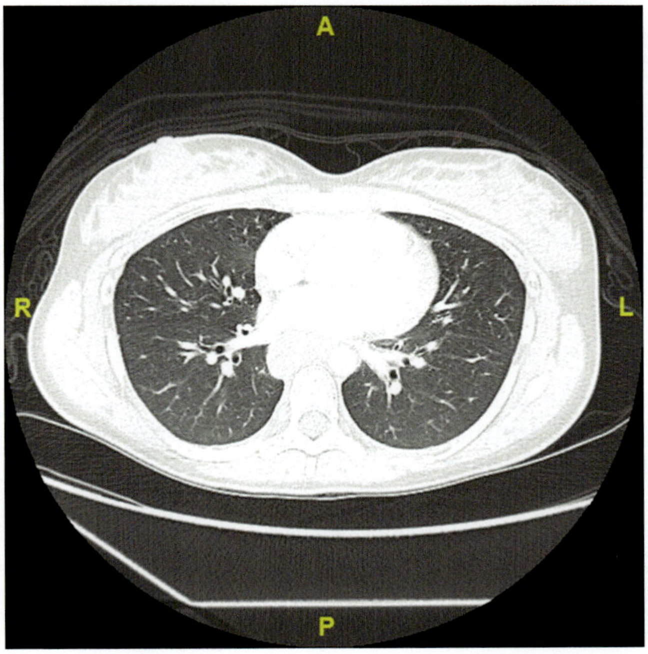

Fig. 53.1 Chest CT showing diffuse patchy infiltrates, most prominent in the para-hilar region, with associated lymphadenopathy

J. A. Mays
Department of Laboratory Medicine and Pathology, University of Washington Medical Center, Seattle, WA, USA

Department of Pathology, Massachusetts General Hospital, Boston, MA, USA
e-mail: jamays@mgh.harvard.edu

J. A. Lieberman · H. Xu (✉)
Department of Laboratory Medicine and Pathology, University of Washington Medical Center, Seattle, WA, USA
e-mail: joshuaal@uw.edu; xu8@uw.edu

H. Xu et al. (eds.), *Practical Lung Pathology*, Practical Anatomic Pathology, https://doi.org/10.1007/978-3-031-14402-8_53

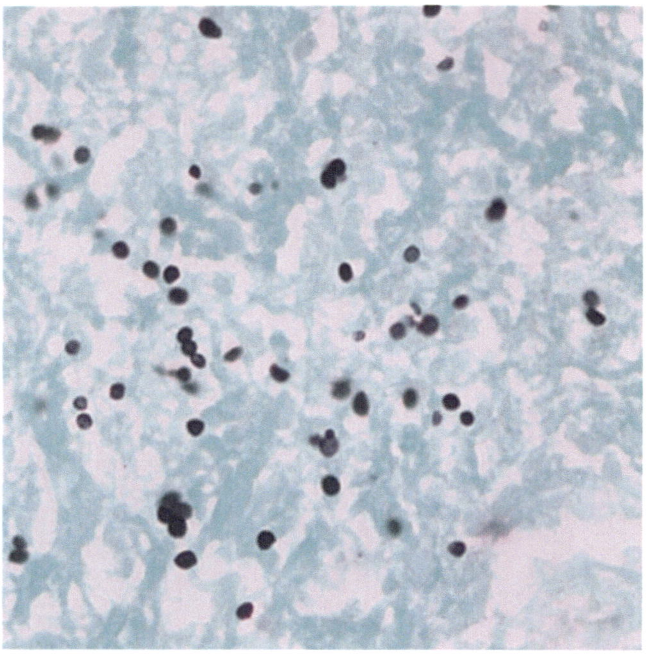

Fig. 53.2 Typical morphology of histoplasmosis. The organisms are small, ovoid yeast forms with narrow-based budding, as contrasted with the folded, umbilicated forms with an argyrophilic dot as seen in *P. jirovecii*

Final Diagnosis: Small Yeasts with Narrow-Based Budding

Comment: These findings are suggestive of *Histoplasma capsulatum* but may be confused with other small yeasts such as *Candida glabrata*, *Pneumocystis jirovecii*, and others. Correlation with microbiology studies is necessary to identify the infectious organism.

Clinical Considerations

Histoplasma capsulatum is an invasive endemic pulmonary fungal pathogen that infects immunocompetent hosts and is seen as narrow-based budding yeast on histologic examination. In North America, *Histoplasma* is most frequently found in the distribution of the Ohio and Mississippi rivers [1], but it is globally distributed and prevalent in sub-Saharan Africa [2, 3] The clinical presentation of histoplasmosis has a wide range of clinical severity: most frequently it is asymptomatic and self-limiting [4] but can produce an acute presentation, a chronic infection akin to mycobacterial disease, or disseminated disease.

P. jirovecii, previously characterized as a protozoan, is now classed as a fungus. It is present worldwide, and although it is overwhelmingly a disease of the immunocompromised, at least one study has found a carrier rate of up to 20% in healthy, immunocompetent adults [5]. *Pneumocystis* pneumonia is one of the most commonly encountered lung infections in people with impaired cell-mediated immunity, such as those with advanced HIV [6], organ transplants, or hematological malignancy. Unlike *Histoplasma* spp. and other fungi, *P. jirovecii* cannot be grown by microbiologic culture [7].

Radiologic Features

Typical radiographic findings in *Pneumocystis* pneumonia are bilateral, diffuse alveolar, and interstitial infiltrates that are typically either lower lobe or hilar predominant but may diffusely involve the lungs. However, multiple atypical radiographic patterns have been reported and include nodular lesions, lobar consolidation, unilateral involvement, cystic spaces, and hilar lymphadenopathy [8]. Up to 20% of patients with AIDS may present with no radiographic abnormalities on chest radiographs, although they will likely have ground-glass opacities on subsequent CT [9]. The key message is that *Pneumocystis* pneumonia is compatible with a wide array of radiographic findings.

In acute histoplasmosis, radiographs most often show patchy consolidation in one or more lobes, frequently with prominent hilar or mediastinal lymph nodes [10]. Severe disease can show diffuse reticulonodular infiltrates, and resolved cases may have calcified nodules. However, a substantial portion of cases may have normal chest radiographs [4, 10]. The variety of radiographic findings reflects the diversity of pathologic manifestations: histoplasmosis can produce an acute presentation, chronic infection akin to mycobacterial disease, disseminated disease, mediastinitis, or a circumscribed nodule of largely resolved infection.

Histologic Features

The diagnosis of *Pneumocystis* pneumonia can be accomplished by recognition of characteristic histomorphologic features of the organism and intra-alveolar exudates (Fig 53.3a). Four developmental forms of *P. jirovecii* are described, in keeping with its former protozoan classification: trophozoites, precysts, cysts, and sporozoites (also known as intracystic bodies). For the purpose of pathologic identification, cysts and trophozoites are the most relevant. The cyst is the largest, most easily recognized stage, and is easily demonstrated with GMS stain. The vegetative forms of *Pneumocystis*, trophozoites, are 1–5 μm in diameter and characteristically attach to type I pneumocytes. The cyst is 5–7 μm in diameter and most contain up to eight intracystic bodies (sporozoites), each 1–2 μm in diameter. These sporozoites have a single nucleus. Some cysts will contain internal

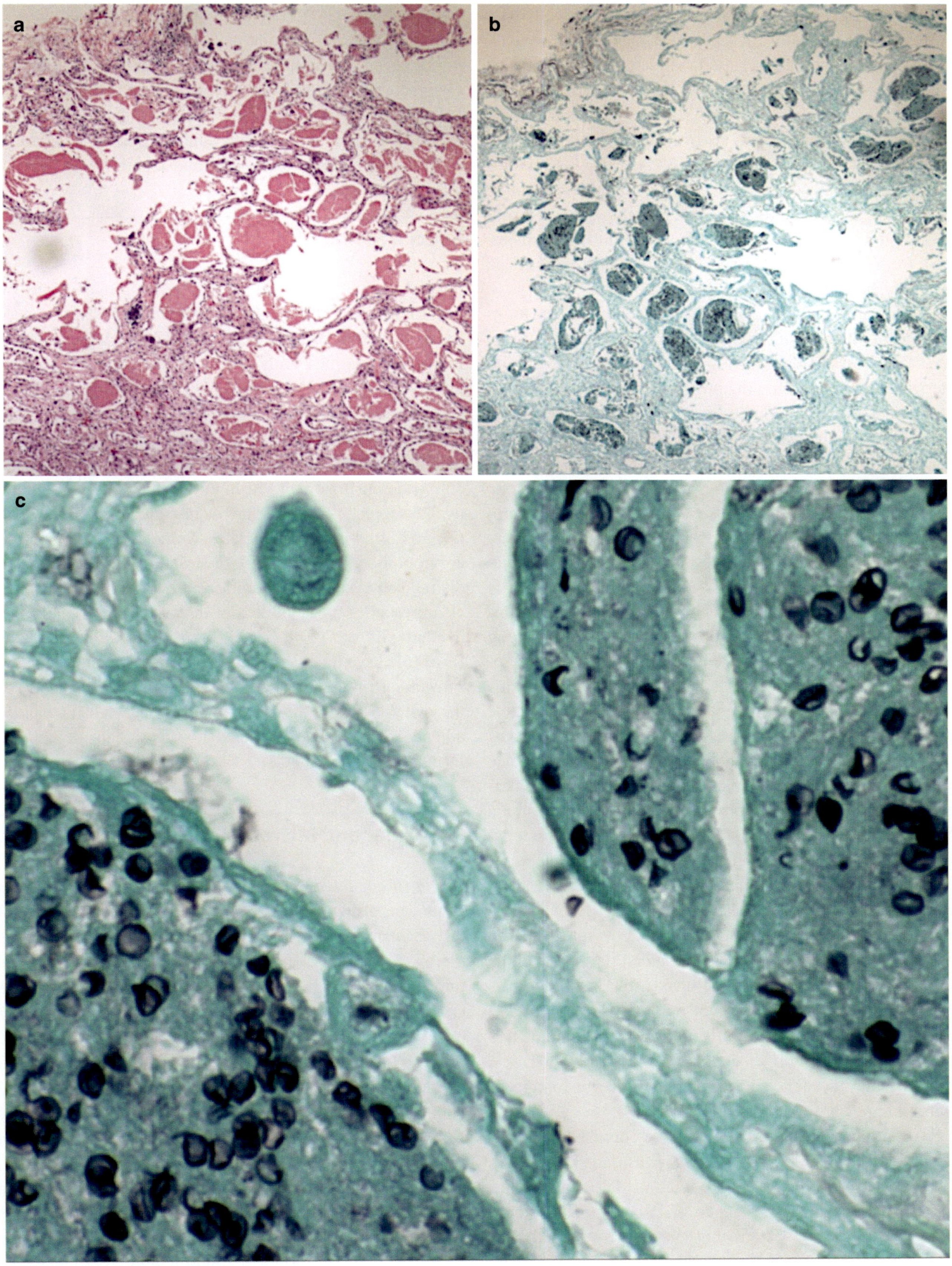

Fig. 53.3 Typical morphology and alveolar filling pattern of *P. jirovecii* pneumonia. Low (100×) magnification sections of a postmortem lung stained with H&E (**a**) and GMS (**b**) demonstrate an alveolar filling pattern with eosinophilic, proteinaceous exudate typical for *P. jirovecii* pneumonia. The opportunistic pathogens are abundant within intra-alveolar exudates and easily seen with a silver stain (**b**, **c**). Note the central umbilication and slightly folded appearance of the organisms at high (400×) magnification (**c**)

comma-shaped structures, either singular or in pairs, that are localized thickenings of the internal layer of the cyst wall. Ruptured cysts that have released their sporozoites will have a characteristic cup or crescent shape when collapsed. Intracystic sporozoites are not visible on histopathologic stains. The cysts are round to oval, focally curved, with crushed "boat" forms present (Fig. 53.3c). These structures are useful in identifying *P. jirovecii* as compared to budding yeast pathogens. When found separately from the cysts, sporozoites and trophozoites are difficult to identify and distinguish from background debris or tissue, but they can have an amoeboid appearance in tissue sections.

Grossly, in patients with *P. jirovecii* pneumonia, the lungs are typically heavy with a gray or tan consolidated cut surface. The most typical histologic features are that of mild interstitial mononuclear inflammation, type II pneumocyte hyperplasia, and eosinophilic foamy intra-alveolar exudates that expand the alveolar spaces (Fig. 53.3a). On higher magnification, the exudates can be punctuated by round basophilic dots that correspond to sporozoite and trophozoite nuclei. These help to distinguish the findings from pulmonary edema or alveolar proteinosis. In tissue sections, there is often characteristic retraction of the exudate from the adjacent alveolar wall.

Although the above features are the most common histologic pattern, *P. jirovecii* can provoke essentially any lung injury reaction pattern. In chronic infection, interstitial fibrosis may be seen. In an acute and progressive infection, diffuse alveolar damage, hyaline membranes, and reactive epithelial proliferation can be seen. There is often robust lymphoplasmacytic inflammation and type II pneumocyte hyperplasia that can be misinterpreted as lymphocytic interstitial pneumonia (LIP) or nonspecific interstitial pneumonia (NSIP). In one study, 19% of patients lacked the characteristic alveolar exudates, and many showed atypical features such as interstitial inflammation (63%), fibrosis (50%), numerous alveolar macrophages resembling desquamative interstitial pneumonia (9%), granulomatous inflammation (5%), hyaline membranes (4%), and interstitial pneumonitis (3%) [11]. Due to this multitude of possible histologic patterns, the differential diagnosis of opportunistic lung infections frequently includes both *Pneumocystis* pneumonia and endemic mycoses such as *H. capsulatum*. In such cases, diagnosis may be delayed without definitive histologic or microbiologic evidence of organisms.

Several infectious etiologies could be confused for *P. jirovecii*. These include *Histoplasma capsulatum*, *Candida glabrata*, and *Cryptococcus* spp. Each of these entities has characteristic findings to suggest it. *H. capsulatum* has small, ovoid yeast forms (2–5 μm) that show narrow-based budding, which is absent in *Pneumocystis*. Yeast forms of *H. capsulatum* typically stain poorly in routine preparations but stain well with GMS (Fig. 53.1). In addition, *H. capsulatum* is primarily an intracellular pathogen, whereas *P. jirovecii* is primarily an extracellular organism within alveolar spaces. *Cryptococcus* yeasts (5–15 μm) are larger than either *H. capsulatum* or *P. jirovecii* and typically have a capsule. Pseudohyphae production by a small yeast, like *C. glabrata*, would argue strongly against the above pathogens.

Special Stains

Special stains for *Pneumocystis* can be grouped into two general categories: those that highlight the cyst wall and its internal structures and those that stain the nuclei of trophozoites and sporozoites. Only cytologic specimens are usable in the case of the latter, and multiple stains, including Giemsa, Wright, and Diff-Quik, can highlight the vegetative state nuclei. More commonly used in clinical practice are stains that highlight the cyst wall. Of these, GMS is the most reliable and sensitive and will highlight the walls of round to oval 5–7 μm cysts and any "crescent" or "boat" forms (Fig. 53.3b) within the exudates. Some cysts have a unique argyrophilic peripheral dot-like structure and are helpful to distinguish cysts from budding yeast forms. This feature is also present as a basophilic dot in cyst forms when seen on hematoxylin and eosin (H&E) preparations. Taken together (Fig. 53.3a), these findings are highly suggestive of *Pneumocystis* pneumonia. In cases where *Cryptococcus* is in the differential diagnosis, a mucicarmine stain is a useful adjunct to visualize capsule; however, capsule-deficient forms exist.

Molecular and Microbiologic Features

While *H. capsulatum* grows reliably in culture, *P. jirovecii* cannot be grown on cell-free media. The inability to culture *P. jirovecii* underlines the importance of clinical suspicion, awareness of key morphologic features, and importance of ancillary detection methods when *P. jirovecii* pneumonia is suspected. Both *H. capsulatum* and *P. jirovecii* can be detected and distinguished from each other by broad-range fungal PCR with sequence-based identification or species-specific PCR. Species-specific assays employ primer sets optimized to bind the target organism's DNA, such as the *Pneumocystis jirovecii* gene *cdc2*, a conserved species-specific cell division cycle2 [12, 13]. Optimized primer binding is thought to have higher analytical sensitivity than broad-range PCR assays. Clinical sensitivity is influenced by pretest probability of infection, tissue volume [14], organism burden, and target gene copy number.

Some microbiology laboratories continue to offer direct fluorescent antibody (DFA) staining of respiratory fluids for *Pneumocystis* detection, although a lack of control material threatens the continued use of these assays (personal communication). The clinical sensitivity of DFA staining is also subject to organism burden and sample volume but performs well in high-prevalence populations, with sensitivity ~55% in HIV-infected patients with suspected PJP [15]. DFA is therefore an excellent assay when PJP is suspected; however, the addition of a species-specific PCR increases sensitivity [12, 13] and should be considered when clinical suspicion is high but DFA is negative. PCR is of particular value when cytopathology or histopathology specimens are the only available diagnostic material.

Key Points for Differentiating *P. jirovecii* and *H. capsulatum*

Both *Pneumocystis jirovecii* and *Histoplasma capsulatum* Cause Pulmonary Infections in Overlapping Patient Populations. What Histopathologic Features Help Distinguish Between *P. jirovecii* and *H. capsulatum*?

Two important differences are very helpful in distinguishing these two infections: tissue distribution and tissue reaction pattern. *P. jirovecii* is predominantly found in the alveolar spaces and is often accompanied by a "frothy" eosinophilic exudate that fills the alveolar space. *H. capsulatum*, on the other hand, germinates from inhaled conidia inside alveolar macrophages and is primarily intracellular with lymphatic dissemination. Eosinophilic exudates in the alveoli are not a typical feature of *H. capsulatum*. Confusion in diagnosis can arise when the typical alveolar exudate of *P. jirovecii* is absent, when atypical tissue reaction patterns—such as granulomatous inflammation or interstitial fibrosis—are present, or when the organisms cannot be well-visualized.

What Morphologic Features Help Distinguish These Two Organisms from Each Other?

These two organisms have similar morphology but can often be distinguished from each other using several morphologic features. First, *P. jirovecii* cysts are slightly larger (5–7 μm) than *H. capsulatum* (2–5 μm) and have a characteristic boat- or cup-like forms and perinuclear dot-like structures indicative of sporozoite release. These morphologic features are important to note since the sizes of the organisms are similar. Second, *P. jirovecii* lack the narrow-based budding typical of *H. capsulatum* dividing yeasts.

What Laboratory Tests Are Available to Confirm the Diagnosis?

Culture is always important in the evaluation of infectious diseases, but only *H. capsulatum* will grow in microbiologic culture. Two other types of assays in the clinical microbiology laboratory are both sensitive and specific: PCR (both organisms) and DFA (*P. jirovecii* only).

References

1. Manos NE, Ferebee SH, Kerschbaum WF. Geographic variation in the prevalence of histoplasmin sensitivity. Dis Chest. 1956;29(6):649–68.
2. Houston S. Tropical respiratory medicine. 3. Histoplasmosis and pulmonary involvement in the tropics. Thorax. 1994;49(6):598–601.
3. Oladele RO, Ayanlowo OO, Richardson MD, Denning DW. Histoplasmosis in Africa: an emerging or a neglected disease? PLoS Negl Trop Dis. 2018;12(1):e0006046.
4. Goodwin RA, Loyd JE, Des Prez RM. Histoplasmosis in normal hosts. Medicine (Baltimore). 1981;60(4):231.
5. Medrano FJ, Montes-Cano M, Conde M, de la Horra C, Respaldiza N, Gasch A, et al. Pneumocystis jirovecii in general population. Emerg Infect Dis. 2005;11(2):245–50.
6. Roux A, Canet E, Valade S, Gangneux-Robert F, Hamane S, Lafabrie A, et al. Pneumocystis jirovecii pneumonia in patients with or without AIDS, France. Emerg Infect Dis. 2014;20(9):1490–7.
7. Liu Y, Fahle GA, Kovacs JA. Inability to culture Pneumocystis jirovecii. MBio. 2018;129(3):e00939–18.
8. Kuhlman JE, Kavuru M, Fishman EK, Siegelman SS. Pneumocystis carinii pneumonia: spectrum of parenchymal CT findings. Radiology. 1990;175(3):711–4.
9. Kennedy CA, Goetz MB. Atypical roentgenographic manifestations of Pneumocystis carinii pneumonia. Arch Intern Med. 1992;152(7):1390–8.
10. Gurney JW, Conces DJ. Pulmonary histoplasmosis. Radiology. 1996;199(2):297–306.
11. Travis WD, Pittaluga S, Lipschik GY, Ognibene FP, Suffredini AF, Masur H, et al. Atypical pathologic manifestations of Pneumocystis carinii pneumonia in the acquired immune deficiency syndrome. Review of 123 lung biopsies from 76 patients with emphasis on cysts, vascular invasion, vasculitis, and granulomas. Am J Surg Pathol. 1990;14(7):615–25.
12. Wilson JW, Limper AH, Grys TE, Karre T, Wengenack NL, Binnicker MJ. Pneumocystis jirovecii testing by real-time polymerase chain reaction and direct examination among immunocompetent and immunosuppressed patient groups and correlation to disease specificity. Diagn Microbiol Infect Dis. 2011;69(2):145–52.
13. Church DL, Ambasta A, Wilmer A, Williscroft H, Ritchie G, Pillai DR, et al. Development and validation of a Pneumocystis jirovecii real-time polymerase chain reaction assay for diagnosis of Pneumocystis pneumonia. Can J Infect Dis Med Microbiol. 2015;26(5):263–7.
14. Gomez CA, Budvytiene I, Zemek AJ, Banaei N. Performance of targeted fungal sequencing for culture-independent diagnosis of invasive fungal disease. Clin Infect Dis. 2017;65(12):2035–41.
15. Choe PG, Kang YM, Kim G, Park WB, Park SW, Kim HB, et al. Diagnostic value of direct fluorescence antibody staining for detecting Pneumocystis jirovecii in expectorated sputum from patients with HIV infection. Med Mycol. 2014;52(3):326–30.

The Differential Diagnosis of Invasive Mold Infections in the Lung

54

James A. Mays and Joshua A. Lieberman

Case Presentation

A 51-year-old woman with a past medical history of lymphangioleiomyomatosis, status post bilateral orthotopic lung transplant 3 years earlier and complicated by chronic lung allograft dysfunction, presented to the intensive care unit with increasing dyspnea and oxygen requirement. She had multiple prior hospitalizations in the previous 3 months, and the clinical team judged her dyspnea to be predominantly due to progression of chronic lung rejection. Although not currently febrile, she had persistent leukocytosis since admission, and her chronic immunosuppression put her at high risk of opportunistic lung infection. A computed tomography (CT) scan with contrast (Fig. 54.1) showed previously known bilateral upper lobe bronchiectasis, scarring, and cystic changes, in addition to newly found right upper lobe consolidation, bilateral patchy ground-glass opacities, and a fluid-filled bulla in the right upper lobe, raising concern for a cavitary lung lesion. Fungal cultures of sputum failed to grow fungal pathogens, but clinical suspicion for fungal infection was nonetheless high. Her empiric antifungal coverage, voriconazole, did not cover some potential pathogens including some species of Zygomycetes.

The patient received a second lung transplant due to her refractory dyspnea and oxygen requirements. On gross examination, both explanted lungs contained multiple patchy areas of firm yellow-white discoloration. The right upper lobe has a 5.0 cm tan-white, circumscribed area with central necrosis and purulent material; fungal culture of the explanted lungs grew *Aspergillus fumigatus* species. On microscopic examination, the right lung showed marked mixed inflammation, abscess formation, and scattered branching septate fungal hyphae without angioinvasion (Fig. 54.2a). The patient completes a 3-month course of voriconazole without recurrence of *Aspergillus* in her new allograft lungs.

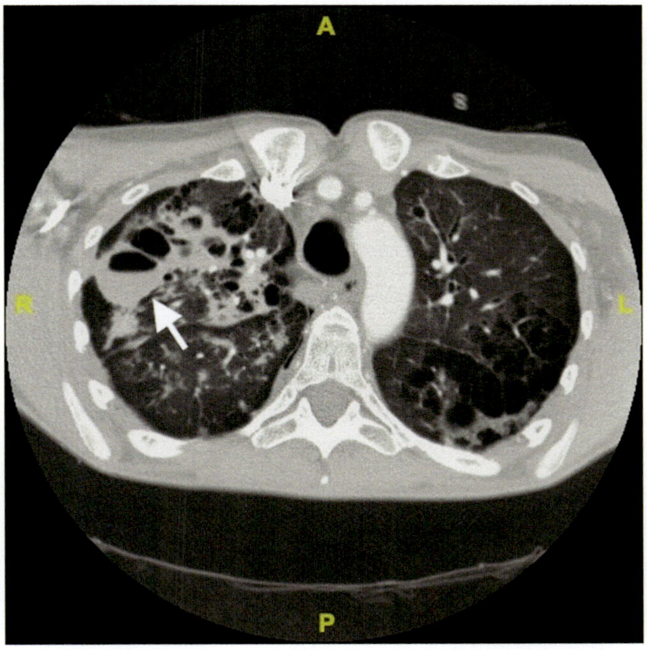

Fig. 54.1 CT scan showing bronchiectasis, scarring, and cystic changes (posterior left lung). Other findings included bilateral patchy ground-glass opacities and a fluid-filled bulla in the right upper lobe concerning for a cavitary lung lesion (arrow)

J. A. Mays
Department of Laboratory Medicine and Pathology, University of Washington Medical Center, Seattle, WA, USA

Department of Pathology, Massachusetts General Hospital, Boston, MA, USA
e-mail: jamays@mgh.harvard.edu

J. A. Lieberman (✉)
Department of Laboratory Medicine and Pathology, University of Washington Medical Center, Seattle, WA, USA
e-mail: joshuaal@uw.edu

H. Xu et al. (eds.), *Practical Lung Pathology*, Practical Anatomic Pathology, https://doi.org/10.1007/978-3-031-14402-8_54

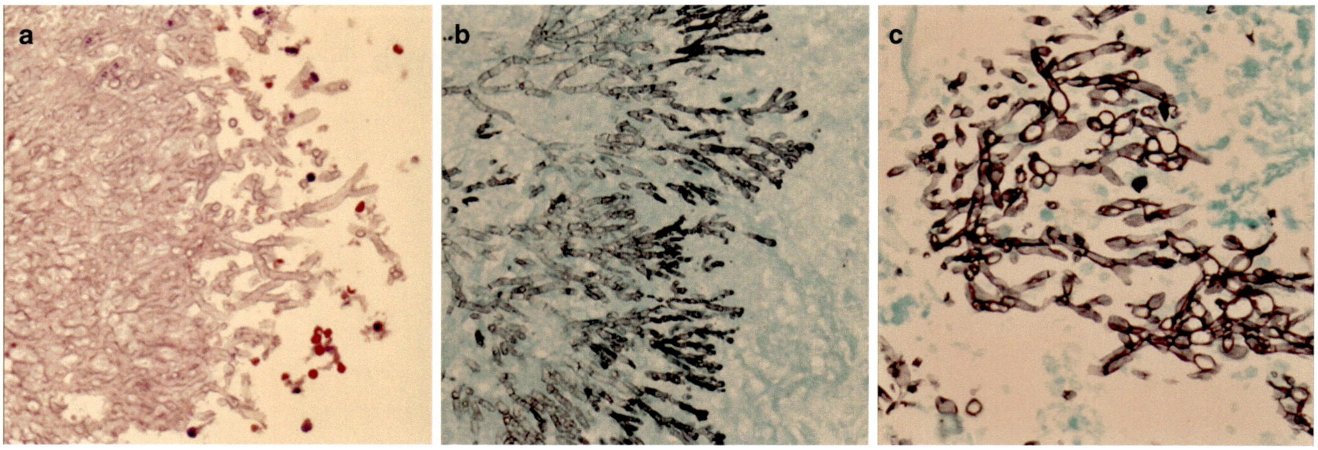

Fig. 54.2 (**a**) Dense colony of *Aspergillus* spp. in an aspergilloma. On the periphery of the colony, septate hyphae with acute-angle branching can be identified. Less characteristic forms are present in the center of the lesion (left), highlighting the concept that different growth conditions will affect the morphology of a given fungus. (**b**) GMS stain of *Aspergillus* spp. Regular, septate hyphae with acute-angle, "militaristic" branching. The organism was identified as *Aspergillus fumigatus* by PCR on a BAL specimen. (**c**) GMS stain of *Aspergillus* spp. Swollen, globose varieties can be present, as can degenerated atypical forms in lesions exposed to antifungal therapy. The organism was identified as *Aspergillus fumigatus* by PCR on a BAL specimen

Final Diagnosis

Septate, hyaline (nonpigmented), hyphae present; see Comment.

Comment: Histopathology is not specific for mold identification. The findings are consistent with a variety of molds, including *Aspergillus* spp., *Fusarium* spp., *Scedosporium* spp., and *Paecilomyces* spp. The absence of visible pigment makes dematiaceous molds less likely. Correlation with microbiology studies is necessary for definitive classification.

Clinical Considerations

Identification of fungi in tissue is a challenging histopathologic problem. While not all fungal processes in respiratory sites are invasive, invasive fungal disease (IFD) is a potentially fatal complication for immunosuppressed patients, particularly neutropenic patients (e.g., hematopoietic stem cell transplant, HSCT) and should be treated as a critical result. The primary role of the histopathologist is to (1) identify whether fungal organisms are present and to report if tissue invasion and/or angioinvasion are observed; (2) classify the fungal forms (Table 54.1); and (3) ensure that appropriate microbiologic cultures or molecular diagnostic assays are performed with haste, as prompt treatment reduces mor-

Table 54.1 Reporting descriptive categories for fungal hyphae observed in tissue is considered best practice given the similarities of many fungal pathogens. Adapted from Guarner J, Brandt ME. Histopathologic diagnosis of fungal infections in the twenty-first century. Clin Microbiol Rev. 2011 Apr;24(2):247–80 [1]

Morphology	Description, diagnostic category, and comment
Hyaline septate hyphae:	Description: Nonpigmented, septate hyphae with acute angle branching
Aspergillus spp., *Fusarium* spp., *Scedosporium* spp., et al.	Diagnosis: "Nonpigmented, septate hyphae"
	Differential: Morphology consistent with *Aspergillus* species and others. If chlamydoconidia present, consider leading the differential diagnosis with *Fusarium* and including *Scedosporium* and *Lomentospora*. Also consider careful examination for pigment. Mucorales can sometimes have occasional septations
Hyaline pauciseptate hyphae	Description: Nonpigmented, pauci-septate hyphae right angle branching
Mucorales genera	Diagnosis: "Nonpigmented pauci-septate hyphae"
	Differential: Consistent with Mucorales genera; however, *Aspergillus* spp. and other hyaline septate molds can sometimes have this morphology
Pigmented hyphae:	Description: Pigmented irregular septate hyphae and yeast-like structures
Dematiaceous fungi, e.g., *Alternaria*, *Madurella*, *Fonsecaea*, and *Phialophora*	Diagnosis: Pigmented yeasts and hyphae with septations
	Differential: Consistent with dematiaceous fungi

tality [2]. It is important to remember that histopathological identification of molds has a diagnostic error rate of at least 20% [3–5], even to the level of genus and within "*Aspergillus*-like" organisms [4]. Therefore, organism identification should not be attempted but rather pathogens categorized into broad groups based on published guidelines [1] (see also Table 54.1).

The genus *Aspergillus* is large and contains multiple sections—a phylogenetic division between genus and species—including sections Fumigati, Terrei, Usti, Nigri, Flavi, Terrei, and others [6] within which important treatment differences exist [6, 7]. Initial treatment with triazole antifungal agents such as voriconazole improves survival in *Aspergillus* infections [8]. The members of the genus *Aspergillus* are histopathologically classified as nonpigmented (hyaline), septate molds and should be reported as part of this broad grouping [1]. The term hyalohyphomycosis describes infection with a nonpigmented (hyalo-) mold (hypho-), as opposed to a phaeohyphomycosis which refers to pigmented mold infections [9]. Within this broad group, comprising not only *Aspergillus* but also other common pathogens, a few gross and microscopic features may suggest an *Aspergillus* or another hyalohyphomycotic pathogen.

The Zygomycota are a diverse mixture including several pathogenic genera that represent a broad section of relatively ancient organisms (800 million years since divergence) within the kingdom fungi [10]. Unlike *Aspergillus* spp., liposomal amphotericin B is the mainstay of therapy [2]. Genera within this group that are pathogenic to humans include *Mucor*, *Rhizomucor*, *Rhizopus*, *Cunninghamella*, *Lichtheimia*, and others [11]. Similar to *Aspergillus*, these organisms do not produce melanin and are thus nonpigmented molds. There, however, the similarities stop: the key histopathologic feature uniting this group is the paucity of hyphal septations.

Immunosuppressed patients are most at risk of IFD, particularly HSCT patients, for whom the incidence of IFD ranges from 5.8% to 8.1% of recipients of non-autologous transplants [12]. In addition, otherwise immunocompetent patients with traumatic injuries, including combat wounds, burns, and environmental exposures, are also at risk. Diabetic patients are also at increased risk for zygomycete infections [11].

The distribution of fungal pathogens varies by practice location. For example, in Western Europe, *Aspergillus* spp. are frequent pathogens, constituting 40–60% of invasive mold infections in some studies [13]. In the Northwest United States, *Aspergillus* spp. represent ~27% of fungi identified in the nasopharynx, and *A. fumigatus* represents 11–18% of pulmonary and sinus infections [14]. At our institution, polyfungal infections were identified in ~16% of sinonasal samples [14]. In our local datasets, two common histopathologic mimics of *Aspergillus* spp.—*Fusarium* and *Pseudallescheria*/*Scedosporium*—accounted for 8–18% of samples, while Zygomycota represented 6–15%. A large multisite study from 23 centers across the United States identified that 43% of IFD cases were due to any *Aspergillus* spp. and 8% attributed to Zygomycota [12].

The diagnosis of zygomycosis is often difficult to establish. Culture is negative in at least 50% of cases, even when hyphae are observed by histopathology [11, 15] and even angioinvasive cases essentially never yield positive blood cultures [16]. Serologic assays and antibodies for immunohistochemistry are not specific, and DNA hybridization (ISH/FISH) assays are limited to experimental use [16]. While liposomal amphotericin B is the initial treatment of choice, some of these organisms (e.g., *Rhizopus*, *Cunninghamella*) have elevated minimum inhibitory concentrations [11, 16]. Therefore, definitive organism identification helps guide clinical decision-making, similar to the case of hyalohyphomycoses.

Radiologic Features

The European Organization for Research and Treatment of Cancer and the National Institute of Allergy and Infectious Disease Mycoses Study Group (EORTC/MSG) have released definitions for establishing a diagnosis of proven, probable, and possible IFD. Probable IFD requires the presence of a host factor (i.e., immunosuppression), a mycological criterion (e.g., culture or microscopic detection), and a clinical criterion [17]. In the case of lower respiratory tract disease, this clinical criterion is usually fulfilled by the presence of one of three findings on CT scan: dense, well-circumscribed lesion(s) with or without a halo sign, an air-crescent sign, or the presence of a cavity. The "halo sign" is a region of ground-glass attenuation surrounding a pulmonary nodule, whereas an "air-crescent sign" contains a radio-opaque mass surrounded by a crescentic and radiolucent cavity, classically associated with aspergilloma. Most immunocompromised patients with invasive pulmonary aspergillosis do not have diffuse infiltrates and rather have focal ones, which are frequently associated with at least one micronodule [7]. Invasive fungal infections can also appear on imaging as lobar or segmental consolidation or wedge-shaped infiltrates. As imaging findings are only one criterion in making a diagnosis of probable invasive fungal disease, none of these signs are by themselves pathognomonic. Similarly, once a presumptive clinical diagnosis of invasive fungal disease is made, no radiological findings are sufficiently specific to rule out one fungal pathogen versus another.

Histologic Features

There are multiple clinical presentations of aspergillosis, including an allergic process, colonization of preexisting cavities (aspergilloma), chronic necrotizing bronchial aspergillosis, chronic necrotizing pulmonary aspergillosis, and an invasive pulmonary aspergillosis. Therefore, the microbiologic detection of *Aspergillus* in an immunocompromised patient does not indicate severe invasive disease. Histologic findings of angioinvasion and infarction indicate invasive pulmonary aspergillosis and have important clinical ramifications which should be communicated to the treating physician.

The histologic diagnosis of aspergillosis depends on the identification of *Aspergillus* hyphae with characteristic appearance; these hyphae are 3–6 μm in width, uniform in shape, septate, and hyaline, with parallel walls with acute angle branching from the parent hypha in a progressive and dichotomous fashion [4]. The hyphae are visible on H&E but are better seen with a GMS or PAS stain (Fig. 54.2b). *Aspergillus* can exhibit atypical or degenerative features under varying circumstances; in aspergillomas, they may form swollen, globose or varicose forms with hyphal diameters of up to 15 μm (Fig. 54.2c). Polarizable calcium oxalate crystals are frequently seen in aspergillus infection [18, 19], particularly in association with *Aspergillus niger* [18]. Microscopically, the hallmark of invasive pulmonary aspergillosis is hyphal invasion of the arteries and veins causing a nodular pulmonary infarct. An occluded or necrotic artery can frequently be identified in association with these lesions. The feature, however, is not specific for invasive pulmonary aspergillosis and may be seen with other angioinvasive opportunistic mycoses. The histologic differential diagnosis for *Aspergillus* includes *Fusarium* spp. and *Scedosporium apiospermum*/*Pseudallescheria boydii*, both being septate hyphae that can cause both angioinvasive pulmonary infection and fungus balls, as well as Zygomycetes.

The clinical presentation of zygomycosis can be similar to angioinvasive aspergillosis, and there is overlap in the defining pathologic process: aggressive invasive hyphae that penetrate bronchial walls, grow into adjacent blood vessels, and cause thrombosis of blood vessels and infarction and hemorrhage in the surrounding lung parenchyma. This can be seen either in the hilar region or the periphery of the lung. Microscopically, this appears as hemorrhagic or nodular infarcts and suppurative pneumonitis. Zygomycetes can also track along nerve fibers; this neurotropism impedes effective surgical control of the infection. Fungal hyphae will be most conspicuous in the walls of blood vessels and in vessel thrombi. The hyphae are pleomorphic and broad (6–25 μm) with thick walls; they branch at various angles, including 90°; and rare septa may be present [20, 21]. The hyphae often have a folded, irregular appearance with uneven contours and width (Fig. 54.3). The branching pattern is irregular and frequently at a much wider angle than *Aspergillus* species. The hyphae are visible on both H&E and GMS stain, but the intensity of silver staining is often less than in *Aspergillus* [20]. Occasional thick-walled, round chlamydoconidia and sporangia may be found in combination with the invasive hyphae. The presence of chlamydoconidia, while arguing against *Aspergillus* spp., does not constitute a diagnosis of Zygomycosis; both *Scedosporium apiospermum* and *Fusarium* spp. can also form similar these asexual reproductive structures. *Aspergillus* hyphae are narrower, more regularly septate, and have a more orderly and dichotomous branching pattern than Zygomycetes hyphae. However, mimics of characteristic *Aspergillus* hyphal morphology and branching pattern exist (e.g., Fig. 54.4), and caution is warranted even in cases with characteristic morphology.

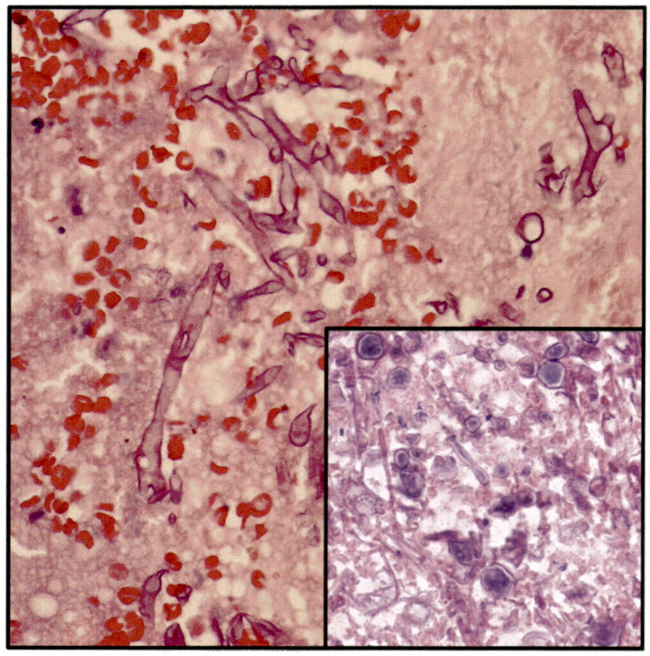

Fig. 54.3 H&E stain. Members of the order Mucorales have wide, irregular, pauciseptate hyphae. Inset: Large, round pseudochlamydoconidia/chlamydoconidia are present; these should not be confused with yeast which are generally smaller and more regular and do not produce broad, pauciseptate hyphae. This organism was identified as *Mucor* spp. by PCR on a tissue specimen

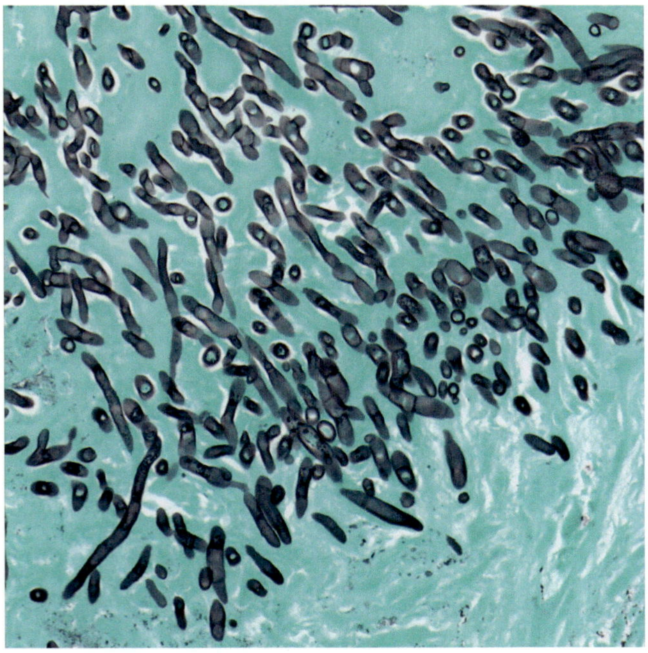

Fig. 54.4 GMS stain of *Alternaria* spp. with narrow septate hyphae with areas of acute angle branching and "militaristic" radial growth giving a low-power impression of *Aspergillus* spp. However, the presence of irregular swellings (chlamydoconidia), faint melanin deposition, and a single "copper penny" (sclerotic) body strongly suggested a dematiaceous mold. A Fontana-Masson stain would highlight melanin pigment in a dematiaceous mold such as this one. The pathogen was identified by broad-range fungal PCR

Immunophenotypic Features

Immunohistochemistry is not routinely available for fungus. Although both polyclonal and monoclonal antibodies are commercially available for aspergilli, the specificity and sensitivity depend upon the antibody [22, 23]. In situ hybridization (ISH) has demonstrated relatively high specificity in distinguishing *Aspergillus* spp. from other hyaline molds such as *Fusarium* spp., *Pseudallescheria boydii* [24, 25], and Zygomycetes [26]. However, ISH has not been widely adopted.

Special Stains

General hyalohyphomycoses stain well with H&E, GMS, and often PAS. Zygomycoses take up stain less reliably. Histopathology lore teaches that PAS is better than GMS for staining zygomycoses; however, while staining with both GMS and PAS may be weak [20], to our knowledge, there is no published evidence demonstrating superiority of either stain.

Approximately 60–70% of dematiaceous molds have melanized cell walls that are best visualized with Fontana-Masson and are more likely to stain strongly for melanin than other molds [27]. However, 40–50% of hyaline molds including *Aspergillus* spp. and *Fusarium* spp. are also positive for cell wall melanin [27]. At least 50% of zygomycetes stain positive for melanin [27, 28].

Molecular Features

Molecular methods for the identification of pathogenic fungi have emerged as essential diagnostic tools from a variety of substrates, including FFPE. Furthermore, data from our institution suggest that histopathologist-selected FFPE blocks as likely to yield an organism identification by PCR than fresh tissue [14]. The available molecular tools include both targeted PCR assays for single organisms such as *A. fumigatus*-specific PCR [29] and broad-range fungal detection [30, 31]. These assays typically amplify genomic DNA within the ribosomal locus, such as 28S or the internal tandem spacer (ITS) regions. Identification is possible due to species-specific differences in the DNA sequence, which are identified either in a second-round (nested) PCR reaction for single-target assays or by amplifying high-diversity regions flanked by conserved, pan-fungal primer binding sites.

While molecular results have not been adopted as diagnostic criteria by the EORTC/MSG due to lack of standardization across diagnostic platforms, the reported sensitivities and specificities are quite high. Sensitivities have been reported as high as 90% in FFPE and >96% for all specimen types compared to culture, with an overall diagnostic yield of 62.9% [31]. The volume of tissue submitted for DNA isolation appears to be an important predictor of diagnostic yield [31]. Assay specificity ranges from 96.4% to >99% and is derived from species-intrinsic sequence variation [30, 31]. Molecular assays are thus critical tools in making a diagnosis of IFD when microbial culture is negative or unavailable.

Key Points for Differentiating Zygomycosis from Hyalohyphomycosis

What Are the Key Morphologic Features that Distinguish Zygomycetes (Mucorales) from Molds Like *Aspergillus* spp.?

IFD is a potentially fatal infection primarily of severely immunocompromised patients. Distinguishing Mucorales is critical as these organisms are treated with liposomal amphotericin B, while most hyaline and dematiaceous molds are treated with triazoles such as voriconazole. The key features of Zygomycota include rare or absent hyphal septa and broad, ribbon-like hyphae. Both hyaline molds like *Aspergillus* spp. and dematiaceous molds produce septate hyphae. Members of the genera *Aspergillus* and *Mucor* are important pathogens that represent two main organism groupings best described as "septate, nonpigmented molds" or "pauciseptate, nonpigmented molds" respectively.

What Are Important Pitfalls in Distinguishing Zygomycetes (Mucorales) from Molds Like *Aspergillus* spp.?

Recent or concurrent antifungal therapy, necrosis/degradation of fungal hyphae, and natural variation in morphology are all important confounders that may lead to atypical morphology. Large, globose, and irregular forms may occur with hyphae of both organisms and typically represent conidia. To avoid confusion with yeasts, size measurements may be helpful (see Chap. 52).

How Reliable Is the Identification of Fungal Hyphae in Tissue?

Recognition of the presence of hyphae is important as it may guide surgical management and should prompt submission of a specimen for culture. Similarly, identification of any Mucorales member justifies treatment with amphotericin B. However, identification beyond broad categories (Table 54.1; see also [1]) is strongly discouraged as many species of fungi may be pathogenic, and the treatment is based on definitive organism identification by culture or molecular identification. Histopathologic identification beyond broad groups is highly error prone, on the order of 20%. The presence of mid-hyphal swellings (chlamydoconidia) in septate molds should prompt consideration of organisms other than *Aspergillus* spp., such as *Fusarium* spp., *Alternaria* spp., *Scedosporium* spp., among others.

What Is the Role of Frozen Section in Evaluating for Invasive Fungal Disease?

In addition to identifying whether a mold is present and, if the histology is sufficiently clear, determining whether the hyphae if are pauci/aseptate (mucormycosis), frozen section offers an important opportunity for the pathologist to "triage" tissue for downstream studies. The pathologist should encourage the surgeon to submit aseptically collected tissue for culture and/or fungal PCR from an area where fungus was identified by frozen histopathology. Alternatively, most microbiology labs can quickly inoculate a fungal culture and then return tissue to the pathology lab for gross evaluation, fixation, and tissue processing.

What Are the Next Steps Beyond Histology for the Characterization of Molds?

Culture is essential, particularly as successful microbial growth allows phenotypic antifungal susceptibility testing. In addition, molecular assays are key methods for organism identification in IFD and readily applied to both fresh and formalin-fixed tissue, as well as body fluids. Molecular methods are especially relevant to Mucorales, which may not grow if damaged by tissue processing for culture or when the diagnosis of fungal infection was not suspected and thus tissue was not submitted for culture.

References

1. Guarner J, Brandt ME. Histopathologic diagnosis of fungal infections in the 21st century. Clin Microbiol Rev. 2011;24(2):247–80.
2. Chamilos G, Lewis RE, Kontoyiannis DP. Delaying amphotericin B-based frontline therapy significantly increases mortality among patients with hematologic malignancy who have zygomycosis. Clin Infect Dis. 2008;47(4):503–9.
3. Sangoi AR, Rogers WM, Longacre TA, Montoya JG, Baron EJ, Banaei N. Challenges and pitfalls of morphologic identification of fungal infections in histologic and cytologic specimens. Am J Clin Pathol. 2009;131(3):364.
4. Shah AA, Hazen KC. Diagnostic accuracy of histopathologic and cytopathologic examination of Aspergillus species. Am J Clin Pathol. 2013;139(1):55–61.
5. Challa S, Pamidi U, Uppin SG, Uppin MS, Vemu L. Diagnostic accuracy of morphologic identification of filamentous fungi in paraffin embedded tissue sections: correlation of histological and culture diagnosis. Indian J Pathol Microbiol. 2014;57(4):583–7.
6. Van Der Linden JWM, Warris A, Verweij PE. Aspergillus species intrinsically resistant to antifungal agents. Med Mycol. 2011;49(Suppl 1):S82–9.
7. Sabino R, Carolino E, Veríssimo C, Martinez M, Clemons KV, Stevens DA. Antifungal susceptibility of 175 Aspergillus isolates from various clinical and environmental sources. Med Mycol. 2016;54(7):740–56.
8. Herbrecht R, Denning DW, Patterson TF, Bennett JE, Greene RE, Oestmann J-W, et al. Voriconazole versus amphotericin B for primary therapy of invasive aspergillosis. N Engl J Med. 2002;347(6):408–15.
9. Wong EH, Revankar SG. Dematiaceous molds. Infect Dis Clin N Am. 2016;30(1):165–78.
10. Muszewska A, Pawłowska J, Krzyściak P. Biology, systematics, and clinical manifestations of Zygomycota infections. Eur J Clin Microbiol Infect Dis. 2014;33(8):1273–87.
11. Skiada A, Lass-Floerl C, Klimko N, Ibrahim A, Roilides E, Petrikkos G. Challenges in the diagnosis and treatment of mucormycosis. Med Mycol. 2018;56(Suppl 1):93–101.
12. Kontoyiannis DP, Marr KA, Park BJ, Alexander BD, Anaissie EJ, Walsh TJ, et al. Prospective surveillance for invasive fungal infections in hematopoietic stem cell transplant recipients, 2001-2006: overview of the Transplant-Associated Infection Surveillance Network (TRANSNET) Database. Clin Infect Dis. 2010;50(8):1091–100.
13. Kuster S, Stampf S, Gerber B, Baettig V, Weisser M, Gerull S, et al. Incidence and outcome of invasive fungal diseases after allogeneic hematopoietic stem cell transplantation: a Swiss transplant cohort study. Transpl Infect Dis. 2018;20(6):e12981.

14. Lieberman JA, Bryan A, Mays JA, Stephens K, Kurosawa K, Mathias PC, et al. High clinical impact of broad-range fungal PCR in suspected fungal sinusitis. J Clin Microbiol. 2021;59(11) e0095521. https://doi.org/10.1128/JCM.00955-21.
15. Parfrey NA. Improved diagnosis and prognosis of mucormycosis. A clinicopathologic study of 33 cases. Medicine (Baltimore). 1986;65(2):113–23.
16. Walsh TJ, Gamaletsou MN, McGinnis MR, Hayden RT, Kontoyiannis DP. Early clinical and laboratory diagnosis of invasive pulmonary, extrapulmonary, and disseminated mucormycosis (zygomycosis). Clin Infect Dis. 2012;54(Suppl 1):S55–60.
17. De Pauw B, Walsh TJ, Donnelly JP, Stevens DA, Edwards JE, Calandra T, et al. Revised definitions of invasive fungal disease from the European Organization for Research and Treatment of Cancer/Invasive Fungal Infections Cooperative Group and the National Institute of Allergy and Infectious Diseases Mycoses Study Group (EORTC/MSG) Consensus Group. Clin Infect Dis. 2008;46(12):1813–21.
18. Farley ML, Mabry L, Muñoz LA, Diserens HW. Crystals occurring in pulmonary cytology specimens. Association with Aspergillus infection. Acta Cytol. 1985;29(5):737–44.
19. Payne SJ, Mitzner R, Kunchala S, Roland L, McGinn JD. Acute invasive fungal rhinosinusitis: a 15-year experience with 41 patients. Otolaryngol Head Neck Surg. 2016;154(4):759–64.
20. Ribes JA, Vanover-Sams CL, Baker DJ. Zygomycetes in human disease. Clin Microbiol Rev. 2000;13(2):236.
21. Lass-Flörl C. Zygomycosis: conventional laboratory diagnosis. Clin Microbiol Infect. 2009;15(Suppl 5):60–5.
22. Challa S, Uppin SG, Uppin MS, Pamidimukkala U, Vemu L. Diagnosis of filamentous fungi on tissue sections by immunohistochemistry using anti-aspergillus antibody. Med Mycol. 2015;53(5):470–6.
23. Schuetz AN, Cohen C. Aspergillus immunohistochemistry of culture-proven fungal tissue isolates shows high cross-reactivity. Appl Immunohistochem Mol Morphol. 2009;17(6):524–9.
24. Montone KT. Differentiation of fusarium from Aspergillus species by colorimetric in situ hybridization in formalin-fixed, paraffin-embedded tissue sections using dual fluorogenic-labeled LNA probes. Am J Clin Pathol. 2009;132(6):866–70.
25. Hayden RT, Isotalo PA, Parrett T, Wolk DM, Qian X, Roberts GD, et al. In situ hybridization for the differentiation of Aspergillus, Fusarium, and Pseudallescheria species in tissue section. Diagn Mol Pathol. 2003;12(1):21–6.
26. Hayden RT, Qian X, Procop GW, Roberts GD, Lloyd RV. In situ hybridization for the identification of filamentous fungi in tissue section. Diagn Mol Pathol. 2002;11(2):119–26.
27. West KL, Proia AD, Puri PK. Fontana-Masson stain in fungal infections. J Am Acad Dermatol. 2017;77(6):1119–25.
28. Sundaram C, Shantveer GU, Umabala P, Lakshmi V. Diagnostic utility of melanin production by fungi: study on tissue sections and culture smears with Masson-Fontana stain. Indian J Pathol Microbiol. 2014;57(2):217–22.
29. Avni T, Levy I, Sprecher H, Yahav D, Leibovici L, Paul M. Diagnostic accuracy of PCR alone compared to galactomannan in bronchoalveolar lavage fluid for diagnosis of invasive pulmonary aspergillosis: a systematic review. J Clin Microbiol. 2012;50(11):3652–8.
30. Rakeman JL, Bui U, Lafe K, Chen Y-C, Honeycutt RJ, Cookson BT. Multilocus DNA sequence comparisons rapidly identify pathogenic molds. J Clin Microbiol. 2005;43(7):3324–33.
31. Gomez CA, Budvytiene I, Zemek AJ, Banaei N. Performance of targeted fungal sequencing for culture-independent diagnosis of invasive fungal disease. Clin Infect Dis. 2017;65(12):2035–41.

Primary Pulmonary Arterial Hypertension Versus Secondary Pulmonary Hypertension

55

Jose G. Mantilla

Case Presentation

A 46-year-old nonsmoker man presents with a 10-year history of progressive dyspnea on exertion with an accelerated decline in the most recent months. At the time of evaluation, his activity is limited, and he requires supplementary oxygen at night. On physical examination, he appears ill, with bilateral edema of his legs. His oxygen saturation at rest is 80%. Auscultation demonstrates a systolic murmur. Echocardiogram shows a severely increased mean pressure in his pulmonary artery (109–114 mmHg; normal 8–20 mmHg). Pulmonary function testing, however, was normal. A chest computed tomography (CT) scan demonstrates enlarged and tortuous pulmonary arteries, and subtle mosaic attenuation of the lung parenchyma, with no significant interstitial fibrosis (Fig. 55.1).

Given the patient's clinical decline, he received a bilateral lung transplant. Histologic examination of the explanted lungs demonstrates marked arterial medial hypertrophy, concentric intimal thickening, and conspicuous plexiform and dilation lesions (Fig. 55.2). No parenchymal lung disease was identified. The overall histologic findings, in the absence of additional pulmonary disease, support the diagnosis of pulmonary arterial hypertension.

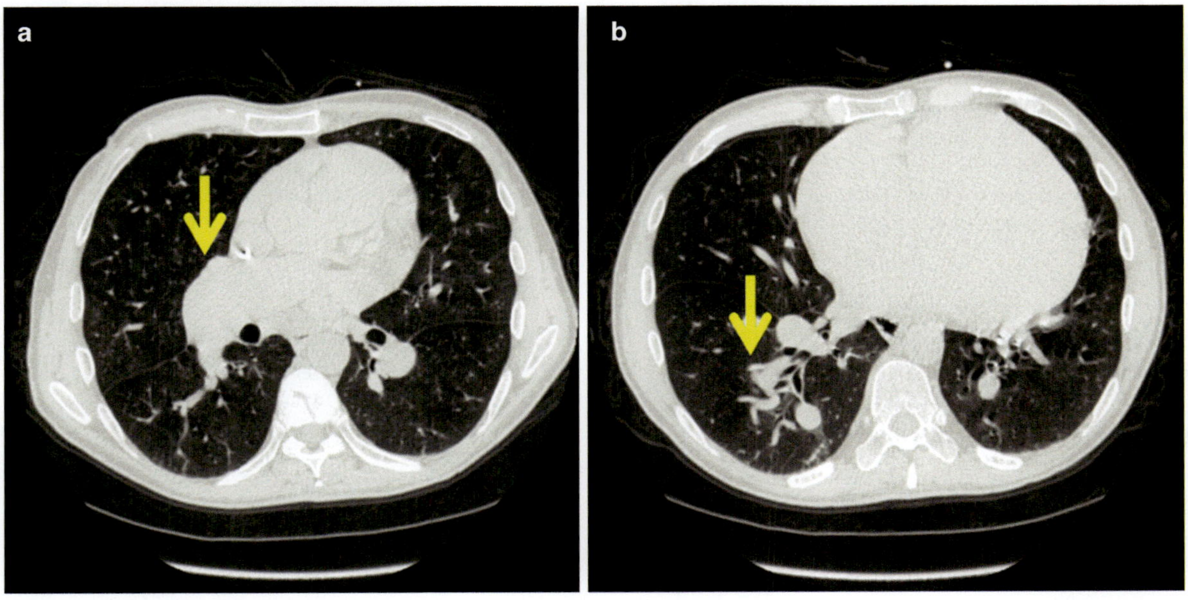

Fig. 55.1 CT features of pulmonary arterial hypertension. (**a**) Severe enlargement of the main pulmonary arteries. (**b**) Thickening and tortuosity of the distal arteries (arrow), as well as right ventricular enlargement. Notice the absence of significant underlying parenchymal lung disease

J. G. Mantilla (✉)
Department of Laboratory Medicine and Pathology, University of Washington Medical Center, Seattle, WA, USA
e-mail: mantilla@uw.edu

H. Xu et al. (eds.), *Practical Lung Pathology*, Practical Anatomic Pathology, https://doi.org/10.1007/978-3-031-14402-8_55

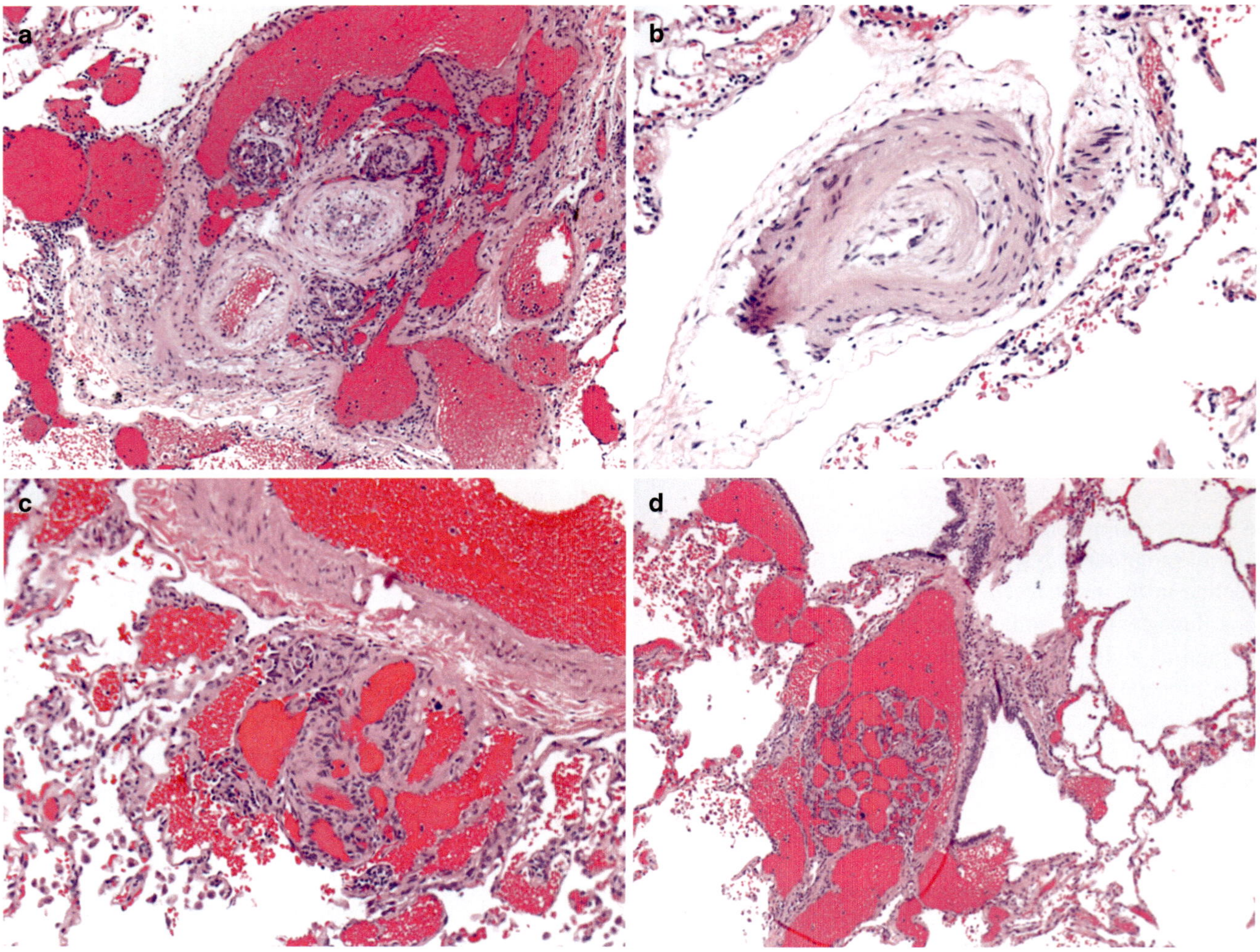

Fig. 55.2 Histologic changes in pulmonary arterial hypertension. (**a**) Typical changes of PAH include the concentric intimal hyperplasia, plexiform lesions, and dilatation lesions (H&E, 100×). (**b**) High-power view of a small artery with prominent concentrically intimal thickening (H&E, 200×). (**c**) High-power view of a plexiform lesion. These lesions are typically located adjacent to arteries and composed of proliferating vessels with a capillary-like architecture (H&E, 200×). (**d**) Dilatation lesions are characterized by aneurysm-like dilated arteries, usually located adjacent to plexiform lesions and/or thickened arteries. They can be associated with pulmonary hemorrhage (H&E, 100×)

Pathologic Diagnosis: Idiopathic Pulmonary Arterial Hypertension

What Is Pulmonary Hypertension?

Pulmonary hypertension is a heterogeneous clinical syndrome, defined by an elevated mean pulmonary artery pressure (≥25 mmHg), and measured at rest during right heart catheterization [1]. Clinical manifestations are nonspecific mostly related to right ventricular dysfunction. These typically include dyspnea on exertion, fatigue, weakness, angina, and syncope. In clinically severe disease, these symptoms may be seen at rest [1].

Which Etiologies Are Associated with Pulmonary Hypertension?

Pulmonary hypertension is a heterogeneous clinical syndrome with varied etiologies, which have been separated in five different groups by the World Health Organization [2] to include the following:

1. Pulmonary arterial hypertension: This includes idiopathic pulmonary arterial hypertension (IPAH), familial pulmonary hypertension (FPAH), and other etiologies discussed below.
2. Left heart disease: This group includes left ventricular diastolic and/or systolic dysfunction, valvular disease,

and other cardiomyopathies. This is the most common etiology of pulmonary hypertension, which is seen in 60–70% of patients with heart failure, as well as a large proportion of patients with valvular disease [3].

3. Lung disease and/or hypoxia: This group includes multiple pulmonary conditions, including chronic obstructive pulmonary disease (COPD), interstitial lung disease, sleep-disordered breathing, alveolar hypoventilation disorders, chronic exposure to high altitude, and developmental lung diseases.
4. Chronic thromboembolic pulmonary hypertension
5. Unclear/multifactorial mechanisms: These include pulmonary hypertension secondary to hematologic malignancies; metabolic disease (e.g., Gaucher's disease, glycogen storage diseases); systemic diseases, such as sarcoidosis and lymphangioleiomyomatosis; and other causes, such as fibrosing mediastinitis or obstruction of the pulmonary vasculature by tumors.

What Do We Understand About the Causes of Primary Pulmonary Arterial Hypertension?

Primary pulmonary arterial hypertension (PAH) is rare, with an estimated prevalence of 7–22 cases per million adults [3–5]. The causes of PAH can be varied, including idiopathic (IPAH), in a proportion ranging from 39% to 92% [4–7] of cases, familial disease (FPAH) in 4–5% [4–7], drug-related in 2–9.5% [4–6], and associated with collagen vascular disease in up to 8% [8]. Other causes include portal hypertension, left-to-right circulatory shunts, and in association with human immunodeficiency virus (HIV).

Mutations in multiple different genes have been implicated in FPAH, the most common of which is the bone morphogenetic protein receptor type 2 (*BMPR2*). Heterozygous mutations in this gene have been described in 50–70% of cases of FPAH, with an autosomal dominant pattern of inheritance, and in 10–40% of cases of IPAH [9]. Patients with mutations in this gene have shown to have a younger age at presentation and more severe disease, compared to patients without it [10]. Other genes less commonly implicated in FPAH include *KCNK3* encoding TASK-1 potassium channel [11] and *ABCC8* encoding the SUR1-a K_{ATP} channel subunit [12]. Mutations in other genes associated with PAH include *ACVRL1*, *ENG*, *CAV1*, and *TBX4* [13].

The connective tissue diseases associated with PAH include most commonly systemic sclerosis, where PAH has been described in 10–12% of patients [8, 14, 15], as well as systemic lupus erythematosus [8, 16], Sjögren syndrome [17], and rarely in dermatomyositis and rheumatoid arthritis [14]. These patients have been shown to have worse clinical outcomes compared to those with IPAH [18].

Lastly, multiple drugs have been associated with the development of PAH, including cocaine, anorexigens such as aminorex, fenfluramine, benfluorex, and amphetamines, chemotherapeutic agents like dasatinib, and interferon alpha and beta [19, 20].

How Can Radiologic Studies Be Used to Diagnose and Classify Pulmonary Hypertension?

Although direct measuring of the main pulmonary artery pressure through right cardiac catheterization remains the gold standard in the diagnosis of pulmonary hypertension [1], multiple noninvasive techniques have been used to diagnose and classify pulmonary hypertension. Among these modalities, transthoracic echocardiography is widely used as an initial screening and evaluation method as well as to evaluate potential associated heart disease [1, 21].

CT imaging is useful, given the capacity to detect, in addition to pulmonary vascular changes, subjacent parenchymal lung disease (e.g., interstitial fibrosis, emphysema), or other intrathoracic lesions, allowing the identification of underlying etiologies [22]. Lastly, ventilation/perfusion (V/Q) scans are considered the preferred method for evaluation of chronic thromboembolic pulmonary hypertension, given its higher sensitivity to detect perfusion defects associated with thrombosis [1, 23].

Typical changes of pulmonary hypertension on routine chest X-rays include right atrial and right ventricular enlargement, as well as enlarged central pulmonary arteries with attenuation of the peripheral vasculature [24].

CT imaging typically demonstrates an increase in the diameter of pulmonary arteries compared to their neighboring airways. In this setting, a pulmonary trunk diameter equal or greater than 2.8 cm has a sensitivity of 69–87% and specificity of 89–100% in the diagnosis of pulmonary hypertension. An increase in the artery to bronchus ratio in at least three lobes has also been demonstrated to be a reliable diagnostic indicator of pulmonary hypertension [24]. Ground-glass opacities, with a predominantly centrilobular pattern, have also been described in up to 40% of patients with PAH [22].

Can Histologic Findings Help Distinguish Between Primary and Secondary Pulmonary Hypertension?

Some common histologic features are present in pulmonary hypertension, regardless of etiology. These include arterial intimal thickening, medial hypertrophy, pulmonary arterial dilation and atheromas, as well as right ventricular hypertrophy [25]. Findings more specific to pulmonary arterial hypertension comprise a spectrum of lesions that involve arteries, including concentric laminar intimal thickening, plexiform lesions, dilation lesions, arteritis, and fibrinoid necrosis (typically associated with severe disease) [25–27]. The morphologic features of these lesions are characterized in Fig. 55.2.

In the case of chronic thromboembolic pulmonary hypertension, the presence of complex lesions similar to those seen in PAH, including plexiform lesions, has been described in areas proximal to the thrombi [28, 29]. However, the presence of multiple intravascular thrombi with recanalization can help exclude primary causes of pulmonary hypertension.

In cases of pulmonary hypertension secondary to parenchymal diseases, it should be possible to identify the underlying disease in association with non-specific vascular changes, while primary cases of PAH often have no associated parenchymal disease. However, it is worth considering that PAH in the setting of collagen vascular disease can be accompanied by interstitial fibrosis in a subset of patients [8]. Ultimately, a thorough clinical and pathologic correlation is fundamental in the distinction between PAH and pulmonary hypertension secondary to other causes.

References

1. Hoeper MM, Bogaard HJ, Condliffe R, Frantz R, Khanna D, Kurzyna M, et al. Definitions and diagnosis of pulmonary hypertension. J Am Coll Cardiol. 2013;62(25 Suppl):D42–50.
2. Simonneau G, Gatzoulis MA, Adatia I, Celermajer D, Denton C, Ghofrani A, et al. Updated clinical classification of pulmonary hypertension. J Am Coll Cardiol. 2013;62(25 Suppl):D34–41.
3. Goldberg AB, Mazur W, Kalra DK. Pulmonary hypertension: diagnosis, imaging techniques, and novel therapies. Cardiovasc Diagn Ther. 2017;7(4):405–17.
4. Jansa P, Jarkovsky J, Al-Hiti H, Popelova J, Ambroz D, Zatocil T, et al. Epidemiology and long-term survival of pulmonary arterial hypertension in the Czech Republic: a retrospective analysis of a nationwide registry. BMC Pulm Med. 2014;14:45.
5. Ling Y, Johnson MK, Kiely DG, Condliffe R, Elliot CA, Gibbs JS, et al. Changing demographics, epidemiology, and survival of incident pulmonary arterial hypertension: results from the pulmonary hypertension registry of the United Kingdom and Ireland. Am J Respir Crit Care Med. 2012;186(8):790–6.
6. Humbert M, Sitbon O, Chaouat A, Bertocchi M, Habib G, Gressin V, et al. Pulmonary arterial hypertension in France: results from a national registry. Am J Respir Crit Care Med. 2006;173(9):1023–30.
7. Peacock AJ, Murphy NF, McMurray JJ, Caballero L, Stewart S. An epidemiological study of pulmonary arterial hypertension. Eur Respir J. 2007;30(1):104–9.
8. Kahler CM, Colleselli D. Pulmonary arterial hypertension (PAH) in connective tissue diseases. Rheumatology. 2006;45 Suppl 3:iii11–3.
9. Hong KH, Lee YJ, Lee E, Park SO, Han C, Beppu H, et al. Genetic ablation of the BMPR2 gene in pulmonary endothelium is sufficient to predispose to pulmonary arterial hypertension. Circulation. 2008;118(7):722–30.
10. Evans JD, Girerd B, Montani D, Wang XJ, Galie N, Austin ED, et al. BMPR2 mutations and survival in pulmonary arterial hypertension: an individual participant data meta-analysis. Lancet Respir Med. 2016;4(2):129–37.
11. Cunningham KP, Holden RG, Escribano-Subias P, Cogolludo A, Veale EL, Mathie A. Characterisation and regulation of wild type and mutant TASK-1 two pore domain potassium channels indicated in pulmonary arterial hypertension. J Physiol. 2019;597(4):1087–101.
12. Bohnen MS, Ma L, Zhu N, Qi H, McClenaghan C, Gonzaga-Jauregui C, et al. Loss-of-function ABCC8 mutations in pulmonary arterial hypertension. Circ Genom Precis Med. 2018;11(10):e002087.
13. Girerd B, Lau E, Montani D, Humbert M. Genetics of pulmonary hypertension in the clinic. Curr Opin Pulm Med. 2017;23(5):386–91.
14. Galie N, Manes A, Farahani KV, Pelino F, Palazzini M, Negro L, et al. Pulmonary arterial hypertension associated to connective tissue diseases. Lupus. 2005;14(9):713–7.
15. Young A, Nagaraja V, Basilious M, Habib M, Townsend W, Gladue H, et al. Update of screening and diagnostic modalities for connective tissue disease-associated pulmonary arterial hypertension. Semin Arthritis Rheum. 2019;48(6):1059–67.
16. Tanaka E, Harigai M, Tanaka M, Kawaguchi Y, Hara M, Kamatani N. Pulmonary hypertension in systemic lupus erythematosus: evaluation of clinical characteristics and response to immunosuppressive treatment. J Rheumatol. 2002;29(2):282–7.
17. Launay D, Hachulla E, Hatron PY, Jais X, Simonneau G, Humbert M. Pulmonary arterial hypertension: a rare complication of primary Sjogren syndrome: report of 9 new cases and review of the literature. Medicine. 2007;86(5):299–315.
18. Hassoun PM. Pulmonary arterial hypertension complicating connective tissue diseases. Sem Resp Crit Care Med. 2009;30(4):429–39.
19. Seferian A, Chaumais MC, Savale L, Gunther S, Tubert-Bitter P, Humbert M, et al. Drugs induced pulmonary arterial hypertension. Presse Med. 2013;42(9 Pt 2):e303–10.
20. Garg L, Akbar G, Agrawal S, Agarwal M, Khaddour L, Handa R, et al. Drug-induced pulmonary arterial hypertension: a review. Heart Fail Rev. 2017;22(3):289–97.
21. Rengier F, Melzig C, Derlin T, Marra AM, Vogel-Claussen J. Advanced imaging in pulmonary hypertension: emerging techniques and applications. Int J Card Imaging. 2019;35(8):1407–20.
22. Rajaram S, Swift AJ, Condliffe R, Johns C, Elliot CA, Hill C, et al. CT features of pulmonary arterial hypertension and its major subtypes: a systematic CT evaluation of 292 patients from the ASPIRE Registry. Thorax. 2015;70(4):382–7.
23. Ohira H, Beanlands RS, Davies RA, Mielniczuk L. The role of nuclear imaging in pulmonary hypertension. J Nucl Cardiol. 2015;22(1):141–57.
24. McCann C, Gopalan D, Sheares K, Screaton N. Imaging in pulmonary hypertension, part 1: clinical perspectives, classification, imaging techniques and imaging algorithm. Postgrad Med J. 2012;88(1039):271–9.
25. Pietra GG, Capron F, Stewart S, Leone O, Humbert M, Robbins IM, et al. Pathologic assessment of vasculopathies in pulmonary hypertension. J Am Coll Cardiol. 2004;43(12 Suppl S):25s–32s.
26. Tuder RM, Marecki JC, Richter A, Fijalkowska I, Flores S. Pathology of pulmonary hypertension. Clin Chest Med. 2007;28(1):23–42, vii.
27. Stewart S, Rassl D. Advances in the understanding and classification of pulmonary hypertension. Histopathology. 2009;54(1):104–16.
28. Piazza G, Goldhaber SZ. Chronic thromboembolic pulmonary hypertension. N Engl J Med. 2011;364(4):351–60.
29. Ackermann M, Gaumann A, Mentzer SJ, Hinrichs JB, Warnecke G, Hoeper MM, et al. Plexiform vasculopathy in chronic thromboembolic pulmonary hypertension. Am J Respir Crit Care Med. 2017;196(8):e48–51.

Pulmonary Capillary Hemangiomatosis Versus Congestion

56

Jose G. Mantilla

Case Presentation

A 50-year-old woman with a remote history of systemic lupus erythematosus presented with a 20-year history of progressively worsening dyspnea on exertion, associated with hypoxemia and a markedly decreased DLCO. An initial transthoracic echocardiogram demonstrated an elevated pulmonary artery pressure (90 mmHg), while CT imaging showed enlarged pulmonary arteries and diffuse patchy mosaic attenuation throughout the lungs (Fig. 56.1).

Initial treatment with pulmonary vasodilators showed no clinical improvement, and the patient ultimately received a lung transplant. Histologic examination of the explanted lungs demonstrated patchy areas of capillary proliferation, highlighted by a CD34 immunohistochemical stain (Fig. 56.2). These changes were accompanied by intimal thickening and medial hyperplasia of the pulmonary arterioles and focal chronic alveolar hemorrhage. Her final pathologic diagnosis was pulmonary capillary hemangiomatosis.

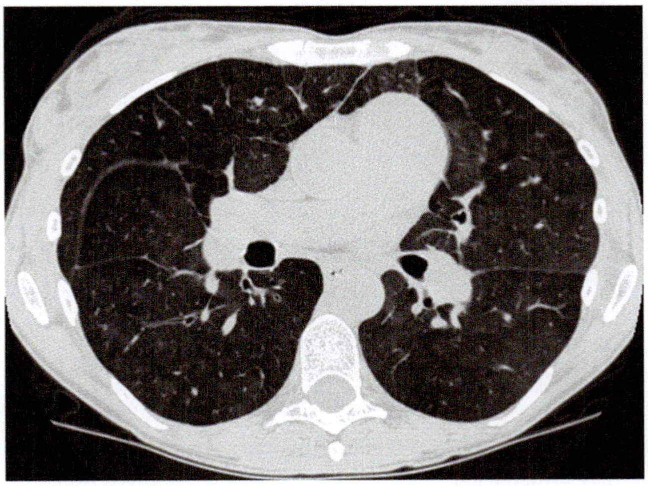

Fig. 56.1 CT imaging of a patient with pulmonary capillary hemangiomatosis, demonstrating bilateral patchy ground-glass opacities and enlargement of the main pulmonary artery, consistent with history of pulmonary hypertension

J. G. Mantilla (✉)
Department of Laboratory Medicine and Pathology, University of Washington Medical Center, Seattle, WA, USA
e-mail: mantilla@uw.edu

H. Xu et al. (eds.), *Practical Lung Pathology*, Practical Anatomic Pathology, https://doi.org/10.1007/978-3-031-14402-8_56

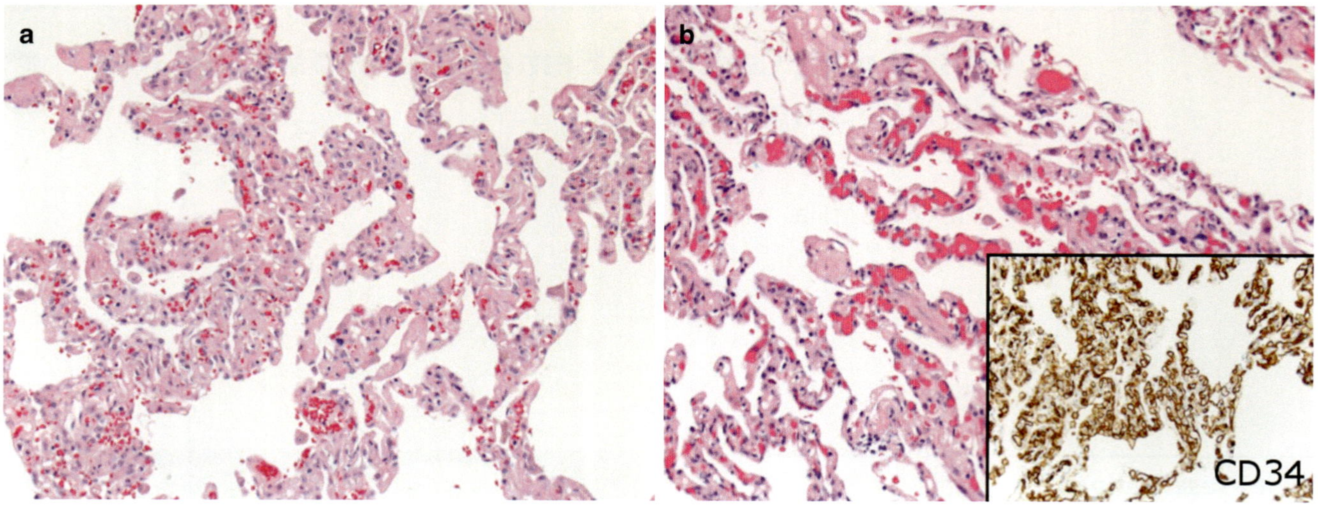

Fig. 56.2 Histologic appearance of pulmonary capillary hemangiomatosis, consisting of patchy areas of proliferating capillary vessels in the lung interstitium, forming multiple layers (**a**, **b**, H&E, 100× and 200×). The capillary endothelium is highlighted by a CD34 immunohistochemical stain (insert, IHC DAB, 100×)

Pathologic Diagnosis: Pulmonary Capillary Hemangiomatosis

What Is Pulmonary Capillary Hemangiomatosis?

Pulmonary capillary hemangiomatosis (PCH) is a rare and poorly understood cause of primary pulmonary hypertension [1]. Clinically, PCH presents with similar clinical symptoms as pulmonary arterial hypertension (PAH). It is commonly associated with hemoptysis and hemorrhagic pleural effusions [2] and often has an aggressive clinical course with limited response to medical therapy. Given the absence of adequate medical therapy, these patients often require lung or lung-heart transplantation.

Although the etiology of PCH has not been well defined, it has been observed in multiple settings, including pulmonary veno-occlusive disease (PVOD) [3], autoimmune diseases such systemic lupus erythematosus [4] and CREST syndrome [5], chemical exposures [2], and rare familial cases [6–8].

There is a significant overlap between PCH and PVOD, which has led to the consideration that these two entities represent different histologic findings of the same disease process. This is supported by the multiple similarities seen in the genetic, clinical, radiologic, and histologic presentation of these entities [2, 3].

On the other hand, PCH has also been postulated to represent a nonspecific reactive process in the setting of pulmonary hypertension [3], given the fact histologic findings of PCH have been reported in association with other entities such as autoimmune disease, hereditary hemorrhagic telangiectasia [9], and in the setting of congenital heart defects [10].

Are There Imaging Features Specific for PCH?

The typical imaging findings of PCH and PVOD are similar and not entirely specific; these include vascular signs of pulmonary hypertension, such as enlargement of the pulmonary arteries and right ventricular hypertrophy. Characteristic parenchymal findings include septal (Kerley B) lines and ground-glass opacities with diffuse, geographic, mosaic, perihilar, patchy, or centrilobular patterns [11–13]. Other findings described include enlarged mediastinal lymph nodes and pleural and/or pericardial effusions [11, 12].

How Can PCH be Histologically Distinguished from Vascular Congestion?

Histologically, PCH is characterized by the proliferation of capillary vessels involving the pulmonary interstitium, with at least two layers in thickness. This proliferation has a typically patchy distribution with well-defined nodules visible at low magnification [2]. At higher magnification, this capillary proliferation can infiltrate larger bronchial and vascular structures and, in rare cases, pleura and/or pericardium, and mediastinal lymph nodes [2].

PCH can histologically mimic vascular congestion, particularly in small specimens. However, the findings in PCH are typically patchy, and capillary proliferation is at least two

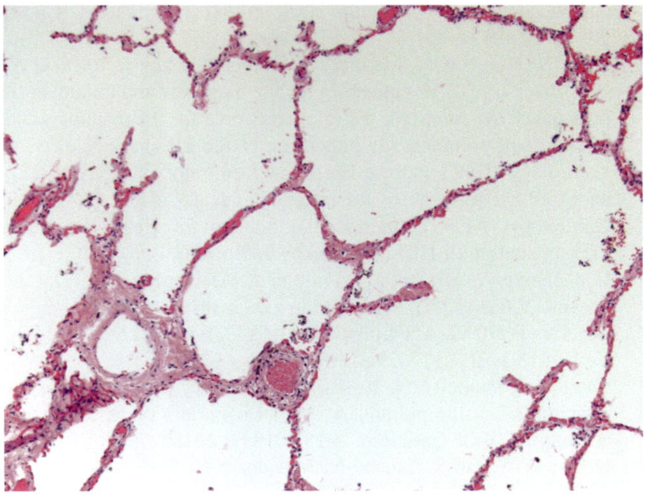

Fig. 56.3 Pulmonary vascular congestion in a patient with acute pneumonia. In comparison to pulmonary capillary hemangiomatosis, vascular congestion typically involves the entirety of the affected lobe, and the capillary vessels, although prominent, are only one layer in thickness (H&E, 200×)

layers in thickness [2]. Other histologic changes that may be seen in PCH include secondary changes of pulmonary hypertension and features also seen in PVOD, such as venous obstruction (described in 80% of cases of PCH), interlobular septal fibrosis (seen in 100% of cases), and a mild lymphocytic inflammatory infiltrate (seen in 71% of cases) [3].

On the other hand, vascular congestion is a diffuse reactive process, consisting of dilatation of preexisting alveolar capillaries, rather than a proliferative process. Histologically, it consists of a single layer of dilated alveolar capillaries, which do not extend into larger bronchial and/or vascular structures (Fig. 56.3).

Are Genetic/Molecular Findings Useful in the Diagnosis and Treatment of PCH?

Biallelic mutations in *EIF2AK4*have been described in a number of cases of hereditary PCH, including both familial and sporadic cases; the former are characterized by an autosomal recessive pattern of inheritance [6, 14]. Mutations in this gene have also been described in patients with clinical diagnoses of PVOD and pulmonary arterial hypertension (PAH) [15, 16].

Current European guidelines for the diagnosis of pulmonary hypertension suggest that detection of biallelic *EIF2AK4* mutations is sufficient to establish a diagnosis of PVOD/PCH without the need for biopsy confirmation [17].

EIF2AK4 (formerly *GCN2*) encodes for a protein involved in adaptation to amino acid restriction, with its activation leading to increased angiogenesis via downstream VEGF expression [18]. This mechanism may explain the abnormal capillary proliferation in the setting of activating mutations in this gene.

What Are the Treatment Modalities Available for PCH?

Unfortunately, no effective medical therapy is currently available in the treatment of PCH, and lung transplant (or heart-lung transplant in cases with secondary heart failure) remains the only viable option in patients with advanced pulmonary hypertension due to this condition [2, 19].

The use of vasodilators typically indicated for pulmonary arterial hypertension (PAH) can lead to fatal pulmonary edema in patients with PCH and/or PVOD, and, therefore, these are contraindicated in this situation [11, 20]. This serious implication highlights the importance of an accurate diagnosis prior to initiation of therapy.

References

1. Almagro P, Julia J, Sanjaume M, Gonzalez G, Casalots J, Heredia JL, et al. Pulmonary capillary hemangiomatosis associated with primary pulmonary hypertension: report of 2 new cases and review of 35 cases from the literature. Medicine. 2002;81(6):417–24.
2. Chaisson NF, Dodson MW, Elliott CG. Pulmonary capillary hemangiomatosis and pulmonary veno-occlusive disease. Clin Chest Med. 2016;37(3):523–34.
3. Lantuejoul S, Sheppard MN, Corrin B, Burke MM, Nicholson AG. Pulmonary veno-occlusive disease and pulmonary capillary hemangiomatosis: a clinicopathologic study of 35 cases. Am J Surg Pathol. 2006;30(7):850–7.
4. Fernandez-Alonso J, Zulueta T, Reyes-Ramirez JR, Castillo-Palma MJ, Sanchez-Roman J. Pulmonary capillary hemangiomatosis as cause of pulmonary hypertension in a young woman with systemic lupus erythematosus. J Rheumatol. 1999;26(1):231–3.
5. Diao XL, Mu XD, Jin ML. Pulmonary capillary hemangiomatosis associated with CREST syndrome: a challenge of diagnosis and treatment. Chin Med J (Engl). 2017;130(21):2645–6.
6. Best DH, Sumner KL, Austin ED, Chung WK, Brown LM, Borczuk AC, et al. EIF2AK4 mutations in pulmonary capillary hemangiomatosis. Chest. 2014;145(2):231–6.
7. Langleben D, Heneghan JM, Batten AP, Wang NS, Fitch N, Schlesinger RD, et al. Familial pulmonary capillary hemangiomatosis resulting in primary pulmonary hypertension. Ann Intern Med. 1988;109(2):106–9.
8. Wirbelauer J, Hebestreit H, Marx A, Mark EJ, Speer CP. Familial pulmonary capillary hemangiomatosis early in life. Case Rep Pulmonol. 2011;2011:827591.
9. Varnholt H, Kradin R. Pulmonary capillary hemangiomatosis arising in hereditary hemorrhagic telangiectasia. Hum Pathol. 2004;35(2):266–8.
10. Aiello VD, Thomaz AM, Pozzan G, Lopes AA. Capillary hemangiomatosis like-lesions in lung biopsies from children with congenital heart defects. Pediatr Pulmonol. 2014;49(3):E82–5.

11. Miura A, Akagi S, Nakamura K, Ohta-Ogo K, Hashimoto K, Nagase S, et al. Different sizes of centrilobular ground-glass opacities in chest high-resolution computed tomography of patients with pulmonary veno-occlusive disease and patients with pulmonary capillary hemangiomatosis. Cardiovasc Pathol. 2013;22(4):287–93.
12. Frazier AA, Franks TJ, Mohammed TL, Ozbudak IH, Galvin JR. From the archives of the AFIP: pulmonary veno-occlusive disease and pulmonary capillary hemangiomatosis. Radiographics. 2007;27(3):867–82.
13. El-Gabaly M, Farver CF, Budev MA, Mohammed TL. Pulmonary capillary hemangiomatosis imaging findings and literature update. J Comput Assist Tomogr. 2007;31(4):608–10.
14. Navas Tejedor P, Palomino Doza J, Tenorio Castano JA, Enguita Valls AB, Rodriguez Reguero JJ, Martinez Menaca A, et al. Variable expressivity of a founder mutation in the EIF2AK4 gene in hereditary pulmonary veno-occlusive disease and its impact on survival. Rev Esp Cardiol (Engl Ed). 2018;71(2):86–94.
15. Hadinnapola C, Bleda M, Haimel M, Screaton N, Swift A, Dorfmuller P, et al. Phenotypic characterization of EIF2AK4 mutation carriers in a large cohort of patients diagnosed clinically with pulmonary arterial hypertension. Circulation. 2017;136(21):2022–33.
16. Best DH, Sumner KL, Smith BP, Damjanovich-Colmenares K, Nakayama I, Brown LM, et al. EIF2AK4 mutations in patients diagnosed with pulmonary arterial hypertension. Chest. 2017;151(4):821–8.
17. Galiè N, Humbert M, Vachiery JL, Gibbs S, Lang I, Torbicki A, et al. 2015 ESC/ERS guidelines for the diagnosis and treatment of pulmonary hypertension: the joint task force for the diagnosis and treatment of pulmonary hypertension of the European Society of Cardiology (ESC) and the European Respiratory Society (ERS): endorsed by: Association for European Paediatric and Congenital Cardiology (AEPC), International Society for Heart and Lung Transplantation (ISHLT). Eur Respir J. 2015;46(4):903–75.
18. Longchamp A, Mirabella T, Arduini A, MacArthur MR, Das A, Trevino-Villarreal JH, et al. Amino acid restriction triggers angiogenesis via GCN2/ATF4 regulation of VEGF and H2S production. Cell. 2018;173(1):117–29.e14.
19. Sharma A, Pandey NN, Kumar S. Pulmonary capillary haemangiomatosis causing pulmonary arterial hypertension: a clinician's conundrum. BMJ Case Rep. 2018;2018:bcr2018227393.
20. Ogawa A, Sakao S, Tanabe N, Matsubara H, Tatsumi K. Use of vasodilators for the treatment of pulmonary veno-occlusive disease and pulmonary capillary hemangiomatosis: a systematic review. Respir Investig. 2019;57(2):183–90.

Pulmonary Veno-Occlusive Disease Versus Pulmonary Arterial Hypertension

57

Omer Abdelaziz Mohammed Saeed and Chen Zhang

Case Presentation

A 65-year-old female presents with worsening dyspnea and chest pain for approximately 2 years. She denies cough, hemoptysis, fever, wheeze, or weight loss. She has a history of smoking and has been diagnosed as chronic obstructive lung disease with pulmonary hypertension. Physical examination shows a mildly stressed woman with clear auscultation in bilateral lungs. Chest X-ray shows patchy bilateral airway opacities and multiple foci of consolidation consistent with multifocal pneumonia. Her chest computed tomography (CT) scan shows diffuse emphysematous changes and nodularity that are thought to represent resolving airway disease (Fig. 57.1). Her pulmonary function test shows mild expiratory airflow obstruction and mild restriction with FVC 2.81 (75%), FEV1 1.97 (68%), and FEV1/FVC 70 (91%). Her cardiac catheterization shows moderate pulmonary hypertension with a mean pulmonary artery pressure (mPAP) of 33 mmHg, elevated pulmonary vascular resistance, and no response to vasodilator therapy. Her left ventricular systolic function is normal. Echocardiography shows moderate right ventricular dilatation and right atrial dilatation. A left upper and lower lobe video-assisted thoracoscopic surgery (VATS) wedge biopsy is performed for a definitive diagnosis.

Microscopic examination of the lung wedge biopsies at low magnification shows preserved alveolar lung architecture with mild emphysematous change and focal fibrous thickening of interlobular septa and pleura (Fig. 57.2a). Patchy areas of alveolar septal capillary congestion are seen.

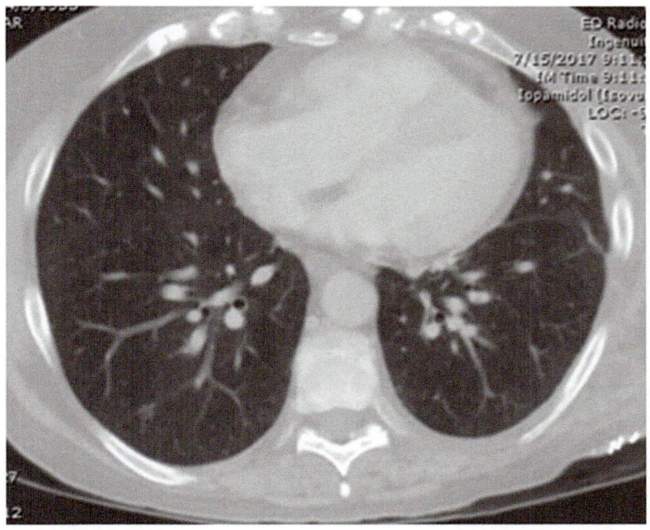

Fig. 57.1 Imaging features of pulmonary veno-occlusive disease (PVOD). Chest CT image shows diffuse emphysematous changes and bilateral patchy ground-glass opacities and nodularity

Higher magnification examination of the fibrous areas within the interlobular septa and pleura reveals narrowing and occlusion of the lumens of small veins by intimal fibrous proliferation (Fig. 57.2b). In some areas, the occluded veins are barely visible within the interlobular connective tissue but are highlighted with elastic stain (Fig. 57.2c). Mild arterial hypertension is also present. Secondary capillary congestion and dilated lymphatics are also seen.

O. A. M. Saeed
Department of Pathology and Laboratory Medicine, Indiana University School of Medicine, Indianapolis, IN, USA

C. Zhang (✉)
Weill Cornell Medicine, Department of Pathology and Laboratory Medicine, New York, NY, USA
e-mail: fjr9007@med.cornell.edu

H. Xu et al. (eds.), *Practical Lung Pathology*, Practical Anatomic Pathology, https://doi.org/10.1007/978-3-031-14402-8_57

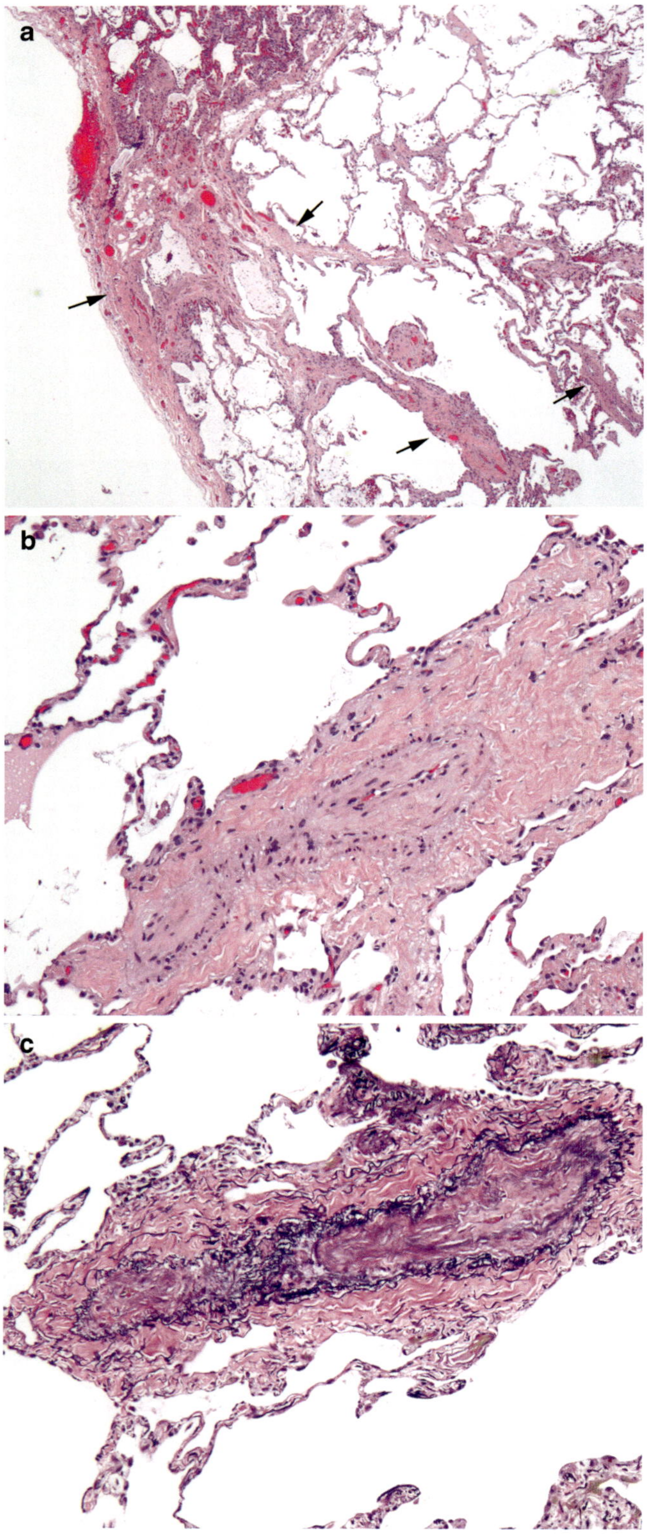

Fig. 57.2 Histological features of PVOD. (**a**) Low-magnification photomicrograph showing emphysematous changes, focal fibrous thickening of interlobular septa and pleura (arrows), and areas of capillary congestion within the alveolar septa (left upper) (H&E, original magnification, ×20). (**b**) Higher magnification of the fibrous area within the interlobular septum demonstrates narrowing and occlusion of the lumens of small veins by intimal fibrous proliferation (H&E, original magnification ×100). (**c**) Elastic stain of the same area in **b** demonstrating a single major elastic layer of the occluded vein (VVG, original magnification ×100)

Diagnosis: Pulmonary Veno-Occlusive Disease (PVOD)

What Is the Definition and Epidemiology of Pulmonary Veno-Occlusive Disease (PVOD) and How Do They Differ from Pulmonary Arterial Hypertension (PAH)?

Pulmonary hypertension (PH) is clinically defined as an increased mPAP of 25 mmHg or more at rest as assessed by right heart catheterization [1, 2]. PH is classified into five groups based on shared clinical features and management [1, 3, 4]. Group 1 includes PAH, with all its subcategories, PVOD and persistent PH of the newborn; group 2 is PH secondary to heart diseases; group 3 includes PH secondary to lung disease or hypoxia; group 4 is chronic thromboembolic PH; and group 5 includes PH with unclear multifactorial etiology [1, 3]. Despite being on the same group as PAH, PVOD has a special designation within this group referred to as group 1′ [5].

PVOD is a rare type of PH that develops as a result of pulmonary venous pathology [5, 6]. Under the current classification (fifth world symposium on PH, 2013), PVOD and pulmonary capillary hemangiomatosis are considered to be on the spectrum of the same disease [4]. Although the true incidence of PVOD is difficult to estimate because many cases are misclassified as PAH, it thought to be around 0.1–0.2 case per million person in the general population [6]. PVOD affects both males and females equally and involves ages from 2 months to the seventh decade [6].

PAH is a chronic disease diagnosed by the presence of PH plus low pulmonary artery wedge pressure <15 mmHg, pulmonary vascular resistance >3 woods unit and the absence of lung disease or thromboembolic phenomenon [7]. The incidence of PAH ranges from 15 to 50 cases per million people in the general population [7]. PAH tends to affect young adults with female predominance [8].

What Is the Etiology and Clinical Presentation of PVOD and How Do They Differ from PAH?

Most cases of PVOD are sporadic and idiopathic, but there are cases reported linking to several risk factors including chemotherapy, occupational exposure to chlorinated solvents, smoking, and autoimmunity [5]. Rare familial cases of PVOD have been reported. PAH can be classified according to etiology into idiopathic, heritable, drug- and toxin-induced, and PAH associated with HIV, connective tissue disease, portal hypertension, congenital heart disease, or schistosomiasis [4].

PAH and PVOD share similar clinical features. Both present clinically as slowly progressive dyspnea and fatigue, starting as exertional and then progress to at rest and finally complicated by symptoms of right-sided heart failure [5, 6].

Many patients present with milder symptoms resembling respiratory infections that progress despite antibiotics therapy [6, 9]. Both PAH and PVOD patients may show mild obstructive and/or restrictive changes on pulmonary function tests. Cardiac catheterization demonstrates increased mPAP but has no value in differentiating PVOD from PAH. Certain clinical findings are thought to favor the diagnosis of PVOD including low transfer coefficient of carbon monoxide, oxygen desaturation after exertion, and pulmonary edema after vasodilation therapy [5, 10]; however, there is considerable overlap in the clinical presentation of PAH and PVOD.

Do PVOD and PAH Look Differently on Radiographic Imaging?

The classical PVOD case shows up in high-resolution CT as centrilobular ground-grass opacities, thickening of interlobular septa, and mediastinal lymphadenopathy [5]. Other findings such as multiple small nodules and pleural effusion can be noted [1, 6]. PAH on the other hand shows pulmonary artery dilatation with decrease of peripheral vasculature, oligemic (hypovolemia) lungs, and depending on the severity might show right atrial and ventricular dilatation [1]. However, the radiographic appearance of PAH and PVOD might overlap, with approximately one third of the cases of PAH show ground-glass opacities characteristic of PVOD [11].

What Are the Pathological Features of PVOD and PAH? What Are the Similarities and Differences?

Given the similar clinical presentation and overlapping radiological findings, lung wedge biopsy is considered the most reliable way telling these two entities apart (Table 57.1).

The pathologic hallmark of PVOD is diffuse involvement of pulmonary venules and veins with fibrosis resulting subtotal or total occlusion [5, 6, 12]. The intima of involved venules and small veins shows significant thickening with loose edematous or sclerotic fibrous tissue resulting in venous occlusion. The findings are often subtle, and the fibrotic occluded veins may be overlooked as nonspecific scarring within the interlobular septa (Fig. 57.2a, b). Elastic stain is especially useful in this situation to highlight the residual elastic layer of the occluded veins (Fig. 57.2c). The media may become arterialized with increased elastic fibers which sometimes have a characteristic calcium deposition [6, 12]. This calcium might elicit foreign body giant cell reaction which is a helpful diagnostic clue. Hemosiderin

Table 57.1 Comparison of histological features of pulmonary veno-occlusive disease (PVOD) and pulmonary arterial hypertension (PAH)

	PVOD	PAH
Location of the lesional vessels	Within the interlobular septa and subpleural	Within bronchovascular bundles, next to bronchioles
Fibrous occlusions of veins	+	–
Capillary congestion	+	–
Hemosiderin-laden macrophages	Common	Uncommon
Arterial intimal/ medial hyperplasia	+/–	+
Muscularization of arterioles	–	+
Plexiform/ angiomatoid lesions	–	+ (in severe form)

deposition in macrophages and pneumocytes is frequently seen [6]. Secondary capillary congestion and/or proliferation indistinguishable from pulmonary capillary hemangiomatosis can be noted [5].

As the names imply, PAH differs from PVOD in that the pathology affects the arterial side of the pulmonary circulation. Characteristically in PAH, the intima of smaller pulmonary arteries show cellular or fibrotic, eccentric, or concentric thickening resulting in vascular narrowing or occlusion [13]. A more peculiar intimal pathology seen in severe PAH usually near arterial branching points is the plexiform lesions which are formed by proliferation of endothelial cells resulting in the formation of multiple vascular channels [12, 13]. Another intimal lesion also seen in severe PAH and commonly in close association with plexiform lesions is vascular dilatation or angiomatoid lesions. The media and adventitia are significantly thickened in PAH with notable inflammatory cuff in the adventitia seen more pronounced in certain subtypes of PAH [13].

Differentiating PVOD from PAH in lung biopsy isn't always straightforward since some venous changes can be seen in cases of idiopathic PAH, while some arterial changes can be seen in PVOD [14]. Generally, the presence of secondary pulmonary capillary congestions and/or hemosiderin-laden macrophages hints on PVOD, whereas plexiform lesion and/or angiomatoid lesions happen almost exclusively in severe PAH. An elastic stain is always helpful to identify lesions and to differentiate between arteries and veins (two elastic layers in the former and one in the latter). However, arterialization of veins may occur during PVOD, and elastic stain will show double layers of elastin, mimicking arteries. In this situation, the venous nature of the vessels can only be confirmed by their interlobular septal/pleural location rather than next to an airway within a bronchovascular bundle.

What Are the Genetic/Molecular Findings of PVOD and How Is It Different from Those Seen in PAH?

Biallelic mutations in translation initiation factor 2 alpha kinase 4 (*EIF2AK4*) are seen in all familial cases of PVOD and in approximately 25% of sporadic ones [1, 5, 14]. In the familial cases, the mutations are thought to be inherited in a recessive manner [14]. These mutations, however, are seen rarely in ~2.2% of the cases diagnosed clinically and/or clinicopathologically as idiopathic PAH [10]. Whether these cases were clinically misclassified as PAH remains to be seen [10].

Mutations involving the bone morphogenic protein receptor 2 (*BMPR2*) are found in approximately 75% of the familial PAH cases and 25% of the sporadic ones [14]. Other rare mutations were also described in cases of PAH including mutations in the Activin A type II receptor like kinase 1 (*ALK1/ACVRL1*), Endoglin (*ENG*), and potassium voltage-gated channel, shaker-related subfamily, and member 5 (*KCNA5*) [1, 15].

What Are the Treatment Modalities and Prognosis for PVOD and PAH?

Unlike PAH, there is currently no targeted therapy that can be used in PVOD [5]. Life-threatening pulmonary edema may occur following the initiation of PAH therapy on patients with PVOD. Lung transplantation remains the only proven therapy to prolong survival in cases of PVOD [5]. The management of patients with PAH is complex and involves complex combination of supportive and targeted therapy [1]. The targeted therapies are usually directed toward three pathways involved in the pathogenesis of PAH, namely, prostacyclin, endothelin 1, and nitric oxide (NO) pathway [1, 5, 7]. Examples of such treatments include epoprostenol and selexipag (prostacyclin pathway), bosentan (endothelin pathway), and sildenafil (NO pathway) [7]. PVOD has a poor prognosis compared to PAH. The disease has a relentless progressive course with mortality rate reaching up to 72% within 1 year [16]. The meantime from diagnosis to either lung transplant or death was reported in one study to be 24.4 months [17]. PAH survival has shown great improvement over the years [5]. According to one of the largest studies of PAH patients, the 5-year survival rate is approximately 57% [18].

References

1. Galiè N, Humbert M, Vachiery J-L, Gibbs S, Lang I, Torbicki A, et al. 2015 ESC/ERS guidelines for the diagnosis and treatment of pulmonary hypertension: the joint task force for the diagnosis and treatment of pulmonary hypertension of the European Society of Cardiology (ESC) and the European Respiratory Society (ERS): endorsed by: Association for European Paediatric and Congenital Cardiology (AEPC), International Society for Heart and Lung Transplantation (ISHLT). Eur Heart J. 2015;37(1):67–119.
2. Hoeper MM, Bogaard HJ, Condliffe R, Frantz R, Khanna D, Kurzyna M, et al. Definitions and diagnosis of pulmonary hypertension. J Am Coll Cardiol. 2013;62(25 Suppl):D42–50.
3. Simonneau G, Robbins IM, Beghetti M, Channick RN, Delcroix M, Denton CP, et al. Updated clinical classification of pulmonary hypertension. J Am Coll Cardiol. 2009;54(1 Suppl):S43–54.
4. Simonneau G, Gatzoulis MA, Adatia I, Celermajer D, Denton C, Ghofrani A, et al. Updated clinical classification of pulmonary hypertension. J Am Coll Cardiol. 2013;62(25 Suppl):D34–41.
5. Montani D, Lau EM, Dorfmüller P, Girerd B, Jaïs X, Savale L, et al. Pulmonary veno-occlusive disease. Eur Respir J. 2016;47(5):1518–34.
6. Mandel J, Mark EJ, Hales CA. Pulmonary veno-occlusive disease. Am J Respir Crit Care Med. 2000;162(5):1964–73.
7. Lau EM, Giannoulatou E, Celermajer DS, Humbert M. Epidemiology and treatment of pulmonary arterial hypertension. Nat Rev Cardiol. 2017;14(10):603–14.
8. Frost AE, Badesch DB, Barst RJ, Benza RL, Elliott CG, Farber HW, et al. The changing picture of patients with pulmonary arterial hypertension in the United States: how REVEAL differs from historic and non-US contemporary registries. Chest. 2011;139(1):128–37.
9. Heath D, Segel N, Bishop J. Pulmonary veno-occlusive disease. Circulation. 1966;34(2):242–8.
10. Hadinnapola C, Bleda M, Haimel M, Screaton N, Swift A, Dorfmüller P, et al. Phenotypic characterization of EIF2AK4 mutation carriers in a large cohort of patients diagnosed clinically with pulmonary arterial hypertension. Circulation. 2017;136(21):2022–33.
11. Rajaram S, Swift A, Condliffe R, Johns C, Elliot C, Hill C, et al. CT features of pulmonary arterial hypertension and its major subtypes: a systematic CT evaluation of 292 patients from the ASPIRE registry. Thorax. 2015;70(4):382–7.
12. Pietra GG, Capron F, Stewart S, Leone O, Humbert M, Robbins IM, et al. Pathologic assessment of vasculopathies in pulmonary hypertension. J Am Coll Cardiol. 2004;43(12 Suppl):S25–32.
13. Tuder RM, Marecki JC, Richter A, Fijalkowska I, Flores S. Pathology of pulmonary hypertension. Clin Chest Med. 2007;28(1):23–42.
14. Eyries M, Montani D, Girerd B, Perret C, Leroy A, Lonjou C, et al. EIF2AK4 mutations cause pulmonary veno-occlusive disease, a recessive form of pulmonary hypertension. Nat Genet. 2014;46(1):65–9.
15. Pousada G, Baloira A, Vilariño C, Cifrian JM, Valverde D. Novel mutations in BMPR2, ACVRL1 and KCNA5 genes and hemodynamic parameters in patients with pulmonary arterial hypertension. PLoS One. 2014;9(6):e100261.
16. Holcomb BW Jr, Loyd JE, Ely EW, Johnson J, Robbins IM. Pulmonary veno-occlusive disease: a case series and new observations. Chest. 2000;118(6):1671–9.
17. Montani D, Achouh L, Dorfmüller P, Le Pavec J, Sztrymf B, Tchérakian C, et al. Pulmonary veno-occlusive disease: clinical, functional, radiologic, and hemodynamic characteristics and outcome of 24 cases confirmed by histology. Medicine. 2008;87(4):220–33.
18. Benza RL, Miller DP, Barst RJ, Badesch DB, Frost AE, McGoon MD. An evaluation of long-term survival from time of diagnosis in pulmonary arterial hypertension from the REVEAL registry. Chest. 2012;142(2):448–56.

58 Lymphangioleiomyomatosis Versus Benign Metastasizing Leiomyoma

Jose G. Mantilla

Case Presentation

A 39-year-old woman with no history of smoking presented to the pulmonary clinic complaining of dyspnea on exertion. Initial pulmonary function tests demonstrated a severely decreased FEV1, FEV1/FVC ratio, and DLCO, indicating a combination of obstructive and restrictive disease. Chest computed tomography (CT) demonstrated multiple evenly distributed thin-walled cysts and scattered ground-glass opacities (Fig. 58.1).

A diagnostic wedge biopsy demonstrated multiple thin-walled cysts and nodules composed of spindle cells with bland nuclear features and abundant eosinophilic cytoplasm (Fig. 58.2a). No features of overt malignancy were identified. Immunohistochemical stains show that the lesional cells are diffusely positive for estrogen receptor, desmin, smooth muscle actin (Fig. 58.2b), and variably for HMB45 (Fig. 58.2c).

After an initial diagnosis, the patient received medical therapy with limited response. Her condition progressively worsened until she received a bilateral lung transplant, with subsequent improvement of her symptoms. The explanted lungs show diffused thin cysts distributed throughout the entirety of the lungs (Fig. 58.3).

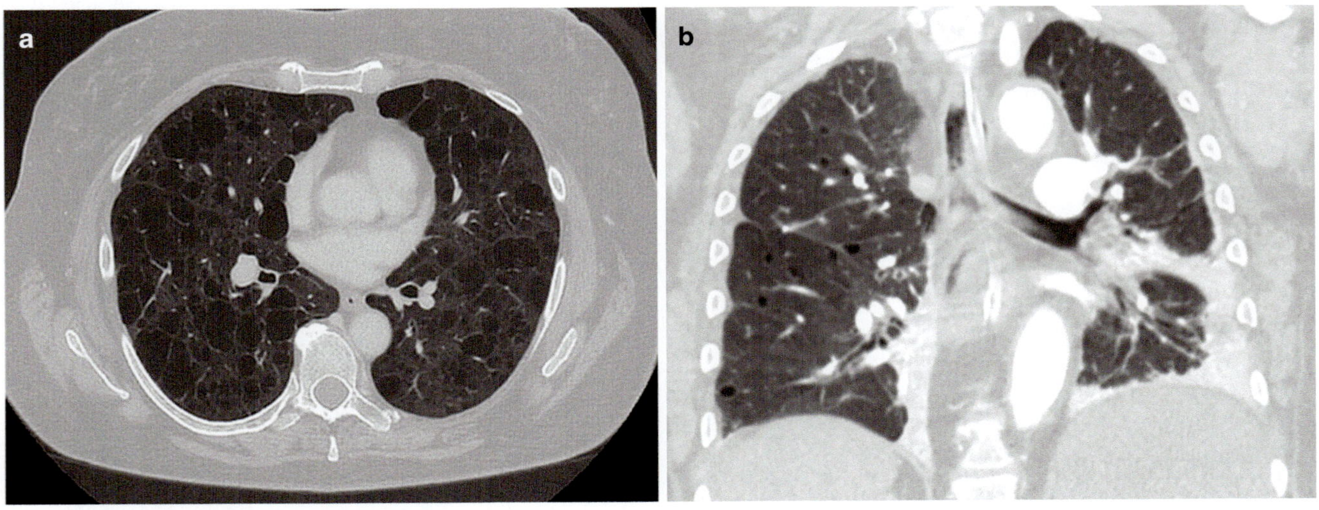

Fig. 58.1 Imaging features of lymphangioleiomyomatosis (LAM). LAM is typically characterized by the presence of multiple thin-walled lung cysts in a homogeneous distribution, as well as associated mediastinal lymphadenopathy. (**a**) Axial view; (**b**) coronal view

J. G. Mantilla (✉)
Department of Laboratory Medicine and Pathology, University of Washington Medical Center, Seattle, WA, USA
e-mail: mantilla@uw.edu

H. Xu et al. (eds.), *Practical Lung Pathology*, Practical Anatomic Pathology, https://doi.org/10.1007/978-3-031-14402-8_58

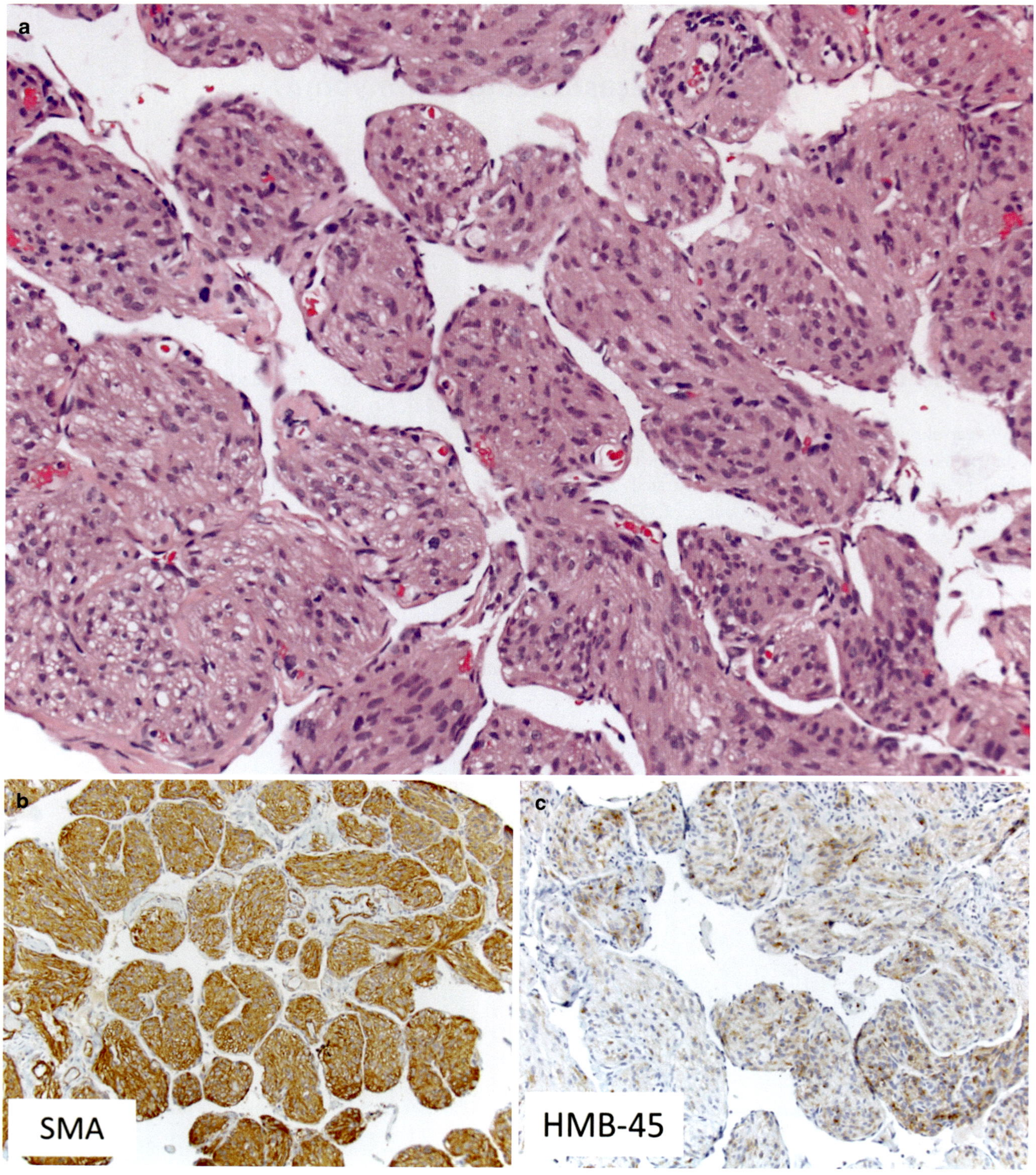

Fig. 58.2 Histologic features of LAM. These lesions are typically composed of cysts with a lymphangitic distribution, composed of cytologically bland myoid cells (**a**), which express smooth muscle actin (**b**) and variably HMB-45 (**c**) (H&E, IHC DAB, 200×)

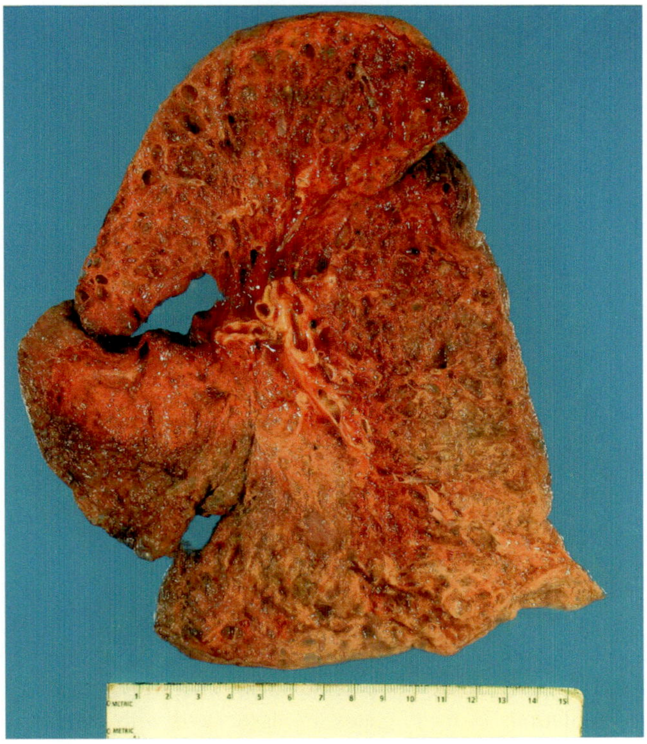

Fig. 58.3 Gross pathologic appearance of LAM. Notice the presence of multiple thin-walled cysts distributed throughout the entirety of the lung

Pathologic Diagnosis: Lymphangioleiomyomatosis

What Are the Clinical and Prognostic Features of LAM and How Do They Differ from Benign Metastasizing Leiomyoma (BML)?

In the setting of multiple lung lesions with smooth muscle differentiation, arising in women of reproductive age, important diagnostic considerations include LAM and benign metastasizing leiomyoma.

LAM is a rare disease which typically presents as multiple thin-walled cystic lesions that replace the lung parenchyma and are clinically associated with dyspnea, spontaneous pneumothorax, and ultimately respiratory failure requiring continuous supplemental oxygen and transplantation [1–3]. Involvement of venous and lymphatic vessels can lead to other less common clinical manifestations, such as hemoptysis, pulmonary hypertension, and chylothorax [1, 2]. Extrapulmonary lymphangioleiomyomas are common, being seen in 19–34% of patients and can often appear in lymph nodes, retroperitoneum, or abdominal and pelvic organs [1, 4, 5].

LAM can be present sporadically, or in the setting of tuberous sclerosis, and patients affected with the latter tend to present symptoms at an earlier age [6]. Given this association, it is worth noting that angiomyolipomas of other organs can be present in up to 90% of patients with LAM and history of tuberous sclerosis, as well as in 30–40% of sporadic forms [1, 7, 8], including bilateral lesions in 13% of all cases [1].

On the other hand, BML is typically detected as asymptomatic pulmonary nodules in women. A history of prior surgery for uterine leiomyomas has been reported in more than 90% of cases, sometimes decades before the detection of pulmonary nodules [9, 10]. These lesions can be solitary or multiple and are not typically associated with respiratory symptoms. BML are known to be responsive to hormonal therapy and decrease in size after menopause [11].

How Can Radiologic Studies be Used to Distinguish LAM from BML?

Multiple air-filled, thin-walled cysts of variable size are identifiable in nearly 100% of cases of LAM when evaluated with high-resolution CT imaging (Fig. 58.1) [12, 13]. These cysts are typically distributed throughout the entirety of the lung parenchyma, without associated air trapping. Other common pulmonary findings include reticulated opacities [14], pneumothorax [13, 14], increased lung volumes, and pleural effusions. Associated cystic lymphangiomas are also seen in the abdomen and/or retroperitoneum in up to 20% of patients [13]. Other extrapulmonary findings described include lymphadenopathy and iliac or retroperitoneal lymphatic vessel dilation [5].

BML typically presents radiologically as solid, well-circumscribed masses which are typically hypointense on T1- and T2-weighted MRI [15]; however, cystic degeneration can be present in a minority of cases [10, 16]. These lesions can be solitary or multiple, have varying sizes, and appear in extrapulmonary sites, including lymph nodes and spine [15, 17], among others (Fig. 58.4).

What Are the Pathologic Features of LAM and BML? How Can Immunohistochemistry be Used to Distinguish These Two Entities?

Histologically, LAM typically consists of solid nodules and cysts composed of cytologically bland spindled to epithelioid perivascular cells (PEC), which surround lymphatic structures in a peribronchial, septal, and subpleural distribution [1, 18]. Immunohistochemically, the neoplastic cells typically express smooth muscle actin and HMB45 in the vast majority of cases, with variable staining intensity [19, 20]. Nuclear expression of estrogen and progesterone receptor has also been demonstrated in most cases, with PR being typically expressed in a greater proportion and intensity [19–21]. In addition, immunoreactivity for beta-catenin in a membranous and cytoplasmic staining pattern has also been described in a majority of cases [19]. Immunohistochemical

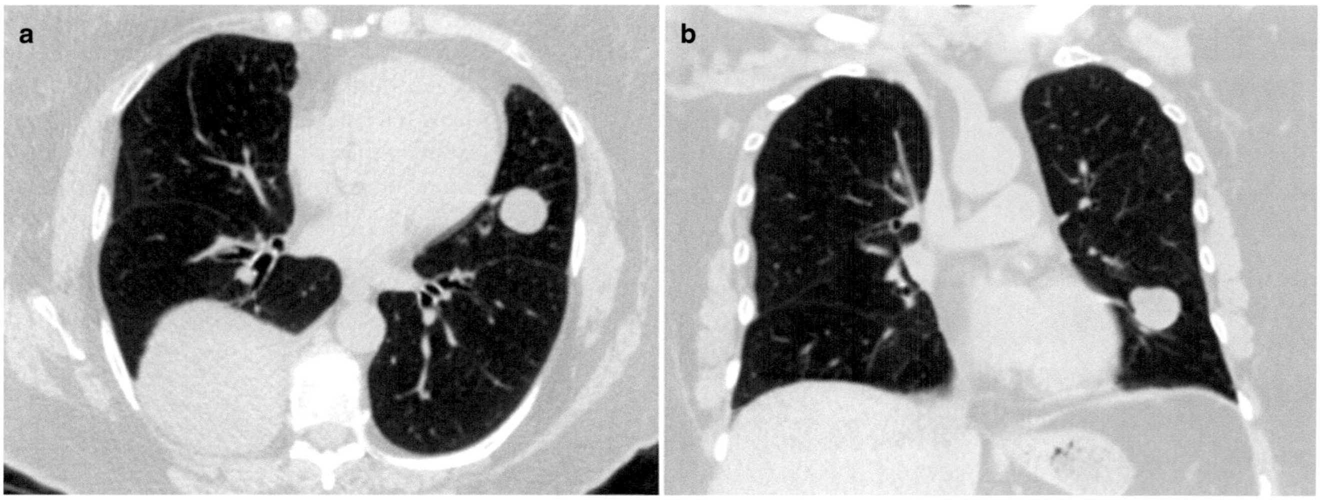

Fig. 58.4 On CT imaging, BML usually demonstrates solid nodules of varying sizes. (**a**) Axial view; (**b**) coronal view

staining for S100 is typically negative. More recently, overexpression of PD-L1 has been described in few cases of LAM, suggesting the potential opportunity for targeted therapy with checkpoint inhibitors [22] (Fig. 58.5).

On the other hand, BML typically consists of solid nodules in a peribronchovascular distribution [10]. These are composed of intersecting fascicles of smooth muscle cells with no prominent cytologic atypia or mitotic activity [10, 11, 16, 17, 23]. Immunohistochemical stains typically demonstrate diffuse expression of markers of smooth muscle differentiation, including desmin, actin, and caldesmon. Strong nuclear expression of estrogen and progesterone receptors has been reported in a majority of cases [17, 23]. Immunohistochemistry studies for HMB-45 and other melanocytic markers are invariably negative (Fig. 58.6).

Are Genetic/Molecular Findings Useful in the Diagnosis and Treatment of LAM?

Approximately 85–90% of cases of LAM are associated with somatic or germline mutations in *TSC1* or *TSC2* [6]. The proteins normally encoded by these two genes, tuberin and hamartin, have an inactivating effect on mTOR, which functions as a promoter of cell division. Therefore, inactivating mutations in these genes are associated with increased mTOR activity and the subsequent development of neoplasms [24]. Based on these observations, the use of mTOR inhibitors, such as sirolimus, has been effective in the medical treatment of LAM and associated with reduction of symptoms and improvement of pulmonary function [7, 24–26].

Are BML Genetically Similar to Their Uterine Counterparts? Are These Truly Metastatic?

Massively parallel sequencing and copy number alteration studies comparing pulmonary BML with their uterine counterparts have demonstrated the presence of identical somatic mutations as well as similar patterns of copy number alterations in paired uterine and pulmonary lesions demonstrating the same clonal origin for these [27–29].

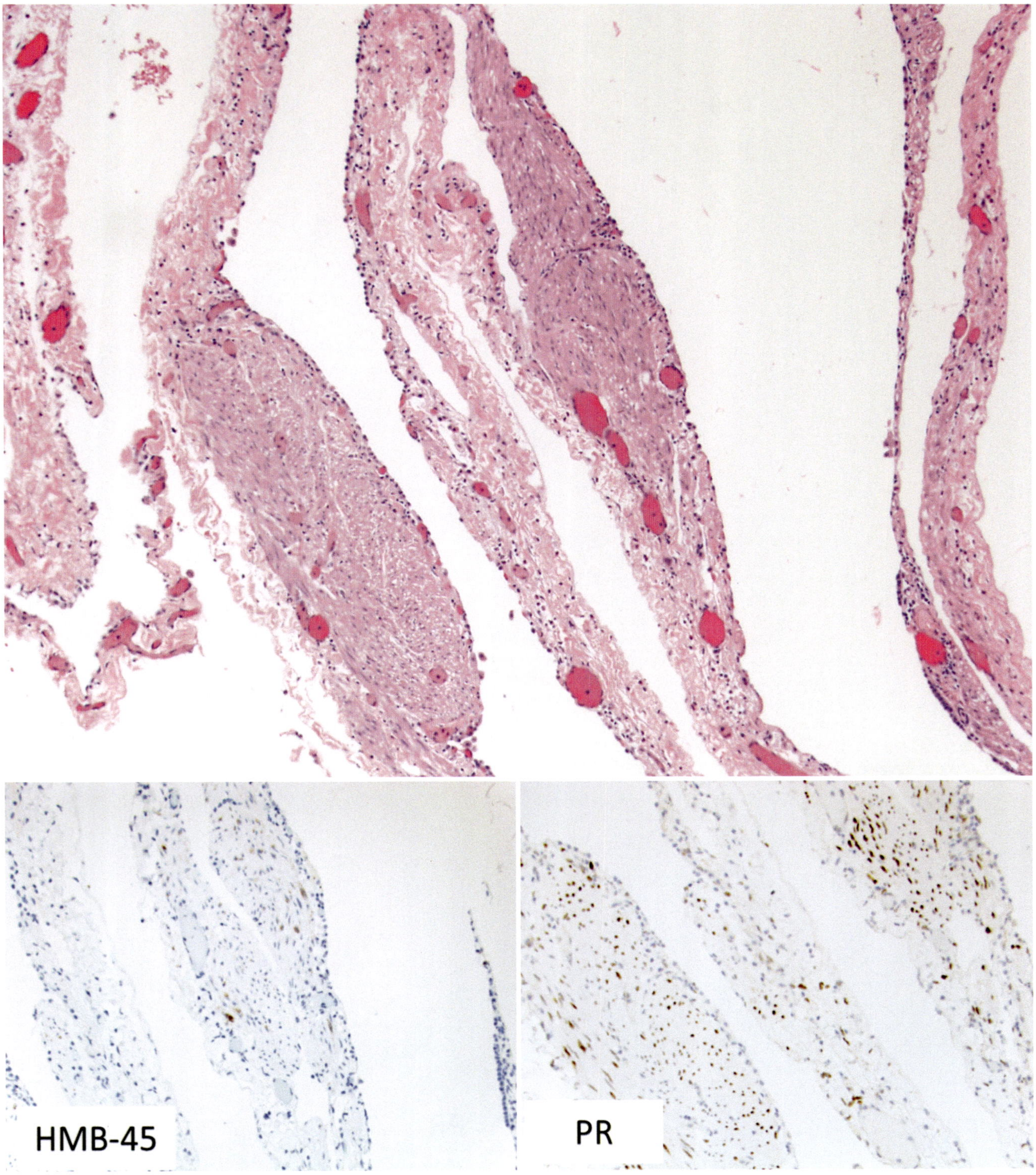

Fig. 58.5 Histologic findings in LAM can be subtle. Notice the presence of myoid cells within the cyst lining (H&E, 100×). In these, expression of HMB-45 can be only focal. Nuclear expression of progesterone receptor can often be helpful for identifying the lesional cells (IHC DAB, 100×)

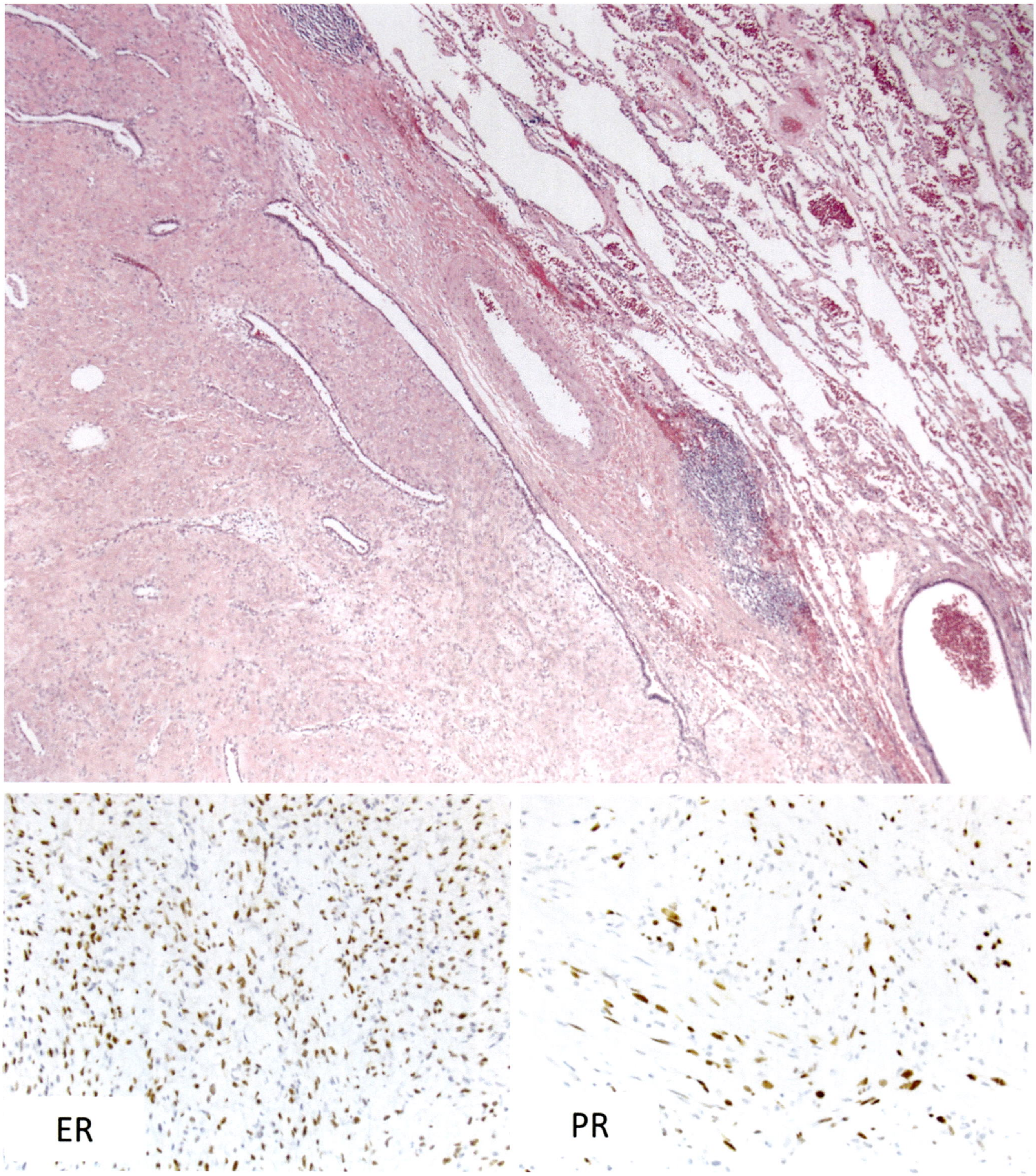

Fig. 58.6 Histologic features of BML. Notice the well-circumscribed smooth muscle proliferation, containing entrapped lung parenchyma (H&E, 40×). Nuclear expression of estrogen and progesterone receptors is typically present (IHC DAB, 100×)

References

1. Johnson SR, Taveira-DaSilva AM, Moss J. Lymphangioleiomyomatosis. Clin Chest Med. 2016;37(3):389–403.
2. Moir LM. Lymphangioleiomyomatosis: current understanding and potential treatments. Pharmacol Ther. 2016;158:114–24.
3. Taylor JR, Ryu J, Colby TV, Raffin TA. Lymphangioleiomyomatosis. Clinical course in 32 patients. N Engl J Med. 1990;323(18):1254–60.
4. Derweduwen AM, Verbeken E, Stas M, Verschakelen J, Coolen J, Verleden G, Wuyts W. Extrapulmonary lymphangioleiomyomatosis: a wolf in sheep's clothing. Thorax. 2013;68(1):111–3.
5. Zhang C, Chen X, Wen T, Zhang Q, Huo M, Dong J, l. Computed tomography lymphangiography findings in 27 cases of lymphangioleiomyomatosis. Acta Radiol. 2017;58(11):1342–8.
6. Murphy SJ, Terra SB, Harris FR, Nasir A, Voss JS, Smadbeck JB, et al. Genomic rearrangements in sporadic lymphangioleiomyomatosis: an evolving genetic story. Mod Pathol. 2017;30(9):1223–33.
7. Xu KF, Tian X, Ryu JH. Recent advances in the management of lymphangioleiomyomatosis. F1000Res. 2018;7:F1000 Faculty Rev–758.
8. Gupta N, Henske EP. Pulmonary manifestations in tuberous sclerosis complex. Am J Med Genet C Semin Med Genet. 2018;178(3):326–37.
9. Esteban JM, Allen WM, Schaerf RH. Benign metastasizing leiomyoma of the uterus: histologic and immunohistochemical characterization of primary and metastatic lesions. Arch Pathol Lab Med. 1999;123(10):960–2.
10. Choe YH, Jeon SY, Lee YC, Chung MJ, Park SY, Lee YC, Kim SR. Benign metastasizing leiomyoma presenting as multiple cystic pulmonary nodules: a case report. BMC Womens Health. 2017;17(1):81.
11. Rizzo V, Parissis H. A rare case of benign metastasizing leiomyoma. J Surg Case Rep. 2017;2017(9):rjx190.
12. Ferrans VJ, Yu ZX, Nelson WK, Valencia JC, Tatsuguchi A, Avila NA, et al. Lymphangioleiomyomatosis (LAM) vs. BML: a review of clinical and morphological features. J Nippon Med Sch. 2000;67(5):311–29.
13. Pallisa E, Sanz P, Roman A, Majó J, Andreu J, Cáceres J. Lymphangioleiomyomatosis: pulmonary and abdominal findings with pathologic correlation. Radiographics. 2002;22:S185–98.
14. Abbott GF, Rosado-de-Christenson ML, Frazier AA, Franks TJ, Pugatch RD, Galvin JR. From the archives of the AFIP: lymphangioleiomyomatosis: radiologic-pathologic correlation. Radiographics. 2005;25(3):803–28.
15. Hur JW, Lee S, Lee JB, Cho TH, Park JY. What are MRI findings of spine benign metastasizing leiomyoma? Case report with literature review. Eur Spine J. 2015;24(Suppl 4):S600–5.
16. Loukeri AA, Pantazopoulos IN, Tringidou R, Giampoudakis P, Valaskatzi A, Loukeri PA, Kampolis CF. Benign metastasizing leiomyoma presenting as cavitating lung nodules. Respir Care. 2014;59(7):e94–7.
17. Zong D, He W, Li J, Peng H, Chen P, Ouyang R. Concurrent benign metastasizing leiomyoma in the lung and lumbar spine with elevated standardized uptake value level in positron-emission tomography computed tomography: a case report and literature review. Medicine (Baltimore). 2018;97(27):e11334.
18. Thway K, Fisher C. PEComa: morphology and genetics of a complex tumor family. Ann Diagn Pathol. 2015;19(5):359–68.
19. Flavin RJ, Cook J, Fiorentino M, Bailey D, Brown M, Loda MF. Beta-catenin is a useful adjunct immunohistochemical marker for the diagnosis of pulmonary lymphangioleiomyomatosis. Am J Clin Pathol. 2011;135(5):776–82.
20. Grzegorek I, Lenze D, Chabowski M, Janczak D, Szolkowska M, Langfort R, et al. Immunohistochemical evaluation of pulmonary lymphangioleiomyomatosis. Anticancer Res. 2015;35(6):3353–60.
21. Gao L, Yue MM, Davis J, Hyjek E, Schuger L. In pulmonary lymphangioleiomyomatosis expression of progesterone receptor is frequently higher than that of estrogen receptor. Virchows Arch. 2014;464(4):495–503.
22. Maisel K, Merrilees MJ, Atochina-Vasserman EN, Lian L, Obraztsova K, Rue R, et al. Immune checkpoint ligand PD-L1 is upregulated in pulmonary lymphangioleiomyomatosis (LAM). Am J Respir Cell Mol Biol. 2018;59(6):723–32.
23. Rege AS, Snyder JA, Scott WJ. Benign metastasizing leiomyoma: a rare cause of multiple pulmonary nodules. Ann Thorac Surg. 2012;93(6):e149–51.
24. Franz DN, Krueger DA. mTOR inhibitor therapy as a disease modifying therapy for tuberous sclerosis complex. Am J Med Genet C Semin Med Genet. 2018;178(3):365–73.
25. McCormack FX, Inoue Y, Moss J, Singer LG, Strange C, Nakata N, et al. Efficacy and safety of sirolimus in lymphangioleiomyomatosis. N Engl J Med. 2011;364(17):1595–606.
26. Gao N, Zhang T, Ji J, Xu KF, Tian X. The efficacy and adverse events of mTOR inhibitors in lymphangioleiomyomatosis: systematic review and meta-analysis. Orphanet J Rare Dis. 2018;13(1):134.
27. Wu RC, Chao AS, Lee LY, Lin G, Chen SJ, Lu YJ, et al. Massively parallel sequencing and genome-wide copy number analysis revealed a clonal relationship in benign metastasizing leiomyoma. Oncotarget. 2017;8(29):47547–54.
28. Jiang J, He M, Hu X, Ni C, Yang L. Deep sequencing reveals the molecular pathology characteristics between primary uterine leiomyoma and pulmonary benign metastasizing leiomyoma. Clin Transl Oncol. 2018;20(8):1080–6.
29. Bowen JM, Cates JM, Kash S, Itani D, Gonzalez A, Huang D, et al. Genomic imbalances in benign metastasizing leiomyoma: characterization by conventional karyotypic, fluorescence in situ hybridization, and whole genome SNP array analysis. Cancer Genet. 2012;205(5):249–54.

Diffuse Pulmonary Lymphangiomatosis Versus Lymphangioleiomyomatosis

59

Jose G. Mantilla

Case Presentation

A 26-year-old woman presented to the emergency room after a motor vehicle collision. Chest computed tomography (CT) performed at that time demonstrated a large pleural effusion, associated with a right upper lobe mass. A wedge excision and pleural decortication demonstrated multiple subpleural and septal lesions composed of prominent, variably dilated and anastomosing lymphatic channels, associated with fibrosis and patchy lymphocytic infiltrates.

On follow-up, the patient had progressive dyspnea associated with restrictive lung disease. Chest CT studies demonstrated bilateral ground-glass opacities, septal and pleural thickening, and recurrent chylous pleural and pericardial effusions (Fig. 59.1). Four years after the initial diagnosis, the patient had a pregnancy during which her pulmonary function severely deteriorated, requiring a cesarean section at 29 weeks. Postoperatively, her respiratory status continued to worsen, ultimately leading to respiratory failure and death.

Autopsy revealed markedly enlarged lungs bilaterally, with extensive areas of pleural scarring. Other findings included marked ascites and additional lesions composed of similarly arranged lymphatic vessels involving the lungs (Fig. 59.2a–c), as well as the mediastinal and retroperitoneal soft tissues (Fig. 59.2d).

Her cause of death was attributed to respiratory failure due to **diffuse pulmonary lymphangiomatosis**.

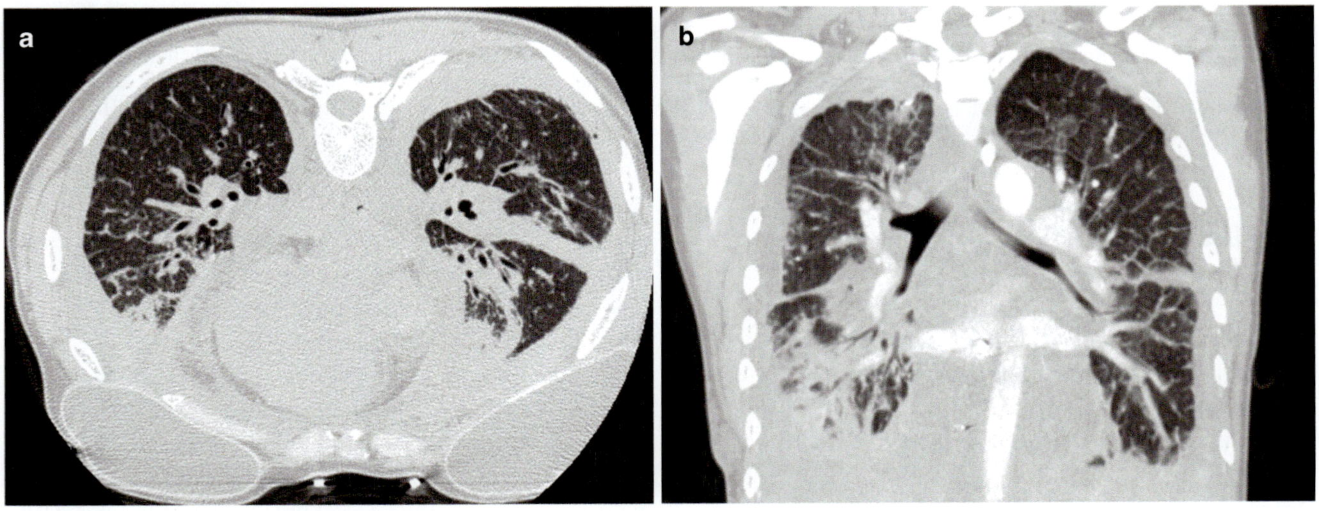

Fig. 59.1 CT imaging findings of diffuse pulmonary lymphangiomatosis commonly include extensive peribronchial/perivascular thickening, scattered ground-glass opacities, and pleural and pericardial effusion. **(a)** Axial view; **(b)** coronal view

J. G. Mantilla (✉)
Department of Laboratory Medicine and Pathology, University of Washington Medical Center, Seattle, WA, USA
e-mail: mantilla@uw.edu

H. Xu et al. (eds.), *Practical Lung Pathology*, Practical Anatomic Pathology, https://doi.org/10.1007/978-3-031-14402-8_59

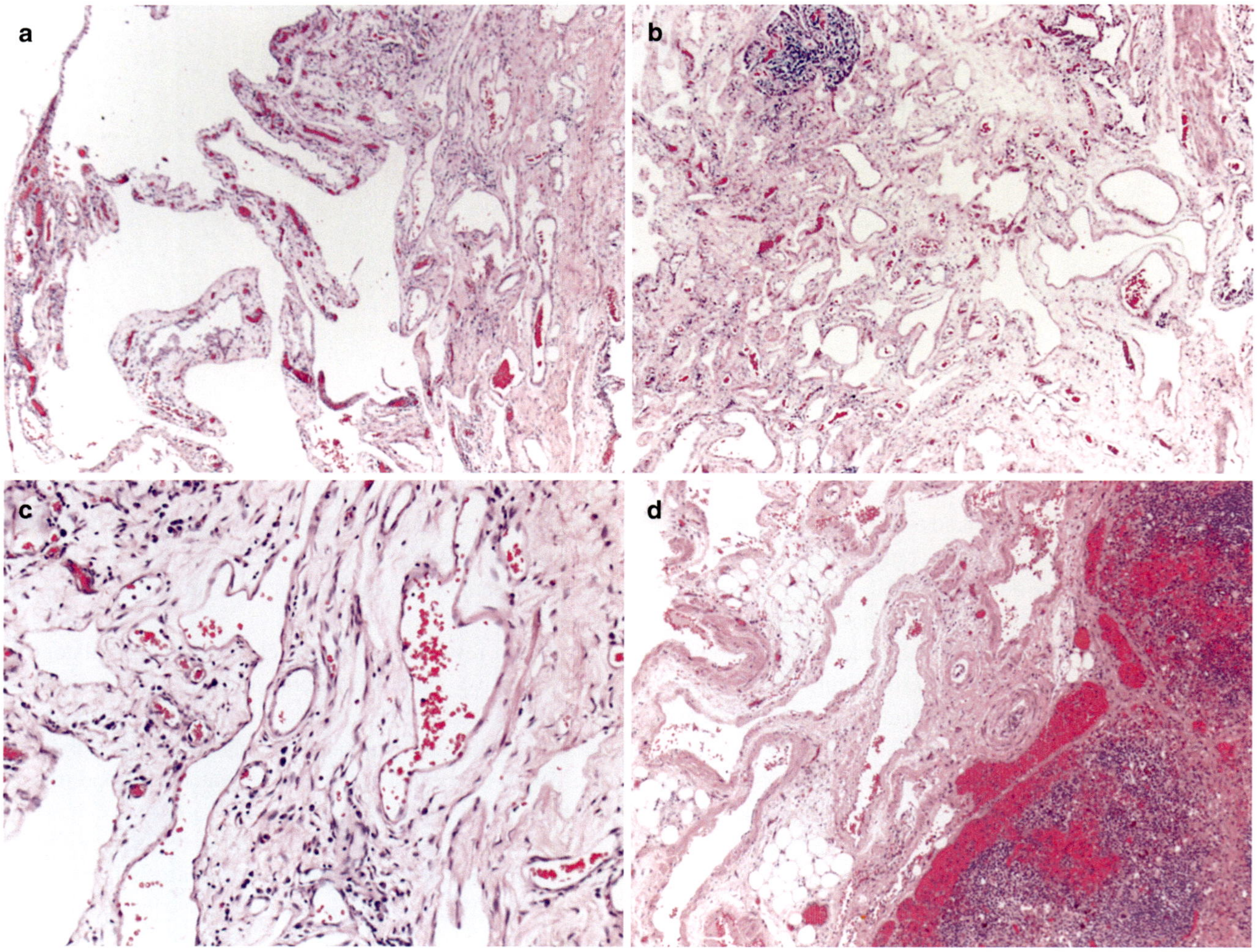

Fig. 59.2 (**a**, **b**) Histologic features of diffuse pulmonary lymphangiomatosis include multiple lesions composed of variably dilated lymphatics with a lymphangitic distribution, accompanied by fibrosis and variable lymphocytic aggregates (H&E, 40×). (**c**) The lesional vessels are lined by cytologically bland lymphatic endothelium (H&E, 200×). (**d**) Extrapulmonary lesions may be seen in DPL; in this particular case in the retroperitoneum, it is associated with lymph nodes (H&E, 40×)

Final Diagnosis: Diffuse Pulmonary Lymphangiomatosis

What Are the Clinical Features of Diffuse Pulmonary Lymphangiomatosis (DPL) and How Do They Differ from Lymphangioleiomyomatosis (LAM)?

Diffuse pulmonary lymphangiomatosis (DPL) is a rare condition characterized by diffuse prominence of lymphatic vessels within the lung parenchyma (lymphangiomas) [1]. It typically arises in children and young adults, with no significant difference between sexes [1, 2]. Rare cases of DPL have been reported in middle-aged adults [3, 4]. DPL is a typically aggressive disease which presents with a wide variety of clinical manifestations; these range from mild wheezing and productive cough to severe respiratory failure associated with infiltrative disease and recurrent pleural effusions [1]. The content of the expectoration and pleural effusion are often chylous [1, 2]. DPL is often associated with other lymphatic abnormalities and involvement of other organs in up to 75% of cases [5]. The clinical prognosis of DPL is poor, and death by respiratory failure is common [2, 6, 7].

On the other hand, LAM shows a marked preference for women of reproductive age. Somewhat similarly to DPL, LAM typically presents with dyspnea, spontaneous pneumothorax, and ultimately respiratory failure. Involvement of venous and lymphatic vessels can lead to other less common clinical manifestations, such as hemoptysis, pulmonary hypertension, and chylothorax [8–10]. This entity is also discussed in Chap. 58 (Lymphangioleiomyomatosis versus Benign Metastasizing Leiomyoma).

How Can Radiologic Studies be Used to Distinguish DPL from LAM?

The most common radiologic manifestations of DPL are distinctive, although not entirely specific. The most CT findings are smooth septal and peribronchovascular thickening and diffusely increased attenuation of mediastinal fat. Other common findings include bilateral patchy ground-glass opacities, pleural and pericardial effusion, pleural thickening, and lymphadenopathy [6, 11]. Representative CT images are seen in Fig. 59.1.

In contrast, the CT imaging appearance of LAM typically consists of multiple air-filled cysts of variable size, distributed throughout the entirety of the lung parenchyma (Fig. 59.3). Other common pulmonary findings include reticulated opacities, pneumothorax, increased lung volumes, and pleural effusions [12–14].

What Are the Pathologic Features of DPL and LAM? How Can Immunohistochemistry be Used to Distinguish These Two Entities?

DPL is histologically characterized by the presence of complex anastomosing thin-walled lymphatic vessels, which are present throughout the lung parenchyma and pleura, with a subpleural, septal, and peribronchovascular distribution (Fig. 59.2a, b). The lesional vessels are lined by cytologically bland endothelial cells (Fig. 59.2c) and may be associated with fibrosis and increased hemosiderin-laden macrophages. True infiltration of the lung parenchyma is usually not seen in DPL [5, 7, 15].

On the other hand, LAM is characterized by the presence of solid nodules or multiple cysts throughout the lung parenchyma, lined by cytologically bland spindled to epithelioid perivascular cells (PEC) (Fig. 59.4). These lesions show a similar anatomic distribution to lymphangiomatosis, given their close association with lymphatic structures, with a peribronchial, septal, and subpleural location [8, 16].

Immunohistochemical stains can be useful to further differentiate DPL from LAM, since the latter has a characteristic immunophenotype, with expression of smooth muscle actin, HMB45 (Fig. 59.4), and estrogen and progesterone receptors (Fig. 59.4) (PR more commonly than ER) in a majority of cases [17–19]. In addition, immunoreactivity for β-catenin in a membranous and cytoplasmic pattern has been described in a majority of cases of LAM [17].

What Other Lesions Should I Consider in the Differential Diagnosis of DPL?

Other lymphatic vascular lesions may be histologically difficult to distinguish from DPL. These include solitary lymphangiomas and lymphangiectasis. The former consist of solitary, typically well-circumscribed lesions composed of abundant lymphatic vessels, lined by cytologically bland endothelial cells, and containing lymph within their lumen. These lesions may be solid or cystic, with capillary and/or cavernous architecture, and are commonly associated with prominent lymphoid aggregates [5]. In small biopsies, and in the absence of clinical and imaging correlation, these lesions may be histologically indistinguishable from DPL.

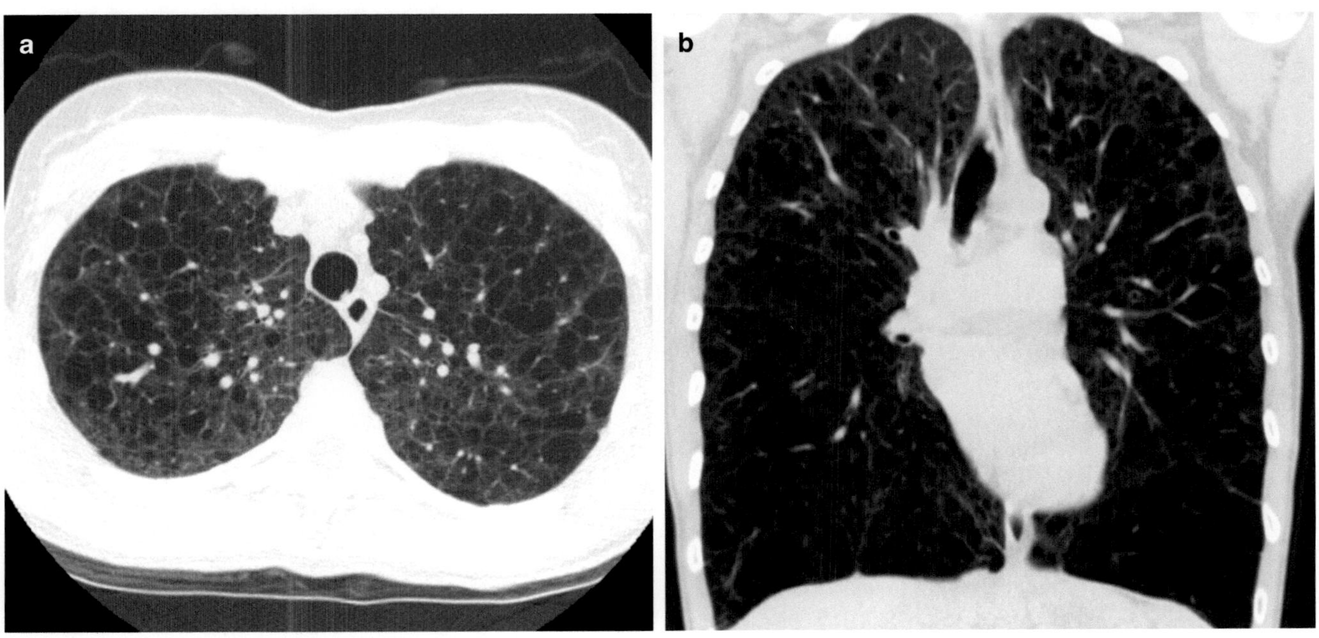

Fig. 59.3 CT imaging findings of lymphangioleiomyomatosis are typically characterized by the variable presence of thin-walled pulmonary cysts, without a predilection for a specific region, and often distributed in a homogeneous manner throughout the lungs. **(a)** Axial view; **(b)** coronal view

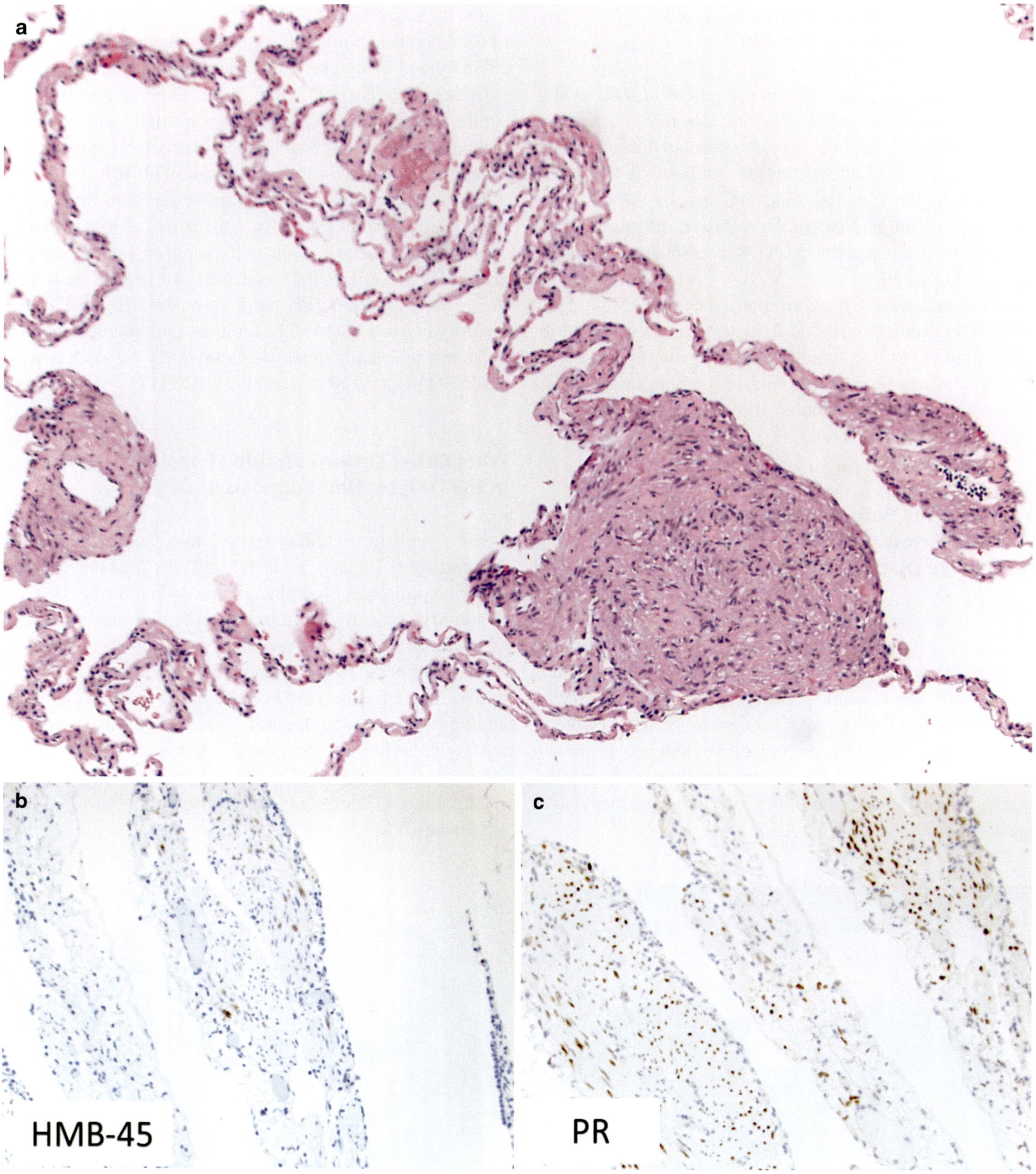

Fig. 59.4 Histologic findings in LAM. (**a**) Notice the presence of myoid cells within the cyst lining (H&E, 100×), which show focal expression of (**b**) HMB-45 and (**c**) variable progesterone receptor (PR) (IHC DAB, 100×)

References

1. Kadakia KC, Patel SM, Yi ES, Limper AH. Diffuse pulmonary lymphangiomatosis. Can Respir J. 2013;20(1):52–4.
2. Ernotte C, Medart L, Collignon L. Diffuse pulmonary lymphangiomatosis. J Belg Soc Radiol. 2018;102(1):64.
3. Lim HJ, Han J, Kim HK, Kim TS. A rare case of diffuse pulmonary lymphangiomatosis in a middle-aged woman. Korean J Radiol. 2014;15(2):295–9.
4. El Hajj L, Mazieres J, Rouquette I, Mittaine M, Bolduc JP, Didier A, et al. Diagnostic value of bronchoscopy, CT and transbronchial biopsies in diffuse pulmonary lymphangiomatosis: case report and review of the literature. Clin Radiol. 2005;60(8):921–5.
5. Faul JL, Berry GJ, Colby TV, Ruoss SJ, Walter MB, Rosen GD, et al. Thoracic lymphangiomas, lymphangiectasis, lymphangiomatosis, and lymphatic dysplasia syndrome. Am J Respir Crit Care Med. 2000;161(3 Pt 1):1037–46.
6. Swensen SJ, Hartman TE, Mayo JR, Colby TV, Tazelaar HD, Muller NL. Diffuse pulmonary lymphangiomatosis: CT findings. J Comput Assist Tomogr. 1995;19(3):348–52.
7. Zhao J, Wu R, Gu Y. Pathology analysis of a rare case of diffuse pulmonary lymphangiomatosis. Ann Transl Med. 2016;4(6):114.
8. Johnson SR, Taveira-DaSilva AM, Moss J. Lymphangioleiomyomatosis. Clin Chest Med. 2016;37(3):389–403.
9. Moir LM. Lymphangioleiomyomatosis: current understanding and potential treatments. Pharmacol Ther. 2016;158:114–24.
10. Taylor JR, Ryu J, Colby TV, Raffin TA. Lymphangioleiomyomatosis. Clinical course in 32 patients. N Engl J Med. 1990;323(18):1254–60.
11. Yekeler E, Dursun M, Yildirim A, Tunaci M. Diffuse pulmonary lymphangiomatosis: imaging findings. Diagn Interv Radiol. 2005;11(1):31–4.
12. Ferrans VJ, Yu ZX, Nelson WK, Valencia JC, Tatsuguchi A, Avila NA, et al. Lymphangioleiomyomatosis (LAM): a review of clinical and morphological features. J Nippon Med Sch. 2000;67(5):311–29.
13. Pallisa E, Sanz P, Roman A, Majo J, Andreu J, Caceres J. Lymphangioleiomyomatosis: pulmonary and abdominal findings with pathologic correlation. Radiographics. 2002;22:S185–98.
14. Abbott GF, Rosado-de-Christenson ML, Frazier AA, Franks TJ, Pugatch RD, Galvin JR. From the archives of the AFIP: lymphangioleiomyomatosis: radiologic-pathologic correlation. Radiographics. 2005;25(3):803–28.
15. Tazelaar HD, Kerr D, Yousem SA, Saldana MJ, Langston C, Colby TV. Diffuse pulmonary lymphangiomatosis. Hum Pathol. 1993;24(12):1313–22.
16. Thway K, Fisher C. PEComa: morphology and genetics of a complex tumor family. Ann Diagn Pathol. 2015;19(5):359–68.
17. Flavin RJ, Cook J, Fiorentino M, Bailey D, Brown M, Loda MF. Beta-catenin is a useful adjunct immunohistochemical marker for the diagnosis of pulmonary lymphangioleiomyomatosis. Am J Clin Pathol. 2011;135(5):776–82.
18. Grzegorek I, Lenze D, Chabowski M, Janczak D, Szolkowska M, Langfort R, et al. Immunohistochemical evaluation of pulmonary lymphangioleiomyomatosis. Anticancer Res. 2015;35(6):3353–60.
19. Gao L, Yue MM, Davis J, Hyjek E, Schuger L. In pulmonary lymphangioleiomyomatosis expression of progesterone receptor is frequently higher than that of estrogen receptor. Virchows Arch. 2014;464(4):495–503.

Intralobar Versus Extralobar Pulmonary Sequestration

60

Jose G. Mantilla

Case Presentation

A 44-year-old woman was referred to the thoracic surgery service with a history of recurrent pneumonia. She reports having approximately one episode per year. Imaging studies demonstrate an intrapulmonary homogenous hypodensity, containing dilated airways that are not connected to the tracheobronchial tree, and a large feeding vessel arising from the thoracic aorta (Fig. 60.1).

Given the presence of symptoms, the lesion was resected. Histologic examination demonstrates lung parenchyma with dilated airways and marked mixed inflammation (Fig. 60.2). The vasculature within the lesion has pronounced intimal thickening and medial hyperplasia. No features of neoplasm were identified. Two years following the resection of her lesion, the patient has been asymptomatic, with no further episodes of pneumonia.

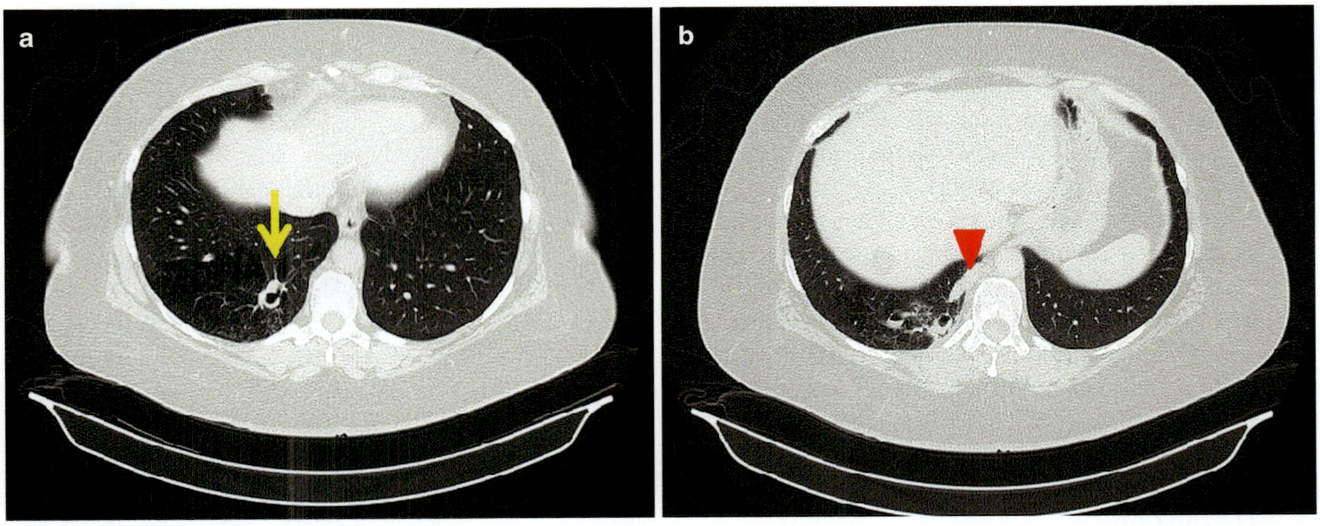

Fig. 60.1 (**a**, **b**) CT imaging findings in intralobar sequestration (yellow arrow). The entirety of the lesion consists of a homogeneous area of hypodensity with smooth contours, containing a large feeding vessel arising from the thoracic aorta (red arrowhead). A distinct pleural envelope is not identified

J. G. Mantilla (✉)
Department of Laboratory Medicine and Pathology, University of Washington Medical Center, Seattle, WA, USA
e-mail: mantilla@uw.edu

H. Xu et al. (eds.), *Practical Lung Pathology*, Practical Anatomic Pathology, https://doi.org/10.1007/978-3-031-14402-8_60

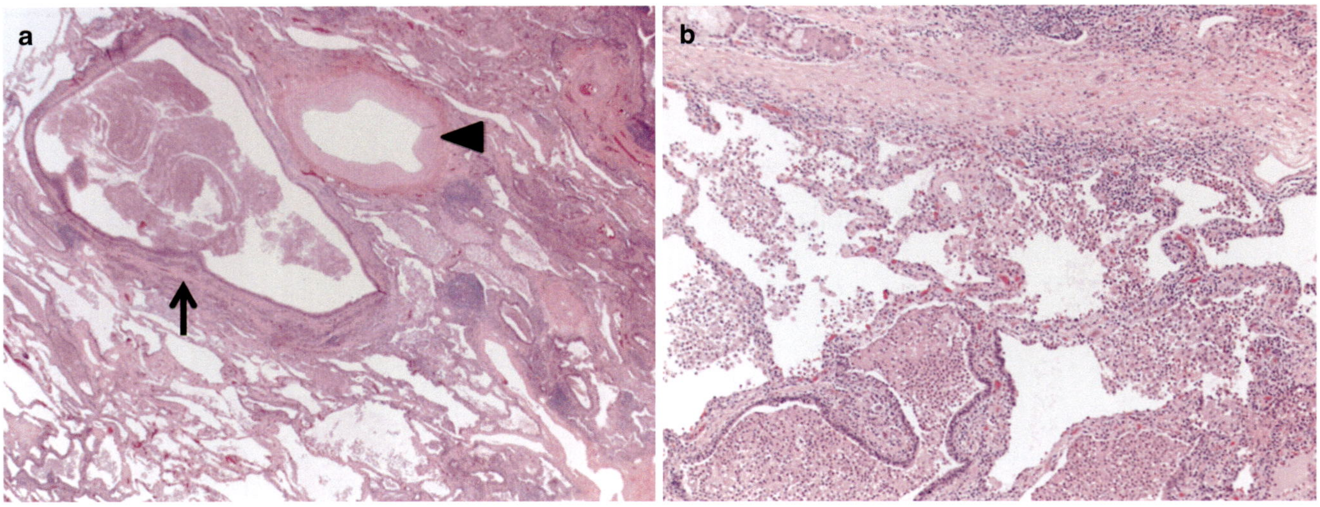

Fig. 60.2 Histologic features of intralobar pulmonary sequestration include lung parenchyma with dilated airway remnants (arrow) and prominent arterial blood vessels (arrowhead) (**a**, H&E, 40×). There is extensive neutrophilic inflammation associated with airway remnants, consistent with the patient's history of recurrent pneumonia (**b**, H&E, 100×)

Pathologic Diagnosis: Intralobar Pulmonary Sequestration

What Is Pulmonary Sequestration?

Pulmonary sequestrations are the second most common malformation of the respiratory system. They consist of portions of the lung that have no direct communication with the bronchial tree, irrigated by an aberrant systemic artery [1, 2]. The venous drainage of these lesions may be connected to the systemic or pulmonary circulation [1, 3].

Based on their pleural covering, pulmonary sequestrations are classified as intralobar, which are contained within the pleura and contiguous with the main mass of the lung, and extralobar, which have their own pleural covering, and are anatomically separate from the lung [1]. The clinical and radiologic manifestations of intralobar and extralobar sequestration typically differ, as discussed below.

How Do the Clinical Findings of Intralobar and Extralobar Pulmonary Sequestration Differ?

Intralobar sequestrations are the most common form of sequestration in both children and adults, representing up to 84% across all ages [2]. When clinically apparent, symptoms typically appear after 2 years of age. The most common presentation in children is recurrent pneumonia, seen in up to 71% of cases [1, 4]. Other less common clinical manifestations include hemoptysis, hemothorax, pneumothorax, and, rarely, cardiac failure [1].

On the other hand, most extralobar sequestrations are detected in the first months of life. They have a distinct male predominance [1] and are associated with other congenital malformations in up to 65% of cases [1, 5]; these most commonly include diaphragmatic abnormalities and other congenital lung lesions [1, 5]. Clinical manifestations typically include respiratory distress, cyanosis, and feeding difficulties. These lesions may also present in utero, in association with polyhydramnios or fetal hydrops [6].

Of the cases of pulmonary sequestration detected in adults, the vast majority are intralobar [7–9]. Adult patients were asymptomatic in 10–47% of cases [7–9], while the most common reported clinical manifestations include cough (34–85%), hemoptysis (9–29%), and fever (16–25%). Infections have also been commonly reported in association with intralobar pulmonary sequestration in adults, in 16–48% of patients [7, 8]. The organisms most commonly isolated include *Aspergillus* sp. and *Pseudomonas aeruginosa* [8, 9]. Given that extralobar sequestrations have a separate pleural envelope, recurrent pneumonia is less common [4, 7].

How Do the Radiologic Findings of Intralobar and Extralobar Pulmonary Sequestration Differ?

Distinction between intralobar and extralobar sequestration relies mainly on imaging findings. Intralobar sequestrations share a common pleural envelope with the lung [10]. They can have multiple associated radiologic manifestations, including areas of consolidation, air-fluid levels, or cystic

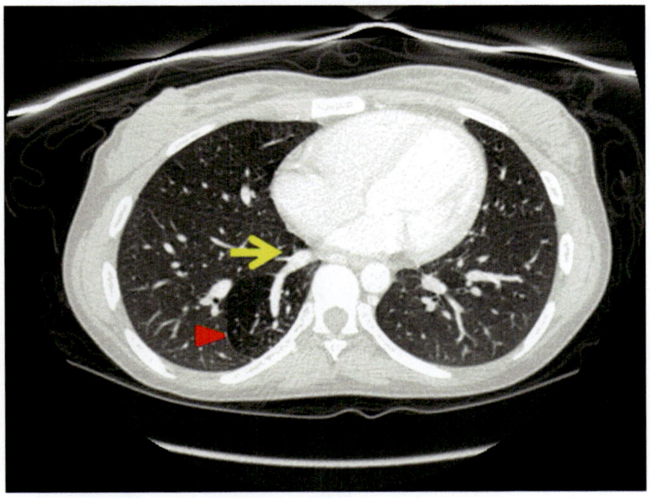

Fig. 60.3 CT imaging findings in extralobar sequestration. Notice the presence of a discrete pleural envelope surrounding the lesion (red arrowhead), as well as the discrete feeding vessel penetrating the lesion (yellow arrow)

change. In their periphery, they may be accompanied by an area of overinflation [11].

Extralobar sequestrations are usually found in the lower lobes, adjacent to the diaphragm. However, extralobar sequestrations have been described in the mediastinum, paravertebral region, and abdomen, among others [6, 11]. In contrast to intralobar sequestrations, these lesions have a distinct pleural envelope, which separates them from the lung (Fig. 60.3).

In both intralobar and extralobar sequestrations, the anomalous blood supply can sometimes be identified on CT imaging. These anomalous vessels most commonly originate from the thoracic aorta (Fig. 60.3) [4].

What Are the Histologic Findings of Pulmonary Sequestration?

Uncomplicated pulmonary sequestrations histologically consist of lung parenchyma containing muscular arterial vessels, which may show hypertensive changes [6, 10]. Remnants of bronchial structures may also be identified. In the case of extralobar lesions, a mesothelial lining may be visible [6]. In contrast, intralobar sequestrations are contiguous with the adjacent lung parenchyma and may sharply abut it or diffusely blend with it [10].

As infectious complications develop, additional histologic changes may be present. These can include fibrosis, prominent inflammation, and cystic degeneration [10].

References

1. Corbett HJ, Humphrey GM. Pulmonary sequestration. Paediatr Respir Rev. 2004;5(1):59–68.
2. Wei Y, Li F. Pulmonary sequestration: a retrospective analysis of 2625 cases in China. Eur J Cardiothorac Surg. 2011;40(1):e39–42.
3. Thilenius OG, Ruschhaupt DG, Replogle RL, Bharati S, Herman T, Arcilla RA. Spectrum of pulmonary sequestration: association with anomalous pulmonary venous drainage in infants. Pediatr Cardiol. 1983;4(2):97–103.
4. Zhang N, Zeng Q, Chen C, Yu J, Zhang X. Distribution, diagnosis, and treatment of pulmonary sequestration: report of 208 cases. J Pediatr Surg. 2019;54(7):1286–92.
5. Savic B, Birtel FJ, Tholen W, Funke HD, Knoche R. Lung sequestration: report of seven cases and review of 540 published cases. Thorax. 1979;34(1):96–101.
6. Rosado-de-Christenson ML, Frazier AA, Stocker JT, Templeton PA. From the archives of the AFIP. Extralobar sequestration: radiologic-pathologic correlation. Radiographics. 1993;13(2):425–41.
7. Alsumrain M, Ryu JH. Pulmonary sequestration in adults: a retrospective review of resected and unresected cases. BMC Pulm Med. 2018;18(1):97.
8. Polaczek M, Baranska I, Szolkowska M, Zych J, Rudzinski P, Szopinski J, et al. Clinical presentation and characteristics of 25 adult cases of pulmonary sequestration. J Thorac Dis. 2017;9(3):762–7.
9. Sun X, Xiao Y. Pulmonary sequestration in adult patients: a retrospective study. Eur J Cardiothorac Surg. 2015;48(2):279–82.
10. Frazier AA, Rosado de Christenson ML, Stocker JT, Templeton PA. Intralobar sequestration: radiologic-pathologic correlation. Radiographics. 1997;17(3):725–45.
11. Zylak CJ, Eyler WR, Spizarny DL, Stone CH. Developmental lung anomalies in the adult: radiologic-pathologic correlation. Radiographics. 2002;22:S25–43.

Index

H. Xu et al. (eds.), *Practical Lung Pathology*, Practical Anatomic Pathology, https://doi.org/10.1007/978-3-031-14402-8

R

GPSR Compliance

The European Union's (EU) General Product Safety Regulation (GPSR) is a set of rules that requires consumer products to be safe and our obligations to ensure this.

If you have any concerns about our products, you can contact us on ProductSafety@springernature.com

In case Publisher is established outside the EU, the EU authorized representative is:

Springer Nature Customer Service Center GmbH
Europaplatz 3
69115 Heidelberg, Germany

Batch number: 10756390

Printed by Printforce, the Netherlands